Studies in Surface Science and Catalysis 34

CATALYST DEACTIVATION 1987

Studies in Surface Science and Catalysis

Advisory Editors: B. Delmon and J.T. Yates

Vol. 34

CATALYST DEACTIVATION 1987

Proceedings of the 4th International Symposium, Antwerp, September 29–October 1, 1987

Editors

B. Delmon
Université Catholique de Louvain, Louvain-la-Neuve, Belgium

and

G.F. Froment
Rijksuniversiteit Gent, Gent, Belgium

ELSEVIER   **Amsterdam — Oxford — New York — Tokyo 1987**

ELSEVIER SCIENCE PUBLISHERS B.V.
Sara Burgerhartstraat 25
P.O. Box 211, 1000 AE Amsterdam, The Netherlands

Distributors for the United States and Canada:

ELSEVIER SCIENCE PUBLISHING COMPANY INC.
52, Vanderbilt Avenue
New York, NY 10017, U.S.A.

Library of Congress Cataloging-in-Publication Data

Catalyst deactivation 1987.

(Studies in surface science and catalysis ; vol. 34)
"Symposium on Catalyst Deactivation"--Pref.
Bibliography: p.
Includes index.
1. Catalyst poisoning--Congresses. I. Delmon, Bernard. II. Froment, Gilbert F. III. Symposium on Catalyst Deactivation (4th : 1987 : Antwerp, Belgium) IV. Series: Studies in surface science and catalysis ; 34.
TP156.C35C379 1987 660.2'995'0289 87-19638
ISBN 0-444-42855-0

ISBN 0-444-42855-0 (Vol. 34)
ISBN 0-444-41801-6 (Series)

Printed in The Netherlands

PREFACE

This Symposium on Catalyst Deactivation came after those organized in different styles successively in Berkeley (1978), Antwerp (1980) and Berkeley again (1985).

For the present symposium, the emphasis was laid on three topics: the techniques used in deactivation studies, the mechanisms of catalyst deactivation, and modelling. With respect to the first, it became apparent that the study of deactivation faces even more difficulties than the characterization of fresh catalysts and the measurement of activity or selectivity. This is due to the multiplicity of interacting processes occurring during deactivation. It was hoped that these points would be clarified in the course of the symposium. Quite substantial progress has been made recently in the understanding of the mechanisms of various processes, particularly coking. It was therefore desirable to accord more time to these topics during the symposium. The third topic corresponds to a problem which is very central to development studies and to the chemical engineering aspect of catalysis: it deals with the representativity of accelerated tests and the modelling of the deactivation phenomena.

We are very grateful to the members of the Scientific Committee whose names appear below, for their help in the difficult task of selecting, from the many submitted contributions, the papers which are assembled in this volume.

Université Catholique de Louvain — BERNARD DELMON

Rijksuniversiteit Gent — GILBERT F. FROMENT

Co-chairmen

SCIENTIFIC COMMITTEE MEMBERS

CONTENTS

Research Papers

B. Delmon and G.F. Froment (Editors), *Catalyst Deactivation 1987*

COKING OF REFORMING CATALYSTS

J. BARBIER

Université de Poitiers, U.A. CNRS 350

40, Avenue du Recteur Pineau

86022 POITIERS - FRANCE

ABSTRACT

The purpose of this review is to link experimental working conditions of reforming catalysts to the quantity, the chemical nature, the location and the toxicity of deposited coke. A discussion of the effect of the metallic and acidic functions brings out that coking is a balanced reaction between production and destruction of coke precursors, nucleation, growth and gasification of more ordered carbon deposits.

INTRODUCTION

Metal based catalysts are used to promote a variety of reactions involving carbon-bearing feedstocks, and coke is deposited on most catalysts. The coking of catalysts containing noble metals has long been of interest, primarily as a result of the industrial importance of reforming process. Most studies have been carried out using a Pt/Al_2O_3 reforming catalyst. In such catalysts, it is well established that total deactivation, as a result of coking, takes many thousands of hours of operation. As a matter of fact the selectivity of reforming catalysts for coking reaction is low, since only one atom of carbon out of 200.000 activated by the catalyst is transformed into a non desorbable deposit of coke under the operating conditions used (1).

The thermodynamics of the reforming reactions are such that it is desirable to work at high temperatures and low pressures (1), but these are the conditions that favor coke formation. In recent years it has been found possible to use multimetallic catalysts supported on alumina to promate reforming. Conbination of Pt-Re, Pt-Ir, Pt-Sn and Pt-Ge have been reported and are now used widely in industry (3)(4). The essential contribution of such catalysts has been greater stability in time. It nevertheless can be seen that the stabilizing effect of additives has not yet received a simple or general explanation. The additives used, however, can at least be grouped into two types (5):

i) additives such as rhenium and iridium which really diminish coke deposit rate

ii) additives such as germanium and tin, for which the coking rate seems at least equivalent, if no higher, than that observed with platinum alone.

It stands to reason that producing less coke under the reaction conditions is not enough to counteract the effects of coking. Indeed the location of this coke and its nature play an important role on its inhibiting effects in various catalytic reactions.

The purpose of this paper is to study the modification of the quantity, the location, the nature and the toxicity of coke induced by a change of the experimental conditions (temperature, pressure), or by a change of the nature of the catalyst (support and metallic phase (dispersion, alloying)). Finally the effect of these different parameters on the coking reaction will be discussed in relation to a described coke build up mechanism.

I) Location, composition and structure of carbon deposits on bifunctional catalysts :

I-1) Location

Coke may be removed by gasification with oxygen. The temperature programmed combustion (TPC) of coked catalysts shows two oxidations, one at around 300°C and the other at around 450°C. These two peaks are particularly well resolved when platinum is supported on non acidic and non microporous alumina. Nevertheless if such is the case, a low oxygen pressure during the TPC analysis, allows a good resolution of the two peaks (figure 1).

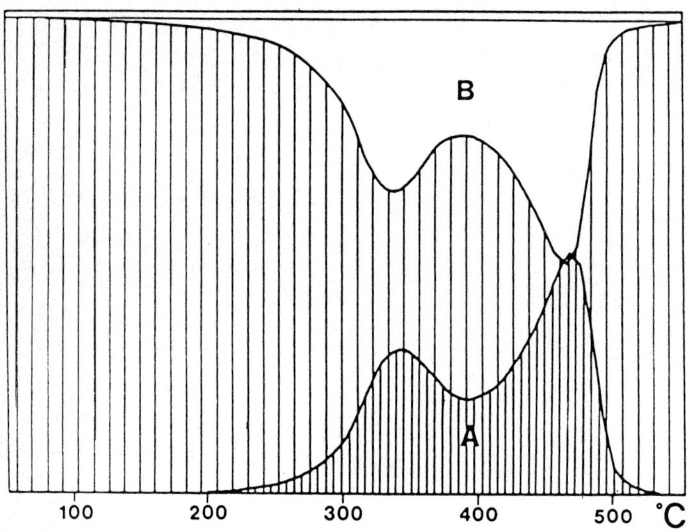

Figure 1 : Temperature programmed oxidation of coked Pt/Al_2O_3 catalyst

(A) CO_2 production (B) O_2 consumption.

A study of these peaks shifting with an increasing temperature shows that the activation energy of coke combustion is equal to 10 kcal for the first peak and 15 kcal for the second one.

Many materials are known to catalyse the gasification of coke, and these include several metals. So it has been found that the low temperature combustion is due to the presence of coke on the metallic phase (6) (7) (8). As a proof, when Pt/SiO_2 catalyst and pure alumina are coked as a mixture and analysed apart by TPC experiments, coke deposited on Pt can be oxidized at 260°C when coke deposited on alumina is oxidized at 550°C (figure 2). Such a difference can be explained by assuming either that platinum catalyses the oxidation of carbon or that coke deposited on the metal is different than coke deposited on the alumina.

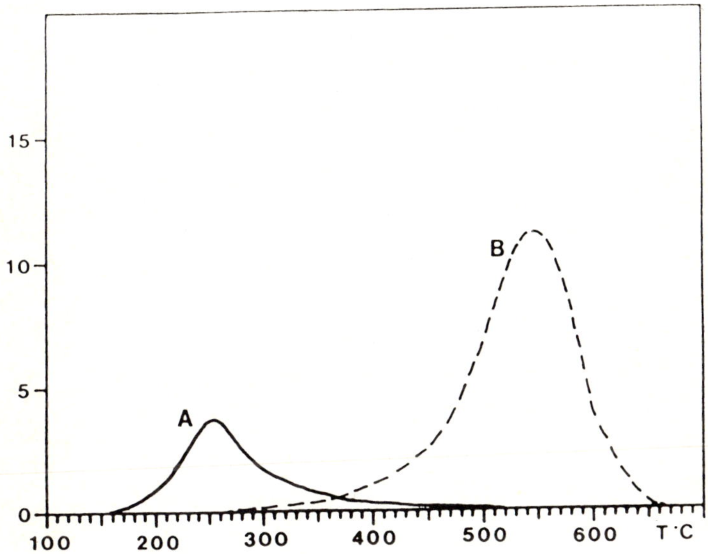

Figure 2 : Temperature programmed oxidation of coke :
(A) deposited on Pt
(B) deposited on Al_2O_3.

The oxidation of coronene deposited on a Pt/Al_2O_3 catalyst proves the catalytic part played by the metal (figure 3).

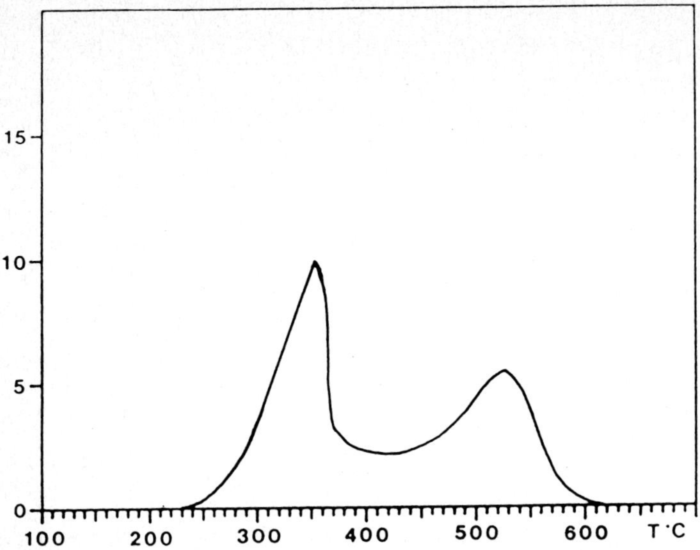

Figure 3 : Temperature programmed oxidation of coronene deposited on Pt/Al_2O_3.

In conclusion, distinction between coke deposited on the metallic surface and on the support can be carried out by temperature programmed combustion. The amount of coke deposited on the metallic phase of a bifunctional catalyst can be determined by combustion at moderate temperature (300°C).

I-2) Composition

Measuring the oxygen consumed and the amount of carbon dioxide produced during temperature-programmed combustion indicates that the coke deposited on Pt/Al_2O_3 corresponds to the formula CH_x. Table 1 shows that coke accumulated on the metal is less dehydrogenated than coke deposited on the support.

catalyst	coking conditions	H/C
Platinum black	cyclopentane + 10% of cyclopentene (400°C)	1.05
Chlorinated Al_2O_3	cyclopentane + 10% of cyclopentene (400°C)	0,5

Table 1 : Comparison of the H/C ratio of coke deposited on pure Pt and pure Al_2O_3 catalysts.

When the coking time increases the hydrogen content of coke decreases (table 2). Comparison of H/C values obtained on coke deposits with those of crude oils (H/C = 1.1-1.6) and of coals (H/C = 0.6-0.8) shows that coke is between polyaromatics and coals.

Time of coking/min	% C	H/C
15	0.61	0.70
60	0.84	0.65
135	1.53	0.63
300	2.53	0.55
600	4.64	0.39

Table 2 : Evolution of the H/C ratio with the coking time

I-3) Structure

Extraction of coke with various organic solvents, after dissolving the inorganic matrix, allows a chemical analysis of the extractable compounds. It has been shown that whatever the experimental conditions and the coking agent may be, extractable coke consists essentially of polyaromatic compounds with a possible branched chain like methyl, sometimes ethyl and uncommonly C_3 or more than C_3 groups.

The unextractable coke can be analysed by X-ray diffraction. Table 3 shows that such deposits are composed of pseudo-graphitic phases with crystallographic characteristics very close to that of pure graphite.

Characteristics of aggregates	coke	graphite
d(A)	3.45	3.35
Lc (A) Thickness of aggregates	17	
La (A) diameter of aggregates	100	
N (mean number of sheets)	6	

Table 3 : characteristics of unextractable coke

II Influence of the nature of the catalyst on the amount of coke deposited

A bifunctional catalyst is defined by the nature of the metallic phase and by that of the support.

II-1) Influence of the nature of the metallic phase :

The amounts of coke deposited on the metal can be determined by combustion at moderate temperature (300°C).

Figure 4 shows the evolution of the variation of the number of carbon atoms deposited on the metal per accessible atom of platinum, as a function of the time on-stream, during the reaction of cyclopentane at 400°C on various catalysts of variable dispersions. The curves obtained show that in the very first moments, when the catalyst is brought into contact with hydrocarbon, the metal attains a coke coverage that will remain constant, whereas the support continues to be charged with coke.

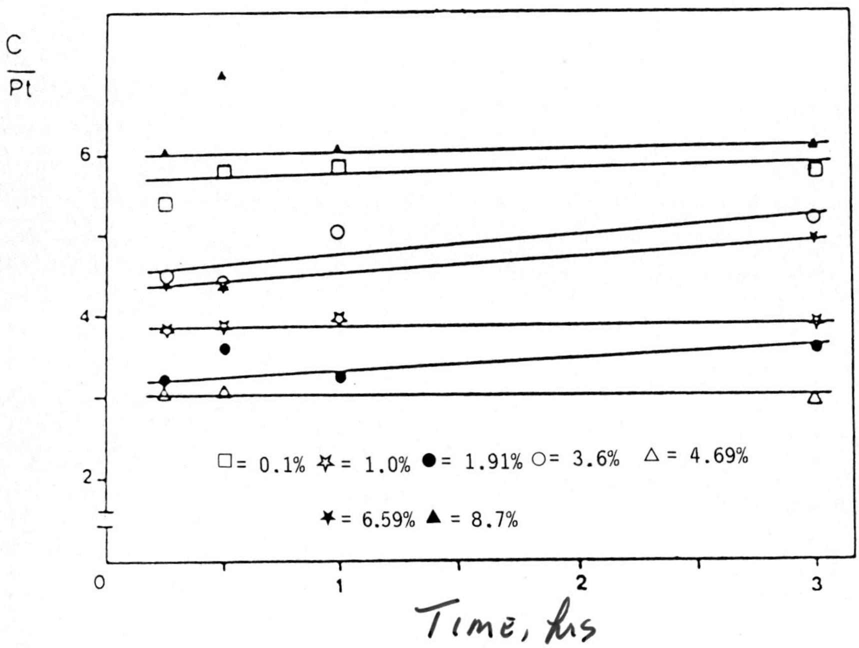

Figure 4 : Effect of the time on stream on the coke coverage of the metallic phase for different Pt/Al_2O_3 catalysts of different metal dispersion.

On the other hand the number of carbon atoms deposited per accessible metal atom varies with the dispersion of the metal. Small platinum particles show a greater resistance to deactivation by coke than do large particles (9). In the same way, Lankhorst et al. (10) showed that the Pt/SiO_2 catalysts with a low metallic dispersion are more sensitive to auto-deactivation than are well dispersed catalyst. This result is in agreement with that of Somorjai and coworkers (11)(12) who proved that coke can settle more easily on planes than on the corners and the edges of metallic crystallites.

The most remarkable progress that has been made in improving the stability in time of reforming catalysts is due to the use, with platinum, of different additives like Re, Ir or S. Figure 5 shows the evolution of the amounts of coke deposited on Re or Ir or S modified Pt/Al_2O_3 catalysts as a function of time-on-stream during coking by cyclopentane at 400°C. The curves obtained show that sulfur will promote the accumulation of coke whereas iridium and rhenium have the reverse effect.

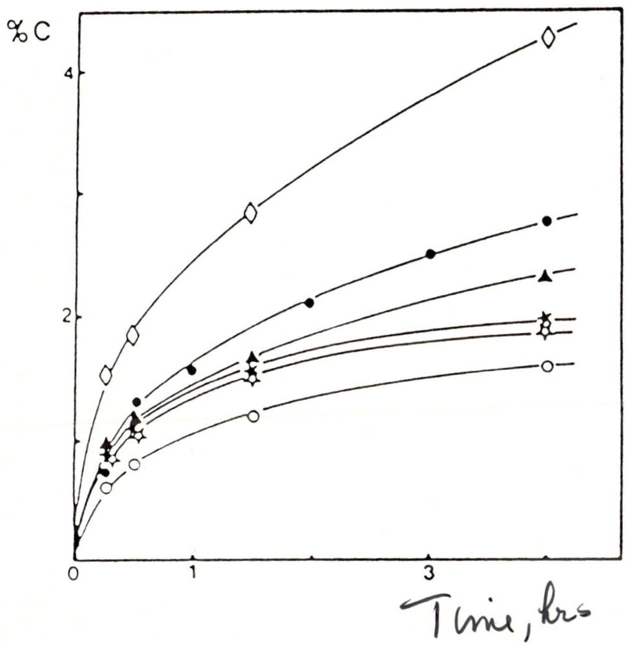

Figure 5 : Effect of the modification of Pt by different additives on the coke formation
Pt/Al_2O_3 (●), $Pt(S)/Al_2O_3$ (◊),
$Pt\text{-}Re/Al_2O_3$ (★), $Pt\text{-}Re(S)/Al_2O_3$ (☆),
$Pt\text{-}Ir/Al_2O_3$ (○), $Pt\text{-}Ir(S)/Al_2O_3$ (▲).

Catalyst	CM = atoms of C deposited on the metal/accessible metallic atom	a/ao relative activity in benzene hydrogenation (a activity of coked catalyst ao activity of uncoked cata)
Pt/Al_2O_3	1.2	0.3
$Pt\text{-}Ir/Al_2O_3$	0.6	0.9
$Pt\text{-}Re/Al_2O_3$	1.0	0.6
Pt-S	0.7	

Table 4 : Influence of Ir-Re-S modified Pt on the amount of coke deposited on the metal (T = 440°C, p = 10 bars H_2/cyclopentane = 2.33)

According to SACHTLER (13) the slowing of the activity of the metallic function could be solely responsible for the reduction in the performances of reforming catalysts. As a proof Table 4 shows that the modification of Pt by Ir, Re or S is able to inhibit the deactivation of the metal and thus to increase the life time of the catalyst though the coke coverage on the whole catalyst can be increased (figure 5).

II-2) Influence of the nature of the support

The nature of the support plays a large part in the rate of coking reactions of supported metallic catalysts. Table 5 gives the amounts of coke accumulated on different platinum catalysts with comparable metallic dispersions but supported on various oxides. The amount of carbon deposited during the reaction of cyclopentane is more important as the acidity of the support is higher

Catalyst	Pt/Al_2O_3	Pt/SiO_2	Pt/TiO_2	Pt/MgO
Amount of C%	2.28	0.09	1.56	0.083

Table 5 : Influence of the nature of the support on the coking reaction of various Pt catalyst by cyclopentane (14)

The same effect can be displayed during the coking by anthracene, at 400°C. of pure alumina modified by chlorine or potassium hydroxide addition. Table 6 shows that the coking level increases with the acidity of the alumina.

Al_2O_3	0.6% K	0.2% K	Pure	0.5% Cl	1% Cl
Thermodesorbed NH_3 (10^2 mole)	7.0	8.2	9.3	10.8	12.20
% C	0.10	0.28	0.50	0.76	1.14

Table 6 : Effect of the acidity of the alumina on the coking rate by anthracene

Similar effects of the acidity of the support were observed during the coking of bifunctional catalysts (16)

Figure 6 compares various temperature programmed combustion curves. Curve (a) corresponds to the combustion of coke deposited on Pt/Al_2O_3. Curve (b) was obtained during the combustion of coke deposited in the same experimental conditions on the Pt/Al_2O_3 catalyst after the basic sites have been neutralized by boric acid. This curve is comparable to curve (a), the only difference being a slight decrease in the amount of deposited carbon. Finally, curve (c), which corresponds to the catalyst neutralized by potassium hydroxide, shows a clearly defined peak at 310°C (coke on the metal) but the high-temperature peak has almost disappeared.

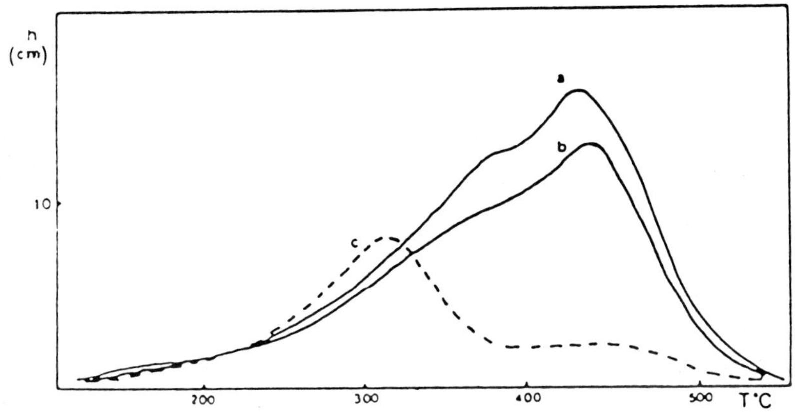

Figure 6 : Envelopes of the CO_2 peaks during the T.P.C. analysis of coked catalysts.

a) 0.59 % Pt/Al_2O_3

b) the same catalyst treated by H_3BO_3

c) the same catalyst treated by KOH.

III) Influence of the experimental conditions on the nature of the deposited coke

III-1) Effect of the pressure

The total amount of coke deposited on a Pt/Al_2O_3 reforming catalyst varies according to the total pressure. (with a constant ratio H_2/cyclopentane = 2.33) following a single relationship :

$$\% \, C = k \, p^{-0.7}$$

However, even if the quantity of coke decreases with an increasing pressure, the location and the nature of coke also are altered. Table 7 shows that an increasing pressure induces, a decreasing toxicity of the coke for the metallic

Coking pressure (bar)	time on	% C	a/ao (relative activity in benzene hydrogenation)	Cm (coke on the metal)
30	900	0.9	0.7	0.8
10	360	1	0.35	1.4
1	60	0.9	0.18	2.8

TABLE 7 : Effect of the operating pressure on the toxicity of coke for the metallic activity.

activity, measured by the benzene hydrogenation reaction.

This result can be explained by table 7 which gives also the temperature programmed combustion results of different samples of catalysts coked at 1, 10 and 30 bars. Increasing coking pressure induces a decrease of the low temperature combustion peak, giving a clear indication of a change of coke location with the coking pressure. At high pressure coke is in preference deposited on the support than on the metal.

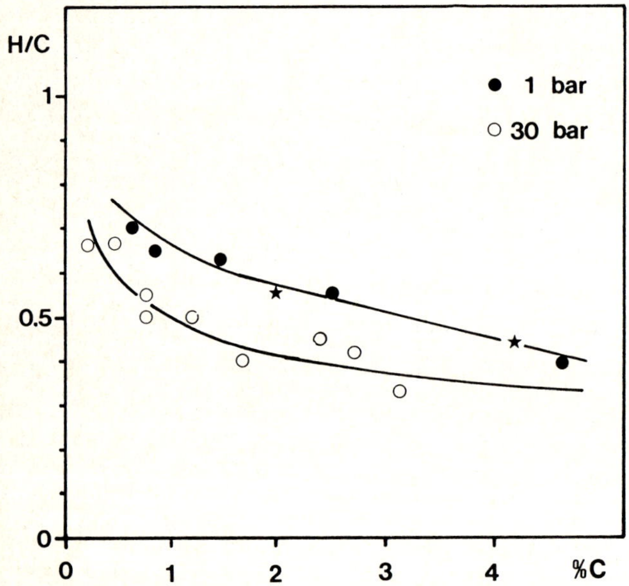

Figure 7 : Effect of the coking pressure on the hydrogen content of coke deposite

● 1 bar 440°C

★ 1 bar 480°C

○ 30 bars 440°C .

The change in coke location is on a pair with a change of the nature of coke. So, coke deposited at high pressure is more dehydrogenated (figure 7) and is a more graphitic one (table 8)

Coking conditions	% C	Extractable coke (%)	graphitic coke
30 bars 440°C 10 hr	0.50	8	92
1 bar 440°C 1/2 hr	0.60	25	75

TABLE 8 : Effect of the coking pressure on the graphitization of coke.

Comparison of curve with tables 7 and 8 suggests that coke deposited on Al_2O_3 is more graphitic than coke deposited on Pt. Such a result is in agreement with a higher hydrogen content of coke deposited on the metal (table 1).

III-2) Effect of the temperature

Different Pt/Al_2O_3 catalysts with different metal loading (1.1%, 0.6% and 0.25%) but with the same metallic dispersions have been coked by cyclopentane at different temepratures. Figure 8 shows that the apparent activation energy of the coking reaction increases with a decreasing metal accessibility. At low temperature the coke coverage increases with an increasing number of accessible metallic atoms. On the other hand at high temperature higner the number of accessible metallic atoms, lower the amount of coke.

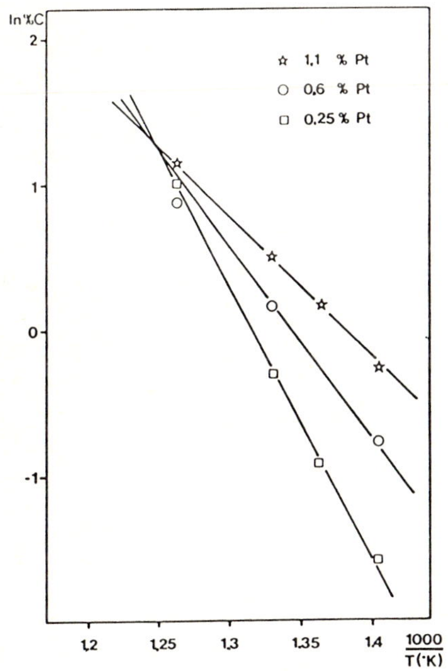

Figure 8 :
Arrhenius plot of the coking reaction on different Pt/Al_2O_3 catalysts.

This result can be explained by assuming that coke accumulation is the resultant of the formation and the elimination of coke on the surface. It appears that an increased number of accessible metal atoms causes, on the one hand, an increase in the production of the precursors of coke, but on the other, an increase in the rate of destruction of this coke. The effect of the accessibility of the metal on the coking reaction of supported metal catalysts will therefore be complex and will vary with the temperature. Activation energy of cracking reactions (destruction of coke) being higher than that of dehydrogenation reaction (production of coke precursors), the production of coke will increase with the number of accessible metallic atoms at low temperature and decreases at higher temperature.

Finally Table 9 shows that the change of the coking temperature do not alter the nature and the location of coke on a Pt/Al_2O_3 catalyst. So, for comparable coke coverage, the hydrogen content of coke and the metallic activity (for benzene hydrogenation) are much the same whatever coking temperatures there may be.

Coking conditions	% C	H/C	a/ao (relative activity in benzene hydrogenation)
440°C	1.9	0.56	0.18
460°C	2.0	0.54	0.20
480°C	1.9	0.55	0.19

TABLE 9 : Effect of the coking temperature on the nature and the location of the coke.

III-3) Effect of the nature of the catalyst :

It has been shown previously that the modification of Pt/Al_2O_3 catalysts by addition of Re or Ir is able to decrease the rate of the coking reaction and to induce a safety of the metallic activity.

The usual explanations are either an increase of the rate of destruction of coke precursors (17) (18) or by assuming that Re or Ir might help to keep Pt atoms in an isolated state, which gives them good resistance to deactivation (19). On the other hand an increasing life time of the catalyst can be explained according to DAVIS et al (11) and DAUTZENBERG et al (19) by the alteration of platinum, which could cause a change in the nature of the deposited coke.

Figure 9 allows a comparison to be made between the temperature programmed combustion of the same quantity of coke deposited on a Pt/Al_2O_3 catalyst and a $Pt\text{-}Re/Al_2O_3$ catalyst. It is worth noting that the low temperature peak is widely decreased by addition of Re to Pt. This result is in good agreement with a lower H/C ratio for the coke deposited on Pt-Re catalyst (figure 10), showing that modification of Pt by Re induces a graphitization of the coke on the support.

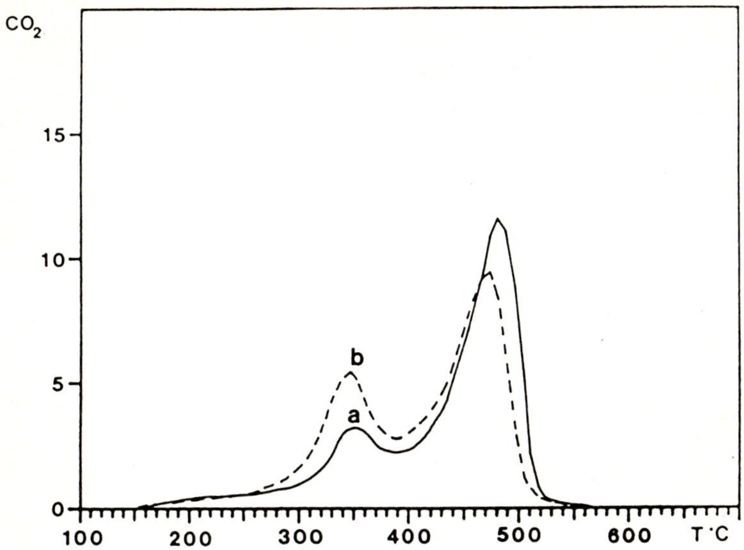

Figure 9 : Temperature programmed oxidation of coke catalysts
a) Pt-Re/Al_2O_3
b) Pt/Al_2O_3.

The same protection of the metallic phase from the coking reaction can be demonstrated by using Pt-Ir/Al_2O_3 catalysts. Figure 11 shows that for such catalysts the low temperature peak of the T.P.C. curves has almost disappeared. The modification of the nature of the coke is obviously demonstrated in table 10 which shows that the modification of Pt by Ir is able to decrease the amount of light hydrocarbon deposits and to promote the graphitization of coke.

Catalyst	% C	% C extractable	% light products M < 202	% graphitic coke
Pt-Ir/Al_2O_3	0.24	5	1	95
Pt/Al_2O_3	0.51	36	68	64

TABLE 10 : Effect of the modification of Pt by Ir on the nature of coke

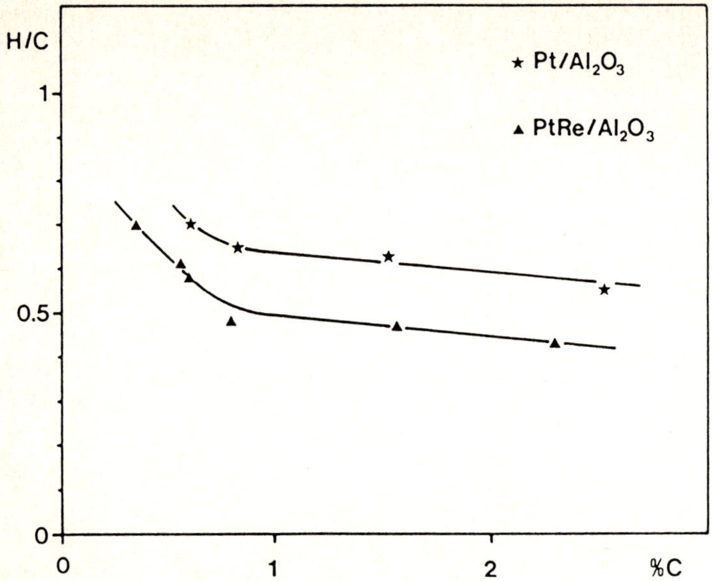

Figure 10 : Effect of the modification of Pt by Re on the hydrogen content of coke deposite.

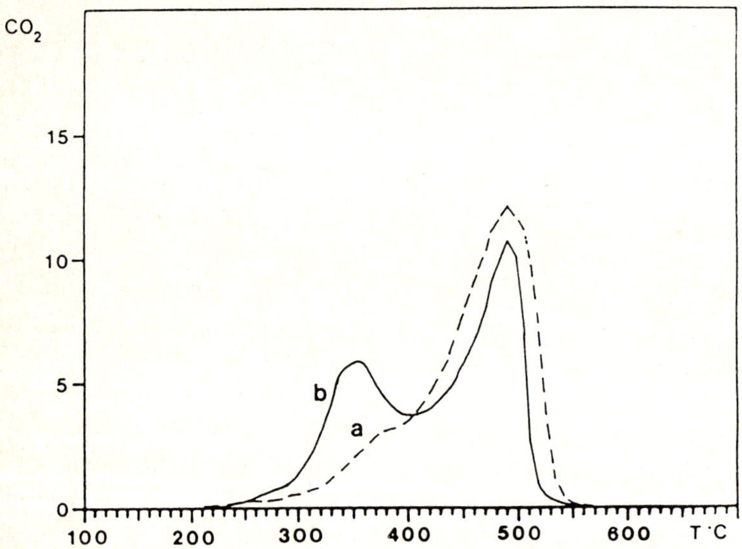

Figure 11 : Temperature programmed oxidation of coked catalysts
a) $Pt-Ir/Al_2O_3$
b) Pt/Al_2O_3.

In conclusion, using bimetallic catalysts like Pt-Re or Pt-Ir brings about a change in the nature of the coke deposited on Pt/Al_2O_3 catalysts. This coke is a more graphitic one, preferentially accumulated on the support. Modification of Pt by Ir or Re has a comparable effect on the coking reaction than on increasing working pressure.

Discussion

Coke deposition on an heterogeneous catalyst is a complex reaction which results partly from the production of coke precursors and also from their destruction. The catalytic properties of the metal are a responsible factor in the coking of bifunctional catalysts by its dehydrogenation properties yielding diolefinic compounds.

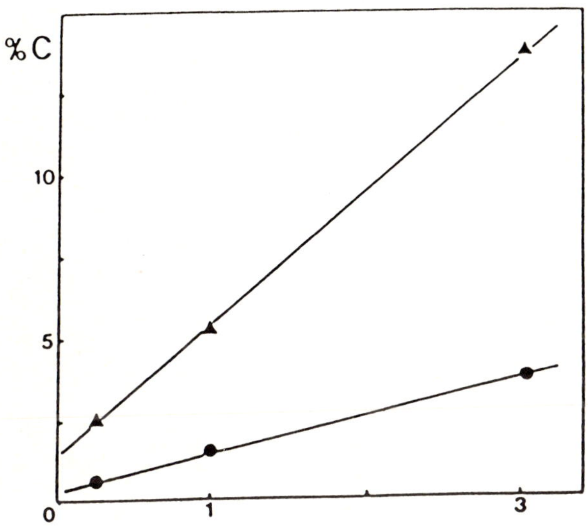

Figure 12 : Coking by a mixture of cyclopentane, cyclopentene and cyclopentadiene in thermodynamical equilibrium ●Al_2O_3, ▲Pt-Al_2O_3.

In fact, in the case of reforming conditions, the dehydrogenation reactions reach as often as not their thermodynamical equilibrium. Besides this production of olefinic coke precursors figure 12 shows that the metal can act in a second way on coke deposition. A chlorinated alumina and a Pt/Al_2O_3 catalyst were coked at 400°C with a mixture of cyclopentadiene, cyclopentene and cyclopentane at thermodynamic equilibrium concentrations. Under such conditions the dehydrogenation properties of platinum are unable to explain the increased coke deposition onPt/Al_2O_3 in comparison with the coke deposited on Al_2O_3. Such a result can be explained by assuming that the metal promotes coke accumulation, for exemple by elimination of hydrogen, yielding very stable dehydrogenated carbonaceous deposits. Finally at high temperature, precursors of coke can be destroyed by the metal. The rate of this destruction is increased by an increasing metallic accessibility.

On the other hand,the prominent effect of the neutralisation of acidic sites shows that the latter play an essential part during the transformation of olefinic compounds into coke. These acidic sites could be responsible for the polymerization and rearrangement reactions necessary for the polymer formed to be stabilized. A mechanism can be proposed to explain the formation of polyaromatic compounds. Cyclopentane can thus lead to naphtalene or to polyaromatic compounds through the following sequence of reactions :

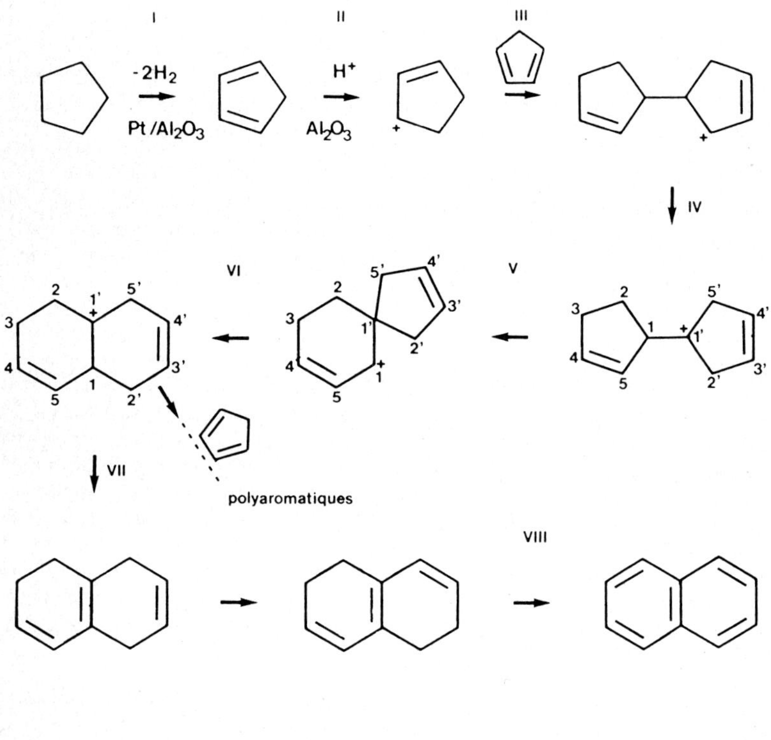

Combinations of Pt-Re, Pt-Ir or Pt-S can reduce deactivation by coking of the metallic phase of reforming catalysts. The protection of the metal from coking reaction can be easily explained by an enhancing destruction of coke precursors in the case of Pt-Re or Pt-Ir catalyst (17). Such an explanation is unlikely for sulfided reforming catalysts (20) but such protection can be said to be the consequence of the heterogeneous metallic surface, if ones assume that coke formation reaction, and sulfur adsorption take place on the same metallic reactive sites (6). On the other hand, the same protection of the metal can be explained by assuming that coke production, like the hydrogenolysis reaction require large ensembles of sites. Sulfur adsorption or Ir-Re addition could be able to break up the periodicity of the surface and as a result prevent coke formation on the metal (19). Alternatively, changes in the activity and selectivity of modified metallic catalysts can be attributed to a "ligand effect" which involves the assumption that the nature and the strength of a chemical bond between an adsorbate like a coke precursor and a metallic surface atom is influenced by the neighbours of that surface atom.

However that may be, modification of platinum by Ir or Re is able to induce a change in the nature and the location of coke. This coke is more heavy, more dehydrogenated, more graphitic and less toxic for the metallic activity (Table 4). An increasing total working pressure has a comparable effect on the nature of the coke and this result agrees with the greater stability of Pt-Re and Pt-Ir catalysts at lower pressures.

However it is worth noting that an increasing temperature does not modify the nature and the location of coke deposited on a bifunctional catalyst. This result can be explained by assuming that the rate limiting step in the transformation

$$\underset{\text{(on the metal or the support)}}{\text{coke precursor}} \longrightarrow \underset{\text{(on the support)}}{\text{graphitic coke}} + H_2 \quad (I)$$

occurs with a very low apparent activation energy like diffusion and migration reactions have. Such reactions like hydrogen or precursors migration are obviously involved in graphitization of coke.

The exact role of the second component is far from clear, but migration reactions, particularly in the case of hydrogen, are known to be favoured by metals such as iridium (21) or rhenium (22). As a result an increasing rate of migration of coke precursors by Re or Ir addition or by an increasing pressure in hydrocarbons, should increase the probability of precursors polymerization yielding stable graphitic aggregates. Such aggregates deposited on the support and including several hundred of carbon atoms will be less toxic for the metal-

In conclusion, according to SACHTLER (13), under the conditions of catalytic reforming with continuous introduction of chlorine, the slowing of the activity of the metallic function could be solely responsible for the reduction in the performances of the catalysts. The protection of the metal from the coking reaction can be enhanced by an increasing working pressure or by the modification of platinum by different additives. Such modifications induce a change in the location and in the nature of deposits playing an important part on the inhibition effect of coke for various catalytic reactions.

REFERENCES

1 J.P. FANCK and G. MARTINO
Progress in Catalyst deactivation
J.L. FIGUEREDO (Ed).
Adv. Study Institute Series, E. App. Sci 54 (1982) 355.
2 M.J. STERBA and V. HAENSEL
Ind. Eng. Chem. Prod. Res. Dev. 15 (1976) 3
3 S.R. TENNISON
Chem. Br. (1981) 536.
4 D.A. DOWDEN
Publ. Catalysis 2 (1978) 1.
5 J.P. FRANCK and G. MARTINO
Deactivation and poisoning of catalysts
J. OUDAR and H. WISE (Ed) Chemical Industries
M. DEKKER Inc. (1986) 205.
6 J. BARBIER, P. MARECOT, N. MARTIN , L. ELASSAL and R. MAUREL
Catalyst Deactivation, B. DELMON and G.E. FROMENT, Eds,
Elsevier, Amsterdam (1980) 93
7 R. BACAUD, H. CHARCOSSET, M. GUENIN, R. TORRESCAS-HIDALGO
and L. TOURNAYAN
Appl. Catal. 1 (1981) 81.
8 J.M. PARERA, N.S. FIGOLI and E.M. TRAFFANO
J. Catal. 79 (1983) 484.
9 J. BARBIER, G. CORRO, Y. ZHANG, J.P. BOURNONVILLE
and J.P. FRANCK
Appl. Catal. 13 (1985) 245.
10 P.P. LANKHORST, H.C. DE JONGSTE and V. PONEC
Catalyst Deactivation, B. DELMON and G.E. FROMENT (Eds)
Elsevier, Amsterdam (1980) 43
11 S.M. DAVIS, F. ZAERA and G.A. SOMORJAI
J. Catal. 77 (1982) 439.
12 G.A. SOMORJAI and D.W. BLAKELY,
Nature 285 (1975) 580.
13 W.H.H. SACHTLER
Second European Symposium on metallic catalysts Bruxelles (1983)
14 J. BARBIER
Appl. Catal. 23 (1986) 225.
15 H. MARTINEZ, P. MARECOT and J. BARBIER
10è Congrès Ibero-Americain II (1986) 1225
16 J. BARBIER, L. ELASSAL, N.S. GNEP. M. GUISNET, W. MOLINA,
Y.R. ZHANG, J.P. BOURNONVILLE, J.P. FRANCK
Bull. Soc. Chim. France 9-10 (1984) 250.
17 R.W. RICE and K. LU
J. Catal. 77 (1982) 104.

18 J.M. PARERA, N.S. FIGOLI, E.L. JABLONSKI, M.R. SAD and J.N. BELTRAMINI
Catalyst Deactivation, B. DELMON and G.E. FROMENT (Eds) Elsevier, Amsterdam (1980) 571.
19 F.M. DAUTZENBERG, J.N. HELLE, P. BILOEN and W.M.H. SACHTLER
J. Catal. 63 (1980) 119.
20 C. APESTEGUIA and J. BARBIER
J. Catal. 78 (1982) 352.
21 M. BOUDART, A.W. ALDAG and M.A. VANNICE
J. Catal. 18 (1970) 46.
22 J. BARBIER, H. CHARCOSSET, G. DE PEREIRA and J. RIVIERE
Appl. Catal. 1 (1981) 71.

B. Delmon and G.F. Froment (Editors), *Catalyst Deactivation 1987*

MULTIPARTICLE-BASED MODELS FOR SINTERING OF SUPPORTED METAL CATALYSTS

D.B. DADYBURJOR
Department of Chemical Engineering, West Virginia University, Morgantown, WV 26506-6101 (USA)

ABSTRACT
Some models for sintering are reviewed. Early models, using predominantly adatom transfer to describe sintering and assuming that individual particles interact only with a bulk adatom phase, are compared with more recent models. The latter take into account the migration of particles (where appropriate), and consider particle-particle interactions through a non-uniform adatom phase.

INTRODUCTION

Sintering as a form of catalyst deactivation is most significant when the catalytically-active species is distributed over a support or substrate. Under these conditions, it is generally advantageous to have the distributed species present in as small a size as possible, so as to have the largest possible surface area for a given amount of material. As the catalysts are exposed to the high temperatures and vapor phase components present either in the catalytic process or in coke-removal processes, the particles sinter, leading to a net increase in the average particle size and a net decrease in the available surface area. (There may be instances where smaller particles exhibit sites which favor less valuable products; in that case, a certain amount of sintering may lead to improvements in selectivity which could overshadow the drop in activity. Nevertheless, sintering beyond a certain limit is bound to have an economic penalty associated with it.)

Qualitatively, the models of sintering are well understood. They are generally divided into two types: one where single species (adatoms) migrate from one particle to another (refs. 1-2), and the other where particles themselves move over the substrate and coalesce with other particles (ref. 3). These two models are extreme cases of a more general model, in which fragments of all sizes, from adatoms to large particles, move on the substrate with diffusion parameters which are size dependent (ref. 4). The rate of formation of surface compounds (refs. 5-6) and nucleation processes (ref. 7) may influence the rate of sintering. These phenomena have been quantified by a number of approaches, including equilibrium particle size distributions (refs. 8,9), kinetic theory (ref. 10), stochastic processes (ref. 11), and the thermodynamics of wetting and spreading (ref. 12). Good reviews of the models and experimental results up to 1983 exist in the literature (refs. 13,14).

The models mentioned above analyze complicated physical phenomena, but under conditions which may not be realistic for supported metal catalysts. For example, average particle sizes are often obtained from the models, and compared with experimental results and with the results from other models, without considering that different experimental techniques may yield different averages, and that different models may yield grossly different particle size distributions having the same average radius. More importantly, most models assume that the particles are evenly distributed throughout the catalyst, whereas in both industrial and model supported metal catalysts, the particles are found in clumps, at least on the microscopic scale. For the low metal loadings customarily found on these catalysts, of the order of 0.1 weight percent, the assumption of an even distribution of particles over the support implies that the particles are relatively far away from one another. Under these conditions, it would be reasonable to suppose that each particle influences only the adatoms around it, and in turn is not influenced by the relative location and size of any other particle. However, in actual practice, local metal loadings may be an order of magnitude higher than the average value. Here, we must take into account the effect of all other particles on the individual particle, in particular the effect of the particles closer to the one in question. The earlier so-called "mean-field" models have been useful in obtaining preliminary data; it is now necessary to model the details of the particle size distribution using models having a multiparticle basis.

A discussion of the work to date in this direction is given below. We start with a description of sintering by adatom transfer ("Ostwald ripening") for a single particle interacting with the average concentration of adatoms on the substrate, i.e., the "mean-field" approach. We then discuss early attempts to look at the effect of having a large local loading, again using Ostwald ripening. Later, we consider models where the adatoms interact with a set of particles on the substrate, in effect having the particles interacting with one another. We then allow particle migration to occur to varying extents, and observe the relative effects on the loss of surface area. Finally, as the interfacial tension between particles and substrate is an important parameter in all sintering models, we observe the effect on the model results of changing this parameter. On a physical basis, the interfacial tension may be expected to change as particles or substrate interact either with each other or with the vapor phase, forming new compounds either on the surface or in the bulk.

MEAN-FIELD MODEL FOR OSTWALD RIPENING

The physical picture is indicated in Fig. 1. The system consists of

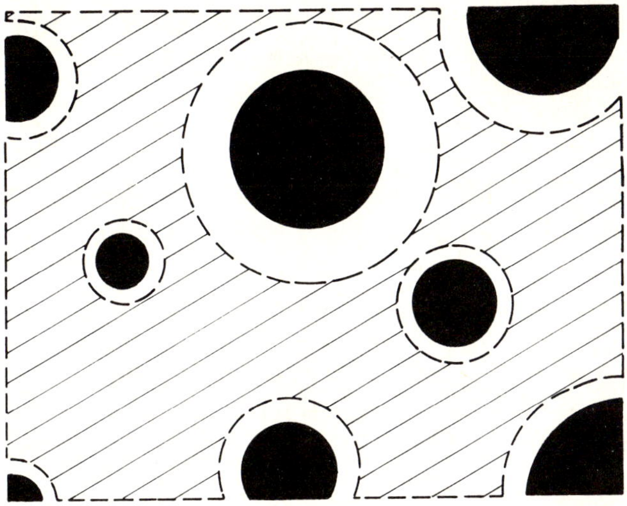

Fig. 1. Physical picture of mean-field model for Ostwald ripening of particles on a two-dimensional support. Filled circles denote particles and the shaded area denotes a bulk phase containing a constant uniform concentration of adatoms. The clear area is a screening region where adatom concentration varies from the interfacial value to the bulk value in a radially symmetric manner (ref. 19). Reprinted with permission from Journal of Catalysis. Copyright by Academic Press.

discrete particles of different sizes located on a two-dimensional surface. The particles may be considered as caps of spheres and are shown as dark circles in the figure. The remainder of the substrate contains adatoms. Most of the adatoms are far from any particle, and are uniformly distributed. This region of the substrate is indicated by the shaded area of Fig. 1. Adatoms in the remaining area of the substrate, i.e., in the clear region of Fig. 1, are sufficiently close to a single particle to be influenced by it alone and not any other particles. The concentration of adatoms at the interface of the particles is related to the size of the particle through the Gibbs-Thomson equation:

$$C_{pi} = C_o \exp [l_c/R_i] \qquad (1)$$

Here C_{pi} is the concentration at the perimeter of particle i, C_o is the adatom concentration in equilibrium with an infinitely large particle (i.e. a flat interface), R_i is the radius of the ith particle, and l_c is a characteristic length given by:

$$l_c = 2\sigma v_m/kT \tag{2}$$

where σ is the interfacial tension between particle and substrate, v_m is the molar volume of a particle, k is Boltzmann's constant, and T is the absolute temperature. Due to the concentration gradient between the particle interface and the bulk phase of the adatoms, the adatoms can either transfer into or away from the particle. When the size of the particle corresponds to the so-called critical radius, i.e., when $C_{pi} = C_1$, the bulk concentration of adatoms, then the diffusion flux for that particle is equal to zero and the particle does not change size. From Eqn. (1), it can be seen that particles larger then the critical size have a diffusion flux towards their interface, and grow in size; analogously, smaller particles decrease in size.

We briefly describe below the Ostwald ripening analysis of Chakraverty (ref. 9) since it forms a useful point of departure for the multiparticle-based models. The concentration of adatoms in the region influenced by a single particle (the clear region in Fig. 1) can be given by the Poisson equation in polar coordinates:

$$\nabla^2 C = 0 \tag{3}$$

with one boundary condition given by Eqn. (1) and the other by:

$$C = C_1 \quad \text{at } r = L \tag{4}$$

where L is a "screening" distance at which the adatom concentration is assumed to be negligibly different from the bulk value. The equation of continuity for a size distribution function f_R is given by:

$$(\partial f_R/\partial t) + (\partial/\partial R)\,(f_R\dot{R}) = 0 \tag{5}$$

where $f_R dR$ is the fraction of particles having size between R and R+dR, $\dot{R}$ is the rate of growth of a particle of size R, and t is the time.

From these relations and a conservation of mass criterion, a time-invariant, or "universal", distribution of sizes can be obtained. For the case when surface diffusion of adatoms is the rate-determining step, the time-invariant distribution is shown by the solid line in Fig. 2. Using some other phenomenon as the rate-determining step changes the details of the curve, but not the general shape. It should be noted that the time-invariant distribution is given in terms of $f_R/\bar{f}$ as a function of $R/\bar{R}$, where $\bar{R}$ denotes the average radius and $\bar{f}$ is the corresponding number of particles. (Rigorously, this relationship should use the critical radius rather than the average radius, but the difference between them is assumed to be relatively

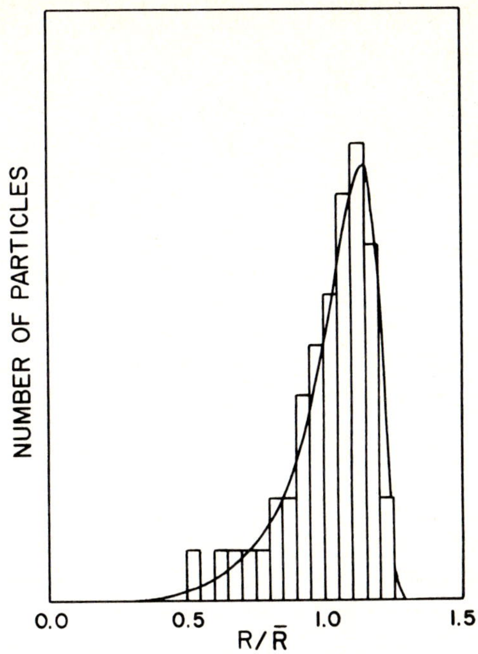

Fig. 2. The curve represents the time-invariant nondimensional distribution corresponding to the mean-field model for Ostwald ripening when adatom diffusion controls the rate. The histograph denotes the approximation used for the initial particle size distribution used in the calculations comparing this model to the multiparticle-adatom interaction model. $\bar{R}$ is the surface-area-averaged particle radius (ref. 19). Reprinted with permission from Journal of Catalysis. Copyright by Academic Press.

small.) Even though the particle size distribution and the average radius or critical radius) of the system change with time during the sintering process, the non-dimensional distribution is not expected to change further with time once the conditions apply that are necessary for the time-invariant distribution to be valid. The required conditions are that an (unspecified) amount of time be allowed to elapse before this "equilibrium" situation occurs; and that the supersaturation of the system, given by the ratio C_1/C_o, be not much greater than unity. This last assumption allows the Gibbs-Thomson relation (Eqn. 1) to be linearized to:

$$C_{pi}/C_o \approx \left\{\exp[l_c/\bar{R}] - l_c/\bar{R}\right\} + l_c/R_i \qquad (6)$$

which results in a considerable simplification in the expression for the adatom flux.

Under these conditions, it is possible to show that the average radius of the particles varies with time according to:

$$\bar{R}^4(t) - \bar{R}^4(0) = K_1 t \tag{7a}$$

where K_1 is a constant. (Again, the rigorous equation requires that the critical radius be used rather than the average radius.) Eqn. (7a) can be recast into the power-law form generally used to describe catalyst sintering. This yields:

$$dS/dt = K_2 S^5 \tag{7b}$$

where S is the total surface area of the metal particles and K_2 is a constant. Again, if other processes are rate-determining, relations analogous to Eqn. (7) can be obtained. For example, if the rate-determining step is the capture or emission of an adatom at the particle interface, then the power index for the average radius in Eqn. (7a) is 2 rather than 4, and the power index for the surface area in Eqn. (7b) is 3 rather than 5.

In summary, Fig. 2 and Eqn. (7) represent the results of Ostwald ripening when each particle interacts only with the bulk phase of adatoms by transferring adatoms through a relatively small "screening" region between the particle interface and the bulk phase of the adatoms. The concentration of the adatoms in the bulk phase is governed by the interactions with each particle individually; in other words, there is an averaging procedure over all of the particles, and the mean adatom concentration interacts with each particle individually. Fig. 2 and Eqn. (7) can be compared with experimental data. If agreement is not found, it could be because the proper rate-determining step was not used, or because sufficient time was not allowed to elapse for the time-invariant distribution to be formed, or because the supersaturation was not small enough for this treatment to be valid. As mentioned earlier, local adatom concentrations can be very much greater than average adatom concentrations; hence, it is likely that local supersaturations may be far from unity even though calculated supersaturations appear to be near this value. In the following sections, we describe techniques which have been used to deal with the case of large supersaturations.

OSTWALD RIPENING WITH LARGE SUPERSATURATION

Lee (ref. 15) quantitatively analyzed the assumption of working with supersaturations that are not too large. He showed that Eqn. (6) is a very good approximation to Eqn. (1) when the value of l_c/R is less than 0.1. However, he noted that errors could be as high as 25% when values of this ratio were increased even to 0.2. Values of this ratio are expected to lie in the range of 0.3 to 0.8 at the temperatures of sintering. Under these conditions, Lee suggests the following approximation, which would be valid for values of l_c/R up to unity:

$$C_{pi}/C_o = \left\{1 - (l_c/\bar{R}) + (l_c/R_i)\right\} \exp\,[l_c/\bar{R}\,] \tag{8}$$

Using Eqn. (8) in place of Eqn. (6) leads to the following analog for the relation of Eqn. (7b):

$$dS/dt = K_3 S^5 \exp[mS/S_o] \tag{9}$$

K_3 is a constant and m is a function of temperature. While in principle K_3 and m are functions of other variables and can be calculated, their values are obtained by fitting experimental data.

Earlier, Ruckenstein and Dadyburjor had introduced the concept of "direct" or "crowded" ripening (ref. 16,17). This was probably the first approach to distinguish between a local metal loading and the average metal loading, and indicated that particle growth (and sintering) could occur even when the system is unsaturated, i.e., when C_l is less than C_o. Under these conditions, Eqn. (1) predicts that the concentration at the particle interface is greater than the bulk phase value, so that particles of all sizes should decrease in size. However, if two particles in Fig. 1 are sufficiently close together that the screening regions (the clear areas) around them actually overlap, then the bulk phase (the shaded region) does not completely surround each of the two particles, so that spherical symmetry is not maintained. In the overlap region, the adatom concentration at the interface of the smaller particle is greater than the value for the larger particle, and therefore adatoms would be transferred "directly" from the smaller to the larger particle without passing through the bulk phase. Depending upon the magnitude of the region of overlap, the large particle could gain more adatoms from this process than it might lose to the bulk phase in the non-overlapped region.

The conditions that have to be satisfied for this process to occur depend upon the sizes of the two particles and the distance between them. For example, if the smaller particle lies entirely inside the screening region of the larger particle, then this process requires that:

$$l_c/R_A > (R_B/R_B-R_A)\ \ln\left[\ln(3.2\tau^{0.4})/\ln(3.2\tau^{0.4}R_A/r_{AB})\right] \tag{10}$$

where R_A and R_B are the radii of the two particles in question ($R_B > R_A$), r_{AB} is the distance between them, and

$$\tau = tD_1/R_A^2 \tag{11}$$

where D_l is the diffusion coefficient of adatoms on the surface. Ordering arguments indicate that if only a partial overlap exists, then the particles are probably sufficiently far apart for crowded ripening to be overshadowed by other phenomena.

Eqn. (10) was obtained for the case of only two particles influencing each other, and was actually intended to explain how sintering could be observed to occur even under unsaturated conditions, when the "mean-field" approach would indicate redispersion rather then sintering. Even so, such an approach would be valid for the case when particles are present in clumps, rather than evenly distributed over the surface, if a way could be found to extend the analysis to allow for several (more than 2) particles interacting with one another. This is the approach taken in the next section. Analogous to the analysis used in this section, where the bulk phase of adatoms is considered not to exist in the region of interest (but is implicitly considered to exist in regions where crowded ripening does not occur), the bulk phase will be considered not to exist at all. Rather, it will be possible to calculate the adatom concentration profile at all positions on the surface, not just in the screening region of Fig. 1. For the region sufficiently far removed from all particles, of course, the adatom concentration should be uniform.

MULTIPARTICLE-ADATOM INTERACTION MODEL

Analysis

The physical picture is indicated in Fig. 3. It is instructive to compare this with Fig. 1, which represents the "mean-field" approach. As mentioned above, the model of Fig. 3 does not hypothesize the existence of a bulk adatom phase of uniform concentration. Instead, the space between the particles contains adatoms at varying concentration levels. Concentration profiles as a function of position can be obtained by following the dashed lines of Fig. 3, representing lines of equal concentrations of adatoms. Note that the lines are not expected to be radially symmetric around each particle (as they would be if they were drawn in the clear region of Fig. 1) due to the presence of the neighboring particles.

The concentration profile of adatoms in the two-dimensional space of Fig. 3 is obtained by considering the collection of particles as a collection of point sources or point sinks of adatoms. The magnitude of the source or sink is a measure of the rate of shrinkage or growth of the corresponding particle. Then the concentration of adatoms is governed by the following relation:

$$\nabla^2 C(\vec{r},t) = -2\pi C_o \sum_{j=1}^{N} B_j(t)\, \delta\left[\vec{r} - \vec{r}_j\right] \qquad (12)$$

for an N-particle system. Eqn. (12) can be compared to Eqn. (3), derived for the case when only one particle (located at the origin) influences the adatom profile. Note the vector form of Eqn. (12), required because the

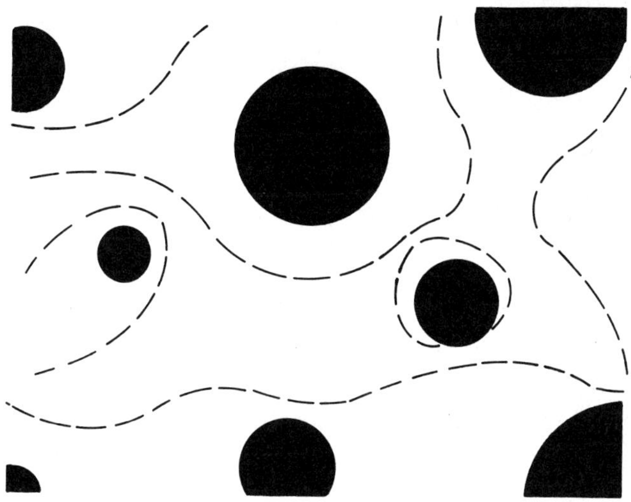

Fig. 3. Physical picture of multiparticle-adatom interaction model for Ostwald ripening. Filled circles denote particles. There is no region of constant uniform adatom concentration. Dashed lines denote points of equal adatom concentration. Note the absence of radial symmetry (ref. 19). Reprinted with permission from Journal of Catalysis. Copyright by Academic Press.

concentration profile is no longer radially symmetric. Note also the change in the righthand side, required now since all particles influence the concentration profile. In Eqn. (12), B_j is a dimensionless source/sink strength; it has a positive value for a growing particle (sink), and a negative value for a shrinking particle (source). The vectors $\vec{r}$, $\vec{r}_j$ represent respectively a location inside the two-dimensional system, and the center of the jth particle. The Dirac delta function indicates that Eqn. (12) is not valid at the locations of the point sources/sinks, $\vec{r}_j$. Physically, this is not significant since our interest ceases at the interfaces of all the particles, and these are always inside the region of interest.

Eqn. (12) can be solved in a manner similar to that devised by Ewald (ref. 18) for the potential field. This has been done both for three-dimensional fields and for two-dimensional fields; we report here only the results (ref. 19) for the case of two-dimensional sintering. The solution requires that the diffusion field be quasistatic, i.e., that the source-sink strengths B_j and the adatom concentration profile C vary reasonably slowly with time. Instead of solving Eqn. (12) directly, the delta function on the righthand side is replaced by three sets of terms. The equation is then solved for each set in turn, and the sum of the three solutions is then the solution of Eqn. (12). The reason for this round-about approach lies in the easier numerical evaluation of the latter solution. Further, the N particles of the system are replaced by a smaller number (N′) of particles in a "basis set", plus the images of the basis set repeated a doubly-infinite number of times in both dimensions. A detailed justification of this approach can be found in the work of Dadyburjor et al. (ref. 19). Here we note that the total number of particles in the system has in fact not decreased but increased; the number N′ is the minimum number required to represent the essentially irregular nature of the particle size distribution. By picking an appropriately large value of N′, we can make negligible the effect of using an image of one of the basis set particles, instead of the actual particle located sufficiently far away. A value of N′ = 50 has been shown to be adequate.

For each particle in the basis set (and its images in both dimensions), the delta function is replaced by the following three terms:

$$\delta_1 = \delta\left[\vec{r} - \vec{r}_j\right] - \left(1/a_o^2\right) \exp\left[- \left(\pi/a_o^2\right) \left|\vec{r} - \vec{r}_j\right| \right] \qquad (13a)$$

$$\delta_2 = \left(1/a_o^2\right) \exp\left[- \left(\pi/a_o^2\right) \left|\vec{r} - \vec{r}_j\right|^2\right] - \left(1/a_o^2\right) \qquad (13b)$$

$$\delta_3 = 1/a_o^2 \qquad (13c)$$

where a_o is the length dimension of the basis set. The first contribution consists of the Diract delta function and a Gaussian sink, the second contribution consists of a Gaussian source and a uniform sink, and the third contribution consists of a uniform source. The overall concentration profile is:

$$(C-C_o)/C_o = B_o + \left(2\pi/a_o^2\right) \sum_j \sum_{\vec{g}}{}' B_j \exp\left[-\left(G^2a_o^2/4\pi\right) + I\vec{g} \cdot \left(\vec{r}-\vec{r}_j\right)\right]/G^2$$

$$+ 0.5 \sum_j \sum_{\vec{\tau}} B_j \,\mathrm{Ei}\left[- \pi \left|\vec{r} - \vec{r}_j - \vec{\tau}\right|^2 /a_o^2\right] \qquad (14)$$

The inner set of summations (over the lattice translation vector, $\vec{\tau}$, and $\vec{g}$, the reciprocal lattice vector relative to $\vec{\tau}$), are the contributions of the images of the jth particle in the basis set. The lattice-translation vector is defined as:

$$\vec{\tau} = h\, a_o\hat{i} + k\, a_o\hat{j} \qquad (15a)$$

where $\hat{i}$, $\hat{j}$ are unit vectors, and h, k are integers. The corresponding reciprocal lattice vector is defined as:

$$\vec{g} = (2\pi h/a_o)\ \hat{i} + (2\pi k/a_o)\hat{j} \qquad (15b)$$

G represents the magnitude of the reciprocal lattice vector. The summations over $\vec{g}$ and $\vec{\tau}$ consist of advancing h and k from $-\infty$ to $+\infty$, but in practice only values from -2 to +2 are needed to obtain a convergent sum. The prime over the summation over $\vec{g}$ indicates that the summation is to exclude $\vec{g} = 0$. The outer summations of Eqn. (14) represent the contributions for all of the particles in the basis set, $j = 1, \ldots, N'$. In Eqn. (14), I represents the imaginary operator and Ei is the exponential integral function.

The source/sink terms B_1 through $B_{N'}$ and the integration constant B_o are parameters which need to be obtained from boundary conditions similar to those used in the solution of Eqn. (3). In the present case, the conservation of mass criterion leads to a local closure condition:

$$\sum_{j=1}^{N'} B_j = 0 \qquad (16)$$

N′ boundary conditions are given by the Gibbs-Thomson equation, one for each particle in the basis set. Since the diffusion field is no longer radially symmetric, the concentration at the perimeter of a particle is no longer a constant. Hence Eqn. (1) can no longer be rigorously used. Instead, an analogous relation is obtained for the perimeter-averaged concentration of adatoms for every particle in the basis set. This yields N′ relations of the type:

$$\exp\left[l_c/R_i\right] = 1+B_o+ B_i\log R_i + \left(2\pi/a_o^2\right) \sum_j \sum_{\vec{g}}{}' B_j\exp\left[-\left(G^2a_o^2/4\pi\right) + I\vec{g}\cdot\vec{r}_{ij}\right]/G^2$$

$$+ 0.5 \sum_j{}'' \sum_{\vec{\tau}} B_j Ei\left[-\pi\left|\vec{r}_{ij}-\vec{\tau}\right|^2/a_o^2\right] + 0.5\ B_i\left(\gamma+\log\left[\pi/a_o^2\right]+\sum_{\vec{\tau}}{}'\ Ei\left[-\pi T^2/a_o^2\right]\right) \qquad (17)$$

Here the double prime (") denotes that j = i is to be excluded from the summation over j, T represents the magnitude of $\vec{\tau}$ and γ is the Euler constant (0.577..).

The solution of Eqns. (14,16,17) yields as a bonus the concentration profile of the adatoms. However, our primary interest is with the sintering rate (growth rate or decay rate) of the individual particles. These can be obtained directly from the values of the source/sink strengths B_1 through $B_{N'}$. Equating the volumetric growth rate of the ith particle with the flux of adatoms to the particle interface yields:

$$d R_i/dt = B_i 1_c D_1/R_i^2 \qquad (18)$$

For a given initial set of values of the location and size of particles in a basis set, therefore, Eqns. (16,17) yield values of the source/sink strengths, B_i. These values are then substituted in Eqn. (18) to obtain the change in size of each particle, which can then be used to obtain the updated values of the B_i terms, and so on. In this manner are calculated the particle size distributions and average sizes of the system as a function of time. Note that the value of B_i required for the growth rate is obtained from Eqns. (16,17), and therefore depends upon the size and location of all particles, and not just upon R_i, the radius of the particle in question.

The effect of particle migration can be taken into account as follows. During each time step in the numerical analysis, each particle of the basis set is considered to move. The distance moved is governed by the size of the particle, and the direction of movement is assumed to be random. A particle which comes into contact with another particle as a result of this motion is assumed to coalesce with it to form a new particle. The size of the new particle is given by adding the volumes of the two contacting particles, and the location is given by that of the larger particle. The new locations and sizes of the particles are used to calculate the source/sink strengths from Eqns. (16,17), and the sintering rate is obtained from Eqn. (18).

The distance moved by the ith particle on the substrate in a time step Δt can be approximated by:

$$\Delta d_i = 2 \ (D_i \Delta t)^{0.5} \qquad (19a)$$

where D_i is the diffusion coefficient of the particle. The size-dependence of the relative migration of particles is factored into the value of D_i by a general equation of the type:

$$D_i = \left(R_1/R_i\right)^n D_1 \qquad (19b)$$

where R_1 is the radius of a single adatom and n is the size-dependence index. As an extreme case, if the diffusion coefficient were to be inversely proportional to the area of the particle base, then $n = 2$. As the other extreme case, $n = 0$ implies that particle migration is independent of size. Finally, values of the angle of particle migration relative to the coordinate system are obtained by using a random number generator between 0 and 2π.

Results

(i) Comparison with mean-field results. The effect of multiparticle interactions with the adatom phase can be obtained by comparing the results from Eqns. (16–18) and from Eqns. (3–6). Note that particle migration effects, i.e., Eqns. (19a,b), are not considered here. As noted earlier, the mean-field results indicate that the particle size distribution of the system approaches a time-invariant distribution (such as in Fig. 2 for the adatom diffusion controlling case) which is then unchanged thereafter. Hence, one way to assess the multiparticle interaction effect is to start with the time-invariant distribution and use Eqns. (16–18). Any deviation from mean-field results will then show up as a change in the suitably-nondimensionalized particle size distribution.

Results using different metal loadings are shown in Fig. 4. The initial particle size distribution is given by the histograph in Fig. 2. The histographs in Fig. 4 correspond to calculated particle size distributions for Pt/alumina catalysts sintered for approximately 22 h. The initial value of the surface-area-averaged radius $\bar{R}(0)$ was chosen to be 10.7 nm. Other parameters of the system can be found elsewhere (ref. 19). The N'(=50) particles of the basis set were initially placed randomly in the unit cell. For the calculations corresponding to Fig. 4a, the metal loading corresponds to an initial fractional surface area coverage, f_s, of 10^{-5}. The initial value of the coverage in the second case is 0.30.

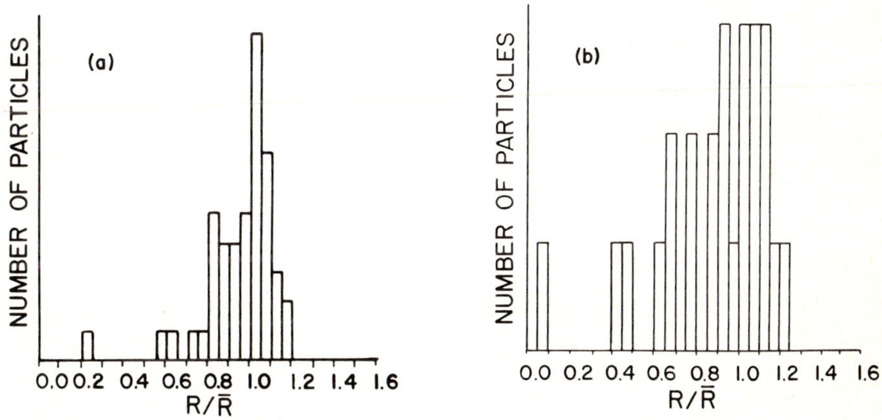

Fig. 4. Results of sintering of Pt/alumina using the multiparticle-adatom interaction model for Ostwald ripening. Initial particle size distributions are given in Fig. 2. (a) Initial fractional surface area coverage is f_s = 10^{-5}, sintering time 21 h. Note similarity of distribution with Fig. 2. (b) f_s = 0.30, sintering time 23 h. Based on (ref. 19). Reprinted with permission from Journal of Catalysis. Copyright by Academic Press.

The histograph of Fig. 4a is only marginally different from the initial histograph, Fig. 2, while the histograph changes appreciably in Fig. 4b. This is consistent with our earlier observation that the mean-field approximation is expected to be valid at low metal loadings, but not when the particles are close to one another. The calculations have been repeated starting with different, random, placement of particles in the basis set. These results (not shown) indicate that the distributions for the low-metal-loading case are not dependent on the initial position, whereas the distributions are only slightly dependent for the extreme case of very high metal loadings. The average particle size for the low-metal-loading case is 11.0 nm, not too far removed from the initial value. Sintering is more pronounced in the calculations for the higher-metal-loading case, the average particle size there being 13.7 nm. Placing the particles in different random positions does not influence the average particle size.

The change in the surface-area-averaged particle size with time of sintering is shown in more detail in Fig. 5. As expected from Fig. 4, values

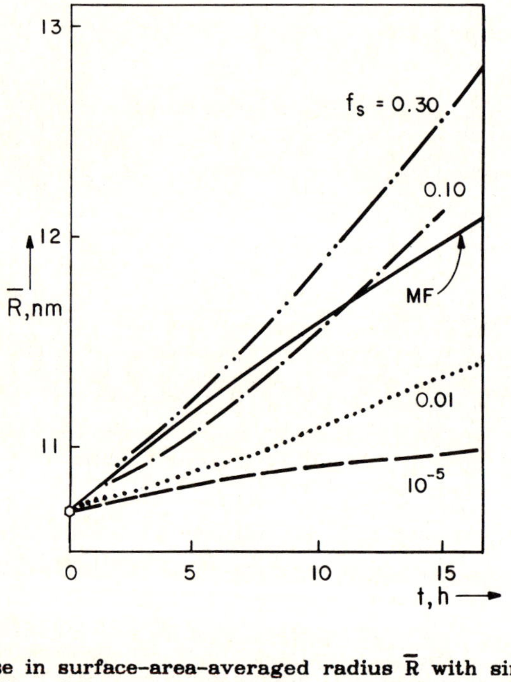

Fig. 5. Increase in surface-area-averaged radius $\overline{R}$ with sintering time t and initial fractional surface area coverage f_s. Solid curve denotes mean-field value from Eqn. (7a). Based on (ref. 19). Reprinted with permission from Journal of Catalysis. Copyright by Academic Press.

of $\overline{R}$ at the same sintering time increase with increasing values of the initial fractional area coverage. Further, the shape of the curves can be seen to change with values of f_s. At small sintering times, the curves are convex with respect to the time axis for the two larger values of f_s, i.e., where multiparticle effects are expected to be significant. The curve corresponding to the lowest value of f_s is concave. Since the area covered by the particles will decrease as sintering progresses, it is expected that the convex curves (of large initial f_s values) will eventually be concave. This transition may perhaps be seen in the curve corresponding to $f_s = 0.01$. The continuous curve in Fig. 5 corresponds to Eqn. (7a), i.e., the mean-field value of the surface-area-averaged radius. As expected, it is concave. The difference between this curve and the curve for $f_s = 10^{-5}$ is approximately 10%. Since Eqn. (7a) is actually a relationship for the critical radius, rather than the average radius, and since these two parameters differ by approximately 10%, the separation of the curves is understandable.

(ii) Contribution of particle migration. Results reported here have been obtained using actual micrographs of model Pt/alumina catalysts for the initial size distribution and location of the particles. The migration of particles is accounted for by using Eqns. (19a,b), along with Eqns. (16-18). The values of the index n in Eqn. (19b) lies in the range 0-2, and the results of the calculation are shown in the upper set of curves of Fig. 6 (l_c = 1.2 nm). For comparison purposes, calculations are also reported when Eqns. (19a,b) are not considered, i.e., for the case when the particles are stationary and only adatoms diffuse on the surface. Details of the calculations can be found elsewhere (ref. 20).

There is no significant or systematic difference between the curve for the stationary particles and the curves for n=1 or 2. However, the curve corresponding to n=0 lies markedly above the other three curves. This implies that when all particles move at a rate which is independent of particle size (and equal to the adatom transfer rate), then sintering can be expected to be enhanced. In this case, there is significant migration and coalescence of the particles. On the other hand, if the rate at which particles move on the substrate is dependent on size to any appreciable extent ($n \geq 1$), then the migration of particles will not play a predominant role in sintering.

(iii) Effect of interfacial tension. The interfacial tension governs the interaction between the particle and support, and is expected to influence the sintering process accordingly. When the particle and support are

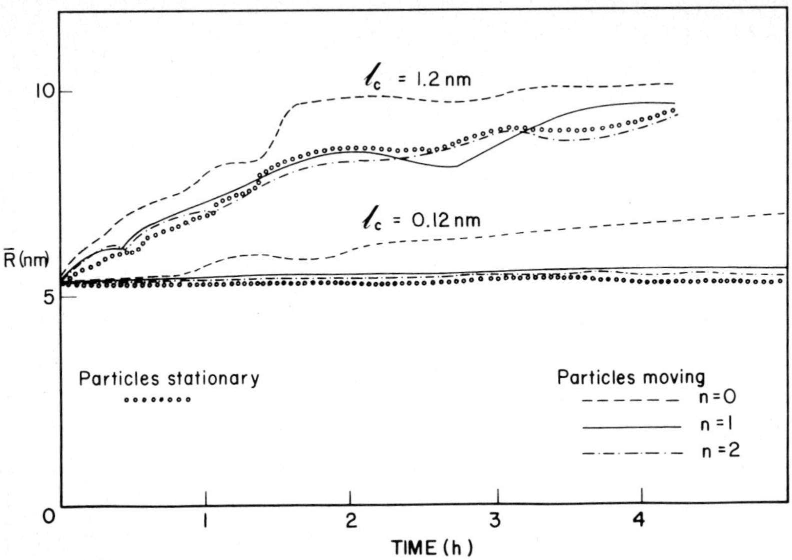

Fig. 6. Effect of particle migration and interfacial tension σ on sintering using the multiparticle-adatom interaction model. The two families of curves correspond to two values of the characteristic length l_c, related to σ in Eqn. (2). Particle migration is excluded in the curves labelled stationary particles. Other curves correspond to increasing dependence of particle migration rate on particle size with increasing values of n; see Eqns. (19a,b). (ref. 20).

similar, e.g., when both are metal oxides, then there is a strong interaction between particle and support, and the value of the interfacial tension is low. Conversely, when the particle and support are dissimilar, e.g., the particle is a metal or hydride, then the interfacial tension is high. In the latter case, the particle may not wet or spread on the support. The interfacial tension σ enters the quantitative model of sintering through the Gibbs-Thomson relation, Eqn. (1), and the definition of the characteristic length l_c in Eqn. (2).

Shown in Fig. 6 are also the results of varying this parameter. Here the value of l_c is decreased by an order of magnitude. When l_c = 0.12 nm, the value of the surface-area-averaged radius, $\overline{R}$, is appreciably less than the value obtained at the larger value of l_c. The rate of sintering is greatly diminished in this case, and this is reasonable on physical grounds. As the interaction between the particle and support increases, the transfer of adatoms (and the migration of particles, if appropriate) is less rapid. Since adatoms have their motion relatively restricted at the low value of l_c, the average particle size is virtually flat for the case of stationary particles. When adatoms and particles both move at the same transfer rate, the motion of particles leads only to sintering. Hence, at the low value of l_c, the average radius is higher for n=0 than when the particles are stationary or move at a size-dependent rate. Comparing the curves for the same value of n and different values of l_c yields the same results as for the stationary particles; i.e., the value of $\overline{R}$ increases to a smaller extent for the lower value of l_c.

CONCLUSIONS

The sintering of supported metal catalysts can be most simply analyzed by assuming that the supersaturation of species comprising the particles is "not too large", i.e., that the metal loading corresponds to two-dimensional saturation. Even for model supported metal catalysts, with care taken to ensure an even distribution of particles on the support, this assumption may not be valid. The problem is further complicated for the case of "real" supported metal catalysts, where the particles are generally distributed in "clumps", at least on the microscopic scale. Early treatments of this problem have led to sintering rate expressions of more accurate form, but which still require experimental data to fit adjustable parameters of dubious physical significance. Other techniques have quantified the regions in which pair-wise particle interactions may be significant. More elaborate methods, described here, treat the general problem of particles interacting with one another through the adatom phase. This model is shown to include the earlier models as special cases, valid at low metal loadings. The present model has been used to show the relative effects of particle migration and particle-substrate interaction on the sintering rate. The results can be explained on physical grounds.

ACKNOWLEDGEMENTS

Portions of the work described above have been supported by the National Science Foundation under Grant CBT 83-20400.

REFERENCES

1. J. M. Lifshitz and V. V. Slyozov, J. Phys. Chem. Solids 19 (1961) 35.
2. C. Wagner, Z. Electrochem. 65 (1961) 581.
3. E. Ruckenstein and B. Pulvermacher, AIChE J. 19 (1973) 356-364.
4. E. Ruckenstein and D. B. Dadyburjor, J. Catal. 48 (1977) 73-86.

5. H. C. Yao, M. Sieg and H. K. Plummer, Jr., J. Catal. 59 (1979) 365-374.
6. R. Gollob and D. B. Dadyburjor, J. Catal. 68 (1981) 473-486.
7. P. Wynblatt and T.-M. Ahn, in G. C. Kuczinski (Editor), Mater. Sci. Res. 10 (Sintering and Catalysis), Plenum, New York, 1975, pp. 83-106.
8. B. Pulvermacher and E. Ruckenstein, J. Catal. 35 (1974) 115-139.
9. B. K. Chakraverty, J. Phys. Chem. Solids 28 (1967) 2401-2412.
10. P. C. Flynn and S. E. Wanke, J. Catal. 34 (1974) 390-399.
11. C. G. Granqvist and R. A. Buhrman, J. Catal. 42 (1976) 477-479.
12. E. Ruckenstein, in J. Bourdon (Editor), Studies Surf. Sci. and Catal. 4 (Growth and Properties of Metal Clusters), Elsevier, Amsterdam, 1980, pp. 57-63.
13. P. C. Flynn and S. E. Wanke, Catal. Rev.-Sci. Eng. 12 (1975) 93.
14. E. Ruckenstein and D. B. Dadyburjor, Rev. Chem. Engg. 1 (1983) 251-355.
15. H. H. Lee, J. Catal. 63 (1980) 129-137.
16. D. B. Dadyburjor and E. Ruckenstein, J. Crystal Growth 38 (1977) 285-287.
17. E. Ruckenstein and D. B. Dadyburjor, Thin Solid Films 55 (1978) 89-99.
18. P. P. Ewald, Ann. Phys. Leipzig 64 (1921) 253-287.
19. D. B. Dadyburjor, S. P. Marsh and M. E. Glicksman, J. Catal. 99 (1986) 358-374.
20. A. Bellare and D. B. Dadyburjor, AIChE J., in press.

B. Delmon and G.F. Froment (Editors), *Catalyst Deactivation 1987*

DEACTIVATION OF MOLYBDENUM CATALYSTS BY METAL AND CARBONACEOUS DEPOSITS DURING THE HYDROTREATING OF COAL-DERIVED LIQUIDS AND HEAVY PETROLEUMS.

A. NISHIJIMA, H. SHIMADA, Y. YOSHIMURA, T. SATO, and N. MATSUBAYASHI

National Chemical Laboratory for Industry, Tsukuba, Ibaraki 305, (Japan)

ABSTRACT

The deactivation of molybdenum catalysts used for hydrotreating coal-derived liquids and heavy petroleums were investigated in order to aid the design of long life catalysts for coal liquid hydroprocessing. Characterization of used catalysts revealed the different features of the metal and carbonaceous deposits derived from coal liquids and heavy petroleums. The changes in the local structure of active metals were also investigated. Regeneration of the catalysts showed that the changes in the active site structure as well as metal and carbonaceous deposits decrease the catalyst activity. Based on the insight gained into the deactivation of these catalysts, new types of catalysts were designed and tested for hydrotreating coal-derived liquids.

INTRODUCTION

Alumina supported molybdenum sulfide catalysts, containing cobalt or nickel promoters, have long been used for hydrodesulfurization of petroleum (refs. 1-6). Recently Co-Mo and Ni-Mo supported catalysts have also been used for upgrading synthetic crudes such as coal-derived liquids. There are, however, fewer commercial scale plants processing synthetic crudes than petroleum crudes, primarily due to severe catalyst deactivation (refs. 6-12). Therefore, there is a strong need for designing better catalysts and processing conditions that will minimize the catalyst deactivation and the need for subsequent catalyst regeneration (refs. 8,9). During the course of development of these new catalysts and processes, the understanding of the process of catalyst deactivation should be the most important feature. A good understanding of the deactivation profile will lead to the development of a new generation of catalysts having a longer life and superior activity. Basic knowledge about active sites and reaction mechanisms of these catalysts will be obtained in the process of deactivation analysis (ref. 8). The main purpose of the present work is to point out both the differences and the similarities in the deactivation behaviors of two types of molybdenum catalysts. One is used for upgrading coal-derived liquid and the other is used for petroleum heavy oil upgrading. The approach involves characterization of used catalysts, model test reactions for evaluating catalyst functions, regeneration of catalysts and developing a concept for design of a long life catalyst based on the understanding of catalyst deactivation. The change in the macroscopic structure of catalysts during use, such as the narrowing of pore diameter caused by the deposition of metals, is an important factor governing the overall activity of catalysts. In the present review, considerations concerning this phenomenon will not be discussed in detail in order to focus attention on the chemical nature of the active sites and their deactivation and regeneration. Some new results as well as a current review are presented. Many excellent reviews describing various aspects of hydrotreating catalysts have provided the background for this paper (refs. 1-6, 8,9, 13-15).

EXPERIMENTAL

Catalysts

Supports prepared and used in this work are alumina, titania, silica, magnesia, zeolites and double oxides such as alumina-titania (ref. 16). Physical and chemical properties of each support, such as pore size distribution and acidity, were controlled by changing preparation conditions. Mo, Ni-Mo and Co-Mo were then loaded on the supports as active species by an impregnation method. Some commercial catalysts were also used to compare catalytic activities and deactivation behaviors with those of the catalysts prepared. Molybdenum catalysts were presulfided before reaction.

Feedstocks

Two kinds of coal-derived liquids obtained from Wandoan (subbituminous) and Yallourn (brown) coals were used as feedstocks (Table 1). The coal-derived liquid(A) from Wandoan coal consists of distillates, while the other one(B) from Yallourn coal includes asphaltene or preasphaltene(refs. 17,18). These coal liquids

TABLE 1
Properties of coal-derived liquids and petroleum feedstocks.

Feed	H/C	530℃+ ★1	Metal	
Coal liquid(A)	1.10-1.25	-	-	
Coal liquid(B)	0.85-0.95	++	++	Na,Ca,Mg,Fe,K
Petroleum(A)	1.6 -1.7	-	-	V,Ni
Petroleum(B)	1.5 -1.6	+	+	V,Ni,Fe

★1 : Residue after distillation at 530℃

were obtained from two separate first stage coal liquefaction processes currently under development in Japan. In some cases, fractions distilled or extracted by toluene or THF were prepared as raw materials for hydrotreating (ref. 16). Petroleum residue and distillates were also used to compare the difference in the deactivation behavior.

Model reactions

Model reactions were performed to clarify basic catalytic functions of the catalysts (ref. 19). 1-methylnaphthalene(1-MN) and diphenylmethane(DPM) were selected as model hydrocarbons for testing hydrogenation(HYG) activity of aromatic rings and hydrocracking(HYC) activity of C-C bonds. The unit used was a batch microreactor. The temperatures selected were 350 and 400℃, respectively. The initial hydrogen pressure was 6.9 MPa and the reaction time 1h.

DEACTIVATION BEHAVIOR OF CATALYSTS

An evaluation of catalyst function as well as the characterization of catalyst properties during catalyst deactivation is necessary to understand the deactivation behavior of the catalyst. Model test reactions are useful to evaluate the degree of the deactivation of each catalyst function such as HYG or HYC activity. Although most model reaction so far proposed and applied are performed under atmospheric pressures (refs. 4,20,21), high pressure reactions are preferred in order to obtain a good correlation between the model reaction and the practical hydroprocessing results (ref. 22).

Some results from the model tests done on fresh and aged catalysts used for hydroprocessing coal liquids and petroleum residue and distillate are summarized in Table 2. Both HYG and

HYC activities of the catalysts decreased to a large extent after long reaction times. The catalysts used for heavier feeds were deactivated to a greater extent than those used for distillates. The catalyst fraction at the exit of the reactor was less deactivated than that at the inlet when the coal liquid(B) was hydrotreated. In contrast, the activity of the catalyst at the exit was less than that of the inlet for petroleum(B) hydroprocessing. This may be due to the different effect of the deposited metals on the activities of the catalysts. For hydrotreating coal liquids, alkaline and alkali earth metals will poison the catalyst activities much more than V and Ni on the catalyst used for residue hydroprocessing. The HYC activities decreased more rapidly than the HYG activities. The used catalyst at the inlet showed no HYC activity after hydrotreating the coal liquid(B). In the case of HYG activities for the model reaction of DPM, the deactivation behaviors were essentially the same as those obtained from the model reactions of 1-MN. Although the degree of deactivation of each function depends on the feed and operating conditions, these results indicate that a

TABLE 2
Evaluation of catalyst deactivation by use of model reactions.

Catalyst	HYG of 1-MN	HYC of DPM	HYG of DPM
Cat A (coal liquid A)			
Fresh	57 (1.0)	8.2 (1.0)	33 (1.0)
Used, Inlet	7.5 (0.13)	1.3 (0.16)	4.5 (0.14)
Outlet	11.3 (0.20)	1.2 (0.14)	5.2 (0.16)
Cat B (coal liquid B)			
Fresh	52 (1.0)	13.3 (1.0)	27 (1.0)
Used, Inlet	1.6 (0.03)	0 (0)	1.2 (0.04)
Middle	8.5 (0.16)	0.5 (0.04)	4.6 (0.17)
Outlet	12.2 (0.24)	0.6 (0.05)	7.3 (0.27)
Cat C (petroleum A)			
Fresh	43 (1.0)	13.7 (1.0)	19.8 (1.0)
Used, Inlet	9.5 (0.22)	1.1 (0.08)	6.1 (0.31)
Middle	17.3 (0.40)	1.4 (0.10)	10.2 (0.52)
Outlet	13.3 (0.31)	1.3 (0.09)	11.0 (0.56)
Cat D (petroleum B)			
Fresh	32 (1.0)	9.1 (1.0)	15.1 (1.0)
Used, Inlet	18.5 (0.58)	0.7 (0.08)	9.0 (0.60)
Middle	14.3 (0.45)	0.6 (0.06)	4.6 (0.31)
Outlet	9.5 (0.30)	0.4 (0.04)	2.5 (0.18)

higher HYC activity is not necessary for catalysts used in heavy feed upgrading because of rapid deactivation of the HYC activity.

CHARACTERIZATION OF USED CATALYSTS

Deposition of carbonaceous material

It is well known that the deposition of carbonaceous materials on molybdenum catalysts is the main cause for the initial catalyst deactivation. There are many similarities in the deactivation by carbonaceous deposits resulting from coal liquids processing and petroleum residue and heavy oil processing (ref. 7,10,23-30). The content of the carbonaceous deposition reaches its maximum steady-state value of about 15-30 wt% in a short period (ref. 9). It generally increases from the entrance to the exit of a fixed bed reactor. The carbonaceous deposit is usually found to be uniformly distributed throughout the catalyst particles for distillates hydroprocessing. While it is concentrated at the external surface of the catalyst extrudate for heavy feeds such as asphaltene or preasphaltene (refs. 30-32). Reaction conditions as well as the feeds used also affect the profile of the deposition (refs. 32,33). The chemical composition of the deposit depends upon the feeds and the operating conditions.

Coal-derived liquids contain larger amount of aromatics and heteroatoms than petroleum. Table 3 shows atomic H/C and N/C ratios for the deposit on the catalyst. Lower H/C ratios for the deposit at the outlet compared to that at the inlet shows the

TABLE 3
Carbonaceous depositions on used catalysts

Catalyst		C (wt%)	H/C	N/C	H/C in feed
Cat A	Inlet	14.8	0.89	0.017	1.10-1.25
	Outlet	19.3	0.76	0.012	
Cat B	Inlet	10.1	1.07	0.024	0.85-0.95
	Middle	10.8	0.90	0.025	
	Outlet	16.5	0.76	0.018	
Cat C	Inlet	11.6	0.89	0.031	1.6-1.7
	Middle	18.9	0.63	0.018	
	Outlet	20.6	0.62	0.017	
Cat D	Inlet	17.6	1.00	0.020	1.5-1.6
	Middle	19.5	0.90	0.019	
	Outlet	27.4	0.77	0.014	

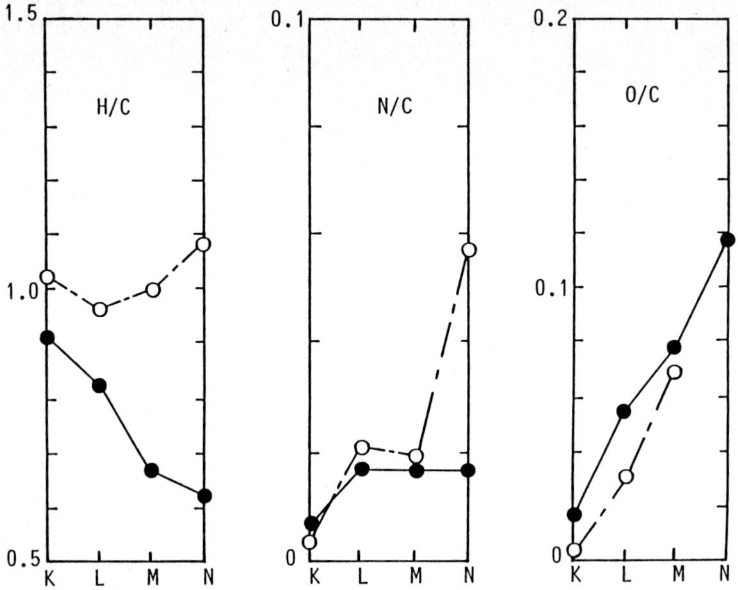

Fig. 1. Elemental analyses of extracts from the catalyst and the feed. K: Hexane-soluble oils, L: Hexane-insoluble and toluene-soluble, M: Toluene-insoluble and THF-soluble, N: THF-insoluble. Elemental analyses of carbonaceous dipositions were obtained on the successive extracts of the spent catalyst. Carbonaceous materials on the catalyst: ○ , Feed: ● .

higher degree of coking at the outlet. The H/C ratio of the deposit on the catalysts used for the processing of coal liquid(B) are similar to those of the feed. On the contrary the H/C ratio of the deposits on the petroleum hydroprocessing catalyst is much smaller than those of the feeds. These phenomena are probably due to the differences in hydrogen donation and solubility of the coke in the feed between coal-derived liquids and heavy petroleum oils. Operating conditions can have some effect on the H/C ratios of the deposition. Coal-derived liquids will reduce the coking of the carbonaceous materials by donating hydrogen and will also remove the carbonaceous materials by dissolving them. Figure 1 shows elemental analyses of each extract of adsorbed and deposited material on the catalysts used for upgrading the coal-derived liquid(B). The atomic H/C ratio of each extract from the catalysts showed a more hydrogenated structure than that of the feed. Higher N/C ratios in the preasphaltene and the THF in soluble carbonaceous deposition indicate that nitrogen-containing compounds also seem to be the precursors for the carbonaceous

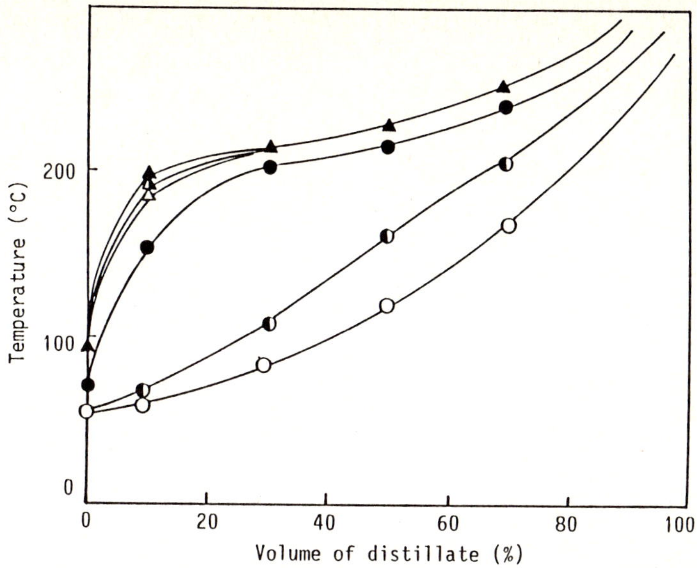

Fig.2. Distillation curves showing effect of nitrogen content on hydrocracking reaction of coal-derived distillates. Three kinds of feeds were hydrotreated over Ni-Mo/zeolite catlyst. These feeds (A,B and C) contain 1100, 340 and 20 ppm of nitrogen, respectively. Feed A: ▲, Feed B: ▲, Feed C: △, Product A: ●, Product B: ◐, Product C: ○ .

deposition. The oxygen-containing compound on the catalyst will affect the chemical states of the active metal.

Figure 2 shows the effect of the nitrogen-containing compounds on the upgrading of middle distillate from Wandoan coal over a Ni-Mo/Y-zeolite catalyst. The hydrocracking activity decreased with the increase of nitrogen content in the feed. These results clearly show that zeolite supported catalysts are easily deactivated by the adsorption of nitrogen-containing compounds and ammonia onto the acid sites. For the upgrading of petroleum distillates, very high hydrocracking activity was achieved.

Figure 3 shows the ^{13}C-NMR spectra of the asphaltene and preasphaltene fractions of the feed as well as the carbonaceous deposit on a THF extracted spent catalyst. The aromatic carbon ratio of the deposition was lower than that of the asphaltene and preasphaltene fractions. This shows that polymerization rather than aromatization is predominant on the catalyst. These results are in keeping with the previous results that the H/C ratio of the deposit is higher than those of the fractions. The peak around 150 ppm also shows that the oxygen-containing aromatic compounds still remain on the catalyst after hydrotreating.

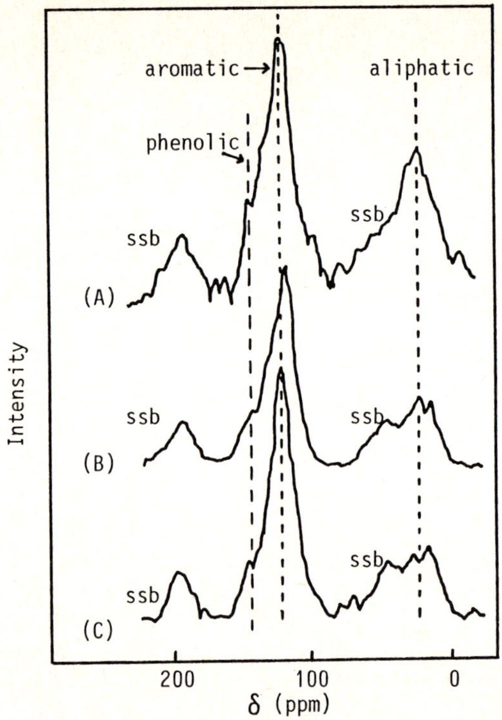

Fig. 3. Magic-angle-spinning solid state ^{13}C-NMR spectra of spent catalyst. Peaks around 30 and 120 ppm indicate methylene bonds in aliphatic carbon and aromatic carbon. The symbol ssb refers to the spinning side bands. (A): Spent catalyst extracted by THF, (B): Asphaltene in feed, (C): Preasphaltene in feed.

Deposition of metals

In coal-derived liquids, the major contaminants are Fe, Ti, Ca, Mg, and Na, while in heavy petroleum Ni, V and Fe are the major metal contaminants. Some features of the deposition of metals from coal-derived liquids and heavy petroleum are quite similar. The deposition of metals are much slower than that of the carbonaceous materials. This results in a slower, but steady deactivation (refs. 7,11,28,30,31,34,35). Metal deposition decreases from the inlet to the exit in a fixed bed reactor (Table 4). The metal deposits are generally found to be concentrated at the external surface of the catalyst extrudate as shown in Fig. 4 and Table 4-B (ref. 11). In large pore catalysts, however, the metal depositions are distributed rather uniformly throughout the

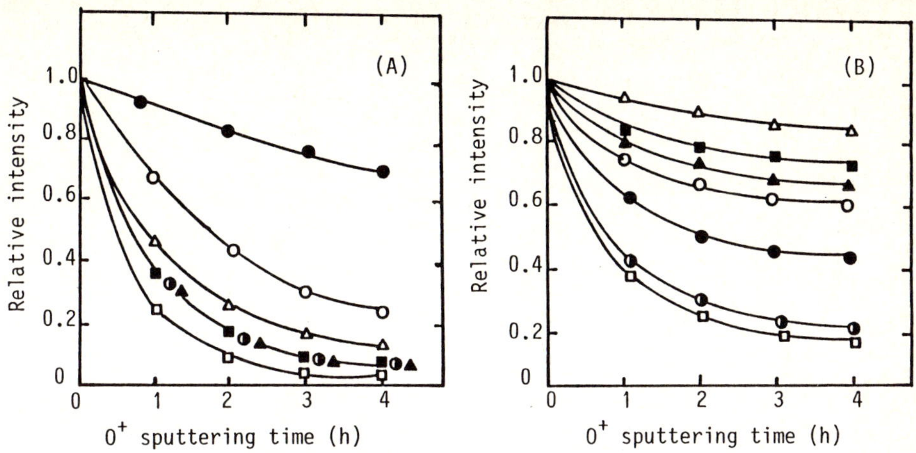

Fig. 4. Depth profiles of metals deposited on outer surface layers of catalyst particles. (A) Unimodal catalyst (pore diameter: 10nm). (B) Bimodal catalyst (pore diameter: 10 and 650 nm). Na: ●, Mg: ■, Si: ◑, K: □, Ca: △, Ti: ▲, Fe: ○.

TABLE 4
Metal depositions on used catalysts

A) ICP and AAS analyses of major metal contaminants on catalysts

Catalyst		Fe	Na	Mg	Ca	V	Ni	Total★1
Cat B	Inlet	4.6	2.4	15.1	1.6	-	-	19.6
	Middle	0.9	1.3	4.1	0.6	-	-	6.9
	Outlet	1.0	1.1	0.8	0.2	-	-	3.3
Cat D	Inlet	-	-	-	-	18.6	4.3	24.5
	Middle	-	-	-	-	5.5	0.9	7.1
	Outlet	-	-	-	-	2.5	0.3	3.5

Figures show the percent values basing on the weight of the fresh catalysts.
★1: Total amounts of metal depositions on the catalysts.

B) XPS analyses of catalyst(B) used for hydrotreating coal liquid

Catalyst		Al	Mo	S	C	Na	Mg	Ca
Sphere	Fresh	100	7	13	110	-	-	-
	Used, Inlet	100	13	43	660	84	100	26
	Middle	100	7.7	28	320	61	61	11
	Outlet	100	9.6	36	440	38	83	24
Powder★1	Fresh	100	6.7	12.2	37	-	-	-
	Used, Inlet	100	6.4	12.3	150	26	33	4.4
	Middle	100	7.0	11.8	140	20	14	2.3
	Outlet	100	7.9	15.0	190	13	9.7	2.2

Figures show atomic ratios of elements basing on Al concentration.
★1: XPS measurements were performed after powdering the catalysts.

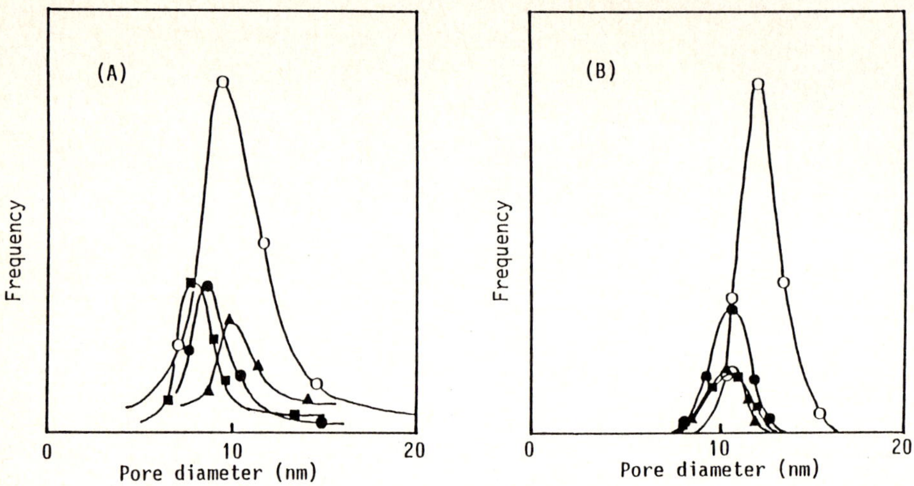

Fig. 5. Changes in pore size distribution of catalysts used for hydrotreating coal-derived liquid and petroleum residue. (A): Hydrotreating of coal-derived liquid with asphaltene. (B): Hydrotreating petroleum residue. Fresh catalyst:○, Used catalysts; inlet: ■ , middle: ● , outlet: ▲ .

catalyst particles after long reaction times (refs. 18,36). The metals are in the form of sulfides on catalysts used in hydroprocessing petroleum residue (ref. 37), while the majority of the metals on the spent catalyst used for hydrotreating coal-derived liquids are present in different forms such as oxides, carbonates and sulfates. This is indicated by the lower amount of sulfur relative to those of other elements as shown in Table 4-B. The metals deposited on the catalysts will affect not only the catalyst deactivation, but also the regeneration of the used catalyst.

Physical properties of used catalysts

The significant decrease in surface area and pore volume for used catalysts after hydrotreating coal-derived liquids and heavy petroleum has already been reported (refs. 7,10,38,39). A catalyst with small micropores loses its surface area and pore volume more rapidly than a catalyst with larger micropores after coal-liquid hydroprocessing (refs. 11,17). The shift of pore size to lower diameters was observed on used catalysts as shown in Fig. 5. However, the behavior of the shift to lower pore diameter was different between the two types of catalysts used for coal liquid and petroleum hydroprocessing. This result indicates the different effect of metal deposition on the physical

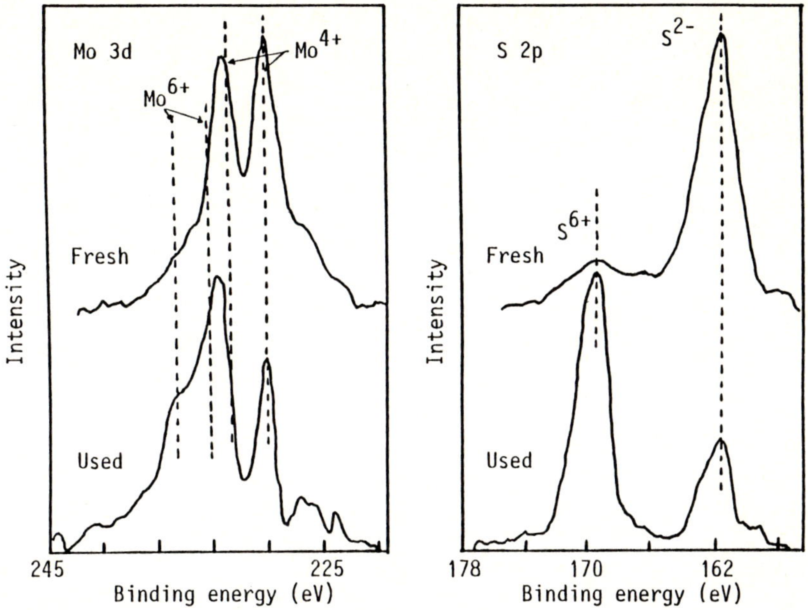

Fig. 6. Mo3d and S2p photoelectron spectra on the catalyst used for hydrotreating coal-derived liquid.

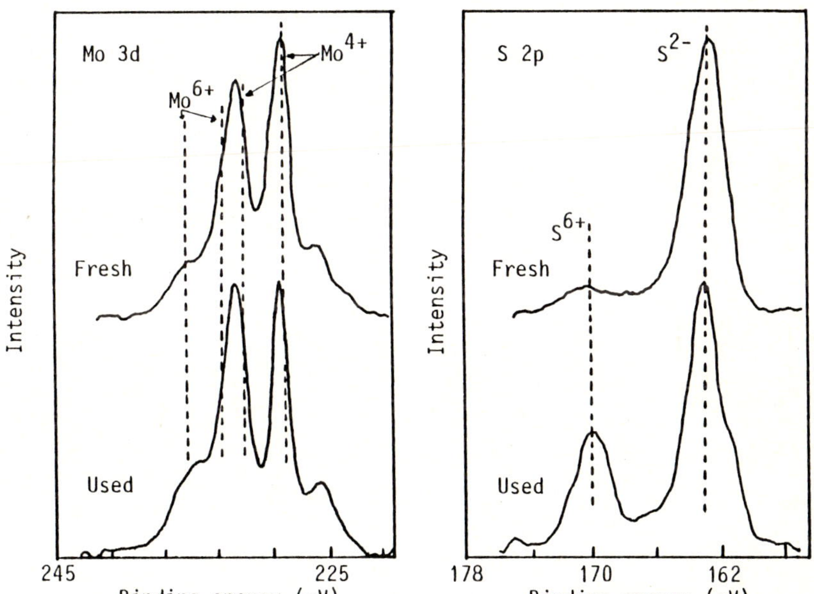

Fig. 7. Mo3d and S2p photoelectron spectra on the catalyst used for hydrotreating petroleum residue.

properties of the catalysts when coal liquids are hydrotreated. The growth of MoS_2 like crystals was observed by TEM analysis of the surface of the spent catalyst, as recently reported (ref. 40)

Chemical properties of used catalysts

Though a lot of discussions have been made concerning the physical properties of used catalysts (refs. 41-44), few studies have been done on the changes in the chemical properties of used catalysts which might occur by migration and gathering of active metals. Quantitative analyses of the molybdenum ions, as measured by XPS, are shown in Table 4-B. Atomic Mo/Al ratios on the surface of the sphere of spent catalysts were larger than that on the fresh catalyst. This indicates that the molybdenum atoms move from the bulk to outer surface layers of the particles during the hydrotreating of coal-derived liquids (ref.45). Figures 6

TABLE 5
EXAFS analyses around molybdenum atoms on used catalysts

Catalyst		O ★1	S ★1	Mo ★1
Standard				
$NaMoO_4.2H_2O$		4.0	-	-
MoS_2		-	6.0	6.0
Cat A	Fresh, Oxide	1.7	-	0.4
	Sulfide	0.8	4.4	2.0
	Used, Inlet	0.9	4.0	2.0
	Middle	0.8	3.9	2.0
	Outlet	0.9	4.3	2.3
Cat B	Fresh, Oxide	1.7	-	0.6
	Sulfide	0.8	4.5	2.0
	Used, Inlet	0.8	3.7	2.1
	Middle	0.8	4.4	2.5
	Outlet	0.9	4.8	2.8
Cat C	Fresh, Sulfide	0.7	4.4	1.8
	Used, Inlet	0.7	4.1	2.0
	Middle	0.9	4.7	2.2
	Outlet	0.9	5.0	2.4
Cat D	Fresh, Sulfide	1.0	3.8	1.3
	Used, Inlet	1.0	5.1	2.3
	Middle	0.7	4.7	1.9
	Outlet	1.0	4.7	2.1

★1: Figures show numbers of coordinated S and O or nearest Mo.

and 7 show Mo3d and S2p photoelectron spectra of molybdenum catalysts used for hydrotreating coal liquid and petroleum residue, respectively. The proportion of Mo^{4+} species attributed to the MoS_2 like species decreased significantly on the outer surface layers after coal liquid hydroprocessing. The decrease in the proportion of Mo^{4+} species occurred because of the low sulfur content of the feedstock. This might be accelerated by the presence of high amounts of oxygen in the feed and by water produced. S2p spectra indicate the change of the electronic state of sulfur from sulfide to sulfate. Considering both the results from the electronic properties of Mo3d and S2p spectra and the surface composition of active species, the changes in the molybdenum structure from sulfide to sulfate are thought to occur during reaction.

EXAFS results for the analysis of molybdenum on the spent catalyst are shown in Table 5. Changes in the concentration of coordinated S and nearest Mo around molybdenum atoms were detected after hydrotreating coal liquids and petroleums. On used catalysts, an agglomeration of molybdenum was found to increase from inlet to outlet in the reactor. The decrease in coordinated sulfur atoms around the molybdenum atoms after coal liquid hydrotreating directly showed the change in the sulfide structure of molybdenum atoms, as previously indicated by the XPS measurement. On the other hand, the coordinated sulfur atoms increased after petroleum hydroprocessing.

REGENERATION OF AGED CATALYSTS

Regeneration of the catalyst is very important not only to the development of practical methods to restore catalyst activity, but also to obtain fundamental knowledge about the cause of catalyst deactivation. This knowledge is invaluable for designing a long life catalyst. In this work, the regeneration of the catalyst was used to give insight into the causes of the catalyst deactivation. Molybdenum catalysts, as already mentioned, are easily deactivated by various means such as carbonaceous or metal deposition. Accordingly, it is necessary to characterize each mode of poisoning and distinguish them from other causes of catalyst deactivation.

Calcining up to 500℃ (in air) and washing with sulfuric acid at different temperatures were used to remove carbonaceous and metal deposits from the catalysts, respectively (refs. 45,46). Resulfiding at 400℃ was carried out in all case in order to reform the sulfides of the active species after burning or washing. Table 6 shows results for the regeneration of the catalysts. With only a few exceptions, the HYG activity for spent petroleum refining catalysts recovered fairly well after calcination. This indicates that the major poisoning is due to carbonaceous deposits. However, when the catalyst was used for hydrotreating the coal-derived liquid(B), HYG activities for the catalyst at the inlet recover only partially after calcining. This indicates catalyst deactivation by metal deposition. Resulfiding of the used catalysts without calcining or washing caused some recovery of HYG activity for the catalyst used in coal liquid hydroprocess-

TABLE 6
HYG and HYC activities observed before and after regenerating catalysts

Catalyst	Regeneration	HYG	HYC
Cat A Fresh		1.0	1.0
Used, Inlet		0.13	0.16
	Sulfiding	0.26	0.63
	Calcining + sulfiding	0.50	1.22
Used, Outlet		0.20	0.14
	Sulfiding	0.40	0
	Calcining + sulfiding	0.66	1.55
Cat B Fresh		1.0	1.0
Used, Inlet		0.03	0
	Sulfiding	0.12	0.03
	Calcining + sulfiding	0.23	0.31
	Washing + calcining + sulfiding	0.85	0.84
Used, Outlet		0.24	0.05
	Sulfiding	0.34	0.05
	Calcining + sulfiding	0.97	0.51
	Washing + calcining + sulfiding	1.07	0.81
Cat C Fresh		1.0	1.0
Used, Inlet		0.22	0.08
	Sulfiding	0.28	0.13
	Calcining + sulfiding	0.54	4.19
Used, Outlet		0.31	0.09
	Sulfiding	0.34	0.04
	Calcining + sulfiding	0.89	2.02
Cat D Fresh		1.0	1.0
Used, Inlet		0.58	0.08
	Calcining + sulfiding	0.58	2.84
Used, Outlet		0.30	0.04
	Calcining + sulfiding	0.95	2.25

Calcining at 500℃, washing with sulfuric acid and sulfiding with H_2S at 400℃ were carried out to refresh the deactivated catalysts.

ing. This result is consistent with the previous result in which the structure of active metals partially changes from sulfide to sulfate or oxide during reaction. The HYG activity of the catalyst deactivated by metal deposition recovered considerably after consecutive acid treatment and burning.

The HYG activity of the catalyst from the inlet was less active than that of the fresh catalyst after the regeneration mentioned above, in spite of the fact that most metal contaminants were removed by acid treatment from the catalysts used for the coal liquid(B). This difference in the HYG activity is probably due to the migration and gathering of molybdenum ions during coal liquid hydroprocessing which were described in the previous characterization of the used catalysts. Few changes in local structures of molybdenum atoms were caused by the moderate temperature calcinations used for regeneration, though some changes occurred during acid washing. The above results indicate that the chemical properties of molybdenum are not restored to their original state by the regenerations and therefore better methods of catalyst regeneration are required.

The HYC activity of the catalyst used for the processing of coal liquid(B) did not recover to the initial level even after washing in sulfuric acid and then calcining. The recovery of the HYC activity of the catalysts used for coal liquid(A) hydroprocessing by calcining and sulfiding shows that carbonaceous deposition decrease HYC activity. This is in good agreement with the deactivation behavior during hydrodesulfurization of petroleum residue. In contrast, the HYC activity of the former catalyst at the inlet remained less active than that at the outlet after the regeneration process of burning and sulfiding. It is evident that metal deposits have a harmful effect on HYC activity in hydrotreating coal liquid(B).

Different phenomena were observed for the HYC activity of the regenerated catalysts used for petroleum and coal liquid(A) hydroprocessing. The HYC activities of the catalysts after calcining and sulfiding were much higher than those of the fresh catalysts. The reason for this strange behavior is not yet clear. Nickel and vanadium contaminants, and an agglomeration and a migration of active ions will affect the catalyst functions. The addition of nickel as promoter onto the catalyst generally increases HYG activity, while an increase in HYG activity for the hydrogenation of DPM was not observed. Accordingly, the major cause for the increase of HYC activity is due to the change in the structure of the active sites. In fact, EXAFS measurements revealed the gathering of molybdenum atoms after hydrotreating petroleums (Table 5). In previous work it was shown that the proper gathering of molybdenum ions can be favorable for HYC activity while a highly dispersed state for the molybdenum ions leads to high HYG activity (refs. 16,47). Therefore, the strange behavior noted above can be explained if the concentration of active sites that are effective for HYG activity do not increase and that of hydrocracking active sites increases because of the gathering of molybdenum ions during the reaction. Thus the change in the structure of active sites can increase HYC activity and decrease HYG activity for the catalyst. Because hydrodesulfurization(HDS) activity generally increases with increasing HYC activity, these results suggest higher recovery of HDS activity. On the other hand, since both higher HYG and HYC activities are necessary for hydrodenitrization(HDN) activity, this suggests that HDN activity recover to a lower extent. The difference in catalyst functions can in turn affect the chemical composition of the carbonaceous deposit formed during the reaction. The elevation of reaction temperature has been observed by some researchers to also have an effect on the nature of the active sites (refs. 24,48-50).

NEW CATALYST DESIGN CONCEPT

Based on a full understanding of the deactivation phenomenon, a new type of catalyst with a longer life can be designed in order to develop a practical process for hydrotreating petroleum and synthetic heavy oils. An easier approach to the prevention of catalyst deactivation can be to pretreat the feeds. Catalytic demetallization and extraction techniques can be used to remove asphaltene and metals from the feed (refs. 23,51,52). Liquefaction processes and operating conditions also affect the deactivation behavior of the catalysts. Two stage liquefaction processes have been demonstrated to impart the advantage of long-term activity to the catalysts (refs. 52,53). Effects of hydrogen pressure, space velocity and reaction temperature on the catalyst deactivation process are now fairly well understood (refs. 27,43,44,54). Physical properties of the catalyst such as pore size distribution and particle size have also been controlled to prevent catalyst deactivation and to increase asphaltene conversion (refs. 39,42,43,55). In the following, the control of chemical properties and function of the catalyst with the aim of designing long life catalysts are discussed in light of the above mentioned findings.

It is known that the interaction between the support and the active metal is different for different supports (refs. 5,16). Therefore, each support gives different local structures to the active ions. This in turn imparts different activities to the variously supported catalysts (ref. 16). For HYC activity the role of acidic sites can be minimal or even disruptive. Acidic sites soon become covered with carbonaceous materials which essentially block their participation in any catalytic reactions. Worse yet, these deposits can grow to the extent that they block off pores where active metals reside. Therefore, the direct participation of the acidic sites of a support are not ultimately important to the HYC activity of the catalyst. More important is the role of the support in modifying and enhancing the activity of the active metals on its surface. The catalyst function required for a particular hydrotreating process defines what needs to be designed into the catalyst. A catalyst with relatively high HYC activity is not suitable for hydroprocessing coal liquid and petroleum with asphaltene, because the HYC activity of the catalyst does not work well in the presence of heavy aromatics. The aromatics can be hydrocracked after hydrogenation of aromatic rings, indicating that a catalyst with higher HYG activity and lower HYC activity will be effective for heavy feeds. Thus the proper control of the HYG and HYC activities of a catalyst seems to be the most important feature in the design of a long life catalyst.

Following from the ideas developed above, two types of catalysts were designed and prepared in this work. For hydrotreating a coal-derived liquid which contains asphaltene, an alumina support was selected because of its high HYG activity among various supports that were evaluated. The chemical properties of the alumina support were then controlled in order to decrease some acid sites as required for HYG activity. In order to give a higher dispersion of active ions, the properties of aluminium hydroxide were controlled during the support preparation. Nickel and molybdenum were then loaded on the support in a highly dispersed state. Although the concentration of active species was much less than that of commercial catalyst, almost the same HYG activity was obtained. On the contrary, this catalyst showed lower HYC activity.

A different type of catalyst having both higher HYC and HYG activities was designed for hydrotreating a coal-derived distillate. Alumina and titania supports gave the highest HYG and HYC activities, respectively, among various supports studied. EXAFS and Raman spectra showed the different degree of agglomeration of molybdenum atoms on titania as compared to that on alumina. The combination of two kinds of different active sites can lead to a synergistic effect. In fact, a synergistic effect for the HYC activity was observed on this double oxides supported catalysts. Accordingly, double oxides of TiO_2-Al_2O_3 were prepared with varying atomic Ti/Al ratios. The molybdenum catalyst prepared showed higher HYC activity than alumina based catalysts. The support which contains titania in it seems to be suitable for reducing carbonaceous deposits due to the lower number of acid sites on titania relative to alumina. Two kinds of catalysts possessing the two types of catalyst functionalities defined above were tested using coal-derived liquids(A and B). The preliminary results indicated that these catalysts showed improvement in activity and initial deactivation.

REFERENCE

1 B. Delmon, Proc. 3rd Int. Conf. Chemistry and Uses of Molybdenum, Climax Molybdenum Co., Ann Arbor, Michigan, (1979) p.73.
2 P. Grange, Catal. Rev. Sci. Eng., 21 (1980) 135.
3 E. Furimsky, Catal. Rev. Sci. Eng., 22 (1980) 371.
4 F.E. Massoth and G. Muralidhar, Proc. 4th Int. Conf. Chemistry and Uses of Molybdenum, Golden, Colorado, (1982) p.343.
5 H. Topsoe and B.S. Clausen, Appl. Catl. 25 (1986) 273.
6 D.S. Thakur and M.G. Thomas, Appl. Catl., 15 (1985) 197
7 D.S. Thakur and M.G. Thomas, Ind. Eng. Chem. Proc. Res. Dev., 23 (1984) 349.
8 B. Delmon, Appl. Catal., 15 (1985) 1.
9 D.S. Thakur and M.G. Thomas, Appl. Catal., 15 (1985) 197.
10 M.G. Thomas and D.G. Sample, Fuel, 60 (1981) 145.
11 A. Nishijima, M. Kurita, T. Sato, Y. Yoshimura, H. Shimada, and N. Todo, Proc. Pan-Pacific Synfuels Conf. Tokyo, Japan, 1982, Vol.2, p.247.
12 M.M. Ahmed and B.L. Crynes, Adv. Chem. Ser., ACS Washington D.C., 179 (1979) 175.
13 G.H. Bartholomew, Chem. Engineering, (1983) 96.
14 J.R. Katzer and R. Sivasubramanian, Catal. Rev. Sci. Eng., 20 (1979) 155.
15 D.L. Trimm, Appl. Catal., 5 (1983) 263.

16 A. Nishijima, H. Shimada, T. Sato, Y. Yoshimura, and J. Hiraishi, Polyhedron, 5 (1986) 243.
17 Y. Yoshimura, T. Sato, H. Shimada, and A. Nishijima, Fuel. Sci. Tech. Int. 4 (1987) 621.
18 H. Shimada, T. Sato, M. Kurita, Y. Yoshimura, and A. Nishijima Chem. Letters, (1983) 181.
19 G.W. Schultz, H. Shimada, Y. Yoshimura, T. Sato, and A. Nishijima, Bull, Chem.Soc. Jpn., 58 (1985) 1077.
20 K. Tanaka, and T. Okuhara, Catal. Rev. Sic. Eng., 15 (1977) 249.
21 F.E. Massoth and K.S. Chung, Proc. 7th Int. Cong. Catal., Elsevier, New York, 1981, p.629.
22 H. Shimada, M. Kurita, T. Sato, Y. Yoshimura, and A. Nishijima Chem. Letters, (1984) 1861.
23 T. Ohtsuka, Catal. Rev. Sci. Eng., 16 (1977) 291.
24 M. Inoguchi et al., Bull. Japan Petrol. Inst., 13 (1971) 153.
25 N. Todo et al., Kogyo Kagaku Zasshi, 74 (1971) 563.
26 A. Nielsen, B.H. Cooper and A.C. Jacobsen, ACS, Div. Petrol. Chem., 26 (1981) 440.
27 J.M. Pazos, J.C. Gonzalez and A.J. Salazar-Guillen, Ind. Eng. Chem. Proc. Des. Dev., 22 (1983) 653.
28 A.J. de Rosset, G. Tan and J.G. Gatsis, Adv. Chem. Ser., 179 (1979) 109.
29 G.J. Stiegel, L.M. Polinski and R.E. Tischer, Ind. Eng. Chem., Proc. Des. Dev., 21 (1982) 477.
30 P.W. Tamm, H.F. Harnsberfer and A.G. Bridge, IEC., Proc. Des. Dev., 20 (1981) 262.
31 J.J. Stanulonis, B.C. Gates and J.H. Olson, AICHE. J., 22 (1976) 576.
32 A.J. de Rosset et al., FE-2010-1 through 9 (1976 and 1977).
33 H.J. Chang, M. Seapan and B.L.Crynes, Proc. 7th Int. Symp. Chem. Reaction Eng., Boston, Mass, ACS Symp. Ser., 196 (1982) 309.
34 Y. Yoshimura, M. Kurita, T. Sato, H. Shimada, Y. Kobayashi, and A. Nishijima, J. Fuel Soc. Jpn., 64 (1985) 68.
35 A.M. Henke, Oil and Gas J., April 68 (1970) 97.
36 J. Wei and R.G. Wei, Chem. Eng. Comm., 13 (1982) 251.
37 T.H. Fleisch, B.L. Meyers, J.B. Hall and G.L. Ott, J. Catal., 86, (1984) 147.
38 H. Beuther, O.A. Larson and A.J. Perrotta, "Catalyst Deactivation", B. Delmon and G.F. Froment (Eds.), Elsevier Publishing Co., Amsterdam, (1980) p.271.
39 L.M. Polinski, G.J. Stiegel and R.E. Tischer, 1980 Status Review, DOE/PETC/TR-81/2 (1981).
40 G.B. Freeman, J. Heink, N.J. Long and B.H. Davis, Appl.Catal., 23 (1986) 309.
41 P.N. Hannerup and A.C. Jacobsen, ACS, Div. Petrol. Chem., 28 (1983) 576.
42 K.L. Riley, ACS, Div. Petrol. Chem., 23 (1978) 1104.
43 C.C. Kang and J. Gendler, Preprints, ACS, Div. Petrol. Chem., 23 (1978) 1421.
44 O. Togari, H. Takahashi and M. Nakamura, J. Jpn. Petrol. Inst., 23 (1980) 256.
45 J.M. Bagdanor and H.F. Rase, Ind. Eng. Chem. Prod. Res. Dev., 25 (1986) 220.
46 US, Patent, 317216 (1981)
47 A. Nishijima, T. Sato, Y. Yoshimura and T. Kameoka, to be published in J. Jpn. Petrol. Inst.
48 D.S. Thakur, F.E. Massoth and M.G. Thomas, Proc. 4th Int. Conf. Chemistry and Uses of Molybdenum, Climax Molybdenum Co., Golden, Colorado, 1982.

49 A. Ocampo, J.T. Schrodt and S.M. Kovach, IEC, Prod. Res. Dev., 17 (1978) 56.
50 M. Ternan and J.F. Kriz, "Catalyst Deactivation", B. Delmon and G.F. Froment (Eds.), Elsevier Scientific Publ. Co., Amsterdam, (1980) p. 283.
51 E. Gorin, C.J. Kulik and H.E. Lebowitz, Ind. Eng. Chem. Proc. Des. Dev., 16 (1977) 95.
52 S.M. Olek and H.S. Sherry, Ind. Eng. Chem. Proc. Des. Dev., 16 (1977) 525.
53 J.W. Rosenthal, A.L. Dahlberg, C.W. Kuehler, D.R. Cash and W. Freedman, Fuel, 61 (1982) 1045.
54 S.W. Weller, Proc. 4th Int. Conf. Chem. and Uses of Molybdenum, Climax Molybdenum Co., Golden, Colorado, (1982).
55 H. Shimada, M. Kurita, T. Sato, Y. Yoshimura and A. Nishijima, Bull. Chem. Soc. Jap., 59 (1986) 2885.

B. Delmon and G.F. Froment (Editors), *Catalyst Deactivation 1987*

CoMo HDS CATALYSTS : SIMULATED DEACTIVATION AND REGENERATION. ROLE OF VARIOUS REGENERATION PARAMETERS

A. ARTEAGA, J.L.G. FIERRO*, P. GRANGE and B. DELMON

Unité de Catalyse et Chimie des Matériaux Divisés, Université Catholique de Louvain, Place Croix du Sud 1, B-1348 Louvain-la-Neuve, Belgium.

* On leave from Instituto de Catalisis y Petroleoquimica, Madrid.

ABSTRACT

The present contribution aims at presenting the essential results obtained in a laboratory study of regeneration. The catalyst was a commercial CoMo/γ-Al_2O_3. We shall briefly recall the findings published in two other publications : the first one investigated the role of coke present in the catalyst before regeneration, and the influence of the number of regenerations. The second dealt with the influence of regeneration temperature.

We present here in more detail a still unpublished part, concerning the influence of steam on regeneration. We simulated regeneration by controlled oxidation at temperature between 400 and 700°C in a 5 % v/v O_2:N_2 mixture containing 6.8 % v/v H_2O. After regeneration the catalysts were resulfided in standard conditions. In contrast with the previous results, activity for hydrodesulfurization (HDS) of thiophene and hydrogenation (HYD) of cyclohexene were markedly diminished after these pretreatments. The catalysts were characterized by infrared spectroscopy of adsorbed NO, XPS and ISS measurements. The sulfur content and the octahedrally coordinated Co species decreased with increasing regeneration temperature, while the $Mo^{\delta+}$ species strongly increased.

Although the results of all the various experiments cannot yet be interpreted in a perfectly consistent manner, we shall indicate the main conclusions.

1. INTRODUCTION

Two of the most valuable properties of HDS catalysts, namely resistance to most catalyst poisons and long-term stability of activity even under quite severe conditions, are unfortunately not unlimited. HDS catalysts are subject to deactivation in the course of use. At the end of an operating cycle, the catalyst must be either discarded or its activity must be reestablished by regeneration. The corresponding decision depends mainly on the causes of the deactivation. If deactivation is primarily due to coking, most of the activity can be recovered by oxidizing the catalyst in a controlled atmosphere of air diluted with nitrogen or steam. However, if a significant amount of deactivation results from ageing or poisoning by metals or other inorganic contaminants (as arsenic compounds, for example), even the most finely controlled and thorough regeneration will still leave the catalyst well below fresh catalyst activity, and regeneration may be uneconomical.

In spite of the importance of the CoMo HDS catalysts, relatively few studies on deactivation and regeneration have been reported in the open literature. This was the reason why we embarked on a detailed study of the regeneration of an industrial CoMo/γ-Al_2O_3 HDS catalyst (1-4). It was confirmed that a regenerated catalyst could possess higher activities than the fresh one (1), as it had been reported for true regeneration in industrial plants (5). The physico-chemical characterization of the regenerated catalyst indicated that an increase of the surface exposure of both Co and Mo ions and a decrease of inactive $CoAl_2O_4$-like species took place. The part of the study which most directly addressed the problem of catalyst damage due to overheating dealt with a series of catalysts regenerated at different temperatures in the presence of a 5 % v/v O_2:N_2 mixture (2,3). At temperatures above 500°C the sulfur content, the number of octahedrally coordinated Co species, hydrodesulfurization (HDS) and hydrogenation (HYD) activities decreased, while exposure of the Mo ions increased. Co ions exposure decreased as a result of diffusion to the subsurface layers of the alumina to form non-sulfidable $CoAl_2O_4$-like species.

Due to the high exothermicity of coke combustion and oxidation of sulfides, the burnoff process of a coked catalyst is generally carried out in the presence of air diluted with nitrogen or steam, which are used as a heat sink. The operation in the presence of steam can be conducted more easily because of its higher heat capacity (6). However, it is believed that steam has a negative influence on the mechanical strength, structure and sometimes even on the activity of the regenerated catalysts. Consequently, the study of the regeneration in the presence of steam constituted an important part of our study.

With the constraints of a laboratory study, our regeneration could only simulate the essential characteristics of that of a catalyst having worked several months or years in a commercial plant. We were forced to limit ourselves to the reoxidation of a precisely reduced-sulfided (activated) catalyst. We reactivated the obtained solid. The essential part of the work is a comparison of the properties of the "regenerated" and reactivated catalysts with those of the fresh catalysts activated for the first time. In some cases, a more detailed simulation of a real regeneration was made; coke was deposited on the catalyst before reoxidation.

In the present communication, we shall summarize very shortly the main findings concerning the influence of deposited coke (1), of the number of regeneration (1) and of regeneration temperature (2).

We shall report in more detail new results concerning the influence of steam during regeneration at different temperatures on the catalytic and physico-chemical properties. The regeneration was simulated as in the other studies (1,2) but H_2O was added to the O_2:N_2 mixture. We compared the HDS and HDY activities of the regenerated catalysts, and their physico-chemical properties (XPS, ISS and IR of NO probe-molecule) with those of the catalysts regenerated in the absence of steam (2), after reactivation in the same conditions.

2. EXPERIMENTAL

2.1. Catalysts

A commercial CoMo/γ-Al_2O_3 catalyst (Procatalyse, HR-306) was used in this study. The extrudates were crushed and sieved to 0.1-0.2 mm size. The chemical composition, as determined by atomic-absorption spectrometry, was 2.9 wt % CoO and 13.8 wt %.MoO_3. The BET surface area of the catalyst in the oxidic form (before activation) was 194 m^2g^{-1}.

2.2. Pre-treatments of the catalyst

The catalyst was subjected to the following pre-treatments :

2.2.1. Activation (A). A 6.5 sample of catalyst was sulfided in a 15 % v/v H_2S:H_2 mixture at 400°C and atmospheric pressure for 3.25 h. For details see refs. (1-4).

2.2.2. Carbon deposition. Accelerated ageing was carried out after activation of the catalyst using an Ar feed containing either 1,3-butadiene or methylcyclopentane at 450°C. For details see ref.(1). Carbon analyses were performed following the method described by Jones et al. (16a). The coke loading of the catalyst was defined by the carbon content expressed as weight percentage (wt %).

2.2.3. Regeneration (Rw). Samples of the sulfided catalyst were heated in N_2 flow at 130°C for 1.5 h. Then a 5 % v/v O_2:N_2 flow containing 6.8 % v/v H_2O (6 dm^3h^{-1}) was introduced and the temperature was progressively increased to the desired value (400-700°C) (average heating rate 5°C min^{-1}) and kept constant for 20 h. Then, dried air was passed over the catalyst for 5 h. Finally, the reactor was allowed to cool to ambient temperature in an N_2 stream. The catalysts obtained in this way will be referred to as A.Rw-T, where T is the temperature of regeneration. Loss of molybdenum and the condensation of large crystallites of MoO_3 at the outlet of the reactor were observed during regeneration at 700°C.

2.2.4. Reactivation (A). The reactivation was carried out in conditions identical to those used in the first activation. After the full pretreatment, the catalysts will be referred to as **A.Rw.A-T** (sulfided catalyst regenerated at the temperature T in the presence of steam and then resulfided).

2.3. Activity measurements

Catalytic activity measurements were carried out at 237°C and 30 bar in a high-pressure reactor (Geomecanique Catatest). The hydrodesulfurization (HDS) and hydrogenation (HYD) activities were measured using a feed charge containing 70 wt % cyclohexane, 29.5 wt % cyclohexene and 0.5 wt % thiophene. The procedure used was the same as that previously reported (1,2). The HDS and HYD activities were defined by the thiophene and cyclohexene conversion on 2 g of catalyst.

2.4. Physico-chemical characterization

The sulfided catalysts were characterized by the following techniques : X-ray photoelectron spectroscopy (XPS), ion scattering spectroscopy (ISS), and infrared spectroscopy (IR) of adsorbed NO. The sulfur content of the catalysts after reactivation was also determined following the method of Jones et al. (16b). The description of apparatus and the working procedure for XPS are given elsewhere (1).

Thanks to the different positions of the IR bands corresponding to NO adsorbed on Mo and NO adsorbed on Co, the intensity of the corresponding bands constitutes a specific measurement of the surface exposition of the various ions. It is actually the only such specific measurement. The method has been described previously (1).

For the ISS measurements, the sulfided catalysts (before catalytic test) were pressed in a sample holder without exposure to air, as for the XPS measurements. A beam of $^4He^+$ ions with an energy of 2 keV, a spot size on the sample of 350 μm and a total current of 7.5 nA were used. Details of the apparatus and the working procedure are given elsewhere (7).

3. RESULTS

3.1. Summary of the previous work

Coke deposited from methylcylopentane or butadiene (1) brought about a decrease of surface area and pore volume (Figure 1). The losses of catalytic activity (HDS and HYD) are reported in Figure 2.

After a first regeneration and reactivation, both activities (HYD and HDS) were substantially higher than those of the fresh catalyst activated for the first time (1). This confirmed the observation (5) concerning industrial off-site regeneration (of a non specified $CoMo/Al_2O_3$ catalyst) with dry gas. Activities in our case decreased slightly after 3 regenerations. A striking finding was that two catalysts with the same HYD and HDS activities could correspond to different quantities of exposed Mo and Co (as indicated by the

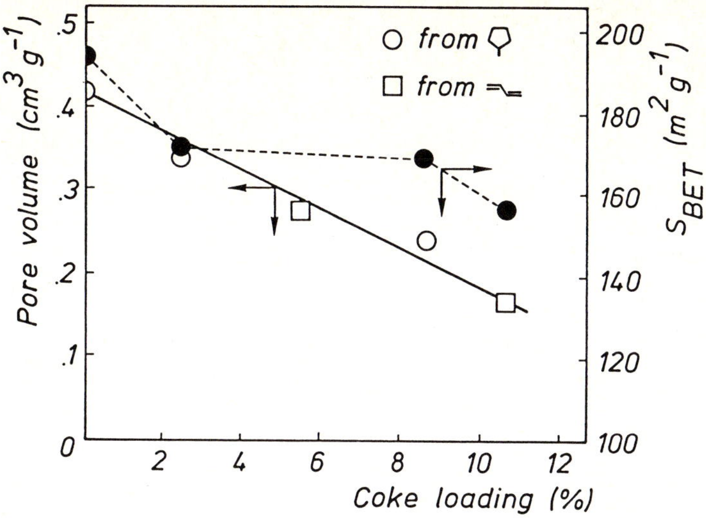

Fig. 1 Pore volume (measured by mercury intrusion) and S_{BET} surface area of the catalyst, as a function of the coke loading.

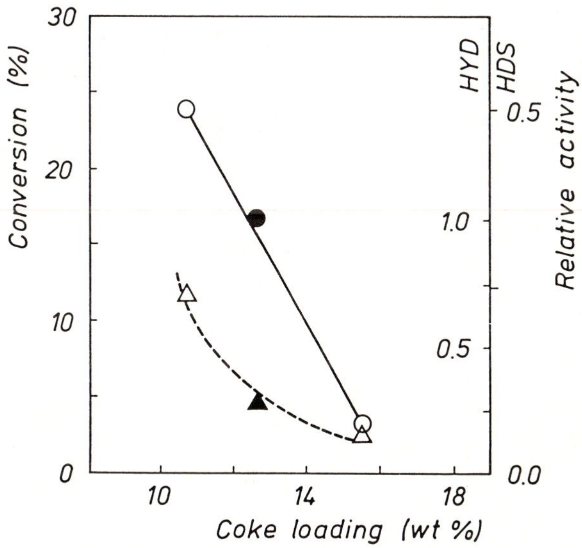

Fig. 2 Influence of the coke loading (1,3-butadiene precursor) on the HDS (○,●) and HYD (△,▲) activities. Relative activities refer to those of the fresh activated catalyst (0.0% C). Full symbols correspond to experimental points obtained at 237°C, 30 bar and LSHV 42 h^{-1}. Open symbols were obtained by linear extrapolation from data at 300°C (ref. 1).

intensities of the IR bands of adsorbed NO). Indeed, we found that the presence of coke deposited before regeneration had an influence on the latter quantities whereas the HYD and HDS activities were the same (Figure 3).

The influence of regeneration temperature (2) will be plotted, together with the new results (steam regeneration) in a subsequent figure (Figure 6); 500°C corresponds to maximum activities. A substantial activity decrease is observed (in HYD and HDS) for regeneration at higher temperatures. XPS measurements indicate an increase of the Mo dispersion with regeneration temperature; the overall Co dispersion is constant. This indeed corresponds to an increase of the surface exposition of Mo. But the number of Co atoms decreases (Figure 4). The correlation between the activities and the intensities of the NO IR bands are presented in Figure 5.

In what follows, we report in detail the results obtained after regeneration in the presence of steam.

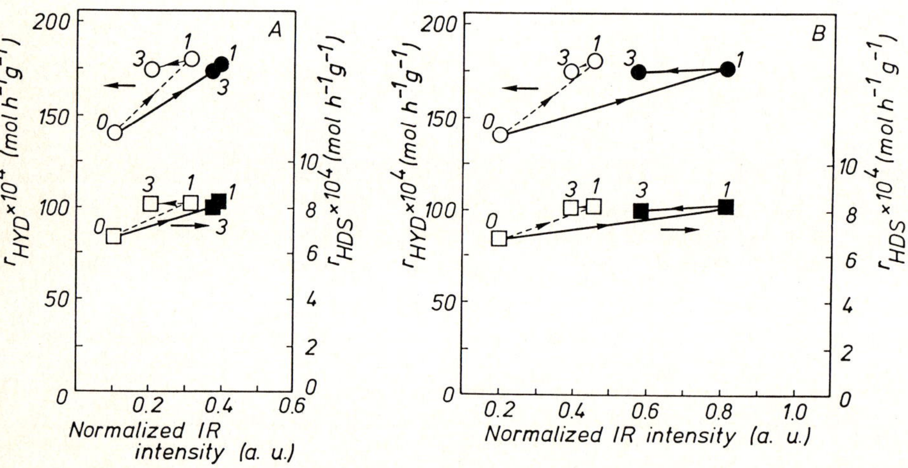

Fig. 3 Dependence of the HDS and HYD activities of sulfided catalysts on IR intensity band of adsorbed NO.
Full and open symbols refer to catalysts regenerated after coking and without coking, respectively. The numbers over the symbols indicate the number of regeneration cycles.

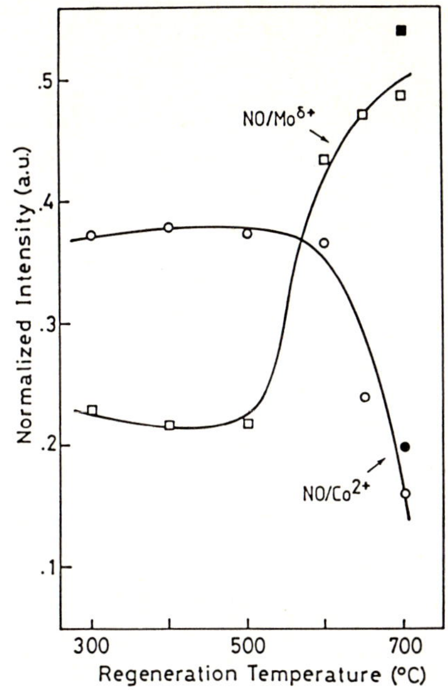

Fig. 4 Influence of regeneration temperature on the normalized IR intensities of NO chemisorbed on Co^{2+} ions (○) (band at about 1850 cm^{-1}) and on $Mo^{\delta+}$ ions (□) (band at about 1680 cm^{-1}).
Full and open symbols refer to catalysts regenerated after coking and without coking, respectively.

3.2. Regeneration in the presence of steam : sulfur analyses

The sulfur content of the reactivated regenerated $CoMo/Al_2O_3$ catalysts are reported in Table 1. This table shows that after the last activation, the sulfur content of the sulfided catalyst varied between 6.8 and 5.9 wt % : the higher sulfur content corresponds to the catalyst regenerated at 400°C, and then decreases with increasing regeneration temperature. The low sulfur content of the A.Rw.A-700 catalyst was not only due to the loss of Mo observed during regeneration, because this loss (0.3 wt % as MoO_3) represents only 0.13 wt % of S calculated as MoS_2.

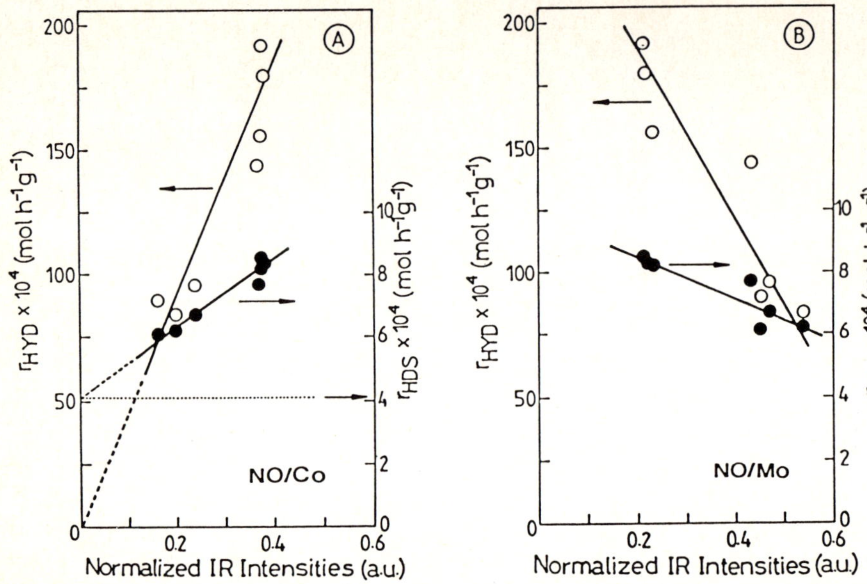

Fig. 5 Correlation between HDS and HYD rates and the normalized IR intensities of NO-probe chemisorbed : (A) on Co^{2+} ions (band at about 1850cm^{-1}) and (B) on $Mo^{\delta+}$ ions (band at about 1680 cm^{-1}).

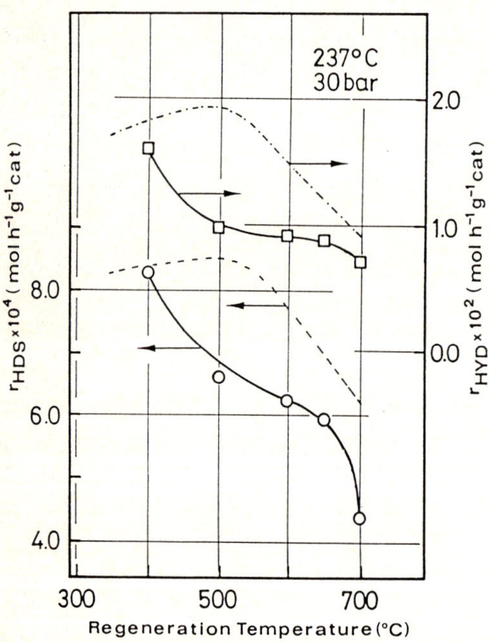

Fig. 6 Influence of the regeneration temperature on the HDS (○) and HYD (□) rates at 237°C and 30 bar. Regeneration carried out in the presence of steam. Dotted lines refer to catalysts regenerated without steam (from ref. 2).

TABLE 1

Molybdenum and sulfur analyses of catalysts

Regenerated non-activated	Mo Content wt % MoO_3	Regenerated and activated	S Content wt %
A.Rw-400	13.8	A.Rw.A-400	6.8
A.Rw-500	ND	A.Rw.A-500	6.4
A.Rw-600	13.8	A.Rw.A-600	6.5
A.Rw-650	13.8	A.Rw.A-650	6.1
A.Rw-700	13.5	A.Rw.A-700	5.9

ND : not determined.

3.3. Regeneration in the presence of steam : Catalytic activity

The thiophene HDS and cyclyhexene HYD rates at 237°C, as a function of the regeneration temperature (400-700°C), are given in Figure 6. For comparison, the results of the catalytic activities for the catalysts regenerated in the absence of steam, are also represented (dotted lines, from ref. 2). The HDS activity of the catalyst regenerated at 400°C in the presence of steam was identical to that observed for the catalyst regenerated in the absence of steam. However, the activity decreased strongly with increasing regeneration temperature. This decrease of HDS activity was more pronounced and more premature than for the catalysts regenerated in the absence of steam. As can seen in Figure 6, cyclohexene HYD activity followed a similar trend, but the activity decrease, relative to the catalyst regenerated in absence of steam at 400°C, was more pronounced for HYD than for HDS.

3.4. Regeneration in the presence of steam : physico-chemical characterization

3.4.1. XPS. Surface composition of the sulfided catalysts (after the catalytic test) is given by XPS. The Mo $3p_{3/2,1/2}$ doublet is shown in Figure 7A for the A.Rw.A-400 and A.Rw.A-650 catalysts. No significant difference, neither in peak position nor in lineshape was found in the A.Rw.A-T catalyst series. The peaks at 395.3 and 412.9 eV are characteristic of Mo^{4+} ions like in the MoS_2 or MoO_2 structures (8-10). Each peak exhibited asymmetric shape, with a shoulder at about 399.0 eV; this is due to some contribution of non sulfided Mo^{6+} (and possibly Mo^{5+}) ions. This phenomenon was more marked in the catalysts regenerated in the presence of steam.

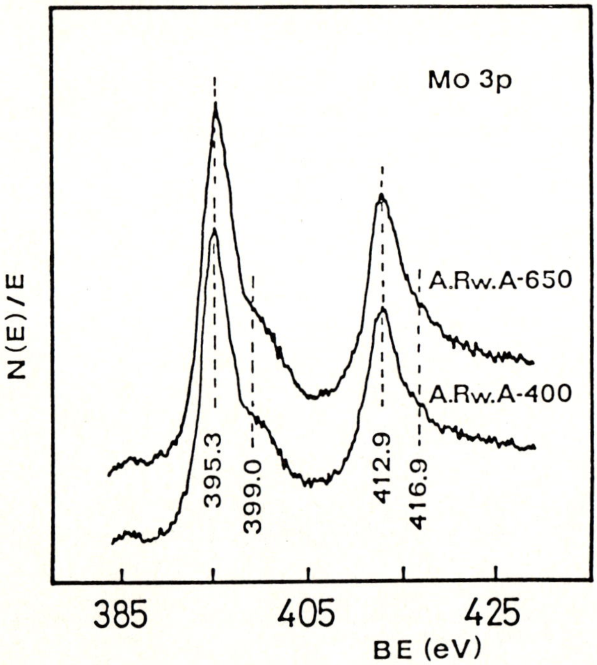

Fig. 7A XPS spectra of the Mo3p levels for the sulfided regenerated catalysts, after catalytic test (A.Rw.A-400 and A.Rw.A-650 catalysts)

The relative intensity, $Mo3p_{3/2}/Al2p$, as a function of the regeneration temperature, is given in Figure 8. The Mo signal increased progressively with increasing regeneration temperature.

In the case of Co, significant differences in the shape of the XPS spectra were found. The spectra of the $Co2p_{3/2,1/2}$ levels are shown in Figure 7B, for the A.Rw.A-T catalysts (T = 400, 500, 650 and 700°C). The most conspicuous feature of these spectra is that increasing the regeneration temperature from 400 to 700°C caused a drastic decrease in the amount of sulfided cobalt (doublet at 779.8 and 794.8 eV), and a simultaneous increase in the amount of non-sulfidable cobalt species (doublet at 782.6 and 795.5 eV) (8, 10-12). In spite of the changes in the nature of the cobalt species detected in Figure 7B, the total Co signal (sulfided + oxidic cobalt) remained virtually constant throughout the explored regeneration temperature range.

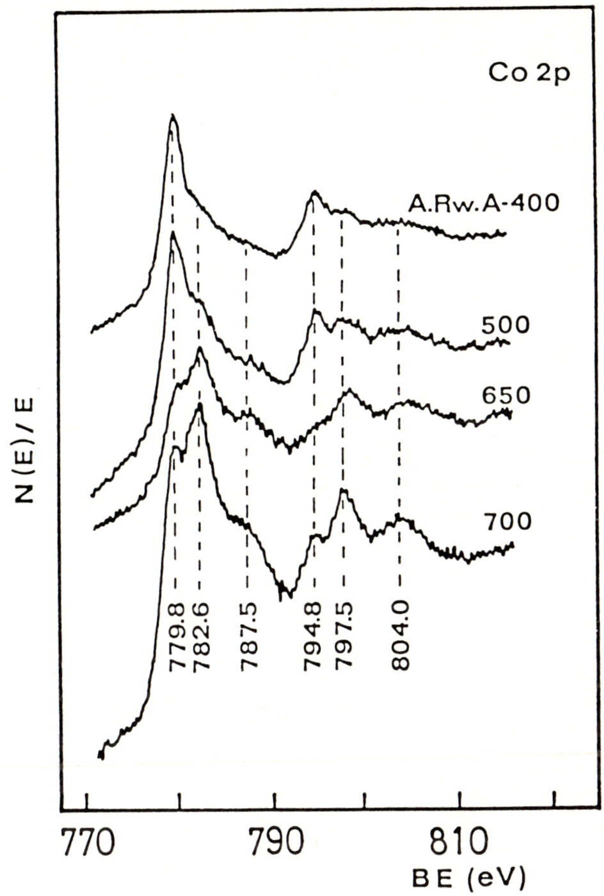

Fig. 7B XPS spectra of the Co2p levels for the sulfided regenerated catalysts, after catalytic test (A.Rw.A-T series)

The S2p photoline of all sulfided catalysts at 162.4 eV (not represented) is characteristic of S^{2-} ions (8). Together with this peak, a second one, much less intense, appeared at about 169.4 eV; it is attributed to sulfate species (1,12,13) strongly held by the support surface. This latter line was absent in the catalysts regenerated above 600°C.

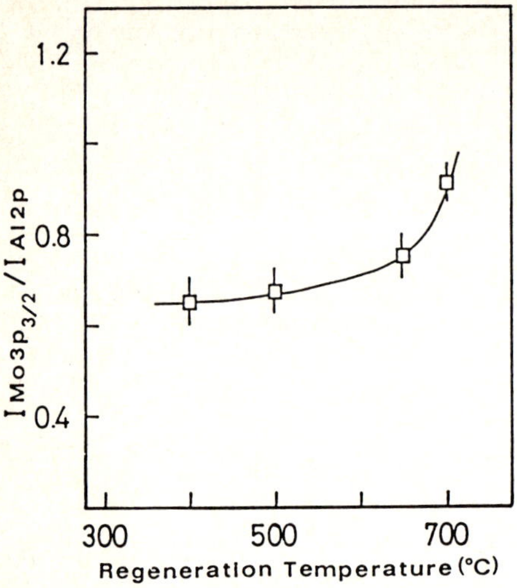

Fig. 8 XPS intensity ratio Mo3p/Al2p for the sulfided regenerated catalysts after catalytic test (A.Rw.A-T series).

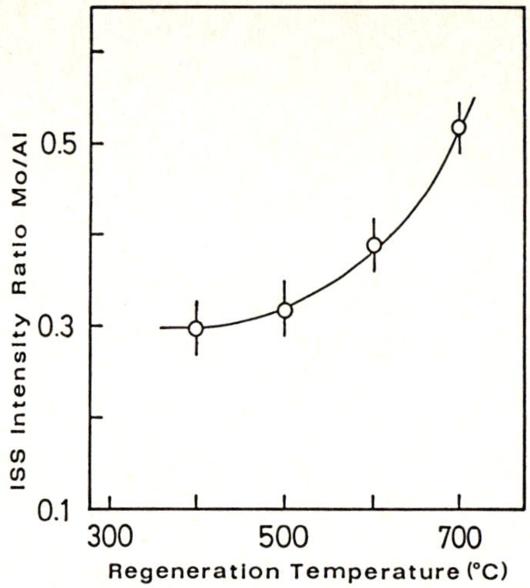

Fig. 10 ISS intensity ratio Mo/Al for the sulfided regenerated catalysts before catalytic test (A.Rw.A-Tseries).

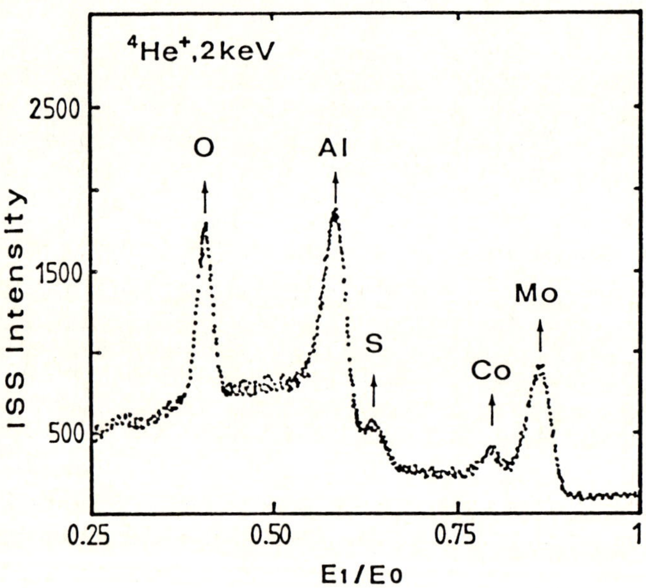

Fig. 9 $^4He^+$ (2 keV) ISS spectrum at 138° scattering angle of a sulfided regenerated CoMo/Al_2O_3 catalyst before catalytic test (A.R.A-700).

3.4.2. ISS. Figure 9 shows a typical ISS spectrum obtained on a sulfided CoMo/γ-Al_2O_3 catalyst (A.R.A.-700). The only observed peaks were due to scattering from O, Al, S, Co and Mo atoms at the catalyst surface, as indicated in the figure. The Mo/Al ISS intensity ratio, as a function of the regeneration temperature, is given in figure 10. This intensity ratio increased strongly with increasing regeneration temperature.

3.4.3. IR of chemisorbed NO. The IR spectra of NO chemisorbed on the sulfided catalysts regenerated at different temperatures (A.Rw.A-T series) are given in Figure 11. The origin of the different bands was described elsewhere (1,2,14,15). Noticeable changes in both lineshape and band intensity as a function of the regeneration temperature were observed.

The normalized infrared intensities of the bands at about 1850 cm^{-1} (symmetric stretching vibration of NO chemisorbed on Co^{2+} in an environment of S^{2-} ions) and 1680 cm^{-1} (antisymmetric stretching vibration of NO chemisorbed on sulfided $Mo^{\delta+}$ ions), as a function of the regeneration temperature, are given in Figure 12. The intensity of the band responsible for sulfided Co^{2+} sites decreased progressively in the 400-700°C temperature range. On the contrary, the intensity of the band responsible for sulfided $Mo^{\delta+}$ sites increased drastically with increasing regeneration temperature.

4. DISCUSSION

The only relevant published results are found in a paper by Ramaswamy et al. (32), who investigated an industrial CoMo/Al_2O_3 catalyst regenerated six times in situ with a water vapor containing gas. Their study did not involve a comparison of the effect of regeneration with and without steam, but the comparison of the physico-chemical properties of a spent commercial HDS catalyst with those of a fresh sample. They observed important changes in the texture (sintering) and structure of the support, and loss of cobalt and molybdenum. They have also observed that the reducibility of the spent catalyst was higher than that of the fresh catalyst.

Our discussion will thus be restricted to our own work. It will mainly concern the new results presented in detail here (regeneration in the presence of steam) and the comparison of regeneration with and without steam. An attempt at a more comprehensive discussion will be made at the end.

4.1. Effect of regeneration on activity

The presence of steam during regeneration of the CoMo/Al_2O_3 hydrotreating catalyst causes unfavorable changes in its properties when subjected to temperatures above 400°C. The HDS activity of the A.Rw.A-500 catalyst (Figure 6) decreased by ca. 20 % with respect to that of the A.Rw.A-400

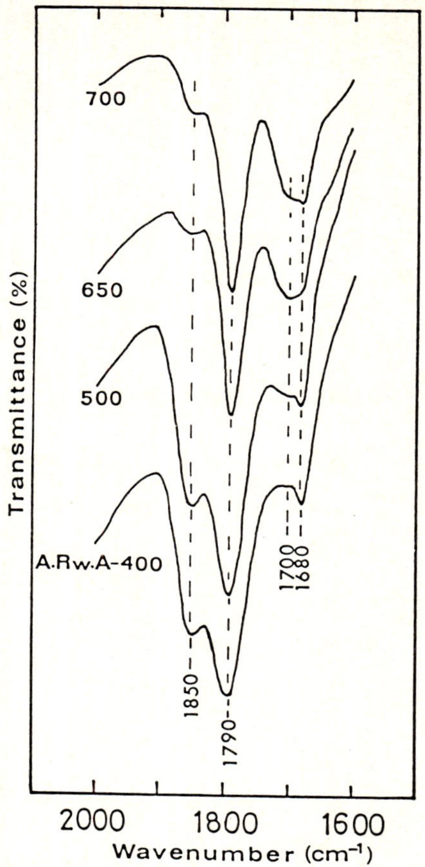

Fig. 11 IR spectra of NO chemisorbed at room temperature on sulfided regenerated catalysts, before catalytic test (A.Rw.A-T series).

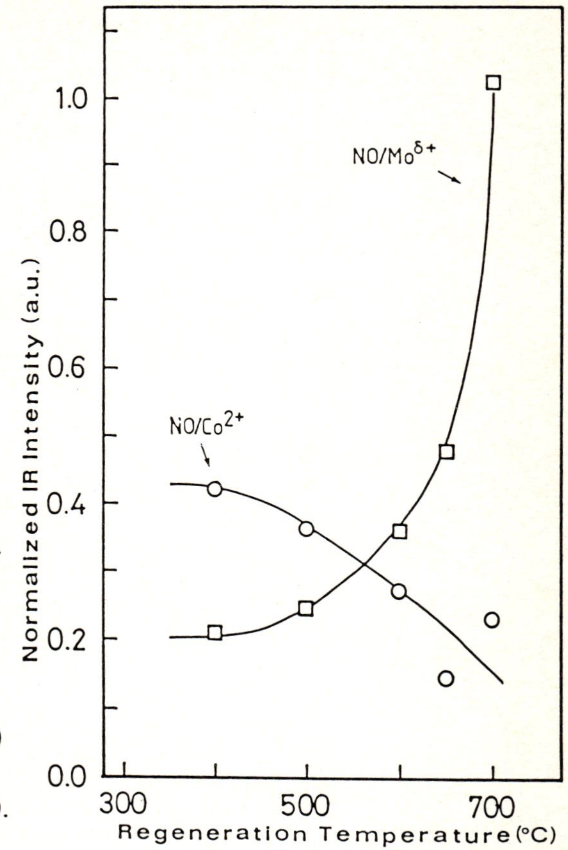

Fig. 12 Influence of regeneration temperature on the normalized IR intensities of NO chemisorbed on :
(○) Co^{2+} ions (band at ca. 1850 cm^{-1})
and
(□) $Mo^{\delta+}$ ions (band at ca. 1680 cm^{-1}).

catalyst, whereas it remained unchanged after regeneration in the absence of steam. This decrease was marked (47 %) when the regeneration was conducted in steam at 700°C. The HYD activity was also drastically affected by the presence of steam. For instance, HYD activity losses of 45 and 60 % were observed on catalysts regenerated at 500 and 700°C, respectively. The difference in the variations of the HDS and HYD functions with the regeneration temperature can be taken as an additional argument to support the hypothesis which assumes that there are different active sites for each reaction. Indeed, the evidence of the existence of different sites for HDS and HYD reactions is very convincing (17,18).

The catalytic activity and selectivity of CoMo HDS catalysts find their origin in the dispersion of the various sulfided phases (MoS_2 or the Co-Mo-S species, and the Co sulfides), the nature of the ions on the surface of these phases (specially Mo or Co on the edges of the MoS_2-like structure) and the spatial relation between the species (proximity of Co sulfides and MoS_2 structure, Co in the MoS_2 edges, etc.). For these reasons, we shall examine in detail the structural changes in the active phase of the sulfided catalysts brought about by regeneration at different temperatures in the presence of steam.

4.2. Effect of regeneration on molybdenum

Two striking effects of regeneration in the presence of steam were observed on the regenerated and reactivated catalysts : one concerns the Mo dispersion and the other, the nature of the Mo superficial atoms.

The XPS and ISS results (Figures 8 and 10) indicate that Mo dispersion increases with increasing regeneration temperatures. This interpretation is supported by the normalized intensity of the antisymmetric stretching IR band of NO-probe chemisorbed on sulfided ionic Mo sites (Figure 12). These results indicate that it is really the $Mo^{\delta+}$ surface concentration which is increased strongly (by a factor of about 5 between A.Rw.A-400 and A.Rw.A-700).

An important change of Mo dispersion has been observed during regeneration at increased temperature in the absence of steam (2,3). However, this phenomenon seems to be enhanced by the presence of steam, especially at the highest temperatures. The concentration of the $Mo^{\delta+}$ sites of the catalyst regenerated at 700°C in the presence of steam (A.Rw.A-700, in this work) was at least twice as high as that of the catalyst regenerated in the absence of steam at the same temperatures (A.R.A-700, in ref. 2). The increase of Mo dispersion has been explained by a redistribution of Mo atoms during oxidation of MoS_2 crystallites (2,3). The vapor pressure of MoO_3 starts to be important in the 600-700°C temperature range. This favors MoO_3 vaporization from MoO_3 crystallites and further readsorption onto the MoO_3-free area of the Al_2O_3. The presence of steam favors this process since MoO_3 reacts with steam to form a volatile $MoO_2(OH)_2$ species (19,20) :

$$MoO_{3\ solid} + H_2O_{\ vap} \longrightarrow MoO_2(OH)_{2\ vap}$$

The above reaction, which is more important at high temperatures, explains the loss of molybdenum observed during regeneration at 700°C. A loss of molybdenum has also been observed during regeneration in the absence of steam (2) or during simple heating, in air, of the oxidic catalysts (28), but only at temperatures as high as 800°C.

The increase of Mo dispersion was accompanied by substantial changes in the nature of exposed $Mo^{\delta+}$ ions after reactivation. This information comes from the antisymmetric stretching mode of NO (band at ca. 1700-1680 cm^{-1}), which is very sensitive to the heterogeneity of the adsorption sites (21). A careful analysis of Figure 11 reveals that there are two overlapping bands in this region of the spectra : one narrow band at 1680 cm^{-1} and another broad one at 1700 cm^{-1}. These bands have been assigned to "sulfidable" and "reducible" but non-sulfidabes (at least at 400°C) $Mo^{\delta+}$ sites, respectively (2). Prada et al. (29) have observed similar bands when the catalyst was first reduced (in a H_2 stream) at temperatures of between 400-800°C and then sulfided (in a H_2S/H_2 stream) at 400 or 530°C. The band at high wavenumber disappeared when the catalyst was sulfided at temperature above 530°C. They proposed that this band was due to NO chemisorbed on MoO_2-like species, which were formed during the pre-reduction step. These species are difficult to sulfide at moderate temperatures and they are inactive towards the HDS reaction (30,31).

If the spectra showed in Figure 11 are compared with those obtained for the catalysts regenerated in the absence of steam (see Figure 4 in ref. 2), it could be noted that the relative intensity of the band at 1700 cm^{-1} (compared with those at 1680 cm^{-1}) is much higher for the catalysts regenerated in the presence of steam. This differences is more marked at regeneration temperatures of 500 and 600°C. This fact seems to indicate that the formation of "reducible" $Mo^{\delta+}$ sites is enhanced by the presence of steam during regeneration. The increase of the surface density of "reducible" $Mo^{\delta+}$ sites with the regeneration temperature might explain the decrease of the sulfur content of catalysts regenerated at high temperatures.

4.3 Effect of regeneration on cobalt

The XPS spectra of Co2p level (figure 7B) suggest a decrease of the surface concentration of sulfidable Co species (peak at 779.8 eV) and a parallel increase of the concentration of oxidic (non sulfided) Co species (peak at 782.6 eV) with increasing regeneration temperatures, whereas the overall Co concentration remains essentially unchanged. The decrease of Co^{2+} ions exposure in an environment of S^{2-} ions is also evidenced by the IR measurements of the NO-probe (figure 12). The normalized IR intensity of the band due to NO chemisorbed on sulfided Co^{2+} ions (symmetric stretching at ca. 1850 cm^{-1}) decreased drastically at regeneration temperatures above 400°C. This phenomenon, which was observed during regeneration in the absence of steam at temperatures above 600°C (2), is explained by Co migration from the surface to the sub-surface layers of the Al_2O_3 to form a spinel $CoAl_2O_4$-like species. Diffuse reflectance spectroscopy (DRS) shows that the formation of $CoAl_2O_4$-like species increases conspicuously between 500 and 600°C (27) : indeed, the Schuster-Kubelka-Munk function, determined at 580 nm from the DRS spectra, increases by a factor of 2 in the samples (the alumina support suffers a drastic sintering at 700°C, which superposes to this $CoAl_2O_4$ formation). These species are difficult to sulfide at 400°C (22) and are catalytically inactive (23). A parallel decrease of the superficial Co was also observed in $CoMo/Al_2O_3$ catalysts subjected to calcination at high temperatures (24-26). The formation of non-sulfidable Co species, together with those of Mo, might explain the decrease of the sulfur content of the catalysts regenerated at high temperatures.

4.4 Activity correlation

In figures 13A and 13B we report the dependence of the HDS and HYD activities of the sulfided catalysts on the normalized IR intensity bands of NO adsorbed on Co and Mo ions. No simple correlation exists between the catalytic activity (HDS and HYD) and the surface density of Co^{2+} ions which adsorb NO (figure 13A). In a previous work (2), we observed a certain linear dependence between HDS and HYD activities and the surface exposure of Co^{2+} ions as determined by IR of NO-probe, for the catalyst series regenerated at different temperatures in the absence of steam (figure 5). However, an enormous scattering of the experimental points is observed, when these results are plotted together with the others presented in figure 13A. A similar result was observed for the same CoMo catalyst subjected to successive deactivation-regeneration cycles (1). In this case (figure 3), catalysts with the same catalytic activity presented large differences in the intensity of the IR bands of NO chemisorbed on superficial Co ions. Therefore, in spite of the linear dependence obtained for a single catalyst series, it is not possible to establish a general correlation between the intensity of the IR band due to NO adsorbed on Co ions and the HDS (or HYD) activity for the $CoMo/Al_2O_3$ catalysts. This is mainly due to the fact that

NO chemisorption measures the total number of the various exposed Co sites (Co in Co-Mo-S, Co_9S_8, CoS_{1-x}, etc...) but does not reflect the specific activity per site.

When the Mo ions are considered, a reverse trend is observed (figure 13B). In other words, catalytic activity decreases when the surface density of Mo ions increases. It must, however, be noted that the intensity values of the IR band due to NO adsorbed on Mo contain the contributions of two different Mo sites. The existence of, simultaneously, a drastic increase of the Mo dispersion and a change of the sulfidability and adsorptive properties of the exposed Mo ions, make even more complicated a full interpretation of these results.

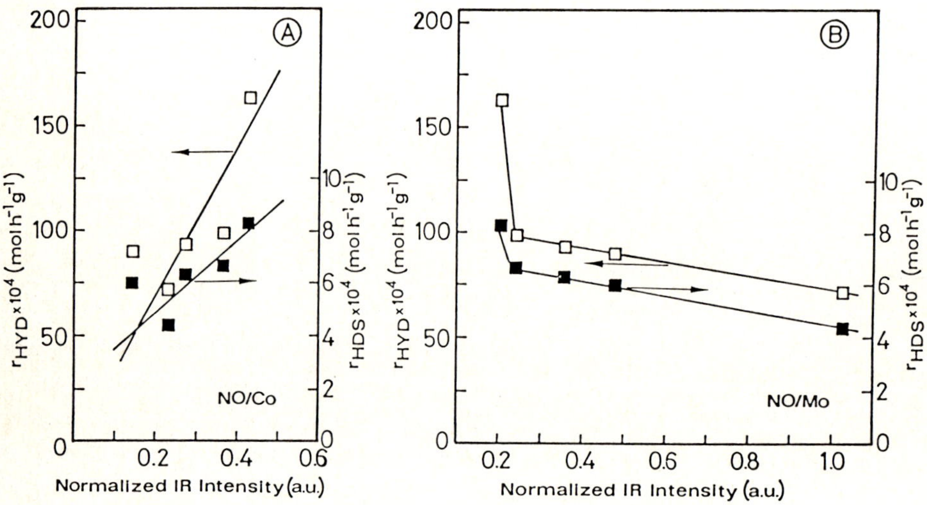

Fig. 13 Dependence of the HDS (■) and HYD (□) activities of sulfided regenerated catalysts on the IR intensity bands of adsorbed NO : (A) : NO/Co ions, and (B) NO/Mo ions (catalysts regenerated in the presence of steam).

5. CONCLUSION

From the data presented above in detail, it can be concluded that infrared spectroscopy of the NO-probe molecule, together with XPS and ISS, are useful techniques for elucidating the nature and changes of the surface species of Co and Mo atoms present in sulfided catalysts subjected to regeneration.

We have shown that the presence of steam during the regeneration of a $CoMo/Al_2O_3$ HDS catalyst at temperatures above 400°C causes unfavorable changes in the catalytic properties. HDS and HYD activities decrease drastically.

The activity loss is accompanied by several physico-chemical changes :

. A drastic increase of Mo dispersion, which is enhanced by the presence of steam;

. The changes in the nature of exposed Mo ions. It is shown that steam enhances the concentration of reducible but non sulfidable Mo sites. This effect is important, even at low regeneration temperatures;

. Migration of the promoter ions to the alumina sub-surface to form a $CoAl_2O_4$-like species.

Although major progress has been made towards the understanding of the changes in the catalyst properties brought about by overheating during regeneration, more research is needed, with the simultaneous use of still more numerous physico-chemical techniques, before a complete interpretation can be arrived at.

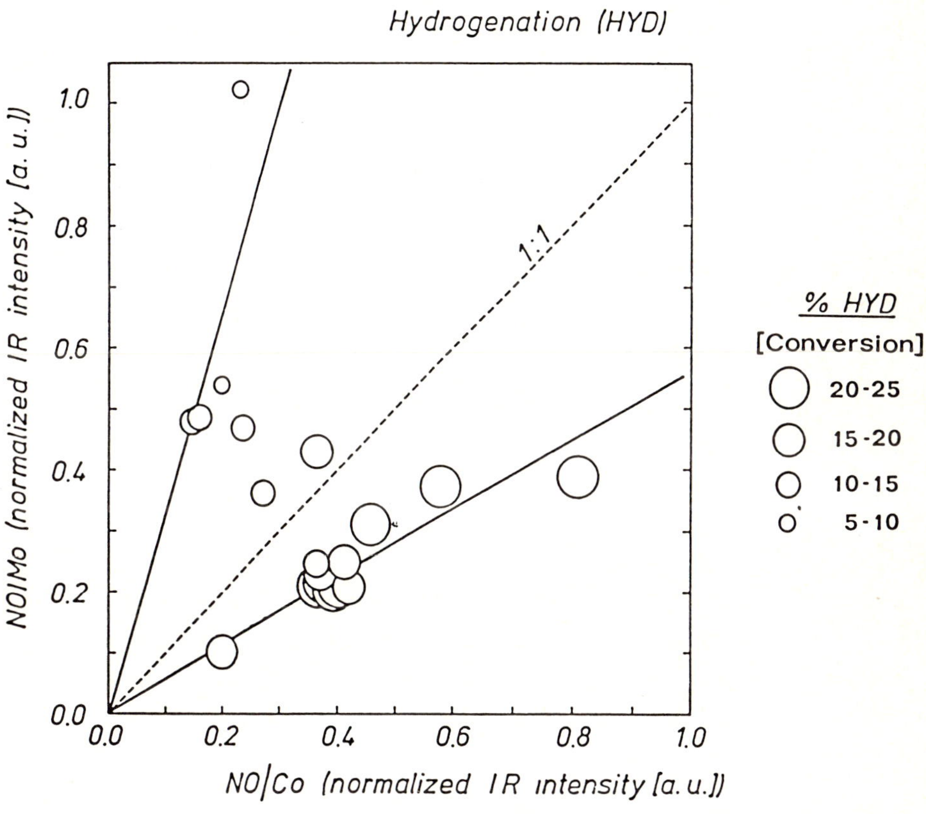

Fig. 14A Correlation between the normalized IR band intensities of NO/Mo and NO/Co, and the HYD activity of regenerated CoMo/γ-Al_2O_3 catalysts.

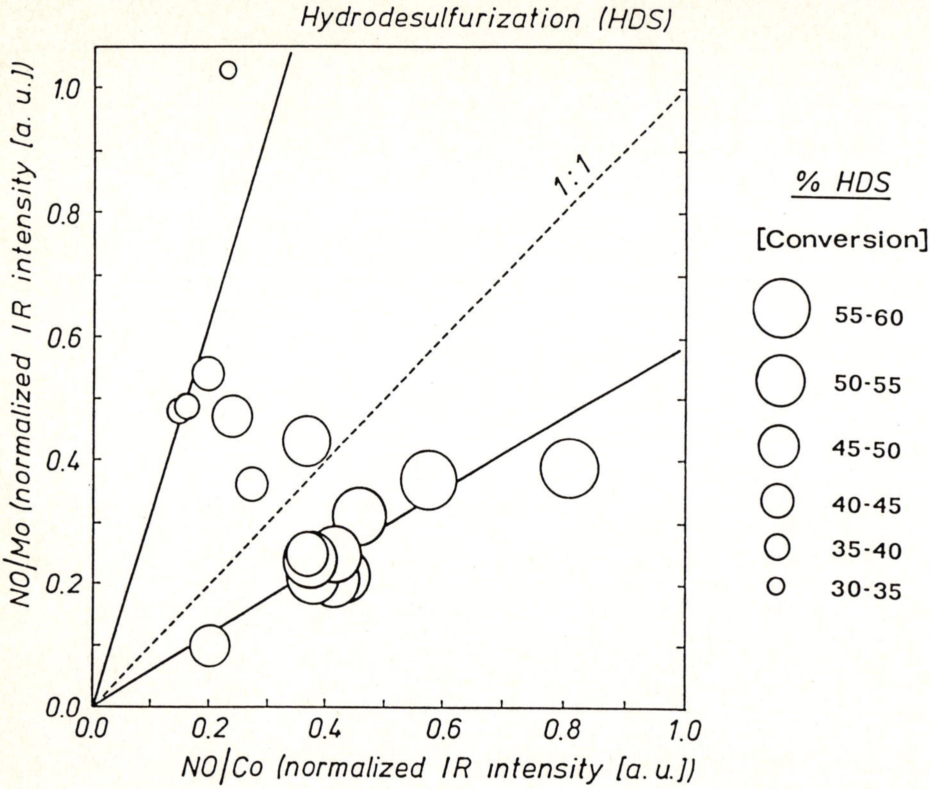

Fig. 14B Correlation between the normalized IR band intensities of NO/Mo and NO/Co, and the HDS activity of regenerated CoMo/γ-Al_2O_3 catalysts.

We have made a surprising observation with our series of catalysts. Let us consider figure 14A (hydrogenation - HYD) or figure 14B (hydrodesulfurization - HDS). The circles are positioned on the figures according to the NO/Mo (ordinate) and NO/Co (abscissa) normalized intensity ratios. Their size represents the magnitude of the activity. It is striking that the most important parameter is the **ratio** of the normalized intensities: the largest circles cluster around a value of (I NO/Co)/(I NO/Mo) of 1.8 for HYD and HDS. Only surprisingly small variations of activities are observed when **both** I NO/Co and I NO/Mo vary in parallel, keeping the above ratio constant. This suggests that a proper balance between the number of exposed Co and the number of exposed Mo is more important that the total number. A similar observation was made by Prada (33) in his study of the activation of the same industrial catalyst as the one used in this study. These new intriguing findings might, together with the use of additional physico-chemical techniques, give clues to more in-depth interpretation.

ACKNOWLEDGEMENT

One of us (A.A.) thanks the "Universidad del Zulia" (Venezuela) for a fellowship. J.L.G.F. thanks the "Instituto de Catalisis", CSIC (Spain) for a sabbatical leave and the "Services de Programmation de la Politique Scientifique" (Blegium) for financial support during that leave. We are indebted to Prof. J. Mercier and Dr J. Devaux of the "Laboratoire des Hauts Polymères" of the UCL for the use of the infrared spectrophotometer. The XPS and ISS equipments were acquired with the financial support of the "Service de Programmation de la Politique Scientifique" and "Fonds de la Recherche Fondamentale Collective" (Belgium), respectively.

REFERENCES

1. A. Arteaga, J.L.G. Fierro, F. Delannay and B. Delmon, Appl. Catal. 26, (1986) 227
2. A. Arteaga, J.L.G. Fierro, P. Grange and B. Delmon, submitted to Appl. Catal.
3. S. Yunes, R. Prada, A. Arteaga, P. Grange and B. Delmon, in "Proc. 3rd Seminary on Catalysis", Salvador (Brazil) (1985) 224
4. A. Arteaga, J.L.G. Fierro and B. Delmon, in "Proc. Xth Iberoamerican Symp. on Catalysis", Merida (Venezuela) (1986) 187
5. G. Berrebi, L'Actualité Chim., October 1983, 29; and unpublished data
6. J.L. Le Page, in "Catalyse de Contact", Edit. Technip, Paris (1978) p 525-528
7. J.M. Beuken and P. Bertrand, Surf. Sci. 162 (1985) 329
8. T. Paterson, J. Carver, D. Leyden and D. Hercules, J. Phys. Chem. 80 (1986) 1700
9. Y. Okamoto, H. Nakano and T. Shimokawa, J. Catal. 50 (1977) 447
10. R.I. Declerck-Grimée, P. Canesson, R.M. Friedman and J.J. Fripiat, J. Phys. Chem. 82 (1978) 885
11. P. Gajardo, P. Grange and B. Delmon, Surf. Interf. Sci. 3 (1981) 206
12. P. Dufresne, J. Grimblot and J.P. Bonnelle, Bull. Soc. Chim. Fr. 3-4 (1980) I-89
13. Y. Okamoto, T. Shimokawa, T. Imanaka and S. Teranishi, J. Catal. 57 (1979) 153
14. J.P. Peri, Preprints Div. Petrol. Chem. ACS, 29 (1984) 889
15. N.Y. Topsoe and H. Topsoe, J. Catal. 84 (1983) 386 and references therein
16. R.F. Jones, P. Gale, P. Hopkins and L.N. Powell, (a) Analyst 90 (1965) 623; (b) J. Iron Steel Inst., May 1966, 505
17. B. Delmon, in "Proc. 3rd Climax Int. Conf. on the Chemistry and Uses of Molybdenum" (H.F. Barry and P.C.H. Mitchell, eds) Climax Molybdenum Co., Ann Arbor, Michigan (1979) 73
18. F.E. Massoth and G. Muralidhar, in "Proc. 4th Climax Int. Conf. on the Chemisty and Uses of Molybdenum" (H.F. Barry and P.C.H. Mitchell, eds) Climax Molybdenum Co., Ann Arbor, Michigan (1982) 343
19. I. Nicolau, A. Aguilo and P.B. De Groot, Ibid., p 234
20. J. Buiten, J. Catal. 10 (1968) 188
21. H.C. Yao and W.G. Rothschild, ref. 18, p 31
22. P. Arnoldy, J.L. de Booys, B. Scheffer and J.A. Moulijn, J. Catal. 96 (1985) 122
23. M.A. Apecetche, J. Lemaître and B. Delmon, Bull. Soc. Chim. Belg. 90 (1981) 419
24. C. Wivel, B. Clausen, R. Candia, S. Morup and H. Topsoe, J. Catal. 87 (1984) 497

25. R. Moné, in "Preparation of Catalysts" (B. Delmon, P.A. Jacobs and G. Poncelet, eds) Elsevier Scient. Publ. Co., Amsterdam, (1979) 381
26. L. Bouyssière, R. Poblete and F.J. Gil-Llambia, in "Proc. 8th Int. Cong. Catalysis" Verlag Chemie, Frankfurt, (1984) 411
27. A. Arteaga et al., to be published.
28. A. Stanislaus and K. Al-Dolama, J. Catal. 101 (1986) 536
29. R. Prada Silvy, J.L.G. Fierro, P. Grange and B. Delmon, in "Preprints 4th Int. Symp. Scientific Bases for the Preparation of Heterogeneous Catalysts" Louvain-la-Neuve, Belgium, 1986, F-9
30. J.M. Zabala, Ph.D. thesis, Louvain-la-Neuve, 1976
31. P. Arnoldy, Ph.D. thesis, Amsterdam, 1985
32. A.V. Ramaswamy, L.D. Sharma, A. Singh and S. Sivansanker, Appl. Catal. 13 (1985) 311
33. R. Prada Silvy, Ph.D. thesis, Louvain-la-Neuve, 1987

B. Delmon and G.F. Froment (Editors), *Catalyst Deactivation 1987*

MECHANISMS OF NICKEL CATALYST POISONING

Calvin H. Bartholomew

BYU Catalysis Laboratory, Department of Chemical Engineering, Brigham Young University, Provo, Utah 84602

ABSTRACT

Poisoning, the strong chemisorption of reactants, products or impurities on active catalytic sites, is an important, difficult deactivation problem in many catalytic processes and particularly in processes involving nickel catalysts. For example, only a few ppm of sulfur impurities can reduce the activity of nickel methanation catalysts by several orders of magnitude within just a few days or weeks; moreover the sulfur thus adsorbed is essentially irreversibly held and cannot be conveniently removed by treatments with air, oxygen, steam, or hydrogen.

Catalyst poisons for nickel can be classified according to chemical species, types of reactions poisoned, and selectivity for active catalyst sites. For example, sulfur in the form of H_2S and organic sulfides is a highly selective, strongly adsorbing poison for nickel hydrogenation, methanation, and steam reforming catalysts. That surface sulfur-nickel bonds are substantially more stable than the corresponding bulk nickel-sulfur bonds is emphasized by the fact that hydrogen sulfide adsorbs dissociatively with a heat of 250 kJ/mole compared to a heat of bulk formation of 75 kJ/mole. Adsorbed sulfur blocks the adsorption of most other species and generally causes a substantial or complete loss of nickel catalyst activity. Whether this loss of activity is a geometric blocking or a longer range electronic effect is somewhat controversial and probably depends on coverage. The evidence is in favor of a combination of geometric and electronic effects at low sulfur coverages and geometric blocking effects at high coverages.

The toxicity of poisons for nickel depends on the stability of the nickel-additive bond as well as the electronegativity of the adsorbing species. Species with a high degree of shielding such as SO_3 are less toxic than poorly shielded species such as elemental sulfur and H_2S. The toxicity of some poisons, e.g. carbonaceous species, depends not only on their strength of adsorption but also on their reactivity with gasifying agents such as hydrogen or water vapor.

INTRODUCTION

Catalyst poisoning (1-6) is one of most difficult deactivation problems in many catalytic processes and particularly in processes involving base metals such as nickel. It is a phenomenon whose global behavior receives extensive study in industrial laboratories for purposes of predicting commercial catalyst life. Yet, a detailed understanding of poisoning mechanisms is, in many important commercial processes, lacking because of the complexity of the poisoning problem and because of the lack of careful, fundamental studies.

One of the most severe and yet commonly encountered poisoning problems is that caused by adsorption of sulfur impurities on metal catalysts (3-5). It is a problem of increasing concern as catalytic processing of sour petroleum feedstocks and coal-derived synthesis gas containing significant concentrations of H_2S and organic sulfides becomes commercially more important. The seriousness of the problem is exemplified in the methanation process in which only a few ppm of sulfur impurities can reduce the activity of nickel catalysts by several orders of magnitude within just a few days or weeks (4); moreover, the sulfur thus adsorbed is essentially irreversibly held and cannot be conveniently removed by treatments with air, oxygen, steam, or hydrogen (4).

During the past decade a number of fundamental catalyst and surface science studies have led to significant advances in the understanding of poisoning mechanisms. Studies up to about 1982 have been summarized in four comprehensive reviews (2-4,6). Many of these previous studies have emphasized the interaction of poisons, particularly sulfur, with nickel. This short review integrates some of the catalyst and surface science studies since 1980 in an attempt to provide the most recent views on the mechanisms of nickel catalyst poisoning with emphasis on poisoning by sulfur. The discussion focuses on several fundamental questions including the following:

o How rapidly and strongly do poisons, especially sulfur, adsorb on nickel?

o What is the mechanism of sulfur poisoning of nickel? Is it due to geometrical blocking or does it involve electronic effects that may propagate many atomic distances from the adsorption site.

o How are poisoning mechanisms affected by the chemistry of the poison? For example, how is poisoning of nickel by arsenic, carbon, chlorine, or phosphorus different from that of sulfur poisoning? How does the chemical oxidation state of the poison affect its toxicity?

In the ensuing section the term poisoning is defined along with important related terms such as selectivity, susceptibility, and toxicity. The effects of shielding, oxidation state, and pore diffusion on poisoning are also discussed. The section thereafter discusses and mechanisms of sulfur poisoning in several important reactions including CO hydrogenation. A comparison of the chemistry of poisoning by different species such as arsenic, chlorine, carbon and sulfur is also made while the role of electronegativity and shielding on toxicity is discussed. Finally the most important conclusions regarding present knowledge of nickel catalyst poisoning are summarized in the concluding section.

DEFINITION OF POISONING

Definition and Kinds of Poisoning

Poisoning (1,2) is the strong chemisorption of reactants, products, or impurities on sites otherwise available for catalysis. Thus, poisoning has operational meaning; that is, whether a species acts as a poison depends upon its adsorption strength relative to the other species competing for catalytic sites. For example, oxygen can be a reactant in partial oxidation of methane to methanol and a poison in ammonia synthesis. In addition to physically blocking adsorption sites, adsorbed poisons may induce changes in the electronic or geometric structure of the surface or result in compound formation (2).

Catalyst poisons can be classified according to chemical species, selectivity for active sites, and the types of reactions poisoned. Table 1 lists three groups of catalyst poisons classified according to chemical origin and their type of interaction with metals. It should be emphasized that interactions of Group VA and VIA elements with catalytic metal phases depend on the oxidation state of the former, i.e., how many electron pairs are available for bonding and the degree of shielding by ligands (1). Thus, the order of decreasing toxicity for sulfur species is H_2S, SO_2, SO_4^{2-}, i.e., in the order of increased shielding by oxygen.

TABLE 1
Common poisons according to chemical origin

Chemical Type	Examples	Type of Interaction with Metals
Groups VA and VIA	N, P, As, Sb O, S, Se, Te	Through s and p orbitals; shielded structures are nontoxic
Toxic Heavy Metals and Ions	Pb, Hg, Bi, Sn Zn, Cd, Cu, Fe	Occupy d-orbitals; may form alloys
Molecules which adsorb with multiple bonds	CO, NO, HCN benzene	Chemisorption through multiple bonds and back bonding

Table 2 lists a number of common poisons for nickel catalysts in several important kinds of reactions. It is apparent that sulfur- and arsenic-containing compounds are typical poisons for nickel in hydrogenation, dehydrogenation, and steam reforming reactions.

TABLE 2
Poisons for selected catalysts in important reactions

Reaction	Poisons
Hydrogenation Dehydrogenation	Compounds of S, Se, Te, P, As, Zn, Hg, halides, Pb, NH_3, C_2H_2
Steam reforming of methane, naptha	H_2S, As, C, coke
CO hydrogenation of coal-derived gases	H_2S, COS, As, HCl

Selective and Nonselective Poisoning

Poisoning selectivity is illustrated in Figure 1, a plot of activity (the reaction rate normalized to initial rate) versus normalized poison

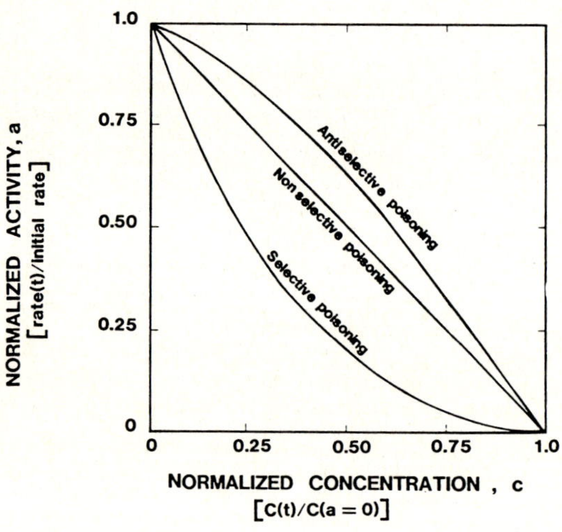

Figure 1. Three kinds of poisoning curves in terms of normalized activity versus normalized poison concentration (Ref 4).

concentration. If poisoning of the most active sites occurs at low concentrations, the poisoning process is "selective." If sites of lesser activity are poisoned initially, the poisoning is "antiselective." An example of selective poisoning is the deactivation of platinum by CO for the para-H_2 conversion while Pb poisoning of CO oxidation on platinum is apparently antiselective (2). If poisoning is nonselective, the linear decrease in activity with poison concentration or susceptibility is defined by the slope of the activity versus poison concentration curve.

Other Important Terms Associated with Poisoning

Several other important terms associated with poisoning are defined in Table 3. Susceptibility, toxicity, poison tolerance and resistance are important concepts that are often encountered in discussions of poisoning including that below.

TABLE 3
Important poisoning parameters

Parameter	Definition
Susceptibility,	Slope of the activity versus poison concentration curve [=(1-a)/C(t)]. Measure of a catalyst's sensitivity to a given poison.
Toxicity	Susceptibility of a given catalyst for a poison relative to that for another poison.
Extent of Poisoning,	The amount of poison required for "complete" deactivation of a catalyst. (Note that a catalyst may not completely deactivate at saturation coverage; see definition of tolerance).
Partition Factor	Amount of poison adsorbed per total amount available. Measure of the reversibility of the poison adsorption at equilibrium.
Resistance	Inverse of the deactivation rate. Property which determines how rapidly a catalyst deactivates.
Tolerance	Activity of the catalyst at saturation coverage (some catalysts may have negligible activity at saturation coverage; see definition of extent of poisoning).

Effects of Pore Diffusion and Associated Experimental Problems

In most processes poisons are strongly and rapidly adsorbed--so rapidly that they are nonuniformly adsorbed to saturation coverage at the entrances to the pores of pellets (i.e. "pore mouth poisoning") as well as at the entrances of fixed bed reactors. The resultant concentration gradients across pellets and reactors seriously complicate the experimental study of poisoning rates and mechanisms. Under these circumstances, fundamental interpretation of the poisoning mechanisms is extremely difficult or impossible. Unfortunately, much of the previous work with real catalysts and some with single crystals were seriously compromised in terms of fundamental understanding by poison concentration gradient. Some experimental considerations for avoiding this and other experimental problems in poisoning studies are discussed by Bartholomew, Agrawal, and Katzer (4). Hegedus and McCabe [2] provide a detailed mechanistic and treatment of intra- and interparticle transport effects.

Smith (7) has treated the effects of pore diffusional resistance of the main reaction and that the poisoning process on activity versus poison coverage behavior. Figure 2 illustrates four cases: (A) slow uniform poisoning and a slow main reaction, (B) slow uniform poisoning and a fast main reaction (in which the pore resistance for the reactants is high), (C) fast nonuniform "pore mouth" poisoning with a slow main reaction (pore resistance for reactants is low), and (D) fast nonuniform "pore mouth" poisoning with a fast main reaction. The functional relationships between activity and

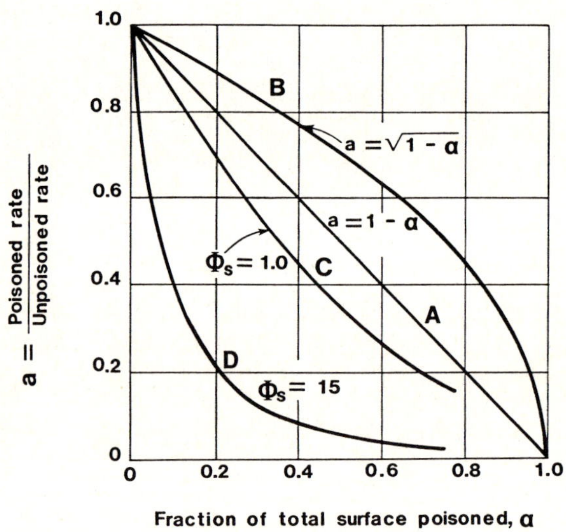

Figure 2. Effects of intrapellet diffusion and poisoning on activity in catalytic reactions: A--Uniform poisoning and slow main reaction, B--Uniform poisoning and fast main reaction, C--Pore-mouth poisoning and slow main reaction, D--Pore-mouth poisoning and fast main reaction (Ref. 7).

coverage in the nonuniform poisoning cases (C and D) involve complex hyperbolic functions resulting in exponential-like declines in activity with coverage (see Fig. 2). Thus, nonuniform poisoning may mimic selective poisoning (compare Figures 1 and 2).

MECHANISMS OF POISONING

Sulfur Poisoning

Because sulfur poisoning is a difficult problem in many important catalytic processes (e.g. hydrogenation, methanation, Fischer-Tropsch synthesis, steam reforming and fuel cell power production it merits separate discussion as an example of catalyst poisoning phenomena. Studies of sulfur poisoning in hydrogenation, CO hydrogenation and steam reforming reactions up to about 1980-2 have been reviewed by Oudar (3), Bartholomew, et al., (4) and Rostrup-Nielsen (5). Most of the previous work dealt with poisoning of metals (particularly nickel) catalysts by H_2S, the primary sulfur poison in most processes of interest.

(i) Sulfur Adsorption on Nickel: Kinetics and Thermodynamics. Previous adsorption studies (4,5,8) indicate that H_2S adsorbs rapidly, strongly and dissociatively on nickel metal surfaces. The high stability and low reversibility of adsorbed sulfur is illustrated by the data in Figure 3, in which most of the previous equilibrium data for nickel (4) are represented on a single plot of log (P_{H_2S}/P_{H_2}) versus reciprocal temperature. The solid line corresponds to the equilibrium data for formation of bulk Ni_3S_2. Based on

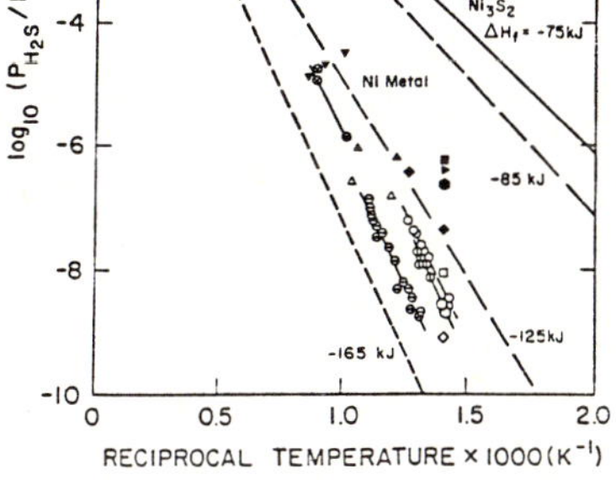

Figure 3. Equilibrium partial pressure of H_2S versus reciprocal temperature (values of ΔH_f based on one mole of H_2S; open symbols, θ = 0.5-0.6; closed symbols, θ = 0.8-0.9) (Ref. 4).

the equation $\Delta G^o = RT \ln (P_{H_2S}/P_{H_2}) = \Delta H - T \Delta S$ the slope of this line is $\Delta H/R$ where ΔH = -75 kJ/mole and the intercept is $-\Delta S/R$. Most of the data lie between the dashed lines corresponding to ΔH = -125 and -165 kJ/mole for coverages ranging form 0.5 to 0.9. Indeed, extrapolation of recent high temperature data to zero coverage (5) yields an enthalpy of adsorption of -250 kJ/mole; in other words surface nickel-sulfur bonds are over a factor of three more stable than bulk nickel-sulfur bonds at low coverage. It is also apparent from Fig. 3 that the absolute heat of adsorption increases with decreasing coverage and that the equilibrium partial pressure of H_2S increases with increasing temperature and decreasing coverage. For instance, at 725 K (450°C) and a coverage of 0.5, the values of P_{H_2S}/P_{H_2} range from about 10^{-8} to 10^{-9}. In other words, half coverage occurs at 1 to 10 ppb H_2S, a concentration range at the lower limit of our present analytical capability! At the same temperature (450°C) almost complete coverage (θ_S >0.9) occurs at values of P_{H_2S}/P_{H_2} of 10^{-7} to 10^{-6} (0.1 to 1 ppm) or at H_2S concentrations encountered in many catalytic processes after the gas has been processed to remove sulfur compounds. These data are typical of sulfur adsorption on most catalytic metals. Thus, we can expect that H_2S (and other sulfur impurities) will adsorb essentially immediately and irreversibly at high coverages in most catalytic processes involving metal catalysts.

(ii) Effects of Sulfur on Adsorptions of Other Molecules. Since one of the necessary steps in a catalytic reaction is the adsorption of one or more reactants, investigation of the effects of adsorbed sulfur on the adsorption of other molecules, (e.g. H_2 and CO) can reveal a great deal about the poisoning process. Previous investigations (4, 9-15) indicate that both H_2 and CO adsorptions on nickel are poisoned by adsorbed sulfur.

Several recent surface science studies of the poisoning by sulfur of CO and hydrogen adsorptions on Ni(100) (9-15) provide insights into the mechanism of sulfur poisoning in CO hydrogenation. Experiments with adsorption of CO on pre-sulfided Ni(100) surfaces by thermal desorption spectrometry (TDS) indicate a weakening of the CO adsorption bond and a rapid, nonlinear decline in the most strongly bound state of CO with increasing sulfur coverage (see Fig. 4); moreover, this CO species is completely poisoned at about 0.3-0.4 ML of sulfur relative to a saturation coverage of 0.5 ML (9-15, Fig. 4). Hydrogen adsorption is poisoned in a similar nonlinear fashion (see Fig. 4).

Some investigators have concluded that the nonlinear drop in CO and hydrogen adsorptions and the weakening of the CO-Ni bond provide evidence for electronic interactions between sulfur and the metal. For example, Goodwin and Kiskinova (11) observed a precipitous drop in the β_2 state of CO on

Ni(100) with increasing sulfur coverage (see Fig. 4a) which at low coverages corresponded to the deactivation of about 8-10 nickel adsorption sites per sulfur atom. This result was attributed to either long range electronic and/or ensemble effects. However, since the decrease in strongly adsorbed CO with addition of various poisons (S, Cl, P, C and N) correlated somewhat with

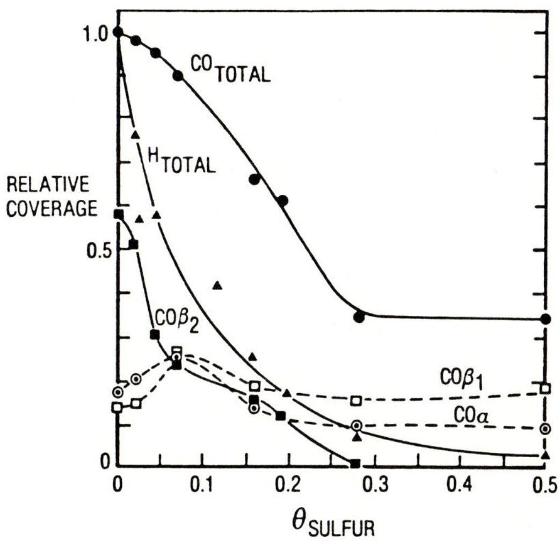

Figure 4. Area under thermal programmed desorption spectra for H_2 and the α, β_1, β_2, as well as total CO curves as a function of sulfur precoverage (Ref. 11).

their electronegativities (see the discussion of the role of electronegativity in poisoning below), it was concluded that electronic interactions over a range of 6-8 a.u. caused a depletion of the Ni3d electron density thereby inducing a weakening of the CO-Ni bond. On the other hand, Madix et al. (13, 14) observed that the decrease in total CO adsorption on Ni(100) with increasing sulfur was linear, except at low coverages and high CO exposures, due to a shift from strongly to weakly bound species; the nonlinear drop at low S coverage was attributed to a local effect, namely the interference by sulfur at low coverages with the ability of CO to form the compression phase characteristic of the sulfur-free surface. Recent careful work by Hardegree et al. (15) confirms that (i) total CO coverage decreases linearly with increasing sulfur coverage, (ii) the coverage by the β_2 state decreases nonlinearly with increasing S coverage, but that one S atoms poisons on the average only two β_2 sites by purely steric (blocking) effects, and (iii) the heat of CO adsorption decreases with increasing S coverage due to a shift from strongly bound to weakly bound species. Thus, the decrease in CO coverage by sulfur is mainly due to site blocking. Nevertheless, the decrease in adsorption strength is consistent with short range electronic effects induced by sulfur either due to electrostatic forces or changes in the local density of state. In other words, the poisoning effects of sulfur on the adsorption of CO (and probably the effect of hydrogen as well) are both geometric and electronic in nature.

That relatively short-range electronic effects operate in the poisoning of adsorption by sulfur is substantiated by theoretical calculations (16-22). Calculations by Lang and coworkers (16-17) to determine the effects of various adsorbates, including sulfur, on a jellium surface indicate that a short-range (3-4 a.u.) electrostatic potential is induced by the adsorbate and can account for the observed destabilization of CO in the presence of sulfur. Although, Feibelman and Hamann (18) demonstrated that sulfur and other adsorbates can induce changes in the local density of states extending over 8 a.u. in Rh atoms, calculations of MacLaren et al. (20-22) indicate that the effects of sulfur and other electronegative atoms on Ni(100) are limited to less than 5 a.u. These authors concluded that electronegative poisons exert a direct effect on the 5σ and 1π levels by increasing their antibonding nature and thereby reducing the interaction of CO with the metal surface while exerting a much weaker influence on the local density of states in nickel compared to rhodium. Calculations by Wimmer et al. (19) indicate that the poisoning of Ni(100) by sulfur involves covalent bonding between S and the Ni surface accompanied by a small transfer of electronic charge from the d state of Ni to S atoms; S atoms also interact directly with adjacent CO molecules to inhibit their dissociation. Accordingly, their work emphasizes that changes in the electronic structure of CO chemisorbed on Ni induced by sulfur are of a complex nature, and thus a simple classification into long-range versus short-range effects may not be meaningful.

(iii) Effects of Sulfur on CO Hydrogenation. Because sulfur adsorbs so strongly on metals and prevents or modifies the further adsorption of reactant molecules, its presence on a catalyst surface usually effects substantial or complete loss of activity in many important reactions (4). This is illustrated by data from Katzer et al. (4) in Figure 5 showing the steady-state methanation activities of Ni, Co, Fe, and Ru catalysts relative to their fresh, unpoisoned activities as a function of gas phase H_2S concentration. These data (obtained in the absence of sulfur gradients) indicate that Ni, Co, Fe, and Ru catalysts all suffer 3-4 orders of magnitude loss in activity at 15-100 ppb of H_2S, i.e., their sulfur tolerances are extremely low! Only at concentrations below 15 ppb H_2S is the poisoning reversible.

Four previous studies (11, 23-25) provide mechanistic information on sulfur poisoning of CO hydrogenation on nickel. One of these (11) involved a surface science study of Ni(100) while the other three (23-25) involved the investigation of real catalysts under conditions in which sulfur was uniformly distributed on the surface. Unfortunately, other studies of sulfur poisoning

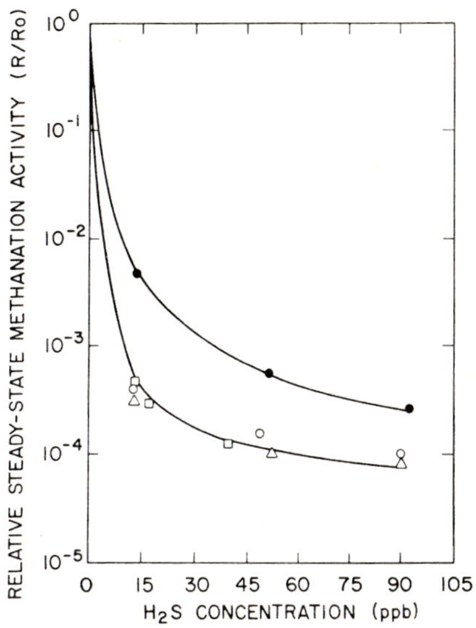

Figure 5. Relative steady-state methanation activity profiles for Ni (●), Co (△), Fe (□), and Ru (○) as a function of gas-phase H_2S concentration. Reaction conditions: 100 kPa, 400°C, 1% CO/99% H_2 for Co, Fe, and Ru, 4% CO/96% H_2 for Ni (Ref. 4).

of nickel in CO hydrogenation (4) involved concentration gradients across the catalyst samples and for that reason do not provide valid mechanistic insights. Each of the four studies is discussed in some detail below followed by a summary comparison of the results.

Differential reaction studies of methanation on a presulfided 25% Ni/alumina catalyst were conducted by Rostrup-Nielsen and Pedersen (23) in the absence of sulfur concentration gradients by sulfiding catalyst samples at 300, 500, and 800°C with H_2S/H_2 ratios varied between 8.4×10^{-9} and 5.7×10^{-6} to obtain a broad range of sulfur coverage. Their results plotted in Fig. 6 as the log of the normalized activity versus $1-S/S_o$, where S and S_o are sulfur coverage and saturation sulfur coverage respectively, show that activity decreases very significantly with increasing sulfur coverage. The slope of the straight line fit of the data of -4.3 was interpreted by the authors to suggest that an ensemble of 4 nickel atoms is required for reaction. They also concluded that since the strong, nonlinear deactivation was accompanied by no change in activation energy that sulfur poisoning in methanation involves site blocking.

Fitzharris et al. (24) investigated in situ the loss of activity of Ni, Ni/alumina and Ni/zirconia catalysts during methanation in a synthesis gas mixture at H_2S levels in the ppb range, using a quartz internal recycle reactor. The reactor and catalyst were configured such that concentration

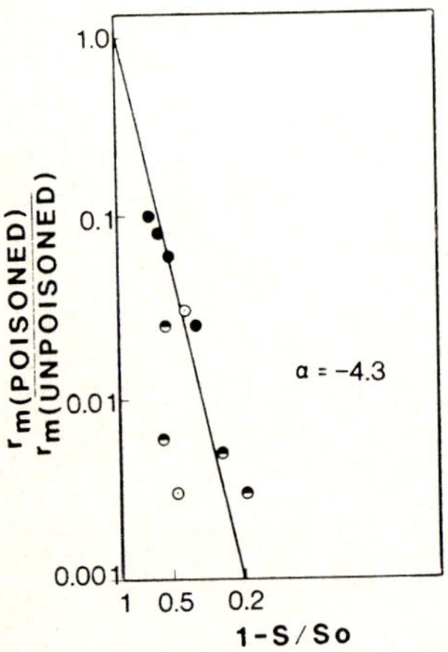

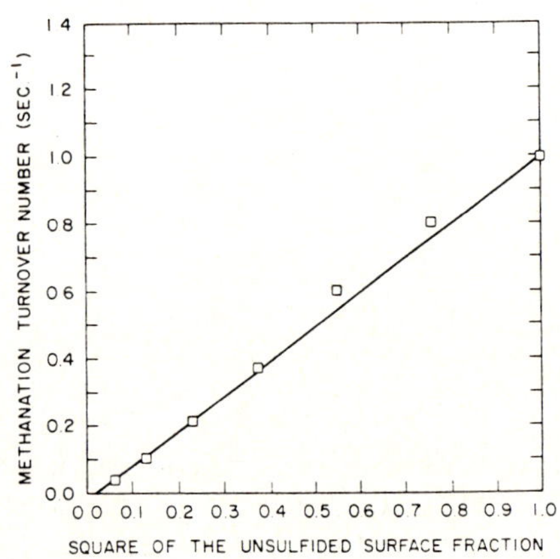

Figure 6. Methanation activity of presulfided catalysts at 300°C, 1 atm, 0.05 g catalyst (0.3-0.5 mm). Sulfidation temperature: filled circles, 800°C; half-filled circles, 500°C; unfilled circles, 300°C (Ref. 23).

Figure 7. Methanation turnover number for Ni/Al_2O_3 as a function of $(1 - \theta_S)^2$. Reaction conditions: 100 kPa, 661 K, 4% CO/96% H_2 (Refs. 4,24).

gradients of both reactants and poison were absent. This approach enabled rates of reaction and deactivation to be measured directly as a function of sulfur coverage. By measuring reaction rate as a function of H_2S adsorbed they were able to obtain a direct relationship between the surface reaction rate and the fractional surface coverage of sulfur. A plot of the rate measured at 388°C and a H_2/CO ratio of 24 versus the square of the unsulfided surface fractions was linear (Fig. 7), suggesting that the number of nickel sites involved in the rate determining step of methanation is two. It should be noted that since these data involved significantly less scatter than those of Rostrup-Nielsen and Pederson (23) they should be considered to be more reliable. The good linear correlation of activity with the square of the unpoisoned surface fraction was interpreted by these authors in terms of a simple blocking of sites; moreover this hypothesis is supported by additional experimental observations by Fitzharris et al. (24), namely that the activation energies and concentration dependencies in the rate expression are the same for fresh and sulfur-poisoned Ni/alumina catalysts.

Erekson and Bartholomew (25) measured the in situ deactivation during methanation of nickel-coated monoliths as a function of sulfur coverage using a quartz, mixed flow microreactor identical to that used by Fitzharris et al. (24). Activity versus sulfur-free fractional coverage plots in Figures 8 and 9 indicate that during reaction at a H_2/CO ratio of 50 in the presence of 0.2 ppm H_2S, 1.0 and 1.5 atoms of nickel are poisoned per adsorbed sulfur atom at reaction temperatures of 525 and 625 K respectively. Combining these data

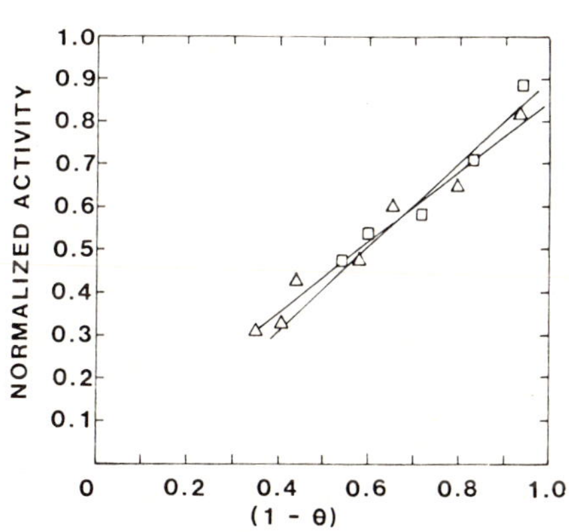

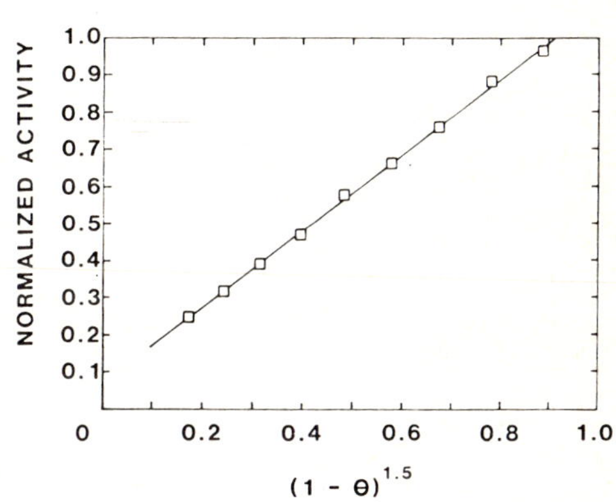

Figure 8. Activity versus sulfur-free area for INCO nickel powder/monolith at 525 K and 575 K. Test conditions: quartz CSTR, 150 cm^3 min^{-1}, 0.2 ppm H_2S, 2% CO in H_2, and 100 kPa (Ref. 25).

Figure 9. Activity versus sulfur-free area to the 1.5 power for INCO nickel powder on a monolith at 625 K; test conditions: quartz CFSTR, 150 cm^3 min^{-1}, 0.2 ppm H_2S, 2% CO in H_2, and 100 kPa (Ref. 25).

with those of Fitzharris et al. (24), indicates a trend of increasing number of nickel atoms (1.0-2.0) deactivated with increasing reaction temperature (525-660 K). Erekson and Bartholomew (25) also observed that the number of nickel atoms deactivated per adsorbed atom of sulfur increased from 0.9 to 4.4 as CO concentration was increased from 2 to 20% (H_2/CO ratio decreased from 50 to 5). This observation was thought to be result of poisoning by both sulfur and inactive carbon at the higher CO concentrations. This hypothesis is supported by previous work (26,27) showing that adsorbed sulfur increases the amount of inactive carbon formed on nickel during methanation. Moreover, the carbon/sulfur synergism could explain the apparent inconsistency between the previous observations by Rostrup-Nielsen and Pederson (23) that four nickel sites are deactivated per nickel atoms at relatively high CO concentrations and by Fitzharris et al. (24) that only two nickel sites are deactivated per adsorbed sulfur atom at low CO concentrations.

Goodman and Kiskinova (11) studied poisoning by sulfur layers of methanation on Ni(100) employing a custom-built surface analysis system to which was attached a retraction bellows enabling the reaction to be conducted at near atmospheric pressures without exposing the sample to air. Sulfur levels were established by exposure of the sample to H_2S at 300 K followed by

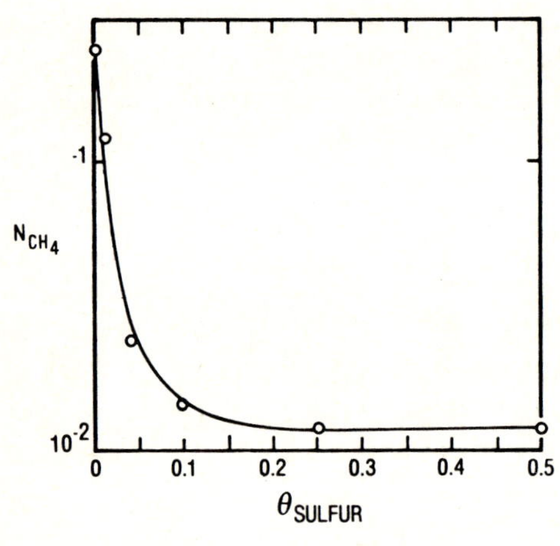

Figure 10. Methanation rate as a function of sulfur coverage on a Ni(100) catalyst. Pressure = 120 Torr, H_2/CO = 4/1, reaction temperature = 600 K (Ref. 11).

heating of the sample to 600 K. The surface coverage of sulfur was determined by Auger Electron Spectroscopy (AES); saturation was found to correspond to 0.5 monolayer (ML). The results plotted (in Fig. 10) as methane turnover frequency (at a total pressure of 120 Torr, a H_2/CO ratio of 4 and a reaction temperature of 600 K) versus sulfur coverage shows a precipitous drop in activity with sulfur coverage; at a fractional sulfur coverage of 0.25 the crystal is completely deactivated. At a fractional S coverage of less than 0.1 the rate was found to be proportional to the partial pressures of hydrogen and CO to the first and zero powers respectively. At a fractional sulfur cover of greater than 0.25 the order of CO becomes unity. Nevertheless, the activation energy at temperatures below 600 K did not change with addition of sulfur. The authors concluded that their data are consistent with electronic effects playing a major role at low sulfur coverages in reducing the reaction rate.

Based on the results presented above for the four catalyst studies involving sulfur poisoning of nickel in CO hydrogenation it is clear that there are some important similarities and differences. Before the results of the real catalyst studies are compared with those of the surface science study, some important differences in the conditions and limitations of these two different approaches should be emphasized. While the surface science study (11) enabled the effects of a known structure of sulfur on the surface of a well-defined metal structure to be determined, one cannot be certain that this sulfur structure determined in the absence of gas phase H_2S is representative of the sulfur structure on a metal crystallite exposed to a finite gas phase concentration of H_2S during reaction. In the case of the real catalysts (23-25) one cannot directly determine the structure of the adsorbed sulfur nor as easily confirm the absence of sulfur concentration gradients.

Table 4 summarizes the results of the four poisoning studies (11, 23-25). In all four studies the activation energy was found to be independent of sulfur level. In two of the studies (24, 25) the concentration dependencies for methanation on nickel were found to be the same for fresh and poisoned catalysts, while the surface science study (11) the order for CO increased after poisoning. The independence of the activation energy and reaction kinetics on sulfur level suggests that poisoning is due to geometric rather than electronic effects. However, the observation by Goodman and Kiskinova (11) that 10 atoms of nickel are deactivated per adsorbed sulfur atom suggests that (i) long range electronic effects or (ii) ensemble effects might be involved; other possible explanations include (iii) a synergistic deactivation

TABLE 4

Effects of sulfur on the activation energy and concentration dependencies for methanation on nickel

	Activation Energy (kJ/mol)		Conc. Dependencies		
Sample	Fresh	Sulfided	Fresh	Sulfided	Ref.
25% Ni/Al_2O_3	90	90	zero	zero	23
Ni/Al_2O_3	100	100	$r = \frac{K_1 P_{CO} X^2}{(K_2 + K_3 P_{CO})^2}$ [a]	same	24
Ni/Al_2O_3	96	96	$r_{CH_4} = kP_{CO}^{-0.3} P_{H_2}^{0.9}$	$r_{CH_4} = kP_{CO}^{-0.4} P_{H_2}^{0.8}$	25
Ni(100)	103	103	$r \alpha P_{H_2}^1$	$r \alpha P_{CO}^1 P_{H_2}^1$	11

[a] x = unpoisoned surface fraction

of nickel by carbon and sulfur (25), (iv) severe poisoning of hydrogen adsorption (see Fig. 4) and (v) steric factors which reduce H or CO mobility or prevent formation of key intermediates (15). The previous discussion in connection with the poisoning of CO adsorption tends to rule out long range electronic effects, while the results of Fitzharris et al. (24) and of Erekson and Bartholomew (25) are not consistent with the existence of large (>2) ensembles. According, explanations (iii), (iv), or (v) are favored; the results of Erekson and Bartholomew (25) showing increasing degree of poisoning with increasing CO concentration favor the synergistic deactivation by inactive carbon and sulfur at high partial pressures of CO.

Effects of Adsorption Strength, Adsorbate Size, Electronegativity, Shielding, and Tendency to Gasify on Poisoning Toxicity

One of the fundamental questions posed at the beginning was: "how is poisoning affected by the chemistry of the contaminant?" It is clear that poisons vary greatly in their toxicities for a given catalyst, reaction and set of reaction conditions (1,6), but it is not generally clear why these large variations exist. Nevertheless, it is a reasonable supposition that there are basic principles that determine poisoning toxicity. Present evidence (1-6) suggests that adsorption strength, adsorbate size, electronegativity, degree of shielding, and tendency for removal by gasification are five properties of poisons that relate to toxicity. Poison toxicity is also affected by reaction type and reaction conditions (4,6). Examples of recent studies that relate toxicity to contaminant properties are described briefly in this section.

(i) Effects of Adsorption Strength. Generally, species that are more strongly bound to a catalytic surface than reactants and products function as poisons. Theoretical calculations (6) indicate that the fraction of surface poisoned and the residence time of the poison on the surface become significant as the adsorption heat of the poison exceeds 150 kJ/mole. Thus, oxygen, sulfur and carbon would predictably function as poisons for reactions involving CO and/or hydrogen since the heats of adsorption or binding energies of these former species are substantially greater than 150 kJ/mole and significantly greater than those of these reactants (8, 28, see Table 5). Indeed this prediction is bourne out by experimental data (1-6), although sulfur is generally the most toxic of these three poisons because of its larger residence time on the surface, for reasons explained below. On the other hand, from the data in Table 5 it is apparent that adsorbed nitrogen should have little poisoning effect on reactions of CO or hydrogen on nickel since its heat of adsorption is significantly less than for these latter species. Indeed, studies of methanation on nickel in the presence of N_2 (29-31) indicate no measurable poisoning effect. It is unfortunate that so little thermodynamic data, other than those shown in Table 5, are available for contaminants on nickel surfaces, e.g. for Cl, As, P, etc.

TABLE 5
Heats of adsorption of various reactants contaminants on Ni (8,28)

Contaminant	Nickel Form	Technique	$-\Delta H_{ads}$(kJ/mol)
O_2	Film	Calorimetry	293-628
S	Ni/Al_2O_3,Nipowder	Equil. Ads. Studies	223-279
C	Ni/Al_2O_3	Equil. Ads. Studies	35-52[a]
CO	Single Crystals		94-138
H_2	Single Crystals	Flash Desorption	84-98
N_2	Film	TD, Cal.	25-59

[a]Enthalpy of segregation from bulk to surface relative to graphite. The binding energy of C(a) relation to C(g) is about 665 kJ/mole.

Besides adsorbing strongly, some poisons react with metal surfaces to form alloys or compounds that are catalytically inactive or they restructure the metal surface (6). Arsenic, for example, is a very severe poison for nickel catalysts in steam reforming; indeed, its effect per mole of uptake is comparable with that of sulfur (32). The evidence indicates that gaseous compounds of arsenic disintegrate very quickly during reaction forming an alloy with nickel that has significantly less activity (32). Sulfur compounds at high concentrations react with nickel to form bulk nickel sulfide (4).

Restructuring of Ni(111) to Ni(100) by adsorbed sulfur at high temperatures is reported by Schmidt and Luss (33). Delescluse (6,34) reports that in the presence of adsorbed sulfur at 600°C the (810) plane of nickel breaks up into the (410) and (100) facets. This restructuring could play an important role in structure sensitive reactions favoring a specific crystallographic plane. For example, in the exchange reaction of benzene with deuterium on nickel, the (111) and 110) planes are most active (35) whereas hydrogenation of benzene is structure-insensitive. Accordingly, sulfur adsorption at high temperatures favoring the (100) plane over (111) and (110) planes will be selectively more toxic for the deuterium exchange.

(ii) Effects of Adsorbate Size. According to Maxted (1) toxicity depends among other things on molecular structure and size. In general, toxicity of a given poison class such as sulfur compounds increases with molecular weight and size of the poison. However, this generalization is most applicable to reactions carried out at relatively low temperatures (e.g., hydrogenations of organic molecules at 300-450 K), since at higher temperatures many organic sulfur compounds decompose on metal surfaces to form two-dimensional sulfides, in which case the poisoning process is independent of the starting compound. There are, nevertheless, several examples of low-temperature hydrogenation reactions in which relationships between toxicity and size have been demonstrated (1,36-39). For example, in their investigation of the hydrogenation of crotonic acid on platinum and nickel at 300 and 433 K, respectively, Maxted and Evans (39) found the relative toxicities to increase in the following order: H_2S, CS_2, thiophene, and cysteine. While thiophene is a strong poison for nickel in hydrogenation of alkenes, Holah et al. (40) found that it was not capable of poisoning more than 75% of the sites in nickel boride or Raney nickel catalysts because the geometric requirements for thiophene restricted easy access to a portion of the catalyst, although this portion was accessible to reactants. This illustrates how diffusional or shape-selective effects in micropores may influence the toxicity of a poison because of its molecular size and/or structure.

(iii) Effects of Electronegativity. Evidence was presented in the discussion above indicating that adsorbed sulfur poisons metal surfaces by both blocking and short-range electronic modification of the metal. If electronic factors are involved in poisoning, it is expected that toxicity might correlate with the ability of the contaminant to electronically modify another atom with which it comes in contact. One measure of such ability is electronegativity.

Kiskinova and Goodman (12, 41) investigated the effects of preadsorbed C, N, P, S, and Cl on the adsorptions of CO and hydrogen on Ni(100) and of preadsorbed P, S, and Cl on the rate of methanation on the same surface. The magnitudes of observed decreases in adsorption capacities and sticking coefficients of CO and hydrogen with increasing poison coverage (Figures 11-13) were found to correlate reasonably well with electronegativity of the poison. For example, the decrease in sticking coefficient for either CO or hydrogen at a given coverage of poison is progressively greater in the order P, S, and Cl having progressively higher electronegativities of 2.1, 2.5 and 3.0 respectively (see Figures 11 and 13). Since atomic and covalent radii for Cl, S, and P are similar (0.99, 1.02 and 1.04 a.u. respectively), and the

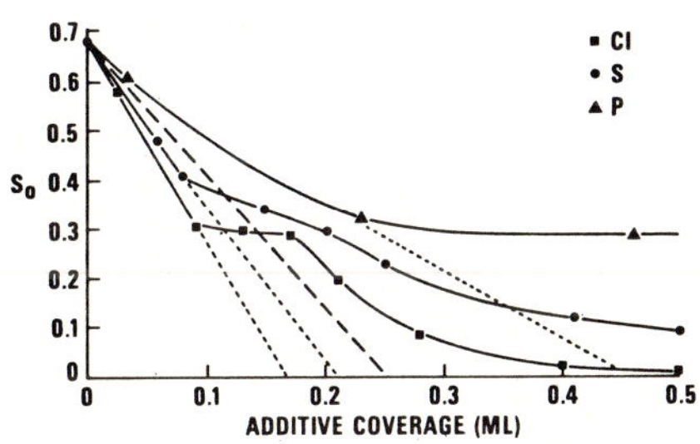

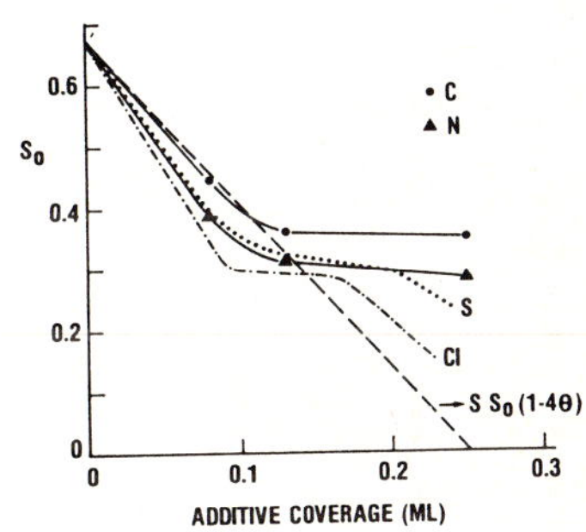

Figure 11. Variation of the CO initial sticking coefficient as a function of additive coverage on Ni(100) (From Ref. 12).

Figure 12. Initial sticking coefficient of CO as a function of additive coverage (Ref. 41).

initial decreases in sticking coefficient for Cl and S were greater than that predicted by simple geometric blocking (see dashed line in Figs 11 and 13), it was concluded that electronegativity plays a major role in the explaining the differences in their poisoning effect (12,38). While C and N have electronegativities (2.5 and 3.0) in the same range as S and Cl their poisoning effects on CO and hydrogen adsorptions are less (see Fig. 12); this is ascribed (41) to their considerably smaller atomic radii (0.77 and 0.75 a.u. respectively) relative to S and Cl (0.99 and 1.02 a.u.). Thus, geometry apparently also plays an important role in poisoning by these contaminants.

The observed greater decrease in methanation rate on Ni(100) due to poisoning by S relative to P also correlates well with the greater electronegativity of S (see Fig. 14). However, in the case of preadsorbed Cl no decrease in methanation rate was observed; subsequent AES showed no Cl remaining on the surface after reaction, apparently as a result of the reaction of Cl(a) with hydrogen to form HCl (41). Accordingly, because of this gasification reaction it was not possible to study the effects of Cl on methanation kinetics.

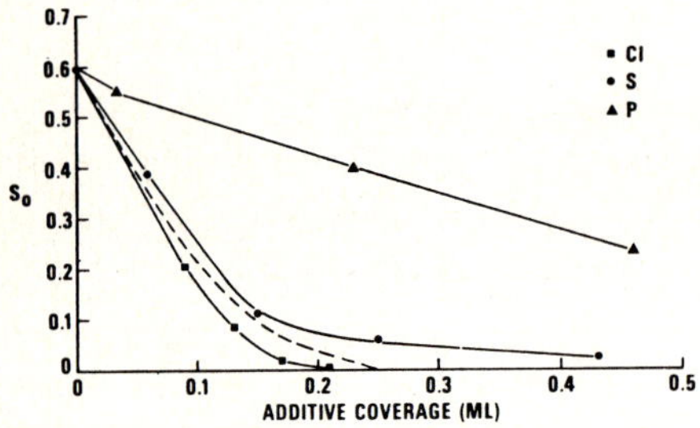

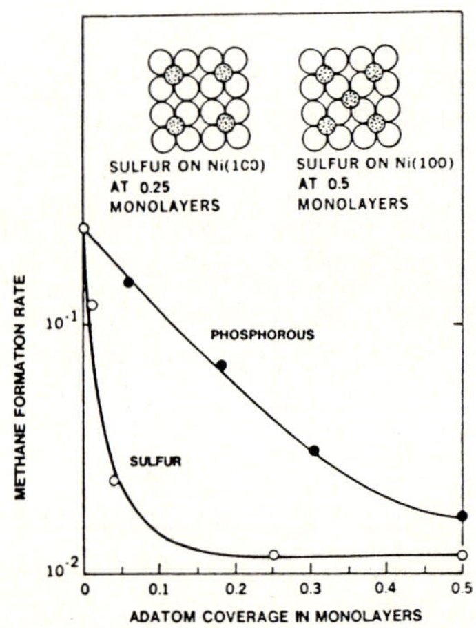

Figure 13. Variation of the sticking coefficient S_0 of H_2 on Ni(100) as a function of additive precoverage. The dashed line represents the theoretical dependence according to the relationship $s = s_0(1 - 4\theta)^2$ (From Ref. 12).

Figure 14. Methanation rate as functions of sulfur and phosphorus coverages on a Ni(100) catalyst. Pressure = 120 torr, $H_2/CO = 4/1$, reaction temperature = 600 K.

(iv) Effects of Shielding. According to Maxted (1) the toxicity of sulfur and nitrogen compounds depends upon their electronic configuration and in particular on the number of ligands surrounding the sulfur or nitrogen atoms, i.e. the degree of shielding of the poison. Shielded structures such as SO_2 and SO_4^{2-} are less toxic than unshielded structures such as S and H_2S; indeed the order of decreasing toxicity for sulfur compounds is S, H_2S, SO_2, SO_3, SO_4^{2-}. Accordingly, it is possible in selected cases to detoxify a poison by oxidation; for example, thiophene which is highly toxic for nickel can be oxidized to sulfone with hydrogen peroxide in the presence of molybdic acid thereby regenerating catalytic activity (1). Similarly, benzene and carbon monoxide which are poisons in olefin hydrogenation reactions can be oxidized; CO can be hydrogenated into nontoxic methane or oxidized to innocuous carbon dioxide. Unfortunately, it is not simple to regenerate sulfur-poisoned catalysts with O_2 because nickel oxide formed simultaneously tends to bury the sulfur layer before it is removed as SO_2 (4). Upon rereduction the sulfur layer returns (4).

(v) Effects of Gasification. Because of their high binding energies with nickel (Table 5) and their high electronegativities, carbon, chlorine, and oxygen might be expected to have toxicities rivaling that of sulfur. Nevertheless, these contaminants are generally less toxic than sulfur in many reactions on metals because of their lower residence times on the metal surface due to gasification reactions. In the presence of reactant hydrogen, for example, carbon, chlorine and oxygen react readily at typical reaction temperatures (400-800 K) to form gaseous methane, HCL and water. In an oxidizing environment carbon and chlorine may react to form gaseous CO_2 and oxides of chlorine. Thus, these gasification reactions serve to detoxify these otherwise poisonous contaminants.

Unfortunately, there is evidence that the presence of sulfur may poison these gasification reactions (4,11,26,27), leading to a synergistic poisoning by sulfur and the other contaminant e.g. sulfur and carbon. Bartholomew and Gardner (26), for example, inferred from an in situ gravimetric study of methanation on nickel/alumina that the adsorption of CO under reaction conditions was reduced by only 50% on the completely sulfided surface; however the reactivity of surface species was drastically reduced. Instead of principally hydrogenatable or volatile surface species observed on the unpoisoned Ni catalyst, a substantial portion (about 80%) of the surface species on the sulfur-poisoned catalyst could not be hydrogenated. Wentrcek et al. (27) obtained similar results in pulse reactor experiments with fresh and sulfur-poisoned Ni/alumina; namely, they observed that the fraction of surface carbon formed by CO dissociation which could be gasified with hydrogen decreased significantly with increasing sulfur coverage. Both sets of data (26,27) are consistent with either (i) a greater poisoning of dissociative hydrogen adsorption than of CO, preventing the gasification reaction of atomic hydrogen with adsorbed carbon species from CO dissociation or (ii) the prevention by geometric or electronic factors of access of adsorbed hydrogen and carbon species preventing formation of key reaction intermediates. The former explanation finds support from the observation that the "completely poisoned" catalyst adsorbs no hydrogen at room temperature (26).

CONCLUSIONS

The discussion in this brief review has focused on several fundamental questions some of which were mentioned at the beginning. The following conclusions form a partial summary of the response to these questions:

1. Poisons such as C, Cl, S, and As adsorb rapidly and strongly on nickel. The binding energies of these contaminants with nickel metal is high relative to those of typical reactants (e.g. CO and hydrogen) and relative to the energies of bonds involved in bulk compounds of nickel with these contaminants, e.g. nickel sulfides and carbides. At sufficiently high concentrations S and C form bulk nickel sulfide and carbide while As reacts with Ni to form an alloy.

2. Poisoning of nickel by S, C, Cl, N and P is due to a combination of geometric (blocking) and electronic effects. The adsorptions of CO and H_2 on the four nearest neighbor Ni atoms are geometrically blocked by adsorbed S, C, Cl, and N. In addition, the adsorption strengths of CO and H_2 on nearest neighbor sites are decreased due the electronic interaction of these contaminants with the nickel surface causing a depletion of the nickel d states; in the case of CO adsorption electronegative poisons exert a direct effect on the 5σ and 1π levels by increasing their antibonding nature and thereby reducing the interaction of CO with the metal surface. Electronic and geometric effects are more pronounced in poisoning of CO and H_2 adsorptions on nickel by S and Cl due to their higher electronegativities and/or sizes relative to C, N, and P. However, the electronic effects in the poisoning of nickel by S or Cl do not extend beyond 4 or 5 a.u., are therefore relatively short range, and involve only nearest neighbor atoms.

3. Poisoning of the methanation reaction by sulfur involves the deactivation of as many as 10 nickel atoms per adsorbed sulfur atom at low sulfur coverages. This observation may be explained by (i) long range electronic effects, (ii) ensemble effects, (iii) a synergistic deactivation by

carbon and sulfur, (iv) severe poisoning of hydrogen adsorption, and (v) steric factors which reduce H or CO mobility thereby preventing formation of key intermediates. The last three explanations are favored by presently available evidence. The independence of the methanation activation energy and reaction kinetics on sulfur level suggests that sulfur poisoning of nickel in this reaction is due more to geometric rather than electronic effects.

4. The toxicity of poisons for a given catalyst in a given raction at fixed reaction condtiions is a function of adsorption strength, adsorbate size, electronegativity, degree of shielding, and tendency for removal by gasification. Generally, poisons of higher adsorption strength, adsorbate size, and electronegativity with a lower degree of shielding (by attached ligands) are more toxic. While carbon, chlorine, oxygen, and sulfur have comparably high binding energies with nickel and high electronegativities, the toxicities of carbon, chlorine, and oxygen in hydrogenation reactions on nickel are significantly lower because of their tendencies to be gasified by reactions with hydrogen to form methane, HCl and water. However, the gasification of these species (particularly carbon) is inhibited by the presence of sulfur.

REFERENCES

1. Maxted, E.B., "The Poisoning of Metallic Catalysts," in Advances in Catal., 3 (1951) 129.
2. a. Hegedus, L.L. and McCabe, R.W., "Catalyst Poisoning," in Catalyst Deactivation, ed. B. Delmon and G.F. Froment, Elsevier, Amsterdam, 1980, p. 471.
   b. Hegedus, L.L. and McCabe, R.W., "Catalyst Poisoning," Catal. Rev.-Sci. Eng., 23 (1981) 377 .
   c. Hegedus, L.L. and McCabe, R.W., Catalyst Poisoning, Marcel Dekker, Inc., 1984.
3. a. Oudar, J., "Sulfur Adsorption and Poisoning of Metallic Catalysts," Catal. Rev.-Sci. Eng., 22 (1980) 171.
   b. J. Oudar, "Modeling Experiments of Poisoning on Metals," in Deactivation and Poisoning of Catalysts, ed. by J. Oudar and H. Wise, Marcel Dekker, Inc., 1985.
4. Bartholomew, C.H., Agrawal, P.K., and Katzer, J.R., "Sulfur Poisoning of Metals," in Advances in Catalysis, 31 (1982) 135.
5. Rostrup-Nielsen, J.R., "Sulfur Poisoning," in Progress in Catalyst Deactivation, ed. J.L. Figueiredo, NATO Advanced Study Institute Series E., No. 54, M. Nijhoff, Boston, 1982, pp. 209-227.
6. J. Barbier, "Effect of Poisons on the Activity and Selectivity of Metallic Catalysts," in Deactivation and Poisoning of Catalysts, ed by J. Oudar and H. Wise, Marcel Dekker, Inc., 1985.
7. Smith, J.M., Chemical Engineering Kinetics, 3rd Ed., McGraw-Hill, 1981, Chaps. 11 and 13.
8. H. Wise, J. McCarty, and J. Oudar, "Sulfur and Carbon Interactions," in Deactivation and Poisoning of Catalysts, ed. by J. Oudar, and H. Wise, Marcel Dekker, 1985.

9. W. Erley and H. Wagner, J. Catal., 53 (1978) 287.
10. K.D. Rendulic and A. Winkler, Surface Sci., 74 (1978) 318.
11. D.W. Goodman and M. Kiskinova, Surf. Sci., 105 (1981) L265.
12. M. Kiskinova, and D.W. Goodman, Surf. Sci., 108 (1981) 64.
13. S. Johnson and R.S. Madix, Surf. Sci., 108 (1981) 77.
14. R.J. Madix, M.Thornberg,and S.B. Lee, Surf. Sci., 133 (1983) L447.
15. E.L. Hardegree, P. Ho, and J.M. White, Surf. Sci., 165 (1986) 488.
16. J.K. Norskov, S. Holloway, and N.D. Lang, Surf. Sci., 137 (1984) 65.
17. N.D. Lang, S. Holloway, and J.K. Norskov, Surf. Sci., 150 (1985) 24.
18. P.J. Feibelman and D.R. Hamann, Surf. Sci., 149 (1985) 48.
19. E.Wimmer, C.L. Fu, and A.J. Freeman, Phys. Rev. Lett., 55 (1985) 2618.
20. J.M. Maclaren, J.B. Pendry, and D.D. Vvendensky, Surf. Sci., 162 (1985) 322.
21. J.M. MacLaren, J.B. Pendry, R.W. Joyner, and P. Meehan, Surf. Sci., 175 (1986) 263.
22. R.W. Joyner and P. Meehan, J.M. MacLaren, and J.B. Pendry, Appl. Catal., 25 (1986) 9.
23. J.R. Rostrup-Nielsen and K. Pedersen, J. Catal., 59 (1979) 395.
24. W.D. Fitzharris, J.R. Katzer, and W.H. Manogue, submitted for publication, 1982.
25. E.J. Erekson and C.H. Bartholomew, Appl. Catal., 5 (1983) 323.
26. D.C. Gardner and C.H. Bartholomew, I&EC Fund., 20 (1981) 229.
27. P.W. Wentrcek, J.G. McCarty, C.M. Ablow, and H. Wise, J. Catal., 61 (1980) 232.
28. I. Toyoshima and G.A. Somorjai, Catal. Rev.-Sci. Eng., 19 (1979) 105.
29. G.A. Jarvi, K.B. Mayo, and C.H. Bartholomew, Chem. Eng. Commun., 4(1980) 325.
30. C.H. Bartholomew, R.B. Pannell, and J.L. Butler, J. Catal., 65 (1980) 335.
31. E.L. Sughrue and C.H. Bartholomew, Appl. Catal., 2 (1982) 239.
32. B. Nielsen and J. Villadsen, Appl. Catal., 11 (1984) 123.
33. L.D. Schmidt and D. Luss, J. Catal., 22 (1971) 269.
34. P. Delescluse, Thesis, Paris 1979.
35. J. Massardier, G. Dalmai-Imelik, and J. Barbier, C.R. Acad. Sci. Paris, Ser. C, 283 (1976) 257.
36. J.L.S. Curtis and M.O. Baker, Anal. Chem., 42 (1970) 278.
37. A. Koppova, V. Zapletal, V. Ruzicka, and J. Soukup, Coll. Czech. Chem. Commun., 38 (1973) 2472.
38. L. Gonzalez-Tejuca, K. Aika, S. Namba, and J. Turkevich, J. Phys. Chem., 81 (1977) 1399.
39. E.B. Maxted and H.C. Evans, J.Chem. Soc., (1937) 603.
40. D.G. Holah, I.M. Hoodless, A.N. Hughes, and L. Sedor, J. Catal., 60 (1979) 148.
41. M. Kiskinova and D.W. Goodman, Surf. Sci., 109 (1981) L555.

B. Delmon and G.F. Froment (Editors), *Catalyst Deactivation 1987*

POISONING OF HYDROGENATION CATALYSTS. HOW TO COPE WITH THIS GENERAL PROBLEM ?

J.P. BOITIAUX, J. COSYNS and F. VERNA.

Institut Français du Pétrole, B.P. 311, 92506 Rueil-Malmaison Cédex, France.

ABSTRACT

The hydrogenation catalysts are deactivated by various impurities contained in the industrial feedstocks. However, the actual effect (inhibition or poisoning) depends notably on the three components system : catalyst-impurity-hydrocarbon. For each system, the deactivation extent is a function of the operating conditions. The effects of various impurities are studied, examples of synergetic effects between two impurities are examined. In each case, possible actions for suppressing or decreasing the harmfull effect are presented.

INTRODUCTION

The hydrogenation is a very widely used reaction in the field of petroleum refining, petrochemistry and chemistry. This reaction operates generally at low temperature, the catalyst is thus very sensitive to various impurities. This general problem of poisoning is so large that it cannot be extensively studied in the range of our paper. We have therefore focused our attention on the hydrogenation of unsaturated hydrocarbons while excluding the compounds with functional groups.

In a first part of this paper, we present the industrial background of the hydrogenation and the complexity of the deactivation problems. Firstly, the word "poisoning" must be accurately defined because it could refer either to a lethal action for which no recovery is possible or to a simple temporary inhibition.

In the following parts, we review the effects of the main impurities present in hydrogenation feedstocks. For some impurities, effects on selectivity are also examined. Some "synergetic" effects obtained with mixtures of two impurities are presented and discussed. Finally, for each impurity, we try to present actions which can be considered for suppressing or decreasing its harmfull effect.

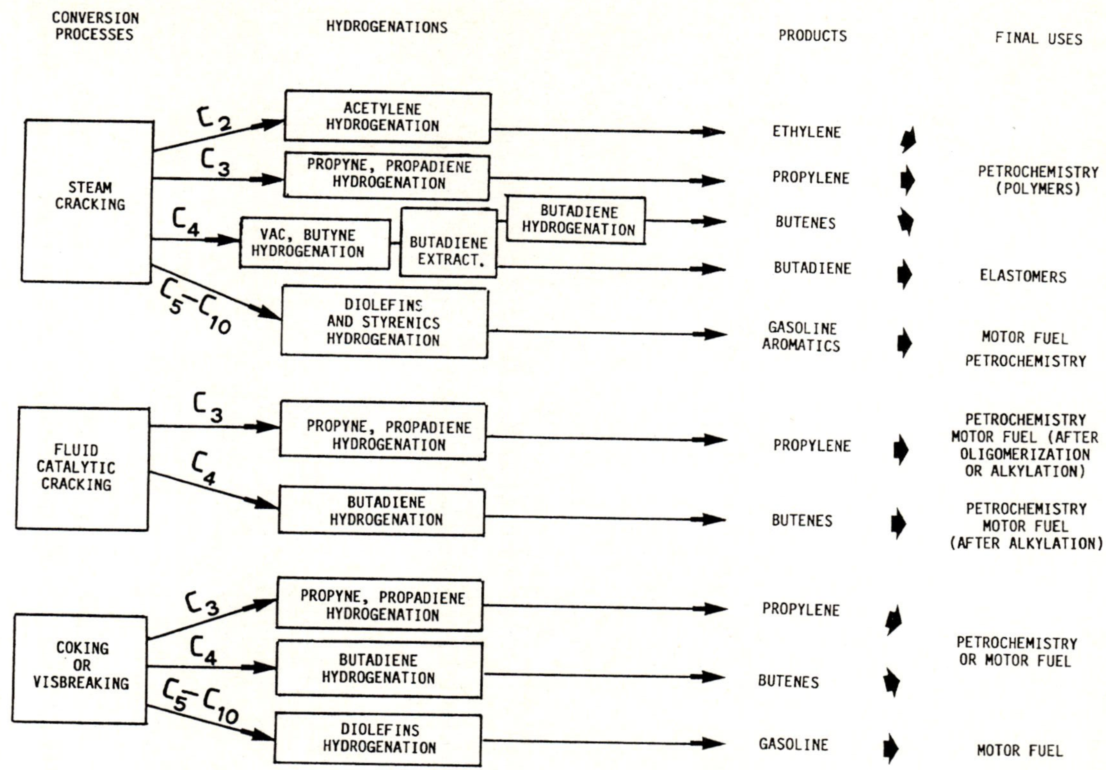

Fig. 1. The various hydrogenation processes.

GENERAL CONSIDERATIONS

The industrial background

The hydrocarbons like acetylenics, diolefins and monoolefins are not present in the natural sources like petroleum and coal ; light aromatics are only present in small proportions. Nevertheless, the chemical industry needs mainly unsaturated hydrocarbons using their reactivities and ability to produce valuable products like for example polymers, elastomers, artificial textiles etc...

Conversion processes have been developed for the production of the above mentioned hydrocarbons. The most important is the steam-cracking which produces from petroleum cuts (light petroleum gas, naphtha, gas-oil) olefins, diolefins and aromatics required by the chemical industry. Other cracking processes have been developed to convert heavy petroleum cuts to more valuable products : fluid catalytic cracking (FCC), coking, visbreaking which produce a lot of unsaturated hydrocarbons.

(a) The role of hydrogenation. All these processes give a mixture of unsaturated hydrocarbons which are not valuable as such. Further hydrogenations are mandatory if one wants to produce usable products for refining and chemical industry.

The figure 1 presents schematically the main conversion processes, the various hydrogenation processes and products obtained. It can be noted that hydrogenation is needed whatever the final use of the product obtained is, i.e. : petrochemistry or motor fuel.

In addition to all these hydrogenations presented in the figure 1, partial or total hydrogenation of aromatics in straight run petroleum cuts are required for production of various refined cuts like for example jet fuels or solvents.

(b) The purity of hydrogenation feedstocks. All the cuts presented in the figure 1 can contain a few ppm or more of various impurities which remain even after purification treatments.

A list of the most frequent impurities present in these cuts is given in the figure 2. The various feedstocks of conversion processes are also given. Nature and concentrations of impurities in the conversion products will depend on the nature of the conversion process feedstock and the efficiency of the purification train. Obviously, the purest cuts are coming from the steam-cracking because this unit is specially designed for production of polymer-grade products.

On the contrary, the other conversion processes, which use much heavier feedstocks, are designed up to now for the production of refined grade cuts and thus can contain higher concentrations of more numerous impurities.

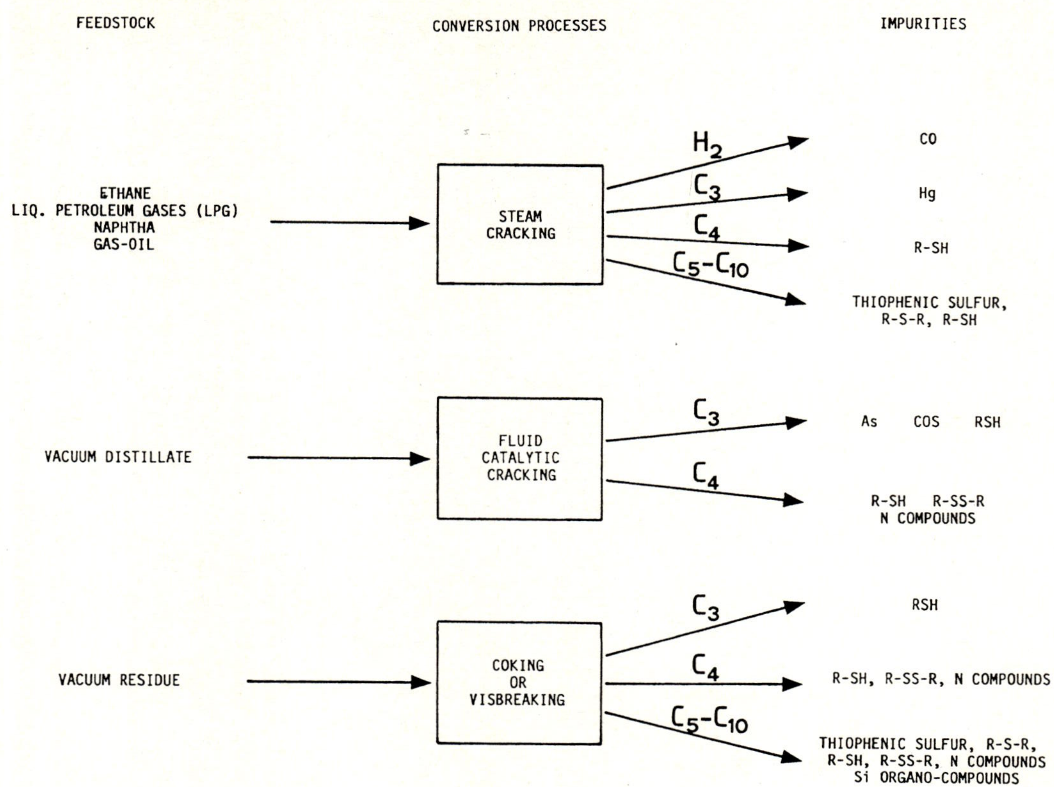

Fig. 2. The impurities in hydrogenation feedstocks.

(c) The hydrogenation operating conditions. Except for steam-cracking C_2 cut hydrogenation, the hydrogenation processes operate in liquid phase at moderate pressures and low temperatures (most generally less than 200 °C). For the hydrogenation of light cuts, the temperatures are generally less than 100 °C.

In these conditions the presence of impurities can be very harmful for the hydrogenation catalyst.

The useful definitions and the comprehensive approach.

For a given catalyst and a given unsaturated hydrocarbon to hydrogenate, it is firstly necessary to determine the kind of effect which is observed. The figure 3 shows schematically the two classes of effect which can be obtained when a given impurity is present in the feed.

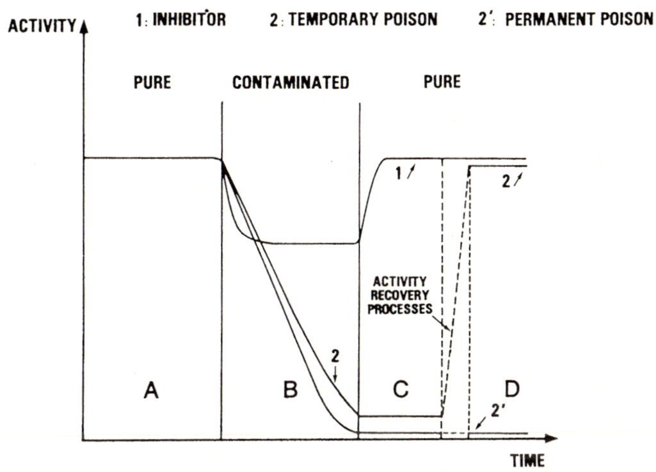

Fig. 3. The two types of effects observed - Inhibitors and Poisons.

In this figure is presented schematically a continuous catalytic test ; the activity is plotted as a function of time. The first part (A) presents the activity obtained with a non contaminated feedstock. After a given time, one switches to a contaminated feedstock (part B), two main effects on activity can be observed : the first one is a rapid deactivation followed by a new steady state of lower but constant activity. After a given time, one switches back to the pure feed (part C) and one observes that the initial activity is fully recovered indicating a reversible effect. The impurity which produces such effect is called INHIBITOR OR ACTIVITY MODERATOR.

Fundamentally speaking, it is generally due to the co-adsorption of the impurity on the catalytic surface resulting in a rapid activity decrease and a new equilibrium depending on the impurity concentration. If the impurity is simply chemisorbed without any dissociation, its effect is fully reversible.

The second possible effect of an impurity is a progressive activity decrease, this latter going down to zero if contaminated feedstock is injected for a sufficient time. The impurity which produces this effect is called POISON. Fundamentally speaking, that is the result of a decomposition of the impurity on the catalytic surface giving a new surface species which is not active.

For a practical point of view, when an industrial operator faces a poisoning of its catalysts, he will firstly try to regenerate it before unloading it and buying a new catalyst load. Two possibilities arise (part D) : the first one is a full recovery of the activity after an appropriate regeneration, the second one is partial or no activity recovery. The impurities giving these results are called respectively TEMPORARY POISON AND PERMANENT POISON.

The complexity of the problem. Here again we have to point out that these definitions are only valid if we consider the effect of an impurity on a given catalyst and with a given hydrocarbon. The kind and extent of deactivation will depend very much on the interaction between these three species. Thus, any realistic study of deactivation requires the consideration of the three components system which is presented in the figure 4.

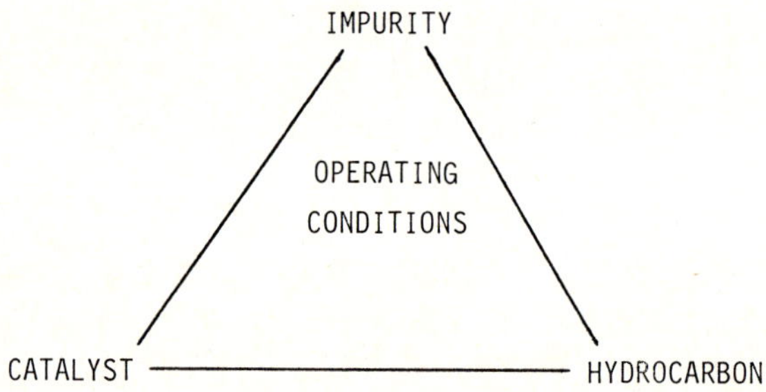

Fig. 4. The triple system.

Moreover the extent of deactivation is also a function of the operating conditions and specifically of the temperature.

Some examples of these triple systems are illustrated on the figure 5. Maximum operating temperatures are indicated inside each triangle. All systems are working under a superatmospheric pressure of hydrogen. These systems are separated in two classes : the first one for which inhibition is observed and the second one for poisoning. We can immediatly notice that some sulfur compounds like thiophene and alkylsulfide can act either as inhibitor or as poison ; the kind of effect observed with these compounds depends on the metal nature and on the hydrocarbon nature. These observations clearly indicate that any conclusive experimentation must be made with the three elements together : the metal, the poison and also the hydrocarbon.

Moreover, the results depend on the experimental conditions and the conclusion is to be restricted to this condition range.

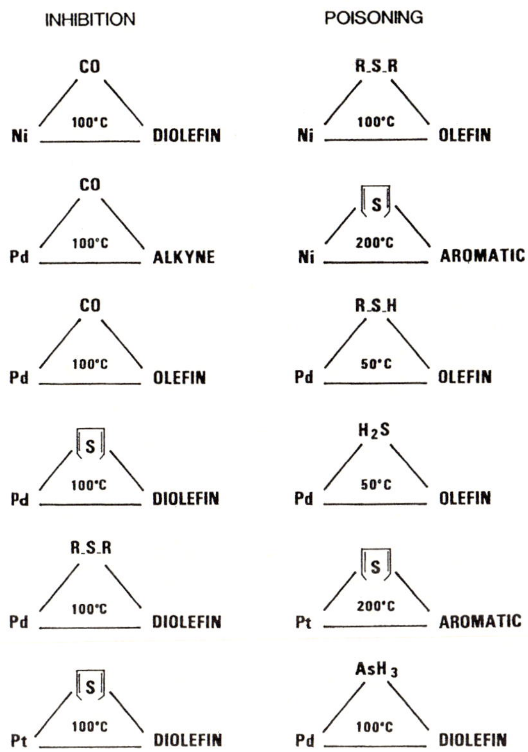

Fig. 5. Several triple systems.

COMPOUNDS WHICH ARE GENERALLY INHIBITORS

Carbon monoxide.

The carbon monoxide is a well known activity moderator ; it is often claimed for its ability to increase selectivy in hydrogenation processes (1) (2) (3) (4). For example, for the selective acetylene hydrogenation of the steam-cracking ethylene cut, industrial practise consists to inject traces of CO. The overall effect of this addition is to decrease the hydrogenation activity while the ethylene yield is generally enhanced. This observation lead often to the conclusion that CO enhances the actual chemical selectivity of the hydrogenation by inhibiting more strongly the ethylene hydrogenation than the one of acetylene. From our point of view, the interpretation seems to be wrong. By taking all necessary precautions for working in the chemical kinetic region while avoiding heat or mass transfer problem, we never observe any selectivity enhancement brought about by CO addition. On the contrary, we observed, for example in the selective hydrogenation of butadiene into 1-butene, that CO does not increase or even decreases the intrinsic selectivity of palladium catalyst (5). The same observation is made with platinum catalyst (6).

An illustration of these facts is given in the figure 6 where we have plotted the relative turnover numbers of 1-butene, 1-3 butadiene and 1-butyne hydrogenation on supported palladium and platinum in absence and in presence of CO. The 1-butene hydrogenation in absence of impurity is taken as the reference (100).

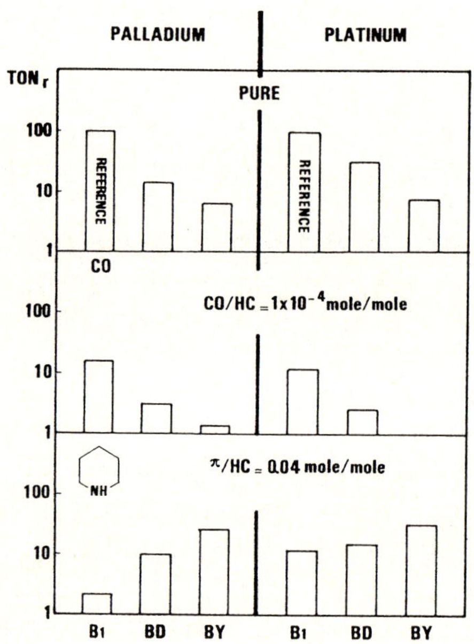

Fig. 6. Relative turnover numbers (TON_r) of 1-butene, 1-3 butadiene (BD) and 1-butyne (BY) on supported Pd and Pt (dispersion = 95 - 100 %) in absence and in presence of CO and piperidine. CO/HC and π /HC are relative concentrations of CO and piperidine to unsaturated hydrocarbon.

We observe on palladium that CO decreases the hydrogenation rates of the three hydrocarbons roughly to the same extent. The same trend is observed for platinum with 1-butene and 1-3 butadiene. Considering these observations, it is not surprising to find that CO has no beneficial effect on the chemical selectivity.

The fact that CO enhances the ethylene yield in industrial acetylene hydrogenation reactor can be explained by the intervention of heat and mass transfer kinetic occuring inside the catalyst pellet. The role of CO is to decrease the activity of palladium free sites which are not fed with acetylene and consequently hydrogenate quickly the adsorbed ethylene (7).

Nitrogen compounds.

Nitrogen compounds are also activity moderator but are mainly used for selectivation of catalysts. They have been widely studied for a long time either in heterogeneous or in homogeneous catalysis (references 8 to 18).

The effect of piperidine on supported palladium was studied by Vasudevan and al. (19) ; the same was done on supported platinum by Robert and al. (6). Some of these results are illustrated in the figure 6 for a catalyst of high metal dispersion.

Contrary to what is observed with CO, the effects of piperidine on palladium are depending very much on the hydrocarbon nature. We observe that hydrogenation rates are influenced in very different ways : severe decrease of 1-butene, roughly no decrease for 1-3 butadiene and a significant increase for 1-butyne. While less pronounced, the same trend is observed on platinum.

These observations help us to understand why selectivity of acetylenic and diolefinic hydrocarbons are enhanced in presence of nitrogen compounds.

Actions against inhibition.

When impurities like carbon monoxyde are incidentally present in the feedstock, the actions which can be done to overcome the problem of deactivation are relatively simple. The most common way used on industrial plants is to increase the temperature in order to recover the same level of activity as the one obtained before occurrence of the impurity.

In case of permanent presence of an inhibitor in the feed, the operating conditions (temperature, contact time) of the hydrogenation reactor can be generally easily designed in order to meet the required conversion.

COMPOUNDS WHICH CAN BE EITHER INHIBITOR OR POISON.

The sulfur compounds belong to this class, and we will see that this approach that considers the triple system catalyst - sulfur compound - hydrocarbon is here particularly useful. An example of this methodology is presented here.

Study of sulfur compounds adsorption on supported palladium.

This study has been performed in the conditions used for the industrial hydrogenation : liquid phase, low temperature and superatmospheric pressure of hydrogen.

We have firstly studied the adsorption of thiophene on palladium supported catalysts. The support is an inert low surface alumina. A first experience is performed in n-heptane under the conditions indicated in the figure 7.

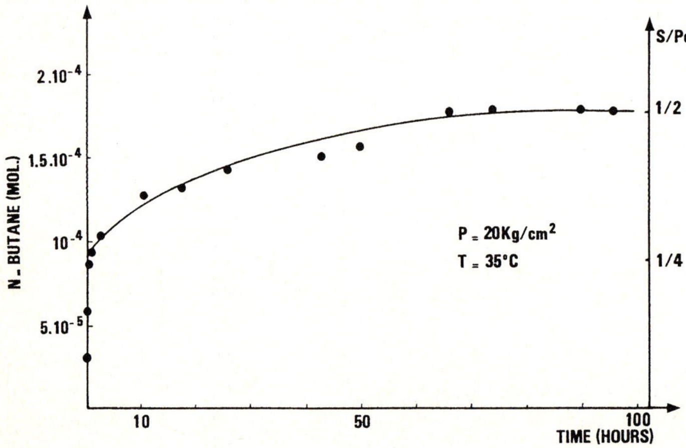

Fig. 7. Dissociative chemisorption of thiophene on a Pd-Al_2O_3 catalyst in heptane.

After addition of thiophene, we observe a rapid formation of butane followed by a slower one which goes finally to a plateau after 65 hours. Neither butadiene, nor butenes, are observed. Moreover, no butylmercaptan and no H_2S are detected in the hydrocarbon mixture ; non-adsorbed thiophene is the only sulfur compound present in the mixture after more than 100 hours.

From this experience, we can infer that a part of the thiophene is dissociatively adsorbed to give butane and palladium sulphide following the reaction :

Thiophene + 3 H_2 $\longrightarrow$ Pd S + butane

By repeating the same experience with several Pd catalysts of various loading and dispersion, we found that the butane formation is directly proportional to the quantity of palladium surface atoms (Pd_s). For each catalyst, a plateau of butane formation is reached which corresponds to a given fraction of surface atoms : 1/2 (see figure 7). The total sulfur content of the catalysts was also measured by X Ray fluorescence on the solid samples after test. The total sulfur quantities was also found to be proportional to the surface atoms and corresponds roughly to one sulfur atom per one palladium surface atom. Adsorption on the carrier was also checked in the same conditions and was found to be negligible.

As a conclusion, it appears that in a paraffinic medium the palladium active surface can be partly sulphided.

A new experience is made in the same conditions with a mixture of thiophene and 3 % mole of isoprene in n-heptane. Evolutions of isoprene, isopentenes (sum of the methylbutenes formed) and isopentane as a function of time are given in the figure 8.

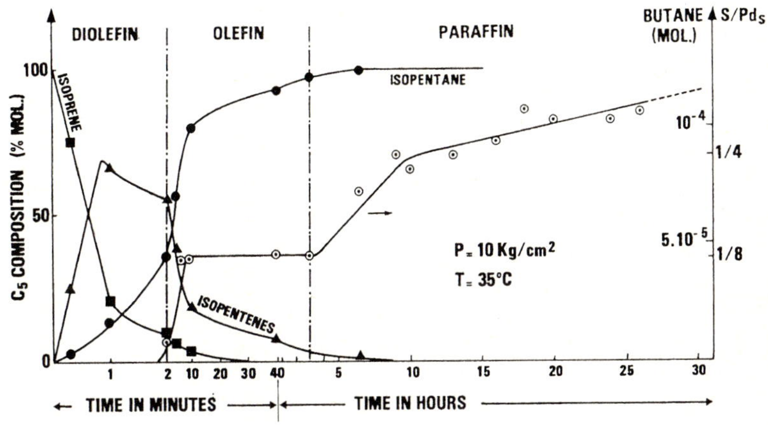

Fig. 8. Dissociative chemisorption of thiophene as a function of the type of hydrocarbon on a Pd-Al_2O_3 catalyst.

The formation of butane from thiophene is also presented. We observe clearly three distinct steps in the figure. The first one corresponds to the state of the catalyst in presence of a diolefin (isoprene) : no butane formation is detected and thus sulphiding of the surface atom does not occur. When isoprene is roughly completely hydrogenated a rapid formation of butane is observed up to a value corresponding to 1/8 of the ration S/Pd_S, this value remains constant as long as olefins (isopentenes) are present in the medium. When olefins have nearly disappeared, the butane formation increases again to reach a value of 1/4 for S/Pd_S, then it slows down, the rate corresponding to the one already observed in the figure 7.

As a conclusion from this experience, it appears that the sulphiding state of the palladium surface depends deeply on the nature of the hydrocarbon thus showing the ambivalent character of sulfur compounds.

Now, if we consider a given hydrocarbon, the extent of surface palladium sulphiding will also depend on the nature of the sulfur compound. We present in the figure 9 a similar experience as the one presented in the figure 8, but using butylmercaptan as sulfur compound.

We observe immediatly very big differences : isoprene hydrogenation rate is drastically reduced and butane formation begins initially. The fraction of sulphided surface palladium reaches a value close to 1/4. Same trend has also been observed when using dibutyldisulfur.

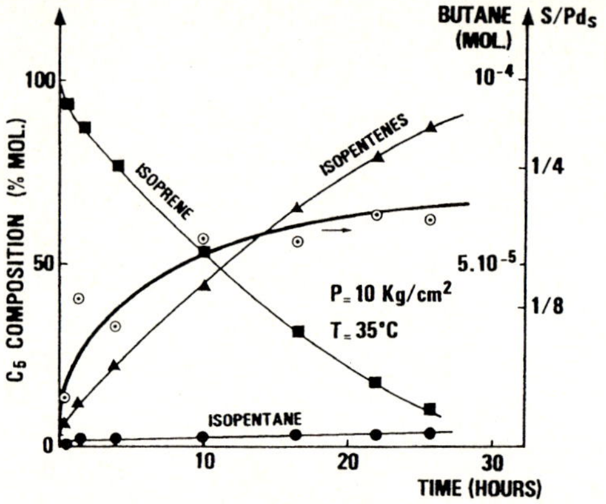

Fig. 9. Dissociative chemisorption of butylmercaptan on a Pd-Al_2O_3 catalyst in n-heptane.

Thus, it appears that the extent of surface sulphiding can vary depending on hydrocarbon and sulfur compounds natures. Therefore, it is now necessary to determine the toxicity of such surface sulfur.

Several samples of a catalyst have been pretreated in the same conditions as the one of figure 7 with thiophene in n-heptane. Thiophene quantity was adjusted to obtain quantitatively a given level of S/Pd_s fraction (from 1/8 up to 1/2). The butane formation and thus the corresponding sulfur fraction on the surface is measured. This value is then compared with the sulfur content of the catalyst after test (measured by X Ray fluorescence). These two values are found to be similar thus indicating that all the sulfur present on the palladium surface corresponds to sulphided palladium atoms without any significant remaining sulfur compounds. The values of turnover number relative to the non sulphided surface are given in figure 10 for 1-3 butadiene and 1-butene hydrogenation as a function of sulfur covering (S/Pd_s).

Firstly, we see that the effect of sulfur is more pronounced on the 1-butene hydrogenation than on the 1-3 butadiene hydrogenation. Secondly, we observe that even with butadiene, the decrease of turnover is not directly proportional to the surface covering. For butadiene 1 atom of sulfur kills roughly 3 atoms of Pd (toxicity = 3) while for 1-butene, toxicity is roughly 5. Thus, the effect of palladium sulfiding appears as a long range action :

presence of sulfur atom does not only affect the metal atom where it is adsorbed.

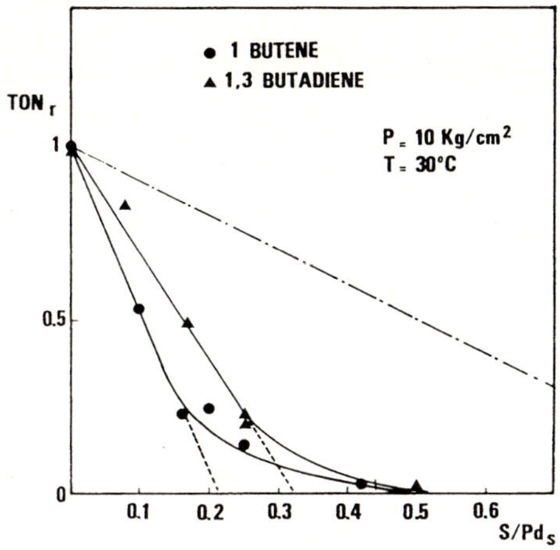

Fig. 10. Toxicity of surface sulfur in the 1-3 butadiene and 1-butene hydrogenation on a Pd-Al_2O_3 catalyst (dispersion = 98 %).

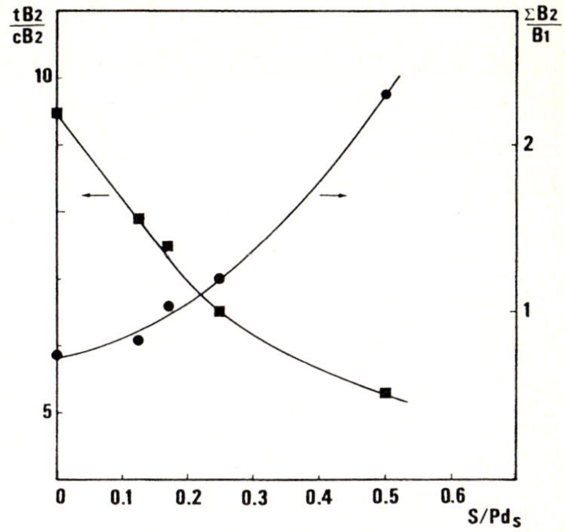

Fig. 11. Selectivities of butenes production (B1 = 1 butene, B_2 = 2 butenes trans + cis) from 1-3 butadiene by hydrogenation as a function of sulfur covering (catalyst of Fig. 10).

The action is not a pure geometric hindrance but it changes either the mechanism (geometry of the adsorption of the hydrocarbon) or the electronic properties of adjacent palladium atoms.

The figure 11 emphasizes the great variation of butenes distribution produced by the sulfiding : the influence of the ratio "sulfur over surface palladium" on the ratio "2 butenes/1butene" (1-4 addition on 1-2 addition) and on the ratio "trans/cis 2 butene" is clear. The distinction between geometric and electronic effect is rather difficult (and not very useful because certainly both exist) but Robert et al. (6) have given some clues in favor to electronic aspect.

Study of adsorption of thiophene on various metals.

We have also studied the chemisorption of thiophene on alumina supported Pt and Rh. The experiments were performed in n-heptane at 20 °C under a pressure of 1 atmosphere of hydrogen. Dissociative adsorption of the thiophene is observed on the two metals and produces exclusively butane like what is observed with palladium. The extent of metal surface sulphiding (S/M_S) is given in the table 1. Results on palladium obtained in the same conditions are given for comparison.

TABLE 1.

Metal	S/M_s
Pt	1/8
Pd	1/4
Rh	1/2

We observe that platinum is much less sulphided than rhodium, the palladium being intermediate. It is interesting to notice that the resistance to sulfur compounds observed empirically is ranked in the same order, i.e. :

$$Pt > Pd > Rh$$

Considering the toxicity of the surface sulfur on platinum, Oudar and Piñol (20) have found in an interesting work on a platinum monocrystal that the deactivation of the butadiene hydrogenation is directly proportional to the sulfur covering, one atom of sulfur killing one atom of platinum (toxicity = 1). This seems to confirm that platinum is more resistant to sulfur than other metals like palladium.

Effect of various sulfur compounds.

In this short review, it is not possible to present a detailed study of the effects of all the sulfur compounds which could be present in the industrial feedstocks.

For diolefin hydrogenation at temperatures less than 100 °C, the deactivation effect of various sulfur compounds on palladium catalysts can be roughly rated as follows :

$$H_2S > RSH \gg R(S_n)R \gg RSSR > RSR > \text{thiophenics}$$

Thiophenic compounds and alkylsulfide (RSR) can be considered as simple inhibitors while H_2S is a poison.

In olefin hydrogenation on palladium, same order can be proposed for temperatures less than 100 °C but the deactivation effects of all the above mentioned sulfur compounds are much more pronounced. On nickel catalysts, the hydrogenation of olefins at temperatures less than 200 °C is completely poisoned by all these compounds.

For aromatic hydrogenation, it is well known that platinum and nickel are the most active metals and can hydrogenate easily aromatics at temperatures lower than 200 °C. But in presence of a few parts per million of sulfur in the feed, these metals are progressively poisoned. In this case, every sulfur compounds can be considered as poisons.

Actions against this poisoning.

The first one is to improve the purification processes, but practically this is not always possible and even with a good purification process, some impurity upsets can occur. Therefore, it appears a strong incentive to design more resistant catalysts.

We have seen here before that platinum appears more resistant to sulfur in the hydrogenation of diolefins but unfortunately, this metal is not selective for the production of olefins. Thus, platinum cannot be used for such a reaction.

A better way is to modify the most active and selective metal, which is palladium, by adding a second metal enhancing its resistance to sulfur. This was described in publication 5 where new bimetallic Pd catalysts are presented and compared with conventional palladium catalysts.

An example is presented in figure 12.

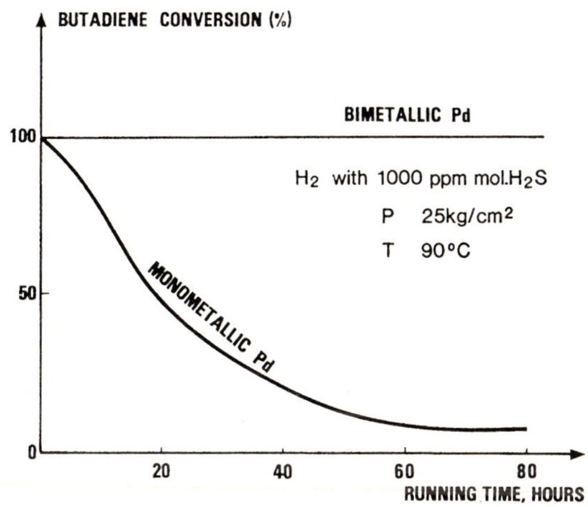

Fig. 12. Comparison of monometallic and bimetallic Pd catalysts in the 1-3 butadiene hydrogenation of a FCC C_4 cut with a H_2S containing hydrogen.

We can see that the butadiene hydrogenation is completely poisoned by H_2S at 90 °C on the palladium catalyst while the conversion remains at 100 % for the bimetallic palladium catalyst.

In the aromatic hydrogenation, new platinum catalysts resistant to sulfur have been developed (21) (22). Dalla Betta and Boudart (23) have suggested that the increased sulfur resistance of platinum supported catalysts is associated with the electro-deficient character of the metal. This interpretation explains the antidote effect of chlorine compounds which is observed on platinum-alumina catalysts (24). In presence of sulfur compounds, the addition of chlorine compounds increases significantly the activity of the metal. This behaviour is interpreted as a variation of sulfiding equilibrium of platinum, the role of chlorine being to decrease the strength of the Pt-S bond.

THE POISONS

Temporary poisons.

Arsenic. The presence of arsenic compounds is very frequent in the catalytic cracking effluents (see figure 2) ; up to now, arsenic is most frequently found in the C_3 cut. Considering the boiling range of this cut, the most probable arsenic compound is AsH_3. Such a compound rapidly poisons the palladium catalyst used in the hydrogenation. It has been shown by using the STEM technique (Scanning Transmission Electron Microscopy) that arsenic present on the used catalyst is entirely localized on the metal particle probably forming a surface bimetallic compound.

Several treatments have been tried to recover the activity of arsenic poisoned catalyst. The most efficient way is a specific regeneration procedure involving an oxydation of the catalyst. We have observed by using STEM that arsenic is moved from the palladium cristallite to the alumina carrier. The probable mechanism of regeneration is the formation of an arsenic oxyde whose high volatility helps the decontamination of the palladium surface. Due to the affinity of the alumina for arsenic oxyde, a recombination occurs with the carrier resulting in a quantitative trapping of the arsenic. This is easily controlled by determining the arsenic content of the whole catalyst : the values obtained are the same on the catalyst before and after regeneration.

Mercury. Mercury is found in natural gaz from several parts of the world. The heavier hydrocarbons associated with methane are often used as feedstock for steam cracking. Mercury has been detected in these feedstocks and is presumably present under metallic form.

The poisoning of active metal is here easily explained by the formation of an amalgam with mercury. The activity recovery by using an appropriate heat treatment is rather easy if we take into account the high volatility of mercury.

While it is possible to cope with arsenic and mercury by using regeneration procedures, it remains the big disadvantage of short cycle lengths and reduced catalyst life. Thus several technics have been developped for removing these contaminants before treatments (25) (26) ; they use specific absorbent materials working generally at low temperature and with an absorption capacity sufficiently high to give long run times.

Permanent poisons.

Silicon. Silicon compounds are often present in the coking effluents due to the use of antifoaming agents in the coker unit. Generally, they are essentially present in liquid effluents as for example gasoline. The poisoning effect is here coming essentially from the hydrogenolysis of the silicon compound on the metal. Here we understand well that activity recovery is impossible. Thus, the only way to decrease the poisoning is to decrease the addition of antifoaming agent. For a given concentration of silicon in the feedstock, it is possible to increase the metal loading of the catalyst. In this case, palladium catalysts should be avoided and nickel, or nickel-molybdenum catalysts would be preferred. The reactor should be designed with a sufficiently high quantity of catalyst such as the top part of the bed can work as an absorbent mass.

Lead. Poisoning by lead is sometimes observed. it is generally due to contamination of feedstocks by tetraethyl lead occuring during transport and storage.

This lead compound is readily hydrogenolyzed on the active metal what results in a rapid poisoning of the catalyst. As for silicon, there is no method for removing the lead from the metal ; the only way to avoid this problem is to prevent the feedstock from being contaminated.

SYNERGETIC DEACTIVATION EFFECT BY SOME IMPURITY MIXTURES

The overall deactivation effect by two impurities present together in the feedstock can be much more pronounced than the simple addition of the individual effects. Such "synergetic" actions can be very numerous and we will here only examine two examples.

COS and H_2O.

We have seen in the figure 2 that carbonyl sulphide is often present in the C_3 cut from catalytic cracking. Generally, due to the up-stream treatment, these cuts contain also a few ten or hundred ppm of water. When such cuts are hydrogenated at low temperature ($<$ 50 °C), a severe poisoning is observed which is similar to the one obtained with H_2S. This can be hardly explained by the action of COS alone ; water alone, if dissolved (no presence of free water), has no significant deactivation effect.

The most probable explanation is that poisoning is coming from the hydrolysis of COS which gives H_2S as follows :

$$COS + H_2O \longrightarrow CO_2 + H_2S$$

This reaction can be easily catalyzed by any active surface and especially the alumina carrier.

One way to solve this problem of poisoning is to improve COS elimination, but the conventional amine and caustic soda washings which are used for H_2S and RSH elimination are not sufficiently efficient for COS complete removal and generally an additional equipment is needed. Therefore, the catalytic treatment has generally to cope with a few ppm of COS present in the C_3 cut. The solution is to use a bimetallic palladium catalyst which can work in presence of H_2S as shown in the figure 12.

Sulfur compounds + nitrogen compounds.

Presence of both types of impurities is detected in some cuts coming from catalytic cracking, and coking or visbreaking processes.

As shown in the paragraph "Nitrogen compounds", a nitrogen compound like piperidine has a very small deactivation effect on butadiene hydrogenation. But, we have observed that if the feedstock contains also sulfur, the deactivation of diolefin hydrogenation brought about by nitrogen compounds is much more pronounced.

Same trend is observed in aromatic hydrogenation on sulfur-resistant platinum catalysts (24). Deactivation by nitrogen alone is not much pronounced, but with a mixture of sulfur and nitrogen compounds, the catalyst is almost completely deactivated. This was explained by a variation of the sulfiding equilibrium : the electrodonor compound (nitrogen compound) reinforcing the metal-sulfur bond contrary to the weakening effect obtained with electroacceptor chlorine compound already mentioned in paragraph "Compounds which can be either inhibitor or poison".

CONCLUSION

We have shown in this paper that deactivation of hydrogenation catalysts is a very complex matter. But people in the Industry continuously face this general problem and have to cope with it. It is thus mandatory for the Research and Development Scientist to study the effect of impurities in realistic conditions i.e. on the working catalyst by considering the triple system catalyst-impurity-hydrocarbon. Determination of the deactivation mechanism is obviously very useful but by far not sufficient. The knowledge of this mechanism must result in the cheapest way to solve the problem.

Sometimes, surpurification will be the best choice, for example by using specific absorbent material working at low temperature. Improvements of catalytic activity recovery processes are also of interest ; but often, development of more resistant catalysts will be the preferred way.

REFERENCES

1 W.T. Mac Gown, C. Kemball, D. Whan and M.S. Scurell, Trans. Faraday Soc., 73 (1977) 632.

2 Yasuhiro Furukawa, Akira Yokogawa, Takashi Yokomizo and Youji Komatsu, Bulletin of the Japan Petroleum Institute, 15 (1973) 56.

3 Dow Chemical Company, U.S. Patent 3,634,536.

4 Maruzen Oil Company, U.S. Patent 3,674,886.

5 J.P. Boitiaux, J. Cosyns, M. Derrien and G. Léger, Hydrocarbon processing, march 1985, 51.

6 J.P. Boitiaux, J. Cosyns and E. Robert, Applied Catalysis, to be published.
7 J. Cosyns, Catalyse par les métaux (1984) CNRS Edition, pp. 371-399.
8 O. Isler, W. Huber, A. Ronco and M. Kefler, Helv. Chim., Acta 30 (1947) 1911.
9 E.N. Marvell and T. Li, Synthesis 8 (1973) 457.
10 E.N. Marvell, T. Gosink and P. Churchley, J. Org. Chem. 37 (1972) 2989.
11 Sokol"skaya, Kinet. Katal. 12 (1971) 525.
12 D.V. Sokol"skii and P. Gadenov, Jsv. Akad. Nauk. Ser. Khim. 20 (1970) 62.
13 H. Lindlar, Helv. Chim. Acta 35 (1952) 446, Org. Synthesis 46 (1966) 89.
14 W. Oroshnik and A.D. Mebane, J. Amer. Chem. Soc. 76 (1954) 5719.
15 W. Oroshnik, G. Karmas and A.D. Mebane, J. Amer. Chem. Soc. 74 (1952) 3807.
16 U.O.P., U.S. Patent 3,433,842.
17 Phillipps Petroleum, U.S. Patent 3,637,877.
18 Phillipps Petroleum, U.S. Patent 3,636,175.
19 J.P. Boitiaux, J. Cosyns and S. Vasudevan, Applied Catalysis 15 (1985) 317.
20 S. Piñol, Y. Berthier and J. Oudar, C.R. Acad. Sc. Paris, T. 301 (1), Serie 2, pp. 17-19 (1985).
21 I.F.P., U.S. Patent 3,954,601.
22 H.R. Debus, R.M. Cahen and R.L. Aga, Hydrocarbon Processing, september 1969, 137.
23 R.A. Dalla Betta, M. Boudart, Proc. Int. Congr. Catal., 5th (Palm Beach, Florida, 1972), vol. 2, 1329.
24 J.P. Boitiaux, J. Cosyns and G. Martino, "Metal-Support and Metal-additive effects in Catalysis", Ed. B. Imelik and Al. Elsevier, 1982, 355-368.
25 N.L. Carr, D.L. Stahlfeld and H.G. Robertson, Hydrocarbon Processing, May 1985, 100.
26 I.F.P., German Patent D.E. 2,656,803.

B. Delmon and G.F. Froment (Editors), *Catalyst Deactivation 1987*

CARBON POISONING OF Pt/SiO_2 CATALYSTS

A. SÁRKÁNY

Institute of Isotopes of the Hungarian Academy of Sciences,
H-1525 Budapest, P.O.Box 77, Hungary

ABSTRACT

Formation of carbonaceous deposits from n-hexane, methane and 1,5-hexadiene has been investigated at 673 K over Pt/SiO2 catalysts of differing dispersion. The measurements with 1,5-hexadiene, 2,4-hexadiene and trans-hexatriene over SiO2 have confirmed the monofunctional behaviour of the catalysts. The initial C/Pt^s value is smaller, the subsequent rate of deposit formation and the fraction of "free" sites are higher on highly dispersed samples than on poorly dispersed ones. On catalysts of high Pt dispersion the C-C bond rupturing activity might impede the transformation of C6 entities into graphitic deposits.

INTRODUCTION

The dispersion of Pt crystallites is known to be one of the factors which affects the activity and the lifetime of reforming catalysts. Hydrocarbon poisoning experiments and kinetic studies have confirmed the larger resistivity of the highly dispersed catalysts (ref. 1). Pt atoms placed at edges and kinks have been proved to be more resistant to the formation of carbonaceous deposits than Pt atoms of high coordination number on the faces of single crystals (refs. 2-3). However, rate data on coke forming processes are scarce and the presented C/Pt^s ratios measured by TPO technique over Pt/Al_2O_3 bifunctional catalysts are in contradiction (refs. 4,5). In a recent paper Barbier et al. have concluded that the C/Pt^s ratio decreases with increasing dispersion over Pt/Al_2O_3 (ref. 5).

The TPO measurements permit the quantitative characterization of the carbon coverage although the unambiguous separation of carbonaceous deposits which are present on the metallic and the acidic sites is not without problem (refs. 4-7). For this reason our attention was focused on SiO_2 supported catalysts. We hoped that with this "inert" support the formation of surface held deposits is peculiar only to the Pt sites. Thus, a study was undertaken using direct gravimetric and TPO measurements over a series of Pt/SiO_2 catalysts. The present work reports on the formation of carbonaceous deposits from n-hexane and the fraction of "free" sites over Pt/SiO_2 catalysts of varying metallic dispersion.

METHODS

Catalysts

Catalysts used in this study are enumerated in Table 1.

TABLE 1

Characterization of Pt/SiO_2 catalysts

Catalyst	Surface area (N_2) m^2/g_{cat}	$Pt^s x10^{18}/g_{cat}$	Platinum Dispersion, %
Pt-black	1.2	11.2	0.37
15 wt% Pt/SiO_2	253	17.07	3.7
10 wt% Pt/SiO_2	288	13.93	4.5
[a]Euro-Pt-1	159	97.92	47.5
1.2 wt% Pt/SiO_2	388	23.52	63.7

[a]6.7 wt% Pt/SiO_2

Pt black was prepared by reduction of H_2PtCl_6 with HCHO in alkaline medium. Aerosil (HS) of Cabot corp. was impregnated by $Pt(NH_3)_4 Cl_2$ using the method of incipient wetness to get catalysts of 10 and 15 wt%/SiO_2 and by $Pt(NH_3)_4(OH)_2$ complex to prepare 1.2 wt% Pt/SiO_2. For the sake of comparison experiments were also performed with a 6.7 wt% Pt/SiO_2 catalyst known as Euro-Pt-1 (refs. 8,9).

The catalyst precursors were reduced at 673 K in a stream of H_2 for 5 hrs. The first TPO measurements with our catalysts indicated that the samples inherited some carbon. For this reason all the samples were oxidized at 623 K for 19 hrs. Then the catalysts were reduced and a few preliminary runs were made with n-hexane/Argon mixtures. After these stabilization treatments the catalysts were characterized.

Characterization

The surface area of the catalysts was determined from N_2 isotherms by the method of BET. The number of surface Pt sites, Pt^s, was inferred from oxygen titration at 293 K using the equations proposed by Benson and Boudart (ref. 10).

Deposit formation

The formation of the carbonaceous deposits was followed by means of a Sartorius (Type 4102) microbalance attached to a gas handling and vacuum system. After hydrocarbon adsorption, the remaining fraction of free sites, 100×f, was determined by CO chemisorption at 293 K. Additional experiments were performed with a n-hexane/argon mixture (3.9 kPa n-hexane) in a single-pass flow reactor. In this system the fraction of the remaining "free" sites was measured by O_2-H_2 titrations. The carbon coverage was determined by TPO in a static circulation system (1.33 kPa O_2, 5 K min^{-1}) collecting CO_2 in a calibrated volume at 79 K and measuring the partial pressure of CO_2 formed at 194 K by a Barocell pressure sensor. A few runs were accomplished in a dynamic system attached via a variable leak to a QMS 511 quadrupole mass-spectrometer (10 K min^{-1}, 1.33 kPa O_2, F $\simeq$ 15 ml min^{-1}). CO chemisorbed at 293 K on free sites measured volumetrically was used as an internal standard.

RESULTS

The carbon forming activity of our support was checked by measuring chemisorption of 1,5-hexadiene, a mixture of 80% 2,4- and 20% 1,3-hexadiene and trans-hexatriene at 623 and 673 K with 1.33 kPa hydrocarbon. The aerosil (HS) sample was treated with 0.1 N HCl and then calcined at 673 K for 5 hrs. The results given in 10^{-6} g hydrocarbon/200 mg support are presented in Table 2.

TABLE 2
Adsorption of dienes and trans-hexatriene on SiO_2

Hydrocarbon	T = 623 K		T = 673 K	
	Adsorbed amount × 10^6 g/200 mg SiO_2			
	[a]total	[b]irrev.	total	irrev.
1,5-HD	12.3	5.6	6.5	3.7
2,4-HD + 1,3-HD	17.7	6.5	7.2	2.5
trans-HT	23.3	7.0	8.9	1.5

1,5-HD: 1,5-hexadiene; 1,4-HD + 1,3-HD: 20% 1,3-hexadiene + 80% 2,4-hexadiene; trans-HT: trans-hexatriene

[a]Adsorbed for 10 minutes; [b]After evacuation for 10 min.

Figure 1 present typical chemisorption results at 673 K with Euro-Pt-1 and 10 wt% Pt/SiO_2, respectively.

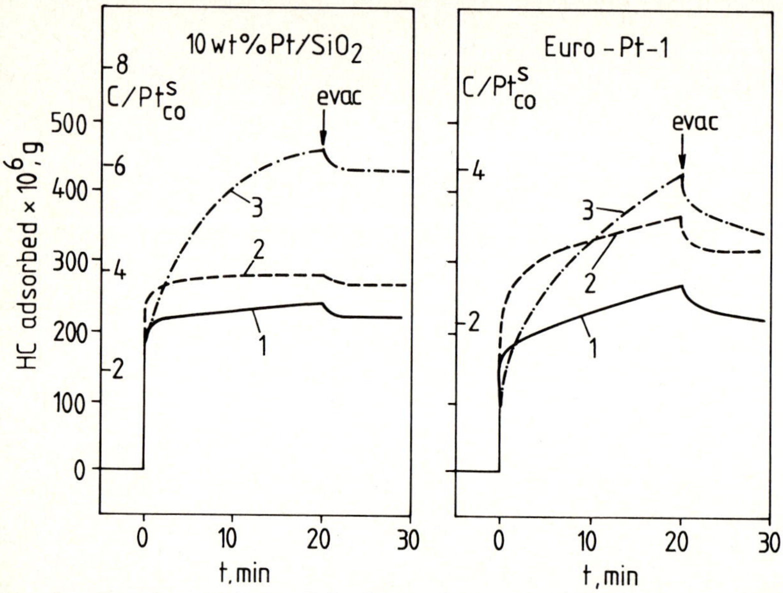

Fig. 1. Chemisorption of hydrocarbons at 673 K on 10 wt% Pt/SiO2 (D = 4.5%) and Euro Pt-1 (D = 47.5%): 1-n-hexane (1.33 kPa); 2-1,5-hexadiene (1.33 kPa); 3-CH4 (7.98 kPa).

With Euro-Pt-1 lower carbon coverages but continuous formation of the deposits, with 10 wt% Pt/SiO_2 higher C/Pt^s values reaching saturation with n-hexane and hexadienes were observed. The 1.2% Pt/SiO_2 showed the behaviour of Euro-Pt-1 whereas Pt-black and 15% Pt/SiO_2 resembled 10 wt% Pt/SiO_2 catalyst.

In Table 3 the initially adsorbed carbon $(C/Pt^s)_i$, the carbon coverage at 20 minutes $(C/Pt^s)_{20}$ and the slope of the deposit formation $(C/Pt^s/min)_{20}$ are collected. After 20 minutes the system was evacuated (10^{-5} Pa) for 10 minutes. The hydrocarbon removed in such a way was expressed as the percentage of the total carbon coverage (100xd). The catalyst was then cooled to 293 K and 0.44 kPa CO was adsorbed for 5 min the CO chemisorbed was recorded after 5 min evacuation. The fraction of free sites ($100xf_{CO}$) is collected in the last column of Table 3.

Characteristic results measured in a single-pass flow reactor are shown in Fig. 2. Here, C/Pt^s and the fraction of free sites, 100xf, are presented as a function of time on n-hexane/Ar stream (4.92 kPa n-hexane).

In Figure 3 the C/Pt^s data for the various catalysts are

TABLE 3

Formation of carbonaceous deposits at 673 K

Catalyst	HC[a]	$(C/Pt^s)_i$	$(C/Pt^s)_{20}$	$(C/Pt^s/min)_{20}$	100xd	$100xf_{CO}$
Pt-black	nH	2.93	3.31	$0.86x10^{-2}$	4.3	5.3
	CH_4	1.93	5.78	$1.93x10^{-2}$	5.6	7.4
15 wt% Pt	nH	3.02	3.43	$1.10x10^{-2}$	3.2	6.2
	CH_4	2.1	6.11	$3.61x10^{-2}$	3.6	4.1
	1,5-HD	3.68	3.99	$1.31x10^{-3}$	1.9	3.5
10 wt% Pt	nH	2,82	3.45	$1.43x10^{-2}$	6.7	7.2
	CH_4	2.12	6.08	$5.48x10^{-2}$	5.3	4.8
	1,5-HD	3.32	3.81	$1.13x10^{-3}$	1.4	2.4
	2,4-HD	3.41	3.67	$1.31x10^{-3}$	1.7	2.6
Euro-Pt	nH	1.54	2,42	$4.73x10^{-2}$	15.4	44.8
	CH_4	0.95	3.68	$6.51x10^{-2}$	10.2	34.0
	1,5-HD	1.65	3.17	$4.83x10^{-2}$	8.8	42.0
	2,4-HD	1.22	2.89	$4.77x10^{-2}$	6.8	40.0
1.2 wt% Pt	nH	1.47	2.13	$4.67x10^{-2}$	16.3	61.2
	CH_4	0.66	3.77	$8.12x10^{-2}$	10.5	46.6
	1,5-HD	1.53	3.46	$5.57x10^{-2}$	10.9	51.1

P, CH4 = 7.98 kPa otherwise 1.33 kPa hydrocarbon.

[a]nH: n-hexane; 2,4-HD: 80% 2,4-hexadiene + 20% 1,3-hexadiene; 1,5-HD: 1,5-hexadiene.

collected in the function of free sites. In Figure 4 the average "thickness" of the carbon islands $C/[Pt^s x(1-f)]$ is shown as a function of free sites.

DISCUSSION

The gravimetric experiments with hexadienes and trans-hexatriene have confirmed that the deposit formation (polimerization) is negligible on SiO_2. Hence, the Pt/SiO_2 catalysts used might be regarded as a monofunctional catalyst on which the deposit formation is governed exclusively by Pt sites.

The experiments with n-hexane - here we refer to $(C/Pt^s)_i$ and $(C/Pt^s)_{20}$ values - have confirmed the lower carbon coverage on the highly dispersed Pt/SiO_2 catalysts. These results support the

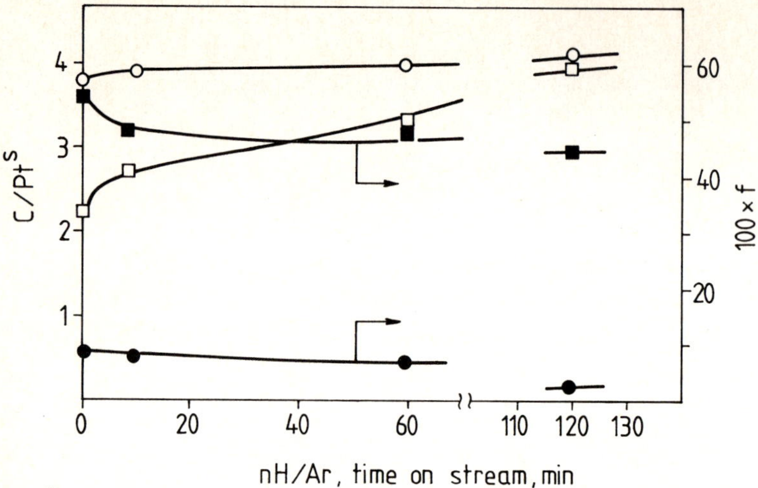

Fig. 2. Formation of carbonaceous deposits from n-hexane and the fraction of free sites at 673 K as a function of time on stream with 10 wt% Pt/SiO2 (O-C/Pts), ● 111×f) and with Euro-Pt-1 (□ -C/Pts, ■ - 100×f); P nH = 4.92 kPa.

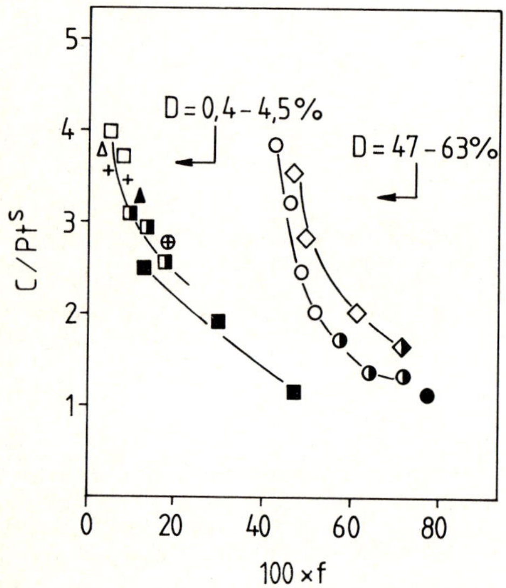

Fig. 3. Deposit formation from 4.92 kPa n-hexane/Ar mixture: the C/Pts ratio as a function of the fraction of free sites: O-Euro--Pt-1, 673 K, 1,10 and 60 min on stream; ◇ -1.2 wt% Pt/SiO2, 673 K, 1,10 and 60 min; ◐-Euro-Pt-1, 623 K, 1,10 and 60 min; ●-Euro-Pt-1, 673 K, 4.92 kPa n-hexane/H2, 60 min; ◆ -1.2 wt% Pt/SiO2, 623 K, 2 min; □ -10 wt% Pt/SiO2, 673 K, 2 and 60 min; ◨ -10 wt% Pt/SiO2, 623 K, 2,10 and 60 min; ■ -10 wt% Pt/SiO2, 553 K, nH/Ar for 9 min then H2 stream for 3 and 15 min; △-Pt-black, 673 K, 2 min; ▲Pt--black 623 K, 2 min; + -15 wt% Pt/SiO2, 673 K, 2,10 min; ⊕-15 wt% Pt/SiO2 nH/Ar for 15 min and then H2 stream for 30 min.

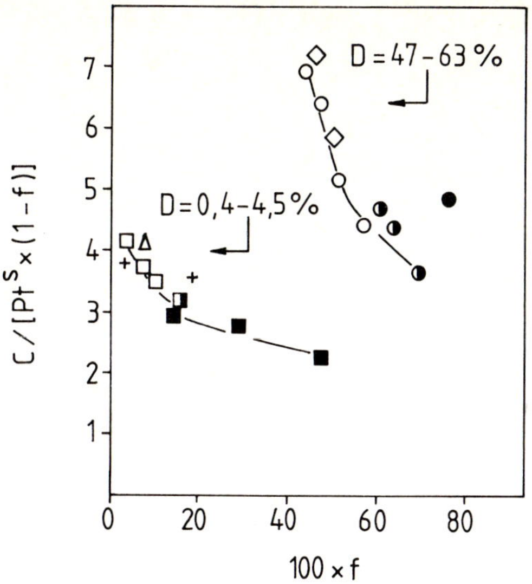

Fig. 4. The average carbon coverage on poisoned Pt^s sites as a function of the fraction of free sites. (For symbols see Fig. 3.).

conclusion of Barbier et al. (ref. 5). The higher resistance of the highly dispersed samples against deposit formation becomes more evident if one regards the carbon coverage as a function of the remaining "free" sites (Fig. 3). The fraction of "free" sites taking identical carbon coverages is higher on small Pt crystallites than on large ones which explains the superior catalytic activity of the highly dispersed catalysts.

The subsequent rate of formation of the carbonaceous deposits from n-hexane $(C/Pt^s/min)_{20}$, is considerably higher on highly dispersed samples than on poorly dispersed ones. The larger mobility of the deposit precursors on Euro-Pt-1 and 1.2 wt% Pt/SiO_2 is also indicated by the $C/[Pt^s \times (1-f)]$ values in Fig. 4. This value represents the average carbon coverage on carbon covered Pt sites.

It follows from the larger subsequent rates of deposit formation on highly dispersed samples that the C/Pt^s ratio might be higher on small Pt crystallites than on large ones. In fact, as shown in Fig. 2 the C/Pt^s observed on Euro-Pt-1 approximates the C/Pt^s value on 10 wt% Pt/SiO_2 after 120 minutes time on stream. It is peculiar, however, that even after 120 minutes the fraction of free sites is still definitely higher on Euro-Pt-1 than on 10 wt% Pt/SiO_2.

The larger rate of the deposit formation is apparently a consequence of the larger fraction of free sites on Euro-Pt-1 and 1.2 wt% Pt/SiO_2. In considering the reasons for the larger fraction of "free" sites on highly dispersed samples the following controlling factors are suggested:

i) The product selectivity pattern of C-C bond ruptures investigated at moderate temperatures ($T < 623$ K) has already confirmed the pronounced hindrance of intermediate product desorption on large crystallites, which indicates that the hydrocarbos are attached to the surface by several carbon atoms (refs. 11-13). On highly dispersed samples even at low H_2/HC ratios localised hydrocarbon interactions have been proposed. The rapid deceleration of deposit formation with n-hexane and hexadienes on our samples of low dispersion might point to the formation of ordered, densely packed carbon layers (ref. 2) which effectively block surface Pt sites producing precursors of coke. As revealed by the results with CH_4, the C_1 entity shows a smaller tendency to form this ordered structure.

ii) The larger reactivity, mobility of the coke precursors on highly dispersed samples is also evident if one regards the fraction of deposits which could be removed by evacuation (Table 3). In general, the larger is the fraction of the deposits which could be removed, the larger is the number of the "free" sites. The larger reactivity of the deposits over Euro-Pt-1 and 1.5 wt% Pt/SiO_2 might stem to some extent from the higher hydrogen content of the surface system. In the course of evacuation the hydrogen required for the desorption of the precursors might be formed by the decomposition of the deposits. The hydrogen on Pt sites might also be evailable by means of the spillover effect. Further experiments are necessary to separate these controlling factors.

iii) In the interpretation of the dispersion effect upon the fraction of "free" sites one should also consider the mechanism of the formation of the carbonaceous deposits. As indicated by the results in Fig. 1 and in Table 3, the rate of deposit formation from hexadiene on catalysts of low dispersion is almost zero at 673 K after 20 minutes contact time. This result confirms that the radical route of the polimerization or the condensation of dienes on the "carbon" surface can be ruled out.

In previous papers $\underline{C}_1$ (refs. 14,15) and polyene routes (refs. 14-18) of coke formation were emphasized on Pt sites. The C_1 route assumes C-C bond rupture and surface migration of C_1 entities. The polyene route has been proposed to involve the condensation reaction of trans-polyenes or cyclopentadienes.

Over catalysts of low dispersion the rate of deposit formation from CH_4 is significantly higher than that from hexadienes. Over highly dispersed samples no significant differences could be observed between the rates of deposit formation with the hydrocarbons investigated. From these observations we suggest that over Pt/SiO_2 catalysts of low dispersion the deposit formation from n-hexane takes place essentially by polyene route whereas over catalysts of high dispersion the C_1 route dominates. This conclusion is also supported by the high fragmentation activity of the latter group of catalysts. The almost identical accumulation rates over Euro-Pt-1 and 1.2 wt% Pt/SiO_2 with the hydrocarbons investigated might indicate that the rate of the deposit formation is limited by the surface transport of the coke precursors.

In conclusion, the presented results have confirmed the structure sensitivity of the formation of carbonaceous deposits over a group of monofunctional Pt/SiO_2 catalysts of differing dispersion. The initial C/Pt^s value is smaller and the fraction of free sites is higher on highly dispersed samples than on poorly dispersed ones. The high C-C bond rupturing activity might impede the transformation of C_6 entities into graphie-like deposits on catalysts of high dispersion. The experimental results in this study might also give some explanation why a second metal like Ir or Re which increases the fragmentation activity is able to ensure the superiority of these bimetallic samples (ref. 19). A different phenomenon of deposit formation appears on $Pt-Sn/Al_2O_3$ catalyst on which the presence of Sn drastically reduces the C-C bond rupturing activity but the PtSn ensembles ensure the mobility of intermediate dienes considered to be responsible for catalyst poisoning. On these samples a very pronounced accumulation of deposits was observed over the acidic support (refs. 14,15).

REFERENCES

1 P.P. Lankhorst, H.C. deJongste and V. Ponec, Studies in surface science and catalysis, Elsevier, Amsterdam, 1980, Vol. 6., pp. 43-52.
2 S.M. Davis, F. Zaera and G.A. Somorjai, J. Catal., 77(1982) 439-459.
3 G.A. Somorjai and D.W. Blakely, Nature, 258(1975)580-586.

4. J. Barbier, P. Marecot, N. Martin, L. Elassal and R. Maurel, Studies in surface science and catalysis, Elsevier, Amsterdam, 1980, Vol. 6., pp. 53-67.
5. J. Barbier, G. Corro, Y. Zhang, J.P. Bournonville and J.P. Franck, Appl. Catal., 13(1985)245-255.
6. J.M. Parera, N.S. Figoli and E.M. Traffano, J. Catal., 79(1983) 481-84.
7. R. Bacaud, H. Charcosset, M. Guenin, R. Torrellas Hidalgo and L. Tournayan, Appl. Catal., 4(1981)81-92.
8. G.C. Bond and P.B. Wells, Appl. Catal., 18(1985)225-30.
9. A. Frennet and P.B. Wells, Appl. Catal., 18(1985)243-57.
10. J.E. Benson and M. Boudart, J. Catal., 4(1965)704-10.
11. J.R. Anderson and Y. Shinoyama, Proc. Int. Congr. Catal., 5th 1972, North-Holland, Amsterdam, Vol. 2., pp. 1111-1120.
12. L. Guczi, K. Matusek, A. Sárkány, P. Tétényi, Bull. Soc. Chim. Belg., 88(1979)497-515.
13. A. Sárkány, J. Gaál and L. Tóth, Proc. Int. Congr. Catal., 7th 1980, Kodansha Ltd. Tokyo, Vol. 1., pp. 291-301.
14. A. Sárkány, H. Lieske, T. Szilágyi and L. Tóth, Proc. Int. Congr. Catal., 8th, 1984, Verlag Chemie, Weinheim, Vol. 2., pp. 613-23.
15. H. Lieske, A. Sárkány and J. Völter, Appl. Catal., in press.
16. C.G. Myers, W.H. Lang and P.B. Weiss, Ind. Eng. Chem., 53(1961) 299-307.
17. Z. Paál and P. Tétényi, J. Catal., 30(1973)350-61.
18. J. Barbier, L. Elassal, N.S. Gnep, M. Guisnet, W. Molina, Y.R. Zhang, J.P. Bournonville and J.P. Franck, Bull. Soc. Chim. France, 9(1984)250-54.
19. V.K. Shum, J.B. Butt and W.M.H. Sachtler, J. Catal., 96(1985) 371-380.

B. Delmon and G.F. Froment (Editors), *Catalyst Deactivation 1987*

COKING ON BIFUNCTIONAL CATALYSTS

J.M. PARERA, R.J. VERDERONE and C.A. QUERINI

Instituto de Investigaciones en Catálisis y Petroquímica -INCAPE-
Santiago del Estero 2654 - 3000 Santa Fe (Argentina)

ABSTRACT

The coking on bifunctional naphtha reforming catalysts was studied to find out which are the coke precursors and the mechanism of their formation. Runs feeding pure hydrocarbons (mainly n-paraffins) and naphtha doped with hydrocarbons were performed at 500°C and various pressures with bifunctional, acidic, and metallic catalysts.

Light paraffins produce small amounts of cyclopentanes which are great coke precursors. With heavy paraffins alkyl aromatics able to form a bicyclic hydrocarbon by cyclization of the alkylic chain are produced. If this bicyclic has an indenic structure (one 5 C atoms ring), it will be a great coke precursor, more reactive than in the case of having two aromatic rings.

The coke formation is a bifunctional process, being the metallic function necessary to dehydrogenate the cyclopentanic ring to a cyclopentadienic ring and the acidic function necessary to condense the cyclopentadienic rings producing polyring compounds. The monometallic catalyst has a greater coke forming capacity than the bimetallics due to its greater dehydrogenating capacity.

INTRODUCTION

In the catalytic processing of hydrocarbons (petroleum refining and petrochemical industry) a carbonaceous deposit called coke is formed on the catalyst surface. This deposit produces catalyst deactivation and changes in the selectivity. Coke formation depends on the catalyst, operational conditions and feed composition. In the case of naphtha reforming, this phenomenon is very important for the economy of the plant because it fixes the length of the cycle between catalyst regenerations by coke burning. For this reason, it is important to know the mechanism of coke formation to act on the parameters in order to decrease its formation.

The composition of the naphtha fed to a reforming unit is generally in the range 55-75% paraffins, 20-40% naphthenes (cyclopentanes and cyclohexanes), and 4-10% aromatics. In virgin naphthas nearly all the paraffins are normal. The naphtha is previously hydrotreated to eliminate sulfur and nitrogen compounds, and -at the same time- the olefins, if present, are hydrogenated. Coke forming capacity of pure hydrocarbons in the range C_6-C_{10} (refs. 1 and 2) and coking capacity of several naphtha cuts (ref. 3) were studied for mono and bimetallic catalysts. Coking capacity of the main constituents of naphtha on mono and two bimetallic catalysts are compared in Fig. 1. Relative coking capacities of the hydrocarbons are plotted as a function of the number of carbon atoms of the

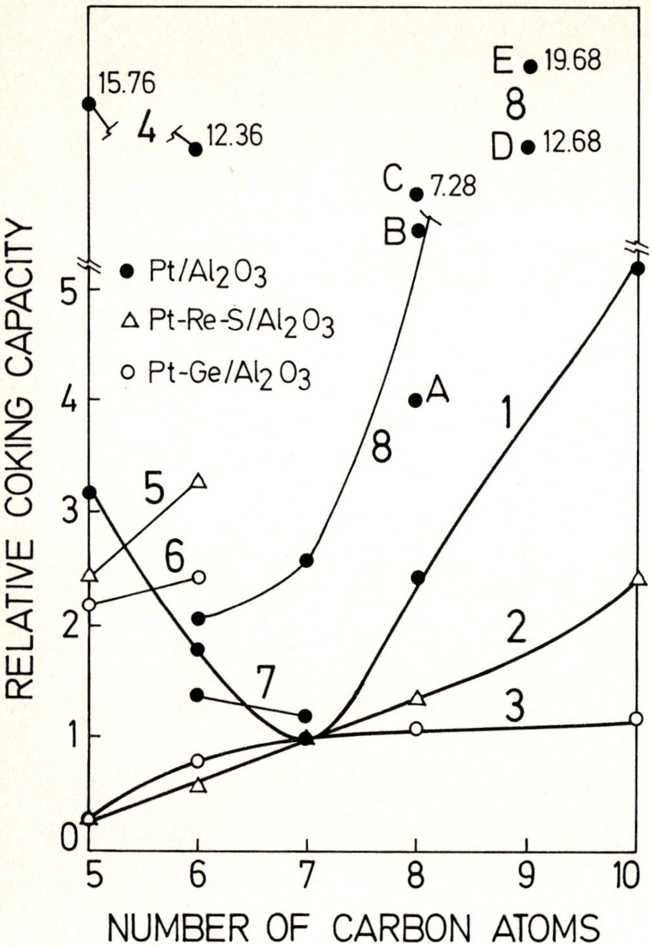

Fig. 1. Relative coking capacity of hydrocarbons on mono and bimetallic catalysts as a function of their number of carbon atoms. For each catalyst the values are relative to the one of n-heptane. Curve 1, n-paraffins on Pt/Al_2O_3; 2, n-paraffins on $Pt\text{-}Re\text{-}S/Al_2O_3$; 3, n-paraffins on $Pt\text{-}Ge/Al_2O_3$; 4, naphthenes of 5 C atoms ring on Pt/Al_2O_3; 5, naphthenes of 5 C atoms ring on $Pt\text{-}Re\text{-}S/Al_2O_3$; 6, naphthenes of 5 C atoms ring on $Pt\text{-}Ge/Al_2O_3$; 7, naphthenes of 6 C atoms ring on Pt/Al_2O_3; 8, aromatics on Pt/Al_2O_3; A, m-xylene; B, ethylbenzene; C, o-xylene; D, i-propylbenzene; E, n-propylbenzene

hydrocarbon fed. Data were taken from (ref. 1) and (ref. 2), and the coke produced by $n\text{-}C_7$ is taken as a unity for each catalyst. The operating pressure used in (ref. 2) for each type of catalyst was the commonest in commercial units -30 kg cm^{-2} for mono and 15 kg cm^{-2} for bimetallic catalysts, and it can be accepted that the trend is the same at both pressures.

Since the main components of naphthas are the n-paraffins, their coking capacity is an important clue to study the coking of the process. As shown in

Fig. 1, on Pt/Al_2O_3 n-C_5 produces a large amount of coke, whereas a smaller amount is produced with n-C_6 and even a smaller amount with n-C_7. From the minimum in coking capacity of n-C_7 there is an increase with the increase in the n-paraffin length. On the other hand, on the bimetallics coke formation always increases with the n-paraffin length. The more striking difference is observed in n-C_5 and n-C_6, being very interesting to explain this difference.

The objective of this paper is to give the reasons of the different coking capacity of mono and bimetallic catalysts studying the differences in catalytic selectivities, different coking capacity of reactants and products, and thus stating a mechanism for coke formation.

EXPERIMENTAL

To see the coking capacity of different hydrocarbons on several catalysts, runs feeding pure hydrocarbons or naphtha doped with 10% wt of pure hydrocarbons were performed. Experiments with doped naphtha are less sensitive to the change of doping agent than in the case of pure hydrocarbons, but have the advantage that the chemical composition of reactants is always nearly the same and is similar to the one of naphtha.

Catalysts

The catalysts used, with weight percentages on sample dried at 120°C indicated between brackets, were the following:

- $Pt(0.35)/Al_2O_3$-Cl(0.88), prepared by impregnation of γ-alumina CK 300 (Ketjen Cyanamid, Amsterdam, Sg = 200 $m^2\ g^{-1}$, Vg = 0.48 $cm^3\ g^{-1}$) with a solution of HCl and H_2PtCl_6 as quoted in (ref. 3).
- Pt(0.33)-Re(0.32)/Al_2O_3-Cl(0.90) of commercial origin and sulfided as indicated in (ref. 2) to 0.03% S. Sg = 168 $m^2\ g^{-1}$, Vg = 0.50 $cm^3\ g^{-1}$.
- Pt(0.37)-Ge(0.24)/Al_2O_3-Cl(0.81) of commercial origin. Sg = 178 $m^2\ g^{-1}$, Vg = 0.46 $cm^3\ g^{-1}$.
- Al_2O_3-Cl(1.03), CK 300 γ-alumina chlorided at 500°C with a stream of HCl-water-air according to (ref. 4).
- SiO_2-Al_2O_3 Grace High Alumina, 24.2% Al_2O_3, Sg = 341 $m^2\ g^{-1}$, Vg = 0.618 $cm^3\ g^{-1}$.
- Pt(0.49)/SiO_2, Sg = 285 $m^2\ g^{-1}$, Vg = 1.2 $cm^3\ g^{-1}$, free of chlorine, provided by Prof. J. Butt from Northwestern University and identified in (ref. 5) as 63.5-SiO_2-Ion X-L.

Feeds

Pure hydrocarbons Carlo Erba RP and hydrodesulfurized naphtha were used as feed. They were dried previous to the run by passage through a bed of 4 A Molecular Sieve. The naphtha had a boiling point range 40-155°C.

Test for catalytic activity, selectivity and coking

A stainless steel bench-scale flow equipment with chromatographic analysis on line was used. The range of pressure was 1-30 kg cm^{-2}, temperature 500°C, hydrogen:hydrocarbon molar ratio = 2, and weight hourly space velocity = 3. Carbon content of catalysts after the runs was determined by combustion-volumetry.

In runs at 15 and 30 kg cm^{-2}, during an intermediate period the pressure was decreased to 3.5 kg cm^{-2} and 10 kg cm^{-2}, respectively, in order to increase the coke deposition (accelerated coking test).

RESULTS

Pure hydrocarbons

n-Pentane. Runs feeding n-C_5 at various pressures and measuring the conversion to CP and the coke deposited on the catalyst were performed on mono and bimetallic catalysts. The results are shown in Fig. 2. For a pressure of 30 kg cm^{-2} the conversion to CP was negligible on the three catalysts. The conversion to aromatics of 8 and 9 C atoms was also measured and the results are shown in Table 1.

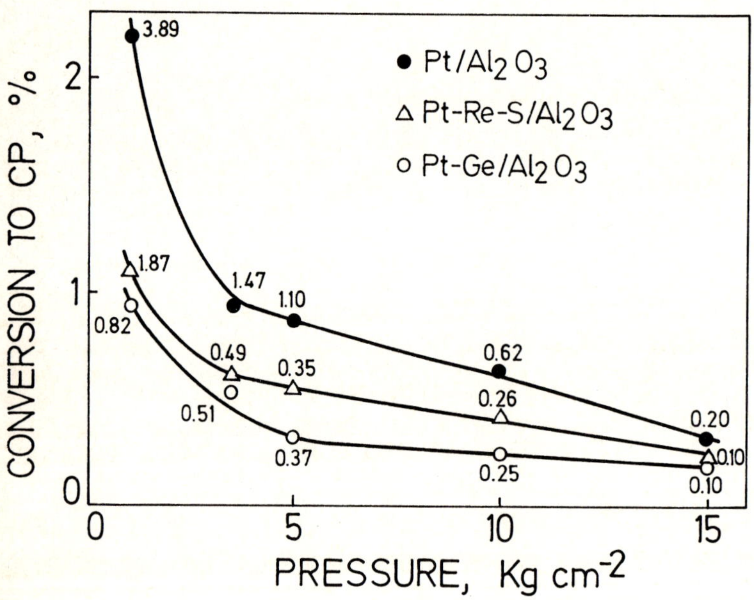

Fig. 2. Conversion of n-C_5 to CP on mono and bimetallic catalysts as a function of pressure. Numbers over the points are the wt% of carbon deposited on the catalyst after the 5 h run

TABLE 1

n-Pentane reforming. Conversion to heavy aromatics

Pressure $kg\ cm^{-1}$	Pt/Al_2O_3		$Pt-Re-S/Al_2O_3$		$Pt-Ge/Al_2O_3$	
	ArC_8 [a]	ArC_9	ArC_8	ArC_9	ArC_8	ArC_9
1	2.59	3.35	4.01	2.07	0.31	0.06
3.5	0.62	0.31	0.59	0.26	0.32	0.00
5	0.33	0.17	0.43	0.16	0.18	0.00
10	0.31	0.11	0.17	0.10	0.04	0.00
15	0.15	0.08	0.06	0.008	0.00	0.00

[a] ArC_8 = aromatic hydrocarbons of 8 C atoms, xylenes and ethylbenzene

n-Hexane. The reforming of $n-C_6$ produces MCP as an intermediate in the bifunctional mechanism leading to benzene. Then, the amount of MCP measured at the reactor outlet is the difference between the amount of MCP produced and the amount transformed into benzene and other products. Table 2 shows the conversion of $n-C_6$ to MCP and the coke deposited on the catalysts at various pressures. To increase coke deposition in the runs at 15 and 30 kg cm^{-2} an intermediate period at lower pressure was intercalated at 3.5 and 10 kg cm^{-2}, respectively. For this reason, the amount of coke can not be compared for different pressures. For each catalyst the conversion of $n-C_6$ into MCP decreases with the increase in pressure, similarly to the case of $n-C_5$. For each pressure, the highest amount of MCP and coke correspond to Pt/Al_2O_3, the intermediate amount to $Pt-Ge/Al_2O_3$, and the lowest amount to $Pt-Re-S/Al_2O_3$. The relative position of the bimetallics is opposite to the position with $n-C_5$.

TABLE 2

n-Hexane reforming, conversion to MCP (%), and coke deposited on the catalyst (wt%)

Catalyst	5 kg cm^{-2} [a]		15 kg cm^{-2} [b]		30 kg cm^{-2} [c]	
	MCP	% C	MCP	% C	MCP	% C
Pt/Al_2O_3	1.90	1.06	1.30	4.85	0.55	0.44
$Pt-Re-S/Al_2O_3$	1.08	0.65	0.42	2.25		
$Pt-Ge/Al_2O_3$	1.11	0.86	0.57	3.90		

[a] Run length 7 h. [b] 7 h at 15 kg cm^{-2}-20 h at 3.5 kg cm^{-2}-7 h at 15 kg cm^{-2}.
[c] 7 h at 30 kg cm^{-2}-20 h at 10 kg cm^{-2}-7 h at 30 kg cm^{-2}

n-Heptane. In the reforming of n-C_7 the 5 C atoms ring naphthenes produced are MCP and DMCP. Table 3 shows the conversion of n-C_7 to these naphthenes, and the coke deposited on the catalyst. Pt-Ge/Al_2O_3 produces the highest conversion to these naphthenes (1.81%) and Pt/Al_2O_3 the lowest (1.20%). The relative position of the bimetallics is the same to that with n-C_6. The production of heavy aromatics is small.

TABLE 3

n-Heptane reforming. Conversion to cyclopentanes and coke deposited on the catalyst on accelerated coking tests

Catalyst	Pressure					
	15 kg cm^{-2} [a]			30 kg cm^{-2} [b]		
	MCP	DMCP	% C	MCP	DMCP	% C
Pt/Al_2O_3	0.20	1.00	4.00	0	0.44	0.25
Pt-Re-S/Al_2O_3	0.80	0.53	3.95			
Pt-Ge/Al_2O_3	0.71	1.10	5.15			

[a]Similar conditions to [b] in Table 2. [b]Similar conditions to [c] in Table 2

n-Octane and n-Nonane. From n-C_7 to n-C_9, increasing the length of the paraffin increases its transformation into aromatics. With n-C_8 and n-C_9 nearly all the intermediates 5 C atoms ring naphthenes are transformed into aromatics. With these paraffins the corresponding aromatics (ArC_8 and ArC_9) are formed, and also bicyclic aromatics -as indene and naphthalene, can be detected. The amount of bicyclics and coke deposition is higher with Pt/Al_2O_3

Methylcyclopentane. The coke formation at 5 kg cm^{-2} in 7 h runs with MCP as feed is the following: 4.60% on Pt/Al_2O_3, 3.70% on Pt-Re-S/Al_2O_3 and 3.95% on Pt-Ge/Al_2O_3. The relative order of coking is the same that the one of n-C_6 (Table 2).

Naphtha doped with hydrocarbons

To see the coking capacity of several hydrocarbons, a naphtha doped with 10% by weight of hydrocarbons was used as feed at 1 kg cm^{-2}. The coke formation after 2 h run is shown in Table 4.

DISCUSSION

Normal paraffins, from n-C_5 to n-C_{10}, are the main components of the naphthas to be reformed and their transformation into aromatics is the objective of the process. Then, the reforming of the n-paraffins and of their products is a useful guide to study the coking produced by naphthas over different catalysts.

TABLE 4

Coke formation on several catalysts fed with naphtha and naphtha doped with 10% of different hydrocarbons

Doping agent	Catalysts					
	Pt/Al_2O_3	$Pt\text{-}Re\text{-}S/Al_2O_3$	$Pt\text{-}Ge/Al_2O_3$	$Al_2O_3\text{-}Cl$	$SiO_2\text{-}Al_2O_3$	Pt/SiO_2
None	3.36(-)	2.55(-)	2.60(-)	0.20(-)	0.70(-)	1.01(-)
CP	3.75(+)	3.08(-)	3.20(-)	0.20(-)	0.68(-)	1.20(-)
CPe	9.20(++)	5.68(+)	5.96(+)	0.54(-)	1.88(-)	2.50(-)
CPde	19.12(+++)	17.10(++)	18.30(++)	11.50(+)	20.28(+)	5.83(-)
MCP	3.50(+)	3.52(+)	3.50(+)	0.20	1.65	
MCPe	7.10(++)	5.13(+)	5.94(+)	1.09	3.15	
MCPde	18.20(+++)	17.06(++)	18.61(+)	8.04	17.38(+)	
CH	3.31	2.87	2.49	0.43	1.47	1.10
CHe	3.40	3.70	4.35	0.99	4.10	
CHde	3.40	3.84	2.61	4.83	6.35	
Bz	3.20	1.94	1.58	0.36	0.80	1.10
$n\text{-}C_5$	4.09	3.15	2.10	0.20	0.80	
$1\text{-}n\text{-}C_5e$	4.35	3.15	2.58	0.22	0.88	
$1,3\text{-}nC_6de$	13.10			6.00	9.21	
n-Propyl Bz	9.75(++)	8.80(+)			1.09	
1,2,4-TM Bz	3.80	3.75			1.00	
Indene	29.78	22.34			24.12	
Indane	9.30	4.45			2.76	
Naphthalene	4.24	4.94			4.37	

CP: cyclopentane, CPe: cyclopentene, CPde: cyclopentadiene, M: methyl, CH: cyclohexane, CHe: cyclohexene, CHde: cyclohexadiene, Bz: benzene, $n\text{-}C_5$: normal pentane, $n\text{-}C_5e$: normal pentene, $n\text{-}C_6de$: normal hexadiene, TM Bz: trimethyl benzene
(+) or (-): positive or negative detection of heavy aromatics (indene, ArC_{10}^+)

Most of the other constituents of naphtha are also products of the n-paraffins reforming. The coking capacity of n-paraffins and other hydrocarbons on mono and bimetallic catalysts was already shown in Fig. 1. For each catalyst, the values are relative to the coking capacity of $n\text{-}C_7$ and the great difference is in the coking capacity of the n-paraffins (curves 1, 2 and 3). It is our aim to explain the different behavior of the catalysts based on a mechanism of coke formation and the different metallic function activity of the catalysts.

Possible reactions of n-pentane on the bifunctional catalysts are the following: hydrogenolysis producing methane and n-butane, hydrocracking producing ethane and propane, isomerization producing iso-pentane, and cyclization producing cyclopentane. Possible types of reactions of $n\text{-}C_6$ are the same to those of $n\text{-}C_5$ with the addition of aromatization leading to benzene. In former papers it was shown that -on mono as well as on bimetallic catalysts, naphthenes with rings of 5 C atoms (CP, MCP) are the greatest coke precursors among the hydrocarbons of the same number of C atoms (refs. 1 and 2), as shown in Fig. 1.

Barbier et al. (refs. 6 and 7), and Parera et al. (ref. 8) showed that coke formation results from the transformation of cyclopentadiene (CPde) produced by dehydrogenation of CP on the metallic function of the catalyst. Then, it is possible to suppose that the difference in coke formation from n-C_5 and n-C_6 on the different catalysts could be due to the different selectivities to CP and MCP and the different dehydrogenation capacities to transform them into CPde and MCPde, respectively. Data in Fig. 2 and Table 2 are in accordance with this supposition: in the reforming of the light paraffins (n-C_5, n-C_6) small amounts of CP and MCP are formed and the coke deposited on the catalysts is related to these amounts, and their dehydrogenation by the catalyst. For instance the amount of CP at 10 and 15 kg cm^{-2} are not much different (Fig. 2), but at the higher pressure the amount of coke is many times smaller because the dehydrogenation is smaller due to the higher hydrogen pressure. Pt/Al_2O_3 is the greatest CP and MCP producer and also the greatest coke producer.

On the three catalysts, the amount of MCP obtained from n-C_6 at 5 kg cm^{-2} is higher than the amount of CP obtained from n-C_5. The decrease in coke formation on Pt/Al_2O_3 passing from n-C_5 to n-C_6 shown in Fig. 1 can be ascribed to the lower coking capacity of MCP compared to the one of CP on this catalyst, as shown in the same Figure. The Figure also shows that on the bimetallics n-C_6 produces more coke than n-C_5, which can be justified by the greater coking capacity of MCP (curves 5 and 6) and its greater production compared to CP.

The different coking capacity of the catalysts with compounds having a cyclopentanic ring depends on the dehydrogenating capacity of the catalyst to form a cyclopentadienic (CPde) ring (refs. 6-8). This ring has a conjugate double bond which is very reactive and can condense with other CPde ring by a diene-dienophile Diels-Alder type condensation giving an indenic structure (ref. 8). When feeding CP in the case of Pt/Al_2O_3, some indene can be detected (Table 4), and when feeding n-C_5 some aromatics of 8 and 9 C atoms are produced (Table 1). The ArC_8 are not great coke producers compared to the ArC_9 which coke production are similar to the ones of cyclopentanes on Pt/Al_2O_3 (Fig. 1). The amount of ArC_9 is small and always the production on Pt/Al_2O_3 is higher.

Feeding with n-C_7 the production of 5 C atoms ring naphthenes on Pt/Al_2O_3 is smaller than the production of MCP from n-C_6, and the coke produced is also smaller. The opposite occurs with the bimetallics (Tables 2 and 3 at 15 kg cm^{-2}), explaining the difference in mono and bimetallics when passing from n-C_6 to n-C_7 in Fig. 1.

Table 4 shows that increasing the dehydrogenation of the ring in the order CP, CPe, CPde, and MCP, MCPe, MCPde, increases the coking on all the catalysts. When the doping agent is CP, because of thermodynamic limitations only a small amount of CPe and even a smaller one of CPde are produced on the metallic function. Doping with CPe, a bit more CPde is produced and also more coke is formed than in the case of CP. When doping with CPde, the greatest production of coke is obtained. Comparing the coke formation on the metal-acid catalysts (Pt/Al_2O_3, Pt-Re-S/Al_2O_3, Pt-Ge/Al_2O_3) with the one on the acid catalysts (Al_2O_3-Cl, SiO_2-Al_2O_3), it can be seen that the presence of the metallic function able to dehydrogenate CP and CPe is necessary for the production of a great amount of coke. The catalyst with only the acid function produced little coke with CP and CPe, meanwhile the coke is as high as on the metal-acid catalysts when feeding MCPde. SiO_2-Al_2O_3 has a stronger acidity than Al_2O_3-Cl, and produces more coke. Comparing the coking capacity of Pt/SiO_2, it is seen that even the metallic function is able to dehydrogenate CP and CPe, the coke formation is not high because of the absence of acidic function where coke precursors can condense. Then, both functions are necessary to produce coke from CP and MCP: the metallic function is necessary to dehydrogenate up to CPde or MCPde and the acidic function is necessary to condense these coke precursors.

It is interesting to compare the coking capacity of the 6 C atoms ring naphthenes on bifunctional and acidic catalysts. It is known (ref. 9) that cyclohexane is rapidly dehydrogenated on the metallic function producing benzene without desorption of the unsaturated intermediates (CHe, CHde). When feeding these intermediates they are also rapidly dehydrogenated in the first part of the catalyst bed, flowing benzene along the bed. Since benzene produces a small amount of coke because of the high stability of the aromatic ring, CH, CHe and CHde produce no much coke on the bifunctional catalysts. On the other hand, the acidic catalysts are not able to dehydrogenate these hydrocarbons. They flow along the catalyst bed and the one more unsaturated, CHde, is able to condense on the acidic function producing an amount of coke greater than that on the bifunctional catalysts. Pt/Al_2O_3 is a more dehydrogenating catalyst than the bimetallics and transform more rapidly the cyclohexanes producing less coke.

Olefins are poor coke producers. Table 4 shows that 1-pentene (1-n-C_5e) has a coking capacity similar to the one of the corresponding paraffin. Diolefins with conjugated double bonds, as 1,3-n-C_6de, have greater coking capacity than paraffins and olefins, but still is smaller than the one of CPde and MCPde. All these results confirm that the coke formation in hydrocarbons of 5 or 6 C atoms is mainly produced by the naphthenes with 5 C atoms ring which are dehydrogenated to cyclopentadienic rings. The conjugate double bond in a 5 C atoms ring is more reactive than in an open chain.

From n-C_7 up, the transformation of n-paraffins into cyclopentanes is negligible and the production of aromatics increases with the length of the chain on all the catalysts. Among the possible products of heavy paraffins reforming, alkyl benzenes and bicyclic aromatics are the greatest coke producers. Then, the selectivity to these products influences the coking capacity of the catalysts. Although the total aromatics production is higher with Pt-Re-S/Al_2O_3 than with

Pt/Al_2O_3 (ref. 2), the amount of heavy and bicyclic aromatics is greater and greater the coke deposition on the last catalyst.

Doping with n-propylbenzene, the coke formation is greater on Pt/Al_2O_3 than on $Pt-Re-S/Al_2O_3$ (Table 4), and a higher amount of indene is detected in the reformate with Pt/Al_2O_3. This can be assigned to the greater dehydrogenating capacity of Pt/Al_2O_3: the alkylic chain of n-propylbenzene can be dehydrogenated and cyclizated producing indane which on Pt can be dehydrogenated to indene which have the cyclopentadienic ring and is very reactive for condensation to coke. Table 4 shows that indane produces more coke on Pt/Al_2O_3 than on $Pt-Re-S/Al_2O_3$, and this could be a consequence of the higher dehydrogenation capacity of Pt/Al_2O_3 to transform indane to indene.

On $SiO_2-Al_2O_3$, indane produces little coke compared to the one produced by indene. This is due to the lack of dehydrogenating capacity to produce the reactive indenic structure from indane.

Naphthalene -though being a bicyclic aromatic, has a smaller coking capacity than indene because of the high stability of the aromatic rings compared to the great reactivity of the cyclopentadienic ring.

CONCLUSIONS

Mechanisms of coke formation on mono (Pt/Al_2O_3) and bimetallic ($Pt-Re-S/Al_2O_3$ and $Pt-Ge/Al_2O_3$) catalysts are similar. The higher coking capacity of Pt/Al_2O_3 is due to its higher dehydrogenating capacity producing more cyclopentadienes from n-C_5 and n-C_6 and more indenic bicyclics from n-C_9 and n-C_{10}. Cyclopentadienic rings are important coke precursors due to the great reactivity of the conjugate double bond. This reactivity is greater than the one of the aromatic ring allowing condensation and leading to polycyclic hydrocarbons.

The proposed mechanism for coke formation from n-paraffins on the reforming catalysts is shown in Fig. 3.

The intermediates are produced from the paraffins and also when using naphtha can enter in the feed. Most part of the monocyclic intermediates leaves the reactor with the reformate, while only a small fraction of the bicyclics leaves it and the other part remains irreversibly adsorbed on the catalyst and is transformed into coke components.

The coke formation is a bifunctional reaction requiring the dehydrogenating capacity of the metallic function and the condensating capacity of the acidic function. The dehydrogenating capacity of the bimetallic catalysts is lower than the one of the monometallic. The bimetallics produce smaller amounts of CP rings and have smaller dehydrogenation capacity to produce CPde rings; nevertheless, these catalysts still have the dehydrogenation activity necessary to produce olefins, which are intermediate in the transformation of n-paraffins into aromatics or i-paraffins. In this way, the second metal improves -regarding coke formation, the catalyst metallic function. Also it is interesting to study changes in the acidic function in order to decrease its condensation capacity keeping unaltered its isomerization capacity.

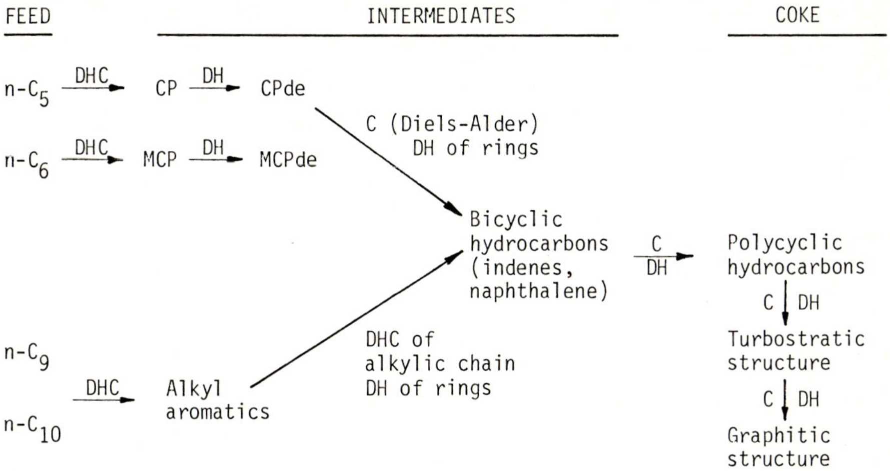

Fig. 3. Mechanism of coke formation from n-paraffins. DHC: dehydrocyclization (metal-acid function), DH: dehydrogenation (on the metallic function) or hydrogen transfer (on the acidic function), C: condensation (acid function)

REFERENCES

1 J.N. Beltramini, E.E. Martinelli, E.J. Churín, N.S. Fígoli and J.M. Parera, Appl. Catal., 7 (1983) 43.
2 J.M. Parera, C.A. Querini, J.N. Beltramini and N.S. Fígoli, submitted for publication.
3 C.A. Querini, N.S. Fígoli and J.M. Parera, submitted for publication
4 A.A. Castro, O.A. Scelza, E.R. Benvenuto, G.T. Baronetti and J.M. Parera, J. Catal., 69 (1981) 222.
5 T. Uchiyima, J.H. Hermann, Y. Inoue, R.L. Burwell, J.B. Butt and J.B. Cohen, J. Catal., 50 (1977) 464.
6 J. Barbier, L. Elassal, N.S. Gnep, M. Guisnet and W. Molina, Bull. Soc. Chim. Fr., I (1984) 245.
7 J. Barbier, L. Elassal, N.S. Gnep, M. Guisnet and W. Molina, Bull. Soc. Chim. Fr., I (1984) 250.
8 J.M. Parera, N.S. Fígoli, J.N. Beltramini, E.J. Churín and R.A. Cabrol, Proc. 8th Int. Congr. Catal., Berlin, July 1984, Verlag Chemie, Berlin, 1984, p. 593.
9 J.E. Germain, Catalytic Conversion of Hydrocarbons, Academic Press, New York/ London, 1969, p. 81.

B. Delmon and G.F. Froment (Editors), *Catalyst Deactivation 1987*

LONG TERM AND SHORT TERM DEACTIVATION ON Pt/Al_2O_3 AND $Sn-Pt/Al_2O_3$ CATALYSTS IN n-HEXANE CONVERSION

J.MARGITFALVI, S.GŐBÖLÖS, E.TÁLAS, M.HEGEDÜS AND P.SZEDLACSEK

Central Research Institute for Chemistry of the Hungarian Academy of Sciences, 1525 Budapest, POB 17, Hungary

ABSTRACT

Deactivation of Pt/Al_2O_3 and different types of $Sn-Pt/Al_2O_3$ catalysts in n-hexane conversion was studied at atmospheric pressure and low conversion. Two terms of deactivation, i.e. short term and long term, were distinguished. Both types of deactivation were very pronounced on catalysts, in which the acidic sites were not blocked by ionic forms of tin or lithium. It was demonstrated that the extent of deactivation in both terms can be different for different reaction products. On monofunctional $Sn-Pt/Al_2O_3$ catalysts the selectivity of the benzene formation increased upon aging. Results obtained in this study are discussed in terms of a generalized reaction scheme, in which poisoning metallic and acidic sites and formation of a carbonaceous surface overlayer have their distinct contribution.

INTRODUCTION

Bifunctional mono- and bimetallic alumina supported platinum catalysts are widely used in hydrocarbon conversion, i.e. reforming, isomerization, aromatization and dehydrogenation (1).

One of the characteristic features of these bifunctional catalysts is their continuous deactivation during the reaction. The formation of carbon deposits, reffered to as "coke", on the catalyst surface is the main reason for the deactivation or aging of these catalysts (2).

The formation of carbon deposits on a working catalysts was observed on both types of active sites, i.e. on the metallic particles and on the acidic support (3). The rate of deactivation and the amount and type of coke deposited on Pt/Al_2O_3 catalysts depend on the size of platinum particles (4), the chlorine content of the catalysts (5), the type and strength of the acidic sites of the support (6) and the texture of the carrier (7). Upon introducing a second metal, i.e. rhenium, iridium, tin, e.t.c. in their metallic or ionic forms, into a supported platinum catalyst not only the selectivity of the Pt/Al_2O_3 catalyst, but the properties towards coking and deactivation are also changed (8-9).

Although many works are devoted to study the deactivation of reforming type mono- and bimetallic catalysts there are still many questions to be answered.

The aim of this work is to demonstrate that rival deactivation routes responsible for the decay in the activity of different types of active sites on Pt/Al_2O_3 and $Sn-Pt/Al_2O_3$ catalysts can be distinguished.

EXPERIMENTAL PART

The base Pt/Al_2O_3 catalyst with 0.5 w% Pt was prepared by impregnation of Ketjen CK-300 type alumina with H_2PtCl_6 in hydrocloric acid solution followed by treatment in hydrogen at 400^oC. Three different types of tin-platinum catalysts were prepared from the base Pt/Al_2O_3 catalyst.

Catalyst Type A, with direct tin-platinum interaction, was prepared via surface reaction between $Sn(C_2H_5)_4$ and hydrogen adsorbed on platinum. Catalysts Type B, with tin-alumina interaction, were prepared form a lithium modified base catalyst Pt(Li) by anchoring $SnCl_4$ or $SnCl_2$ into the alumina (catalysts B1 and B2, respectively). Catalyst Type C, with tin-platinum and tin-alumina interactions, was prepared from catalyst type A via lithiation and subsequent tin introduction. Details on the catalyst preparation can be found elsewhere (10). Surface species of catalysts Type A and B are given Scheme (I). The characteristic features and designation of catalysts used are given in Table 1.

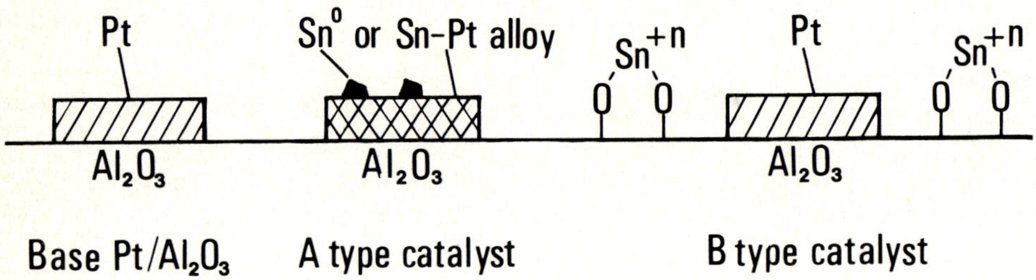

SCHEME (I) Surface species on $Sn-Pt/Al_2O_3$ catalysts

Studies of n-hexane conversion were carried out at 480^oC in an atmospheric catalytic microreactor as described elsewhere (11). In all experiments the n-hexane/hydrogen ratio was 1:5. An emphasize was laid to study the reaction at low conversion. In this way most of the primary reaction products (e.g. 1-hexene, methylcyclopentenes e.t.c.) could be followed. In this study following reaction products will be discussed: methane, propane, light hydrocarbons (C_1-C_5), 2-methylpentane (2MP), 1-hexene (1-$C_6^=$), methylcyclopentane (MCP), its corresponding unsaturated derivatives ($MCP^=$ and $MCP^{==}$) and benzene (B).

TABLE 1

Designation and properties of catalysts used

Catalysts	Type of interaction	Sn %	Li %	Cl %	H/Pt[a]
Pt	-	-	-	1.06	0.30
Pt(Li)	Al-O-Li	-	1.08	1.08	0.23
Pt-Sn(A)	Sn-Pt	0.15	-	1.10	0.19
Pt-Sn(B1)[b]	$(Al-O)_n$-Sn	0.12	1.29	1.53	0.13
Pt-Sn(B2)[c]	$(Al-O)_n$-Sn	0.12	1.04	1.44	0.15
Pt-Sn(C)	Sn-Pt $(Al-O)_n$-Sn	0.15 0.10	n.a.	n.a.	0.11

[a] measured after hydrogen treatment at 550°C
[b] tin precursor: $SnCl_4$;
[c] tin precursor: $SnCl_2$

RESULTS

Typical time on stream curves of n-hexane conversion are given in Figure 1. In this figure the extent of aging of different types of catalysts can be compared. Both A type Sn-Pt/Al_2O_3 and the base platinum catalysts (i.e. bifunctional catalysts) have high initial activity but their deactivation is very fast. Contrary to that the initial activity of catalysts, in which the acidic sites are blocked (Pt(Li), Type B and C Sn-Pt/Al_2O_3, i.e. monofunctional catalysts) is low but these catalysts are very stable as their rate of deactivation is low.

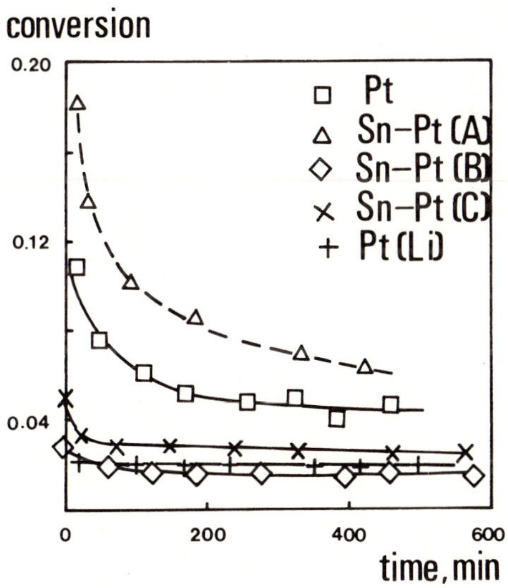

Fig. 1. Deactivation of Pt/Al_2O_3 and Sn-Pt/Al_2O_3 catalysts in n-hexane conversion. Catalyst weight: 0.15 g, flow rate: 90 ml/min.

Catalytic properties of catalysts studied are given in Table 2, where conversion and selectivity values measured on the fresh and aged catalysts are compared. In comparison to the base Pt/Al_2O_3 catalyst the selectivity of monofunctional catalysts (Pt(Li), B1, B2 and C) have been significally altered. On these catalysts selectivities for isomerization (i.e. formation of 2MP and 3MP) and hydrogenolysis (or hydrocracking) were strongly suppressed. On bifunctional catalysts, i.e. on the base Pt/Al_2O_3, and catalyst Type A, the formation of chain lenghtening products (toluene, xylenes, condensed aromatic hydrocarbons, e.t.c.) were observed. Contrary to that on cata-

TABLE 2

Conversion and selectivity data obtained on fresh and aged catalysts

Catalysts	Conversion, %	Selectivities, %						
		CH_4	C_3H_8	$1\text{-}C_6^=$	2MP+ $+i\text{-}C_6^=$	MCP	$MCP^=+MCP^{==}$ $+C_6^{==}$	B
Pt	29.83 (4.57)	0.28 (0.25)	2.80 (2.80)	11.0 (16.3)	20.4 (26.3)	5.5 (9.7)	1.1 (3.3)	43.9 (13.8)
PtLi	2.77 (1.81)	0.43 (0.44)	1.38 (1.07)	20.2) (22.2)	2.0 (0.4)	7.7 (0.9)	17.9 (11.2)	18.4 (26.4)
Pt-Sn(A)	41.24 (6.31)	0.10 (0.19)	1.66 (1.90)	3.8 (14.5)	18.8 (22.5)	4.5 (8.6)	1.3 (4.1)	51.7 (24.3)
Pt-Sn(B1)	2.82 (1.50)	0.34 (0.43)	1.35 (1.13)	20.7 (28.0)	1.7 (0.5)	5.2 (0.9)	22.1 (12.1)	13.2 (22.1)
Pt-Sn(B2)	3.22 (1.92)	0.42 (0.43)	1.72 (1.16)	17.8 (21.4)	2.0 (0.5)	7.8 (1.1)	23.0 (11.2)	14.4 (23.0)
Pt-Sn(C)	5.03 (2.37)	0.10 (0.13)	0.77 (0.56)	22.2 (30.4)	1.0 (0.2)	9.0 (1.0)	14.4 (6.4)	13.3 (9.1)

Fresh catalysts: after 1st minute, aged catalysts: after 500 min on time on stream. For aged catalysts results are given in paranthesis. Experimental conditions: $t_R = 480^oC$, weight = 0.15 g, flow rate: 90 ml/min.
Abbreviations: B: benzene, $1\text{-}C_6^=$: 1-hexene, 2MP: 2-methylpentane, MCP: methylcyclopentane, =: monoene, ==: diene.

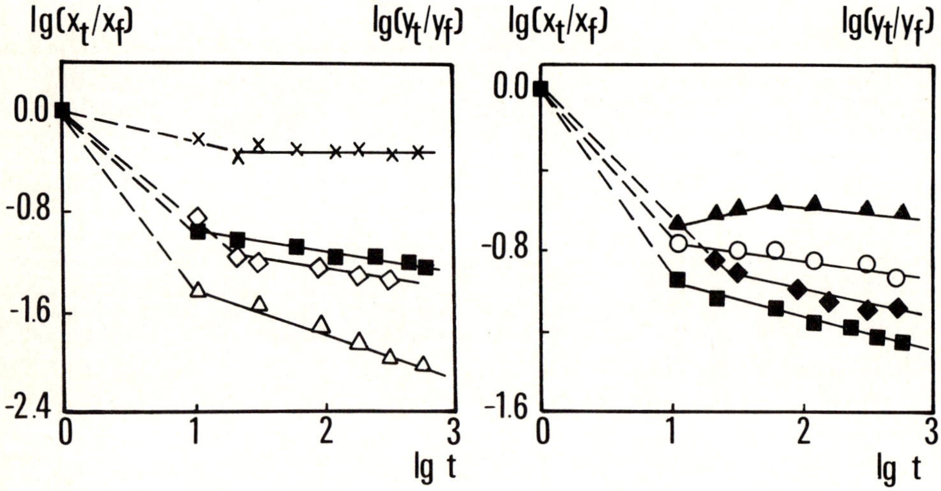

Fig. 2. Deactivation of Pt/Al_2O_3 base catalyst. ■ - conversion, △ - benzene, ▲ - methylcyclopentane, ◇ - CH_4, ◆ - C_3H_8, x -1-hexene, o - 2-methylpentane. Experimental conditions: catalyst weight: 0.05 g; flow rate: 15 ml/min.

Table 3

Activity changes upon aging

Catalysts	Conversion	Relative activities a) CH_4	$1\text{-}C_6^=$	B	C_3H_8	2MP+ $i\text{-}C_6^=$	MCP	$MCP^{==}$	$MCP^=$
Pt	0.15	0.13	0.23	0.05	0.15	0.20	0.27	0.42	0.60
PtLi	0.65	0.68	0.72	1.00	0.51	0.15	0.08	0.55	0.36
Pt-Sn(A)	0.15	0.31	0.89	0.07	0.18	0.18	0.29	0.55	0.41
Pt-Sn(B1)	0.53	0.68	0.72	0.89	0.45	0.15	0.09	0.37	0.26
Pt-Sn(B2)	0.60	0.62	0.74	0.94	0.41	0.14	0.07	0.38	0.25
Pt-Sn(C)	0.48	0.62	0.63	0.33	0.34	0.12	0.05	0.20	0.21

amount of catalysts: 0.15 g, flow rate 90 ml/min,

[a]calculated from conversion and product yields as ratios of x_a/x_f of y_a/y_f, where x_a and y_a conversion and yields measured after 500 minutes on time on stream x_f and y_f are corresponding values measured after the first minute.

TABLE 4

Selectivity changes upon aging

Catalysts	Selectivity changes [a] CH_4	$1\text{-}C_6^=$	B	C_3H_8	2MP+ $+i\text{-}C_6^=$	MCP	$MCP^{==}$	$MCP^=$	$\Sigma(C_1\text{-}C_5)$
Pt	0.88	1.49	0.31	1.00	1.29	1.77	4.00	2.76	1.00
PtLi	1.02	1.10	1.43	0.78	0.22	0.12	0.84	0.55	1.00
Pt-Sn(A)	1.97	3.81	0.47	1.14	1.19	1.92	3.50	2.68	1.01
Pt-Sn(B1)	1.26	1.35	1.67	0.84	0.27	0.17	0.70	0.50	1.03
Pt-Sn(C)	1.32	1.37	0.69	0.73	0.21	0.11	0.43	0.44	1.25

amount of catalysts: 0.15 g, flow rate 90 ml/min;

[a] calculated from selectivity data as the ratio of the selectivity values: $(S_j)_a/(S_j)_f$, where $(S_j)_a$ = selectivity after 500 minutes on time on stream; $(S_j)_f$, selectivity after the 1st minute.

lysts, in which the acid sites were blocked by ionic species (Li^+, or Sn^{+n}) no chain lengthening products were formed.

Characteristic activity and selectivity changes upon deactivation are given in Table 3 and 4. The activity and selectivity changes are expressed as the ratios $(x_j)_a/(x_j)_f$ and $(S_j)_a/(S_j)_f$ where indexes "a" and "f" are denoted to aged and fresh catalysts, respectively. The lower the values of these ratios are the higher the extent of aging process towards the formation of a given reaction product. One of the characteristic behaviour of Pt(Li) and Type B catalysts is the stability of the yield of benzene upon deactivation. On these catalysts the total loss of activity after 500 minutes is only 10 %. Depending on the experimental condition on these catalysts in the short term range deactivation period an increase in the benzene yield was observed. Contrary to that on bifunctional catalysts the loss in the benzene formation is dramatic. On the monofunctional catalysts such of drastic activity loss was observed for methylcyclopentane.

Selectivity changes given in Table 4. indicate that metallic sites responsible for the formation of the primary reaction products, for instance, methane and 1-hexane, are poisoned in less extent on all types of catalysts. Contrary to that products, in the formation of which acidic sites are involved shows different selectivity changes upon aging, i.e. their $(S_j)_a/(S_j)_f$ values are either > 1 or < 1 depending on the type of catalysts used.

In order to characterize the extent of deactivation the equation given by Voorhies (12) was modified to the following form:

$$\lg(x_t/x_f) = \lg A - n \lg t \qquad (1)$$

Where x_t - conversion or yield of a given product in moment t, x_f = conversion or yield measured in the first minute, the ratio x_t/x_f is a measure of deactivation and will be referred to as relative activity values. The rates of long term and short term deactivation can be evaluated by equation (1). The higher the absolute value of n is the higher the rate of deactivation of the reaction studied. The deactivation pattern of the base Pt/Al_2O_3 catalyst is given in Figure 2A and Figure 2B. The corresponding values of "n" can be obtained from the slope of the stright lines. In order to characterize the aging of the metallic and acidic sites the deactivation of different types of reaction products were compared. Figure 2A shows the deactivation of metallic sites, while Figure 2B that of the acidic sites. Two deactivation terms can be distinguished:a fast one in the first ten-thirty minutes, which is followed by a slow one. The former was assigned as short term and the latter as long term deactivation. It can be seen that on the metallic sites the rates of short term and long term deactivations increase in the following order: 1-hexene < methane < conversion < benzene. The rate of short term deactivation of MCP, C_3H_8 and 2MP are identical, but these values are lower than the rate of deactivation of n-hexane conversion. Contrary to that distinct differences can be seen in the long term deactivation where the rate of deactivation increase in the following order: MCP < propane < 2MP < conversion. These results clearly demonstrate that different aging processes are involved in the deactivation of metallic and acidic sites. On different types of catalysts the rates of short term deactivation of n-hexane conversion increased in the following order: B type Sn-Pt < < C type Sn-Pt < A type Sn-Pt < Pt/Al_2O_3 (see Fig.1.). The rates of deactivation of different reaction products increased as follows: Pt/Al_2O_3: MCP < 2MP < < C_3H_8 < conv. < 1-$C_6^=$ < benzene < CH_4; A type Sn-Pt: 1-$C_6^=$ < MCP < 2MP < conv. < < CH_4 < benzene < C_3H_8; B type Sn-Pt: benzene < 1-$C_6^=$ < CH_4 < conv.< C_3H_8 < 2MP<MCP

C type Sn-Pt: CH_4 < 1-$C_6^=$ < conv. < C_3H_8 < 2MP < B < MCP.

These differences show that in the short term deactivation (i) different deactivation processes are involved in the aging of these catalysts, and (ii) on Pt/Al_2O_3 and A type Sn-Pt catalysts deactivation of the metallic sites, on B type Sn-Pt catalysts deactivation of the acidic sites prevails.

On the base Pt/Al_2O_3 catalyst the rate of short deactivation was very sensitive to the changes in the flow rate of the reactants. At constant value of WHSV (equal to 21.5 h^{-1}) the rate of short therm deactivation of n-hexane conversion increased in the following order: 90 ml/min: n = 0.38; 30 ml/min: n = 0.48; 15 ml/min = 0.62. These experimental data indicate that, mass transfer induced effects are also involved in the aging process. Detailed characterization of the short term deactivation would require more experimental data at the very beginning of the experiments. These studies are in progress in our laboratory.

TABLE 5

Long term deactivation parameters

N^o	Catalysts Type	Catalysts weight, g	Flow rate, ml/min	Deactivation parameter, n: Conversion	CH_4	C_3H_8	Benzene	1-$C_6^=$	2MP
1	Pt/Al_2O_3	0.05	90	0.16	0.06	0.16	0.16	0.04	0.19
2	Pt/Al_2O_3	0.15	90	0.31	0.24	0.35	0.48	0.12	0.33
3	Pt/Al_2O_3	0.30	90	0.38	0.32	0.43	0.70	0.19	0.43
4	Pt/Al_2O_3	0.05	30	0.20	0.17	0.31	0.45	0.08	0.13
5	Pt/Al_2O_3	0.025	15	0.11	0.12	0.15	0.28	0.03	0.13
6	Sn-Pt(A)	0.15	90	0.29	0.05	0.18	0.45	0.09	0.24
7	Sn-Pt(B1)	0.15	90	0.08	0.07	0.10	0.08	0.03	n.a[a]
8	Sn-Pt(B2)	0.15	90	0.06	0.06	0.09	0.06	0.02	n.a[a]
9	Sn-Pt(C)	0.15	90	0.13	0.08	0.22	0.12	0.04	n.a[a]

a) on these catalysts formation of 2-methylpentane was strongly suppressed.

Characterization of the long term deactivation was done by using equation (1). Values of "n" are given in Table 5. Upon increasing the amount of the base catalysts, i.e. upon increasing conversion of n-hexane, the rates of deactivation of all products increased. In experiments N^o2, N^o5, N^o4 the same value of WHSV were maintaned varying the amount of catalysts and the flow rate as given in Table 5. It has already been mentioned above that the short term deactivation is strongly affected by the flow rate of the reactants. The pronounced short term deactivation resulted in a significant decrease in the rate of long term deactivation. The lower the flow rate of the reactants is the lower the rate of long term deactivation of all products. Under this experimental condition the long term deactivation pattern of the Pt/Al_2O_3 catalyst strongly reseambled that of the B type $Sn-Pt/Al_2O_3$ catalysts.

The long term deactivation behaviour of the A type Sn-Pt/Al_2O_3 catalyst is only slightly altered in comparison to the base Pt/Al_2O_3 catalyst. On A type catalyst due to the site blocking effect of tin the rates of deactivation of sites responsible for hydrogenolysis and dehydrogenation are less than on the Pt/Al_2O_3 catalyst.

From data given Table 5 it can be seen that catalysts type B have very low rates of deactivation of both active sites, i.e. metallic and acidic one. These data indicate that acidic sites are strongly involved in the deactivation processes taking place on reforming type catalysts.

DISCUSSION

In all reforming type catalysts, due to their bifunctional character, the activity and selectivity are strongly affected by the ratio of free metallic and acidic sites. In our bimetallic catalysts shown in Scheme (I), the number of these sites are strongly controlled. The aging induced activity and selectivity changes observed in this study (see Tables 2-4) can be attributed to different extent of poisoning of the metallic and acidic sites. This poisoning effect can alter the ratio of free metallic to acidic sites.

In order to understand these selectivity changes we have to know how the main routes of n-hexane conversion, leading to different types of C_6 hydrocarbons, are affected by coke formation. In Scheme (II) the main routes for the formation of different types of C_6 hydrocarbons on both types of active sites are given. In addition to C_6 hydrocarbons there are two types of further reaction products: (i) light hydrocarbons, and (ii) higher alkylaromatics and condensed aromatic hydrocarbons. Light hydrocarbons can be formed from all C_6 hydrocarbons given is Scheme (II) by hydrogenolysis or hydrocracking. The source of chain lengthening products has been discussed elsewhere (13-15).

The primary products of n-hexane conversion on catalysts studied are n-hexene and light hydrocarbons. The selectivity of n-hexane conversion on these catalysts strongly depends on the extent of conversion. For instance, on fresh Pt/Al_2O_3 catalyst upon increasing the conversion from 4 to 30 % the initial selectivity of all linear hexenes decreased from 20 to 10 % and the selectivity of benzene increased from 20 to 44 %. On a working catalyst at a given conversion value the selectivity is controlled by thermodynamic factors and by the ratio of free metallic to acidic sites. It means that any decrease in the number of each types of sites by "coke" deposited will result in an alteration in the product selectivity.

Results given in Tables 2-4 strongly indicate that by suppression of the number of acidic sites in a Pt/Al_2O_3 catalyst by introducing Li^+ or Sn^{+n} ions not only the selectivity of the catalysts but their deactivation pattern is also

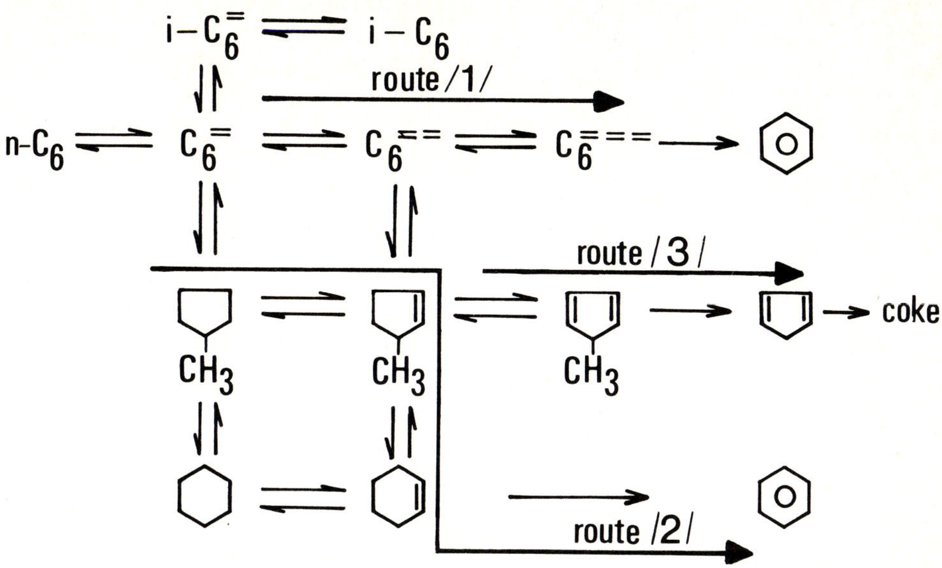

Scheme(II) Routes for the formation of different types of C_6 hydrocarbons.

altered. The strong suppression of acidic sites resulted in a change in the overall reaction route. On B type Sn-Pt/Al_2O_3 and Pt(Li) catalysts the consecutive route for benzene formation (16) prevails (route 1). Characteristic feature of these monofunctional catalysts are as follows: (i) low rate of the overall deactivation, (ii) strong suppression of the formation of MCP upon deactivation, (iii) very slight extent of deactivation towards benzene formation in the long term deactivation period, (iv) an increase in the yield of benzene formation in the short term deactivation range.

Contrary to the B type Sn-Pt catalysts the deactivation pattern of the A type one is very similar to that of the base Pt/Al_2O_3. Due to the bifunctional character of these two catalysts the selectivity of skeletal isomerization, i.e. formation of 2-methylpentane, is high. However, due to the coke formation on the support the number of acidic sites decreases. This decrease can be responsible for the permanent increase in the 1-hexene/2-methylpentane and 1-hexene/ /C_3H_8 product ratios observed on Pt/Al_2O_3 and A type Sn-Pt/Al_2O_3 catalysts upon their deactivation.

One of the characteristic feature of the Pt/Al_2O_3 and A type Sn-Pt/Al_2O_3 catalysts is the strong deactivation of the formation of benzene. This observation can be explained by strong involvement of different types of acidic sites in the formation of benzene. Based on literature data in the formation of methylcyclopentane both metallic (17) and acidic sites (18) can be involved. Our recent finding (19) that MCP is not a primary product of n-hexane conversion it is good agreement with the proposed reaction scheme (II). We suggest that at high temperature different types of acidic sites are involved in the benzene formation via C_5 cyclization of 1-hexene (18) and ring enlargement (20) followed by subsequent dehydrogenation of the C_6 ring on the metallic sites (route 2). This route is very fast, but due to the strong deactivation of the acidic sites, is strongly suppressed on the Pt/Al_2O_3 and A type $Sn\text{-}Pt/Al_2O_3$ catalysts. In addition to route (2), the formed methylcyclopentane can be further dehydrogenated into $MCP^{=}$, and $MCP^{==}$ (route 3), resulting in cyclopentadiene, the strongest coking agent.

On the Pt/Al_2O_3 and A type $Sn\text{-}Pt/Al_2O_3$ catalysts the yield of formation of methylcyclopentane showed a very interesting changes upon long term deactivation. First, it slightly increased and latter on remained either constant or decreased only slightly (see Figure 2.). This can be attributed to the fast poisoning of the acidic sites responsible for consumption of $MCP^{=}$by the ring enlargement. The stability in the formation of MCP and the relatively slow deactivation of sites involved in dehydrogenation reactions (see Figure 2. and Table 5.) can be responsible for the fast deactivation via formation of $MCP^{=}$, $MCP^{==}$, cyclopentadiene and Diels-Adler type coking on the acidic sites (21).

Contrary to that on B and C type $Sn\text{-}Pt/Al_2O_3$ catalysts the rate of deactivation of MCP is the highest among all reaction products (see Tables 2-4). As far as on these catalysts deactivation of the acidic sites prevails, the strong poisoning of the formation of methylcyclopentane is an indirect evidence that acidic sites are involved in its formation.

Let us discuss the differences between B and C type $Sn\text{-}Pt/Al_2O_3$ catalysts. Both catalysts have the same initial benzene selectivity values (see Table 2). However, on the deactivated C type catalyst the benzene selectivity was much lower than on the aged B type one. Characteristic feature of the B type catalysts was a slight increase in the yield of benzene and a significant increase in the benzene selecetivities upon long term deactivation. These increases are attributed to the aging process. From literature data it is known that fast formation of a carbonaceous surface overlayer can take place on the surface of platinum (22). If this overlayer has an ordered structure it can enhance the orientation of the readsorbed diolefins into the most favourable one required for the final dehydrogenation and cyclization into benzene. This ordered overlayer can not be formed on bifunctional catalysts due to strong poisoning of the platinum site by different chain lenghtening products as alkyl aromatic and condensed aromatic compounds.

On the C type catalyst due to the site blocking effect of Pt ensambles by tin the formation of the above mentioned ordered carbonaceous overlayer is hindered. The resulting configuration of the adsorbed C_6 dienes is less favourable for the benzene formation (23). The net results are (i) relatively fast deactivation of the metallic sites in the short term deactivation and the decrease in the benzene selectivity in the long term deactivation range.

From experimental evidences that (i) upon introducing tin into the platinum the characteristic deactivation pattern of the A type Sn-Pt/Al_2O_3 catalyst was not changed with respect to the base catalyst and (ii) the above discussed difference between B and C types of Sn-Pt/Al_2O_3 catalysts we concluded that the metal-metal (Sn-Pt) type interaction could not be responsible for the improved activity maintenance of industrial Sn-Pt/Al_2O_3 catalysts.

CONCLUSIONS

In deactivation of Pt/Al_2O_3 and different types of Sn-Pt/Al_2O_3 catalysts by coke deposition the loss of activity and the observed selectivity changes can be attributed to the alteration in the ratio of unpoisoned metallic to acidic sites. Our results clearly show that coke formation on the support is responsible for the fast deactivation of bifunctional catalysts. The support can not be considered any more as an inert reservoir for the coke formed. Consequently, such kind of recent statement, as for instance: "poisoning of the metal function by carbonaceous residues controls long-term deactivation of a reforming catalysts" (23) should be revised.

REFERENCES

1 B.C.Gates, J.R.Katzer and G.C.A.Schuit in "Chemistry of Catalytic Process", McGraw-Hill, New York, 1979, p. 184.
2 C.G.Myers, W.H.Lang and P.B.Weisz, Ind.Eng.Chem., 53 (1961) 299.
3 J.Barbier, G.Corro, Y.Zhang, J.P.Bournonville and J.P.Franck, Appl.Catal., 13 (1985) 245.
4 P.P.Lankhorst, H.C.De Jongste and V.Ponec, in "Catalyst Deactivation (B.Delmon and G.F.Froment, eds.), Elsevier, Amsterdam, 1980, pp. 43-52.
5 A.G.Graham and S.E.Wanke, J.Catal., 68 (1981) 1.
6 W.L.Callender, S.G.Brandenburger and W.K.Meerbott, Catal.Proc.Int.Cong. 5th 1972, 1 (1972) 1256.
7 M.E.Levinter, G.M.Panchenkov and M.A.Tanatarov, Khim.Tekhnol.Topliv i Masel, 3 (1966) 9.
8 R.L.Jacobson, H.E.Kluksdahl, C.S. McCoy and R.W.Davis, API Div.Refining, Proc. 34th Midyear Meet., Vol.49, Chicago, 1969, pp. 504.
9 J.C.Barbier, P.Duhaut, F.Eschard and J.Guillemat, Rev.Assoc.Techniciens Pét., 220 (1973) 43.
10 J.Margitfalvi, M.Hegedüs, S.Göbölös, E.Kern-Tálas, P.Szedlacsek, S.Szabó and F.Nagy, in Proc. 8th Int.Congress on Catalysis, Berlin (West), July 2-6, 1984, Vol. IV. Verlag Chemie, Weinheim, 1984, pp. 903-914.
11 J.Margitfalvi, M.Hegedüs, P.Szedlacsek and F.Nagy, Acta Chim.Hung., 119 (1985) 213.
12 A.Voorhies, Ind.Eng.Chem., 37 (1945) 318 .
13 J.Margitfalvi, M.Hegedüs, S.Göbölös, E.Kwaysser, L.Koltai and F.Nagy, Acta Chim.Hung., 111 (1982) 573.

14 J.Margitfalvi, M.Hegedüs and F.Nagy, J.C.S. Chem.Commun., 1982, 65.
15 A.Sárkány and P.Tétényi, J.C.S. Chem.Commun., 1980, 525.
16 Z.Paál and P.Tétényi, J.Catal., 30 (1973) 350.
17 F.G.Gault, C.Corolleur and S.Corolleur, J.Catal. 24 (1972) 385.
18 H.Höffkes, E.Baumgarten and D.Hollenberg, J.Catal., 77 (1982) 257.
19 P.Szedlacsek and J.Margitfalvi, to be published.
20 E.Christoffel, F.Fetting and H.Vierrath, J.Catal., 40 (1975) 349.
21 N.Pernicone, F.Lazzerin and G.Lanzavecchia, J.Catal., 10 (1968) 83.
22 S.M.Davis, F.Zaera and G.A.Somorjai, J.Catal., 77 (1982) 439.
23 V.K.Shum, J.B.Butt and M.H.Sachtler, Appl.Catal., 11 (1984) 151.

B. Delmon and G.F. Froment (Editors), *Catalyst Deactivation 1987*
1987 Elsevier Science Publishers B.V., Amsterdam — Printed in The Netherlands

DEACTIVATION OF $Ag_xSb_yO_z/SiO_2$ CATALYST FOR THE CONDENSATION OF ISOBUTENE AND FORMALDEHYDE TO ISOPROPENE

AN Li-Dun, JIANG Zhi-Cheng, YIN Yuan-Gen*

Lanzhou Institute of Chemical Physics, Chinese Academy of Sciences, P.O. Box 97, Lanzhou, P.R. China

* Present Address: Beijing Technical Institute for Chemical Fiber, Beijing, P.R. China

ABSTRACT

The chemical composition, surface distribution of the elements, and crystal structure of fresh and deactivated $Ag_xSb_yO_z/SiO_2$ catalysts were investigated by X-ray Photo-Electron Spectroscopy (XPS), Scanning Auger Microprobe (SAM), the Electron Microdiffraction (EMD) technique in Analytical Electron Microscopy (AEM), Atomic Absorption Spectroscopy (AAS) and the minireaction technique. The active phase of this catalyst and the causes of its deactivation were analyzed in terms of the differences in the composition and distribution of surface elements and the change in chemical composition and crystallographic structure of the active components of fresh and deactivated catalysts as well as by evaluating their activity.

INTRODUCTION

$Ag_xSb_yO_z/SiO_2$ catalysts (1) appears to have higher activity and selectivity for one-step gaseous condensation of isobutene and formaldehyde to isopropene than $Cr_xP_yO_z/SiO_2$ catalyst (2); but its stability is not satisfactory. Yu (3) has investigated the surface acidity of $Ag_xSb_yO_z/SiO_2$ catalyst and proposed that the active sites appear to be proton acid and the cause of the deactivation of the catalyst is the irreversible adsorption of water molecules on them replacing the proton acid sites. Chen (4) did not find any Brönsted acid sites in this catalyst by in-situ IR using the pyridine adsorption method and attributed the deactivation mainly to the decrease in their electron acceptor sites. In this work, fresh and deactivated $Ag_xSb_yO_z/SiO_2$ catalysts were characterized, mainly by means of the XPS, SAM and EMD techniques in AEM, and AAS, to investigate the composition and structure of the active phase in this catalyst. We will discuss the reasons for its deactivation, which could provide useful information for improving the stability of this catalyst system.

EXPERIMENTAL METHODS

Preparation of the samples

(1) Preparation of the catalyst. Silica gel spheres (20-50 mesh, specific

surface area ca. 165 m^2/g) dried at 120^oC for 2 hrs were impregnated with a solution of silver nitrate and antimony chloride (until just wet) dried and washed with warm de-ionized water free from chloride ions, and then dried again and calcined at 500^oC in air for 4 hrs.

(2) Preparation of Sb_2O_4. Sb_2O_3 (A.R., Fourth Factory of Chemicals, Shanghai) was calcined at 800^oC in air for 3 hrs. XRD measurement confirmed its crystal phase as α-Sb_2O_4.

(3) Preparation of $AgSbO_3$. Ag_2O (A.R. Beijing Factory of Chemical Reagents) and Sb_2O_3 (as mentioned above) were thoroughly mixed in an equimolecular ratio and calcined in air at 960^oC for 4 hrs. XRD measurement confirmed the crystal phase as cubic $AgSbO_3$.

Evaluation of the activity of the catalysts

The catalytic behavior of the catalysts was evaluated with the help of fixed-bed minireactor system which had a loading capacity of 14 ml catalyst (ca. 7 g). The molar ratio of isobutene to formaldehyde was 6.6 - 6.8. The reaction was carried out at 300 - 310^oC in periods of 50 min. with a contact time of 0.6 - 0.8 sec. Air was used as the regenerating gas flowing countercurrently against the reactant fluid; the regeneration was carried out at 500^oC in periods of 50 min.

Electron spectroscopy methods

A PHI-550 multiple electron spectrometer (Physical Electron Co., Perkin Elmer) was used to make XPS, AES and SAM measurements. A MgK (1253.6 eV) target was taken as XPS source. The C_{1s} (284.6 eV) of contamination carbon and Si_{2p} (103.4 eV) of the support SiO_2 were designated as the reference standards of binding energy in the pure compounds and the catalyst samples respectively. The charge effect on the sample surface during XPS measurements was neutralized with a flooding electron gun. Because the $Sb_{3d5/2}$ and O_{1s} peaks overlap, the quantitative analysis of the surface elements is carried out according to the following procedure: first, the peak area of the related peaks is measured (i.e. Si_{2p}, $Sb_{3d3/2}$, $Ag_{3d5/2}$ etc.); secondly, $Sb_{3d5/2}$ intensity is calculated with the photoelectron sections given by Scofield (5) and confirmed experimentally (6):

$$I_{Sb_{3d5/2}} = I_{Sb_{3d3/2}} \cdot \frac{\sigma_{Sb_{3d5/2}}}{\sigma_{Sb_{3d3/2}}}$$

then the related atomic ratio is computed using Wagner's atomic sensitivity factor (7). Owing to the charge effect, it is difficult to do AES (and SAM) analysis for the isolated catalyst samples. We controlled the energy of the primary electron beam carefully, thereby controlling the yield of secondary electrons, and the AES spectra and SAM images of the isolated samples were obtained successfully with a lateral resolution of 5 μm.

Transmission electron microscopy (TEM) and the electron microdiffraction (EMD) technique

Both the topographic pictures and electron diffraction patterns were obtained by means of a Hithachi H-600 electron microscope. The support, SiO_2, of the catalysts was dissolved and removed (9), and the residue was transferred into the machine to take the topographic and EMD pictures.

RESULTS AND DISCUSSION

XPS Results

The measurements showing the chemical states of silver and antimony in some typical Ag- and/or Sb-containing compounds and $Ag_xSb_yO_z/SiO_2$ catalysts are shown in Table 1. It is clear that the difference in $Sb_{3d3/2}$ binding energy between Sb(III) and Sb(V) is only 0.7 eV, so XPS is not an ideal method for judging the chemical states of the Sb element (10). Nevertheless, the antimony on the surface of real catalysts (NA-142 and NA-128) can be considered as Sb(V) when we compare the binding energy of their $Sb_{3d3/2}$ peaks with that in typical Sb-containing compounds.

TABLE 1

XPS results of Ag- and/or Sb-containing compounds and $Ag_xSb_yO_z/SiO_2$ catalysts

Name of compounds or catalysts	Binding energy (eV)		
	$Sb_{3d3/2}$*		$Ag_{3d5/2}$
	experim. value	literat. value	experim. value
Ag_2O & Sb_2O_3 (equimol.mix.)	539.7	539.4(11)	368.1
Sb_2O_4	539.3	539.7(12)	
$AgSbO_3$	540.4	540.3(6,10)	
NA-142(F)**	540.7		368.5
NA-142(W)***	540.5		368.4
NA-128(F)	540.2		368.5
NA-128(W)	540.2		368.3

* Owing to the overlap of $Sb_{3d5/2}$ and O_{1s} peaks, the Eb value of the $Sb_{3d3/2}$ peak and its chemical shift were used to determine the Sb-chemical state.

** "F" means fresh catalyst.

*** "W" means "waste" catalyst deactivated in stability experiment.

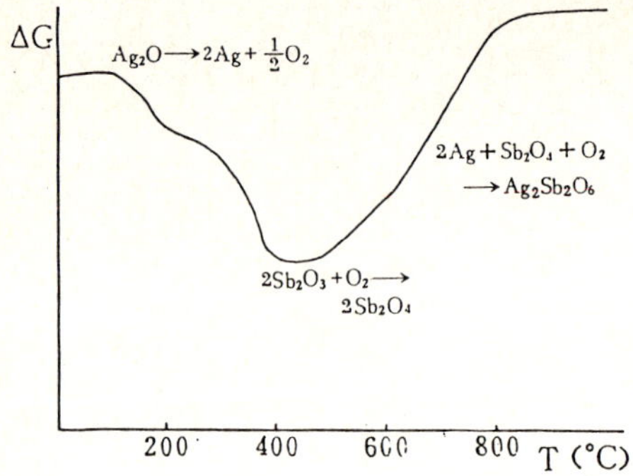

Fig. 1. TG spectrum of the equimolar mixture of Sb_2O_3 and Ag_2O.

Because of the fact that the chemical shift of $Ag_{3d5/2}$ peaks in different compounds is too small for its valences to be distinguished and the AgM_4VV signal is too weak to define the peak position owing to the low Ag-content in real catalyst, it is difficult to determine the chemical state of silver with XPS-Auger parameters. We determined it only in individual fresh catalyst as Ag(I) with the latter method. From the results of thermal analysis of a pure compound system, Sb_2O_3 mixed with equimolar Ag_2O (Fig. 1), it can be seen that Ag(0) and Sb_2O_3 are the major forms at 500-520°C (13), the temperature at which the catalysts are calcined. As a result of that, the summed weight of Ag and Sb in the catalyst is only 2.0% of the total weight, and the highly dispersed active components can transfer electrons to the support SiO_2, so they exist in higher oxidation states.

Table 2 compares the composition of the bulk and the surface of the catalysts, from results obtained by AAS and XPS respectively. The chemical analysis data are close to the ratio of the raw materials used, but in the surface layers silver is always enriched. This surface segregation becomes more striking after about 1750 hrs of the reaction and is accompanied by a serious decrease in catalytic activity.

TABLE 2
Comparison between the bulk and the surface composition of $Ag_xSb_yO_z/SiO_2$ catalysts

Catalyst number	Ag : Sb (atomic ratio)	
	AAS analysis	XPS analysis
NA-142(F)	0.24 : 1.00	1.00 : 1.00
NA-142(W)	0.23 : 1.00	3.00 : 1.00

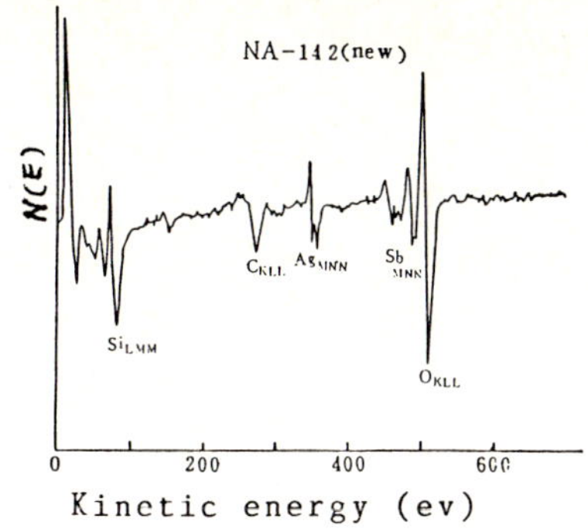

Fig. 2. AES Spectrum of fresh $Ag_xSb_yO_z/SiO_2$ catalyst.

AES and SAM analytical results

The results of repeated measurements for various samples are shown in Figs. 2, 3, 4, 5. Figure 2 presents an AES spectrum for point analysis of the fresh catalyst. Figures 3, 4, and 5 show SAM images of the fresh catalyst, the used catalyst after 10 hrs of the reaction, and the regenerated "waste" catalyst, respectively. It is obvious that the surface distribution of Ag and Sb atoms is "symbiotic" for the first two samples (i.e. where Ag atoms exist, Sb atoms exist too). But for the waste catalyst, which had undergone the reaction-regeneration cycle many times during an acummulated reaction time of 175 hrs and was markedly deactivated, the surface Ag and Sb atoms are non-symbiotic, although the Ag_{mvv} and Sb_{mvv} peaks are significant. When the waste catalyst was not regenerated, a carbon deposit (ca. 2 wt %) would covered the catalyst's surface. In this state the Sb_{mvv} peak was too weak to be detected, but the Ag_{mvv} peak was still sufficiently intense to be measured. This proved further that the surface enrichment of silver is greater in waste catalyst than in fresh catalyst.

TEM and EMD results

From the TEM micrograph in Fig. 6a it can be seen that the active component particles, as concentrated clusters, are spheroidal and of quite a uniform size (0.10 - 0.15 μm o.d.). The EMD pattern (Fig. 6b) is also very clear. Bright points in the pattern show some mono-crystals, which can be seen clearly on the fluorescent TEM screen. By measuring the distance R between the transmission point and diffraction point (cycle), the spacing d between two adjacent crystalline faces can be calculated from the equation

$$L\lambda = Rd$$

where L is the distance (mm) between the crystal and the photographic plate and

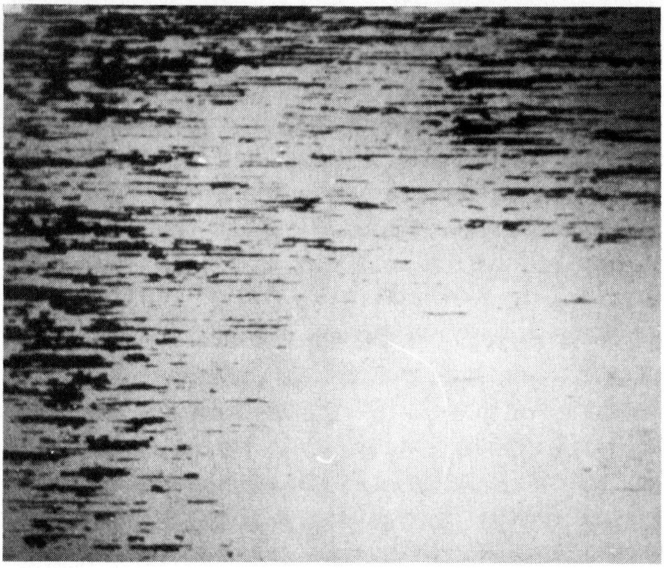

Fig. 3. SAM Image of NA-142(F) catalyst.
(a) Ag_{mvv}.

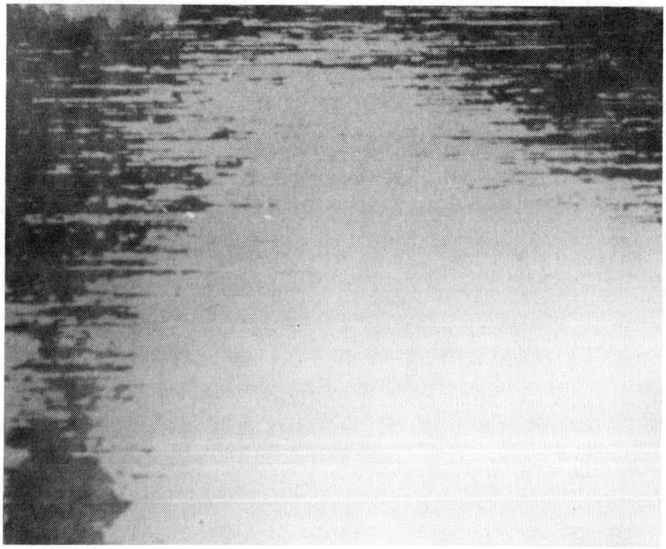

Fig. 3. SAM Image of NA-142(F) catalyst.
(b) Sb_{mvv}.

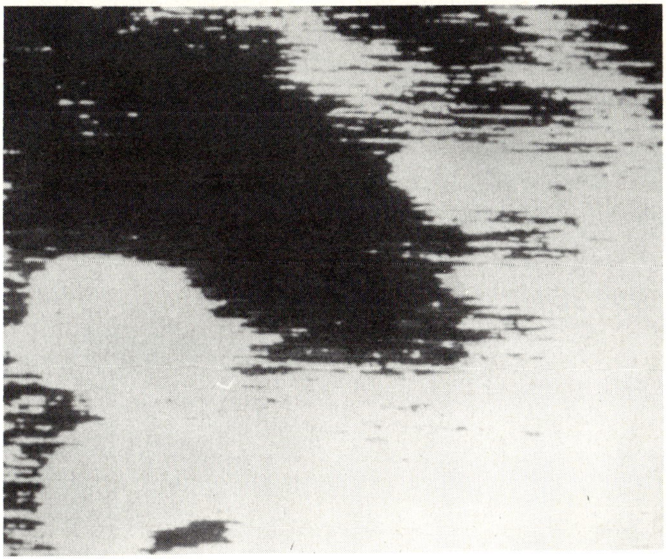

Fig. 4. SAM Image of NA-142 worked for 10 hrs.
(a) Ag_{mvv}.

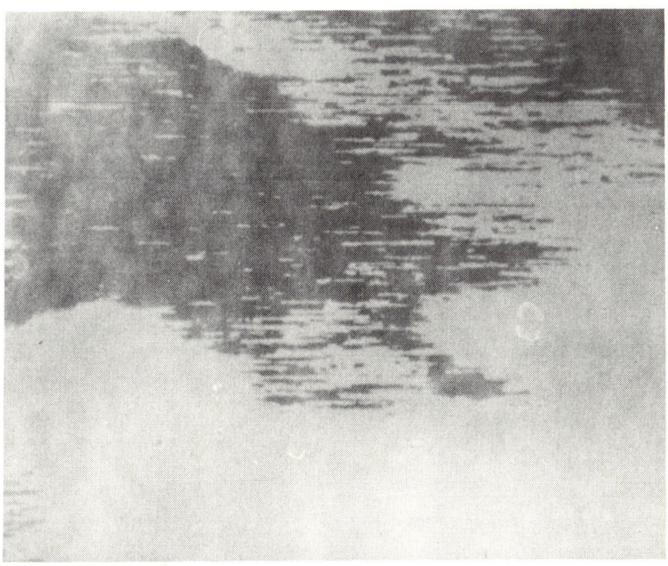

Fig. 4. SAM Image of NA-142 worked for 10 hrs.
(b) Sb_{mvv}.

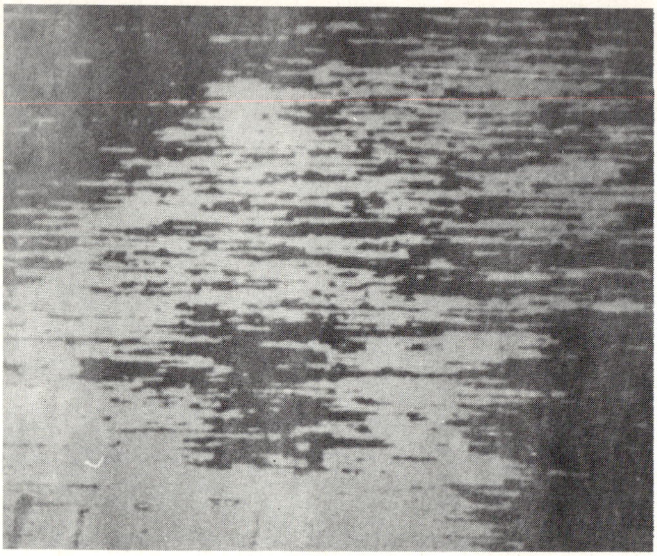

Fig. 5. SAM Image of NA-142(W) catalyst.
(a) Ag_{mvv}.

Fig. 5. SAM Image of NA-142(W) catalyst.
(b) Sb_{mvv}.

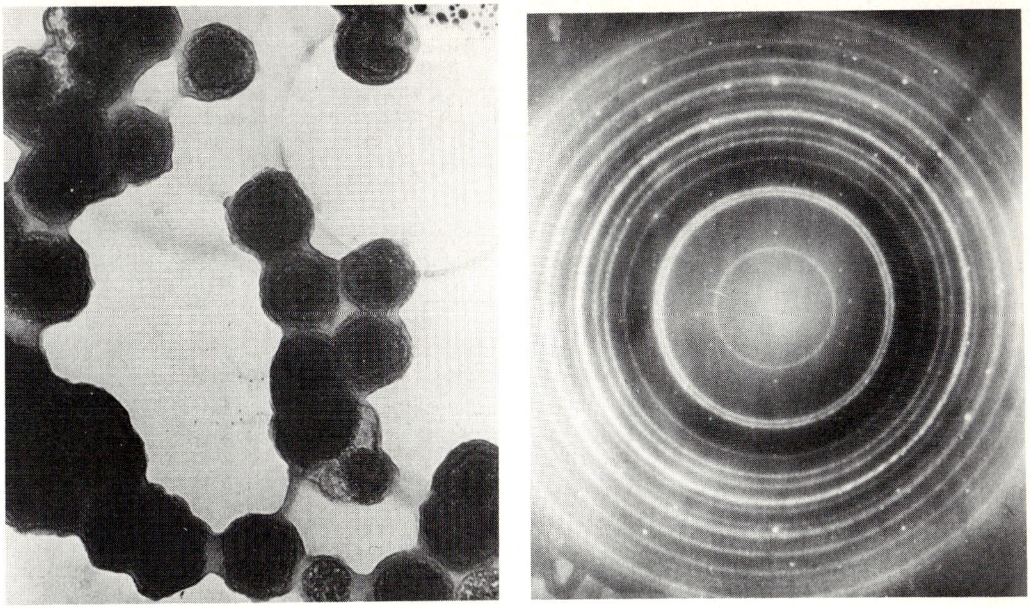

Fig. 6. (a) TEM Micrograph of NA-142(F) catalyst.
(b) EMD Picture of NA-142(F) catalyst.

λ is the wavelength (Å) of the electron beam (for this machine Lλ=29.96 mm·Å). From the d values we can then infer the corresponding crystal phases (Table 3) on the basis of ASTM data.

It is evident that the crystalline phases of fresh catalyst consist mainly of $AgSbO_3$ (cubic system) and Sb_2O_4 (perpendicular system). But for the waste catalyst, both the topography (Fig. 7a) and the crystalline phases (Fig. 7b and Table 4) of the active components varied greatly: the particle sizes are non-uniform, the large ones being 0.15 - 0.50 μm, and the small ones only 25 - 60 Å; the crystalline phases are changed to Sb_2O_3 and Ag metal. It is well worth noticing that the immersion of the metal silver phase will make Ag-surface-segregation easy, because the Ag atom in silver metal possesses the smallest specific surface free energy (14).

Exploration of the active phase in $Ag_xSb_yO_z/SiO_2$ catalyst and analysis of the causes of its deactivation

As mentioned above, the results of XPS and SAM show that the surface enrichment in silver is much more striking in the waste catalyst than in the fresh one. Why is this so? According to basic thermodynamics, the formation of a new surface requires work accompanied by a positive change of free energy. In order to minimize the positive surface free energy, the component which has the

TABLE 3

The results of crystal phase analysis of the active components in NA-142(F) catalyst by EMD.

Spacing, d, (Å)	Relative intensity*	Corresponding crystal phases	
		Sb_2O_4	$AgSbO_3$
5.789	w		
3.034	s	v	
2.902	s	v	v
2.296	vw		
2.045	w		v
1.924	w		v
1.770	vs	v	v
1.678	vw		
1.569	vw		
1.513	s		v
1.397	w		v
1.300	w		v
1.170	vw		v
1.148	w		

* vs = very strong; s = strong; w = weak; vw = very weak.

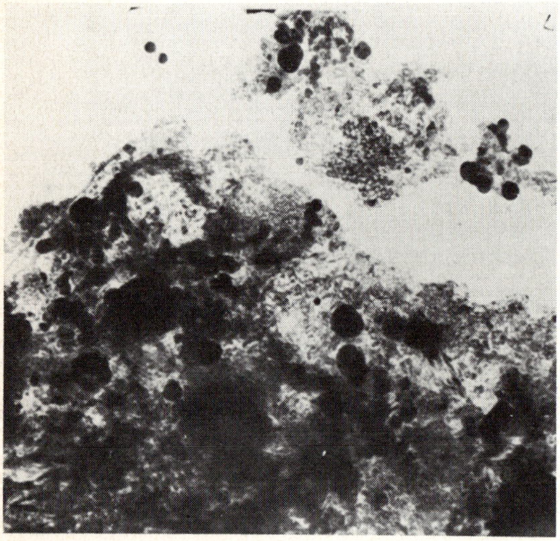

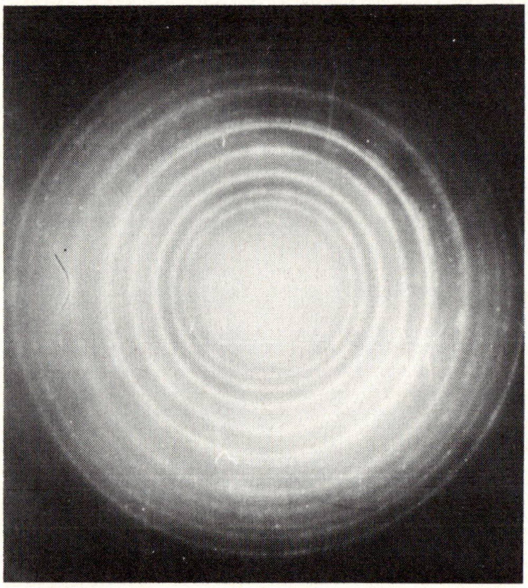

Fig. 7. TEM Micrograph (a) and EMD pattern (b) of NA-142(W) after regeneration.

TABLE 4

The crystalline structure of active components in the waste catalyst, NA-142(W)*

Spacing, d, (Å)	Relative intensity**	Corresponding crystal phases	
		Sb_2O_3	Ag(0)
4.069	w		
3.981	w		
3.179	fs	v	
2.807	fs	v	
2.359	s		v
1.993	s	v	(v)
1.667	s	v	
1.613	w	v	
1.359	w		
1.256	w	v	v
1.180	w	v	v
1.123	w	v	
1.048	w	v	v
0.953	vw		v

* In order to avoid the interference of carbon deposit, the waste catalyst was regenerated

** s = strong; fs = fairly strong; w = weak; vw = very weak.

lowest free energy tends to migrate toward the external surface. In a Sb_2O_3 - Ag(0) - Sb_2O_4 - $AgSbO_3$ - SiO_2 system, the lowest surface free energy is that of silver, which then has the largest probability of migrating to the surface. Since, in order to migrate from the interior of a solid to its external surface, an element must overcome a barrier of activation energy, the migration process can occur only at higher temperatures. As a rule of thumb, the Tammann temperature, approximately 1/2 the melting-point temperature (Kelvin scale) of the metal (or compound) (15), is sufficiently high for the atoms (or ions) in the bulk to migrate to the external surface. As the activation temperature (520°C) for the catalyst preparation and its regeneration temperature (500°C) are both higher than the Tammann temperature of silver, the silver element in the catalyst has not only the potential (i.e. lowest surface free energy), but also finds itself in suitable conditions (500 - 520°C) to migrate towards the uppermost surface layer, leading to surface enrichment in silver. This is coincident with the fact that the decrease in numbers of electron acceptor sites could be clearly measured by ESR. The spin number per gram of the waste catalyst was reduced by 43% in comparison with the fresh one; furthermore, the topography of the waste catalyst changed and silver and antimony on the surface layers of the waste became non-symbiotic. Either the surface enrichment in silver or the non-symbiotic distribution bring about the separation of silver and antimony.

As mentioned above, the main phases of active components in the fresh catalyst are $AgSbO_3$ and Sb_2O_4. We have prepared Sb-containing (no silver) catalyst, Sb_2O_4/SiO_2, in which the active phase is perpendicular Sb_2O_4 established by XRD. Its catalytic activity is very low (formaldehyde conversion is 39%). Xu and Ding (16) have established experimentally that if in Ag- and/or Sb-containing catalyst systems supported on SiO_2, the catalyst has the appropriate surface acid strength distribution and the right amount of electron acceptors, they show better catalytic behavior only when silver and antimony co-exist in the catalysts. Summing up the different results for Ag_xO_y/SiO_2, Sb_xO_y/SiO_2 and $Ag_xSb_yO_z/SiO_2$ catalysts, it is reasonable to infer that a silver-antimony compound functions in the catalytic behavior of $Ag_xSb_yO_z/SiO_2$ catalyst, and the crystalline structure of the Ag-Sb compound appears to be cubic $AgSbO_3$, whose crystal size is too small to be measured by XRD.

The catalyst was reduced in the course of the reaction due to the reactive properties of the reactants, especially formaldehyde, but during regeneration of the catalyst was partly reoxidized. After the repeated reaction-regeneration cycle the active phase would be gradually reduced. The silver element in the catalyst is able, as mentioned above, to migrate to the uppermost surface layer, which makes Ag-Sb separate and destroys the crystal structure of active components, thus varying the electron acceptor number on the catalyst surface. In this way the catalyst is gradually deactivated by the Prins reaction (17).

We also looked at carbon deposition and possible variation of the surface area of the catalyst. The carbon content was nearly constant, ca. 2 wt% of the total weight, and the surface area did not change at all (ca. 180 m^2/g).

These results imply that silver is an unstable factor in the catalyst. Replacing silver by another element whilst retaining the catalytic activity of the Ag-Sb catalyst should be the way to improve the stability of the catalyst system.

There remains one question to clarify: why are there differences in the conditions of $AgSbO_3$ formation for pure compounds and for highly dispersed catalyst?

ACKNOWLEDGEMENTS

The authors wish to express their appreciation to Prof. Ding Shixin for supporting this work, and to Dr. Xu Xianlun, Mrs. Yu Ling, Gu Jinfang, Mr. Yang Dexin and Chen Gexin for supplying some of the samples and catalytic reaction data. We would also like to thank Prof. Zang Jingling (Dalian Institute of Chemical Physics) who performed the TEM and EMD measurements.

REFERENCES

1 Ding Shixin, Xu Xianlun, Personal communication, March 1984.
2 Gue Zhunlu, Xu Xianlun, Petrol. Chem. Ind., (China), 1 (1974).
3 Yu Gentao, ibid, 11(8), (1982) 535.
4 Chen Zhiwen, Dang Zhongyuan, in Proc. 2nd Nation. Conf. Catal., Xiamei, Oct. 1984, Bo57.
5 J.H. Scofield, J. Electron Spectros. Relat. Phenom., 8 (1976) 126.
6 F. Garbassi, Surf. Interf. Anal., 2 (1980) 165.
7 C.D. Wagner, Handbook of X-ray Photoelectron Spectroscopy, Physical Electron Co. 1979.
8 Jiang Zhicheng, An Li-Dun, in Proc. Nation. Conf. Electron Spectros., Wuhan, Dec. 1985, II-7.
9 G. Blanchald, J. Catal., 70 (1981) 168.
J.M. Basset, ibid, 37 (1975) 22.
10 T. Birchall, J. Chem. Soc. Dalton Trans., (1975) 2003.
11 W.E. Morgan, Inorg. Chem., 12 (1973) 953.
12 Y. Boudeville, J.C. Vedrine, J. Catal., 58 (1979) 52.
13 K.J.D. Mackenzie, J. Therm. Anal., 15 (2) (1979) 333.
14 G.A. Somorjai, "Chemistry in Two Dimensions Surface", Cornell University Press, Ithaca and London, 1981.
15 P.G. Menon and T.S.R. Prasata Rao, Catal. Rev. -Sci. Eng., 20 (1) (1979) 97.
16 Xu Xianlun, Ding Shixin, in "Selects of Chemical Engineering" Gansu, China, 1980, pp. 87-93.
17 P.B. Venuto and P.S. Landis, Adv. Catal., 18 (1968) 259.

B. Delmon and G.F. Froment (Editors), *Catalyst Deactivation 1987*
1987 Elsevier Science Publishers B.V., Amsterdam — Printed in The Netherlands

DEACTIVATION OF A V_2O_5 - TiO_2 CATALYST FOR THE OXIDATION OF o-XYLENE TO PHTALIC ANHYDRIDE

V.A. NIKOLOV[1], D.G. KLISSURSKI[2] and K.I. HADJIIVANOV[2]

[1]"G.Genov" Chemical Plants, Russe 7000 (Bulgaria)
[2]Institute of General and Inorganic Chemistry, Bulgarian Academy of Sciences, Sofia 1040 (Bulgaria)

ABSTRACT

The vapour phase partial oxidation of o-xylene to phtalic anhydride over a vanadia-titania catalyst has been investigated under industrial conditions with a view to elucidating the reasons for catalyst deactivation. The catalytic activity and selectivity are tested in an integral pilot-plant reactor,whereas the changes of the catalyst are studied by X-ray analysis, IR spectroscopy, specific surface area measurements, elementary analysis etc. The catalyst deactivation is due to several independent reasons: (i) anatase - rutile transformation, (ii) specific surface area decrease, and (iii) decrease in surface concentration of the promotors. The former two reasons lead to a reduction of activity, whereas the latter one is accompanied by a loss of selectivity. On the basis of the experimental studies and a mathematical model of the process, a more efficient method of charging of the industrial reactor has been proposed.

INTRODUCTION

The vapour phase catalytic oxidation of o-xylene to phtalic anhydride is usually carried out in packed-bed tubular reactors at 630 - 770 K. Among various oxide systems containing V_2O_5, the combination of V_2O_5 and TiO_2 (anatase) exhibits the best activity and selectivity (refs. 1-6). Owing to the fact that the reaction is highly exothermic, the temperature is reduced using a molten salt as a coolant. A sharp rise of temperature ("hot spot" temperature) followed by a drop is observed in the catalyst bed. To prevent rapid catalyst deactivation, the hot spot temperature must be kept within definite limits. However, a high temperature is to be maintained in the remaining part of the reactor to achieve a high degree of conversion. The hot spot is very sensitive to the inlet o-xylene concentration, inlet temperature and the catalytic activity (ref. 7). Under the effect of the reaction mixture and the high temperature, irreversible changes occur in the catalyst and lead to its deactivation, which results in a decrease of the process productivity. According to Galantowicz et.al. (ref. 8), temperatures higher than 733 K cause deactivation due to an anatase-rutile transformation. Wachs and Chan (ref. 9) have reported that X-ray diffraction on 7,0% V_2O_5/TiO_2 samples shows the presence of crystalline V_2O_5 in fresh samples and a significant amount of V_2O_4 in used ones.

The purpose of this paper was (i) to investigate, under conditions close to the industrial, the reasons for deactivation of industrial vanadia - titania catalysts, (ii) to examine the effect of the kind and extent of deactivation on the process productivity, and (iii) to propose a possibility of intensification of the process using the results obtained as well as mathematical modelling.

EXPERIMENTAL

Catalysts

The industrial vanadia - titania catalyst used had a composition of 93,4 wt % TiO_2, 6,0 wt % V_2O_5, 0,2 wt % P_2O_5, 0,1 wt% WO_3 and 0,1 wt % Al_2O_3. The support consisted of porcelain spheres 6 mm in diameter. The catalytic layer thickness was 0,2 mm.

Titanium dioxide (anatase) was obtained by hydrolysis of titanium tetrachloride (ref. 10). Samples of this substance (5g) were suspended in 0,1 M solution of H_3PO_4 and KH_2PO_4, respectively, 300 ml each. After filtering, the samples were dried at 420 K.

Catalytic activity and selectivity measurements

The o-xylene oxidation was carried out in a typical non-isothermal tubular reactor containing one stainless tube. The dimensions of the tube were completely identical with those of a separate tube installed inside the industrial multitubular reactor. The internal diameter and height of the tube were 25 mm and 3500 mm, respectively. The reactor contained about 1,13 l of the catalyst. The temperature in the bed was measured by a movable thermocouple. The experiments were performed under a pressure close to the atmospheric with a relatively high excess of air. The initial o-xylene concentration was varied from about 26 g/Nm^3 to 60 g/Nm^3. Part of the experiments were performed with a water vapour inlet concentration of 30 g/Nm^3. The temperature was varied from 635 to 670 K.

The maleic anhydride content was determined by polarographic analysis, whereas the concentrations of unreacted o-xylene, o-tolualdehyde, phtalide, benzoic acid and phtalic anhydride were determined chromatographically with a Pye Unicam instrument.

Characterization of the catalysts

The phase composition of all samples was determined by a Dron-3 diffractometer using CuK$_\alpha$-radiation. The IR spectra were recorded with UR-20 and Specord-75-IR spectrophotometers, and the electron microscopy patterns were taken with a JEM 100 B apparatus. The specific surface areas were determined by the BET - method. Some surface characteristics were established using mercury porozimetry. To study the surface compounds, the samples were pressed into pellets of 20 - 40 mg/cm^2 and subjected to a repeated heating at 720 K under vacuum and oxygen. A standard vacuum apparatus ensuring a residual pressure less than 10^{-2} Pa was used. The elementary analysis was performed by atomic absorbtion, ESCA, spectrophotometry and chemical methods.

RESULTS AND DISCUSSION

Thermal deactivation

Fig. 1 shows the changes of the temperature profile in the reactor, whereas Table 1 presents the changes in activity and selectivity of the catalyst during its exploitation.

TABLE 1
Changes in activity and selectivity of the catalyst during its exploitation.

Time of exploitation (months)	Selectivity towards: phtalic anhydride (%)	phtalide (%)	Conversion of o-xylene (%)
1	73,6	0,005	99,9
6	72,8	0,10	99,8
15	69,6	0,67	99,7

The temperature profiles show that the activity of the catalyst in the hot spot zone decreases with time. After 15 months exploitation, the hot spot changes its position by 40 cm and its temperature by about 80 K. X-ray phase analysis showed

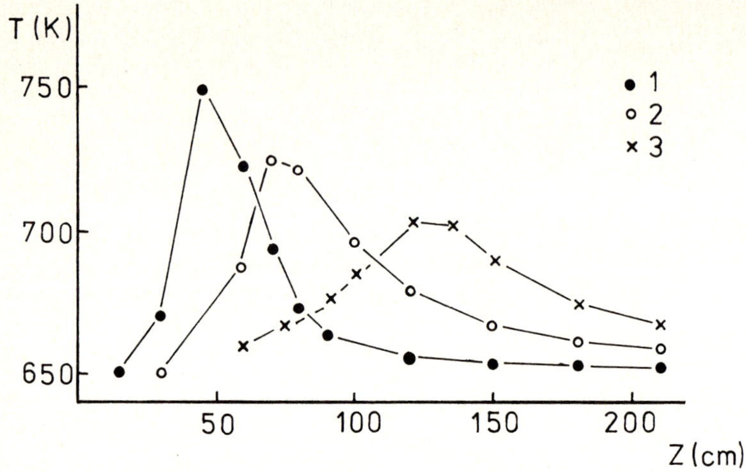

Fig. 1. Changes of the temperature profiles in the reactor during the catalyst exploitation. Inlet o-xylene concentration, 40,0 g/Nm^3; gas rate, 4,5 Nm^3/h for a tube; exploitation time: 1 month (1), 6 months (2), and 15 months (3).

that anatase - rutile transformation occured to a small extent only in the catalyst used in the hot spot zone at temperatures higher than 730 K. The specific surface area of this catalyst decreased significantly (down to 2,6 m^2/g), whereas for a catalyst used in the zone of lower temperatures this value was 8,0 m^2/g, i.e. close to the initial surface area (9,0 m^2/g). No changes in the catalyst composition after its deactivation were observed. Hence, this kind of deactivation is mainly characterized by a surface area loss leading to a decrease of activity per unit mass.

(i) Simulation of the experimental results. An one-dimensional plug flow model of the fixed bed reactor was used for a quantative description of the effect of catalyst deactivation on the kinds of temperature and concentration profiles in an industrial reactor. The following reaction scheme was accepted:

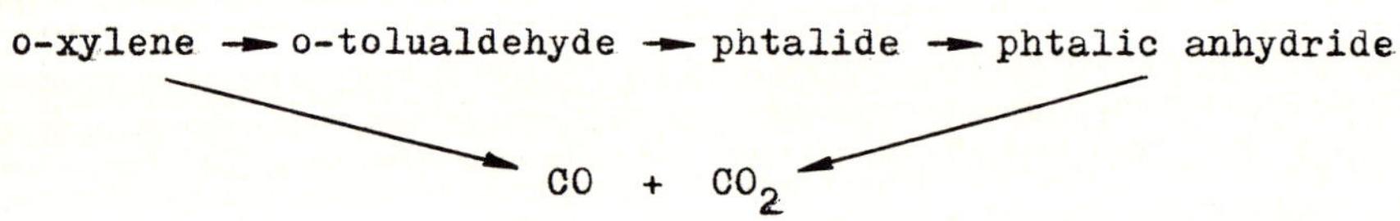

The balance equations are given below:

vapour phase:

$$-u \frac{dC_i}{dZ} = K_f \cdot Q_v \cdot (C_i - C^s_{i,s})$$

$$u \cdot \rho_f \cdot C_p \frac{dT}{dZ} = h_f \cdot Q_v \cdot (T^s_s - T) - \frac{4U}{d_t} (T - T_w)$$

solid phase:

$$\rho_b \cdot r^i_i = K_f \cdot Q_v \cdot (C - C^s_s)$$

$$(-\Delta H) \cdot \rho_b \cdot r^i_i = h_f \cdot Q_v \cdot (T^s_s - T)$$

(The symbols used are given at the end of the paper.)

The kinetic parameters proposed by Calderbank (ref. 11) were used. An important parameter in the model is the catalytic activity factor. The catalytic activity distribution is given by the equation:

$$F_k = 1{,}0 + UF (Z - l)$$

where UF (Z) is the unit step function, and l is the position of the hot spot (cm). Thus, for $Z < l$, $F_k = 1{,}0$ and for $Z \geq l$, $F_k = 2{,}0$. This means that the catalytic activity undergoes a two-fold increase with an axial position at the hot spot ($Z = l$). Hypothetically, this corresponds to a partial catalyst deactivation in the upstream position of the reactor that has occured after several months of operation. A similar factor of the catalytic activity has been used by Pirkle et.al. (ref. 12).

On the basis of this mathematical model, different variants of catalyst "deactivation" were simulated. It was established that the hot spot zone was situated in the first upper 120 cm of the catalyst layer (Fig. 2). The hot spot position determines the place of the thermal catalyst deactivation. This statement offers a possibility of repeated application of a part of the catalyst. Some of the results obtained after such an experiment are given in Table 2. They show that the partial change of the catalyst has no negative influence on the process efficiency: the selectivity toward phtalic anhydride is practically unchanged, whereas the content of the undesirable product, phtalide, is below the admissible percentage (0,1 %).

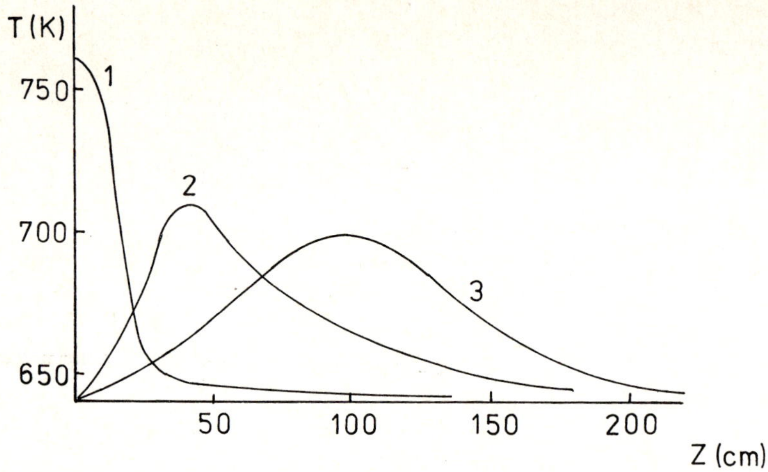

Fig. 2. Simulated temperature profiles. Inlet o-xylene concentra-concentration, 40,0 g/Nm^3; gas rate, 4,5 Nm^3/h for a tube; cooling medium temperature, 653 K; l = 0 cm (1), 40 cm (2), and 100 cm (3).

TABLE 2

Activity and selectivity of the catalyst layer after the complete and partial recharge of the reactor. Exploitation time 3 months.

Reactor type	Recharge of the reactor	Selectivity towards: phtalic anhydride (%)	Selectivity towards: phtalide (%)	o-Xylene conversion (%)
industrial	complete	73,1	0,01	99,8
industrial	partial	73,2	0,025	99,8
pilot	partial	73,4	0,02	99,9

Deactivation by water vapour

The deactivation of the vanadia - titania catalyst may be due to a decrease in surface concentration of the promotors. One of the reasons for this type of deactivation is the high concentration of water vapour in the reaction mixture which is to be found at accident or other extremal conditions. To the best of our knowledge, this type of deactivation has not been reported by other authors.

To elucidate the changes occuring in the catalyst under the effect of the water vapour thermal treatment, 30 g/Nm^3 water were added to the reaction mixture for 150 h. The selectivity of the catalysts obtained as well as some other characteristics of the samples are given in Table 3. The corresponding values for catalyst samples untreated with water vapour are also given for the sake of comparison.

TABLE 3
Some characteristics of catalysts treated or untreated with water vapour.

Catalyst pre-exploitation time (months)	Water vapour treatment (h)	Content of P_2O_5 (%)	Selectivity toward phtalic anhydride (%)
-	150	0,14	58,4
10	150	0,12	63,0
-	-	0,22	71,6
10	-	0,20	70,4

As can be seen, after the treatment the selectivity decreases significantly, whereas the activity remains almost the same. The main change in the catalyst is the decrease of the total phosphorus content which is about twice as low as in the fresh catalyst. The capillarity of the samples also decreases, probably due to the lower phosphorus content.

These results are confirmed by IR spectra. The spectra of our samples, compared with IR spectra of V-P-O systems (ref. 13), indicate a lower phosphorus content in the water vapour treated samples. No changes in the specific surface area and catalyst morphology are observed. Hence, the water vapour treatment decreases the phosphorus content on the catalyst surface, which is accompanied by a loss in selectivity.

Recent studies on the V_2O_5-TiO_2 system by means of IR spectroscopy of probe molecules have shown that part of the coordinatively unsaturated titanium ions remain on the surface even in the presence of 5 wt % V_2O_5 (refs. 14,15). These results are confirmed by HREM studies (ref. 16). Hence, vanadia forms no complete coverage on the anatase support. In view of the fact that titania favour the complete oxidation of some aromatic compounds (ref. 17), the V_2O_5 - TiO_2 system should have a similar effect too. Perheps, in industrial catalysts phosphorus blocks the free

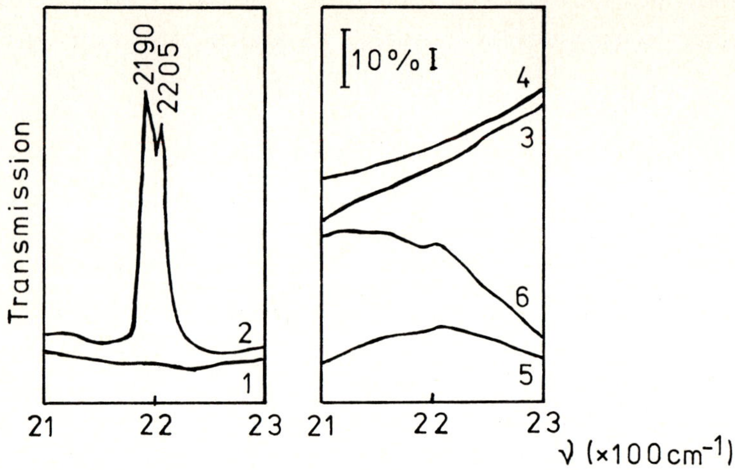

Fig. 3. IR spectra of: anatase (1); after contact with CO, 40 torr (2); anatase modified by H_3PO_4 (3); after contact with CO, 40 torr (4); anatase modified by KH_2PO_4 (5); and after contact with CO, 40 torr (6).

titania surface, thus decreasing the amount of the complete oxidation products.

To check the above hypothesis, some model investigations were carried out. The surface Lewis acidity of pure and phosphate - modified anatase was studied by means of IR spectroscopy of probe molecules. The X-ray phase analysis of all samples showed the presence of anatase only. The phosphorus existence on the surface of the modified samples was detected by ESCA measurements.

The carbon monoxide molecule is very appropriate for the study of the surface Lewis acidity (ref. 18). Fig. 3 presents the IR spectra of pure and phosphate-modified anatase samples before and after their placing in a CO atmosphere (40 torr). According to literature data (refs. 18,19) two types of Lewis acid sites are present on the anatase surface: the frequencies of the corresponding C-O stretching modes are at 2190 and 2205 cm^{-1}, respectively. The surface of the modified samples shows no Lewis acidity. Further studies indicated a stable blocking. Lewis acid sites did not appear even after a thermal treatment at 920 K under vacuum or after reduction with CO (40 torr) at the same temperature. Hence, the phosphate ions are bonded tightly to the anatase surface. The interaction of the surface phosphates with water vapour can be illustrated by the following simplified scheme:

$$\underset{\displaystyle Ti}{\overset{HPO_4}{|}} \quad + \quad H_2O \quad \longrightarrow \quad Ti - O \quad + \quad H_3PO_4$$

This leads to liberation of pure anatase surface and to a decrease in selectivity of the catalyst.

The results obtained show that a catalyst deactivated in this way cannot be used for a partial recharging of the reactor.

CONCLUSIONS

The high temperature and the reaction mixture used cause some irreversible changes in vanadia - titania catalysts for the o-xylene oxidation, which results in their deactivation. The main kinds of deactivation observed are: (i) anatase - rutile transformation, occuring in the hot spot zone, (ii) surface area loss, leading to a decrease in activity per unit mass of the catalyst, and (iii) a decrease of the surface phosphorus concentration, leading to loss of selectivity.

If the deactivation is mainly of the second type, the catalyst changes can be described by a mathematical model of the process by including the factor of catalytic activity. According to this model as well as by experiments the possibility of partial recharging of the reactor has been shown.

ACKNOWLEDGEMENTS

The authors wish to thank Dr. I. Havezov and Dr. G. Tiuliev (Bulgarian Academy of Sciences) for their help in some of the experiments.

SYMBOLS

C_i - concentration of the component "i",
C_p - specific heat,
d_t - reactor tube diameter,
h_f - gas-solid heat transfer coefficient,
ΔH - heat of the reaction,
K_f - gas-solid mass transfer coefficient,
Q_v - specific surface area of the catalyst pellet,
r_i - reaction rate with respect to the component "i",
T - average temperature inside the reactor tubes (K),

T_w - temperature of the cooling medium,
u - superficial velocity of the cooling medium,
U - heat transfer coefficient at the reactor wall,
Z - axial coordinate,
ρ_b - bulk density of the fixed bed,
ρ_f - gas mixture density.

Sub- or superscripts

s - solid interface.

REFERENCES

1 I. Wachs, R. Saleh, S. Chan and C. Chersich, Appl. Catal., 15 (1985) 339-352.
2 M. Wainwright and N. Foster, Catal. rev. - Sci. Eng., 19 (1979) 211-237.
3 V. Nikolov, R. Radkov, B. Djurov, S. Georgiev and G. Georgiev, Chimia i industria (in Bulgarien), 55 (1983) 74-76.
4 BRD Patent No 2,436,009 (1976).
5 A. G. Liubarski, A. G. Gorelic, V. P. Petoian, E. V. Lianin and V. S. Bescov, Kinet. Katal., 14 (1973) 956-961.
6 O. M. Ilinitch, G. K. Borescov, A. A. Ivanov, V. F. Liahova and N. P. Beliaeva, Neftechimia (USSR), 18 (1978) 270-279.
7 G. F. Froment, Adv. Chem. Series, 109 (1972) 1-34.
8 M. Galantowicz, M. Gasior, B. Grzybowska and J. Sloczynski, Przemysl Chemiczny, 62 (1983) 87-89.
9 I. Wachs and S. Chan, J. Catal., 91 (1985) 366-369.
10 G. Brauer (Editor), Handbook of Inorganic Synthesis, Vol. 4, Mir, Moscow, 1985, pp. 1460-1461.
11 P. H. Calderbank, K. Chandrasecharan and C. Fumagali, Chem. Eng. Sci., 32 (1977) 1435-1441.
12 J. C. Pirkle, I. Wachs and J. Sobel, in Foundation of computer-aided Chemical Process Design, Vol. 2; Proc. Int. Conf. held at New England Colledge, Henniker, New Hampshire, July 6-11, 1980, pp. 401-429.
13 B. E. Zaitsev, Z. I. Ejkova and I. I. Ioffe, Kinet. Katal., 7 (1966) 755-759.
14 G. Busca, L. Marchetti, G. Centi and F. Trifirò, J. Chem.Soc., Faraday Trans. I, 81 (1985) 1003-1014.
15 H. Miyata, Y. Nakagawa, T. Ono and Y. Kubokawa, Chem. Soc. Japan, Chem. Lett., (1983) 1141-1144.
16 Z. C. Kang and Q. X. Bao, Appl. Catal., 26 (1986) 251-267.
17 A. J. van Hengstum, J. C. van Ommen, H. Bosch and P. J. Gellings, Appl. Catal., 8 (1983) 383-388.
18 A. A. Davydov, IR Spectroscopy Applied to Surface Chemistry of Oxides, Nauka, Novosibirsk, 1984.
19 G. Busca, H. Saussey, O. Saur, J.-C. Lavalley and V. Lorenzelly, Appl. Catal., 14 (1985) 245-260.

B. Delmon and G.F. Froment (Editors), *Catalyst Deactivation 1987*

DEACTIVATION OF ALKALI PROMOTED MAGNESIA IN OXIDATIVE COUPLING OF METHANE

C. MIRODATOS. V. PERRICHON, M.C. DURUPTY and P. MORAL
Institut de Recherches sur la Catalyse, Laboratoire Propre du C.N.R.S. conventionné à l'Université Claude Bernard, LYON I, 2 avenue Albert Einstein, 69626 Villeurbanne cédex, France.

ABSTRACT

The deactivation of MgO and Li/MgO catalysts during oxidative coupling of methane is studied together with the morphological and chemical changes of the solids. Evidence of different processes through magnesia sintering and loss of alkali are presented and the nature of the active surface is discussed in terms of Li/Mg interface.

INTRODUCTION

Since the pioneering work of Keller and Bhasin (ref.1), the oxidative coupling of methane into ethane and ethylene has attracted much attention and is considered now as an alternative route for methane conversion. An extensive screening of natural or synthetic oxides has revealed that numerous materials were effective catalysts for the methane dimerization (refs.1-7). Due to the high thermodynamic stability of the methane molecule, the reaction has to be performed at temperatures higher than 700 K. This necessarily involves physical and chemical changes in the solid phase, from its initial state as precursor to its final state as the working catalyst. However, although much attention has been devoted to the cataloging of active phases or to the identification of reaction intermediates leading to mechanistic schemes (refs. 5,8), few data are available concerning the ageing process of the catalysts, which may provide key information on the nature of the active site and consequently on the mechanism. Iwamatsu et al. (ref. 7) have recently emphasize the importance of the specific surface area in the oxidative dimerization of methane on magnesia based systems.

Studying the mechanism of the methane dimerization (ref.8) we felt it necessary to follow systematically the chemical and morphological changes of a coupling catalyst during its activation and in the course of the reaction. The selected catalyst is a magnesia promoted by lithium carbonate, similar to the solid studied by J.H. Lunsford et al (refs. 3,5), which was found to be selective towards C_2 hydrocarbons and rather stable after calcination at high temperatures. The unpromoted magnesia is also tested for comparison.

Data of BET measurements, TEM, XRD, micro DTA and chemical analysis are provided and discussed together with the catalytic performances (activity, selectivity, ageing behaviour) of the solids.

EXPERIMENTAL

Catalyst precursor preparation

Magnesium hydroxide was prepared by adding a magnesium chloride solution (0.25 M) to a potash solution (0.5 M), the precipitate being centrifuged, washed and dried under vacuum at 353 K. Magnesium hydroxide and lithium carbonate, were added to deionized water at 273 K and the resulting slurry evaporated under vacuum at 333 K.

Catalytic experiments

The catalytic experiments were carried out in a fixed bed quartz microreactor operated at atmospheric pressure. The precursor samples were activated in the reactor at 723 K under an oxygen flow of 3.6 l h^{-1} for 3 h then the temperature was raised linearly (2 K mn^{-1}) up to the reaction temperature and the reacting mixture (O_2, CH_4, He) admitted. The reaction conditions were typically, unless otherwise specified : P_{CH_4} = 7.8 kPa, P_{O_2} = 4.6 kPa, total flow rate = 1 ml s^{-1}. The catalyst weight was varied between 20-600 mg in order to maintain the total conversion below 30 %. All the gases were analyzed by gas chromatography. In order to obtain catalyst samples for analysis and characterization at various stages of activation and reaction, the reactor was cooled down to room temperature. Each run was carried out following the same procedure and starting from a fresh sample of precursor.

Characterization techniques

BET area and mesoporosity distribution measurements were realized with an automated nitrogen volumetric adsorption equipment constructed at the Institute. The catalysts were outgassed at 423 K for 3 h at a pressure < 0.1 Pa before the completion of the full N_2 isotherm. The distribution of the pores sizes was obtained using the Roberts method (ref. 9).

The examination of the catalysts was made using transmission electron microscopy. The apparatus was a JEOL 100 Cx with a resolving power of 3 Å.

The X Ray diffraction patterns were obtained with a diffractometer equipped with a copper anticathode.

The evolution of the initial catalyst upon heating in flowing N_2/O_2 mixture (5 K min^{-1}) was followed by differential thermal analysis, the reference sample being kieselguhr.

The chemical analysis were performed by atomic emission spectroscopy for lithium and atomic absorption spectroscopy for magnesium, after solubilization in dilute hydrochloric acid.

RESULTS

Ageing phenomena

Typical changes in catalytic activity with increasing temperature obtained with freshly activated samples are depicted in Fig. 1 : with the Li/MgO sample, the total conversion and the C_2 yield (curves a and a' respectively) increase up to around 975 K (with an apparent activation energy of ca 40 kcal $mole^{-1}$) then suddenly decrease in the 975-1020 K range. At higher temperature, the activity increases again with an apparent activation energy near the initial value. This tends to indicate that the previous drop of activity cannot be related to a drastic change of reaction mechanism but much more likely to a process of deactivation of the sample. The unpromoted magnesia behaves much differently since its total activity increases monotonously like the related C_2 yield (curves b and b'). Both phenomena are observed in a temperature range where no significant purely thermal conversion occurs (curve c). Let us note the higher C_2 yield (ethane + ethylene) for the Li/MgO sample by comparison with the unpromoted magnesia, whatever the temperature of reaction is, in accordance with the known performances of this catalyst (refs. 5,7).

In order to better define this deactivation effect specifically observed on the Li/MgO sample, a series of long term catalytic runs have been carried out at given temperature, as shown in Fig. 2.

At 907 K (curve a), a fast initial deactivation is observed, followed by a pseudo-stabilization of the rate of conversion. When the reacting gases are admitted at 1023 K, a lower reaction rate is observed together with a smooth and limited deactivation (curve b). This indicates that, besides the proper deactivation process at a fixed temperature, a drastic alteration of the catalytic surface occurs in the 900-1020 K range during the activation phase. Such a phenomenon is irreversible since the conversion at 907 K after the run at 1023 K is 22 times lower than the initial conversion on the fresh sample (curves c and a).

Fig. 3 reports the changes in C_2 selectivity and activity for sequential runs carried out without changing the catalyst. Thus, there is a substantial difference in the selectivity at 907 K between a fresh catalyst (23 %) and the same catalyst which has been heated meanwhile at 1023 K for 50 h (56 %).

The question arises if the trend to favor complete oxidation on fresh catalyst and methane coupling on 1023 K-heated sample depends mainly on the

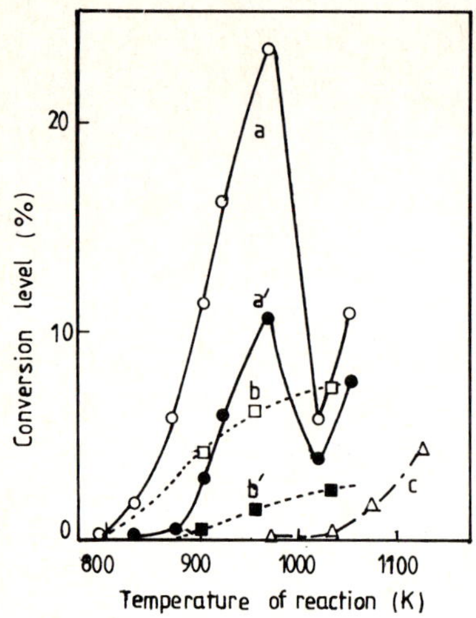

Fig. 1. Activity vs reaction temperature on Li/MgO (a, a'), MgO (b, b') and with empty reactor (c). Total conversion (a, b) ; C_2 yield (a', b') (m_{cat} = 200 mg).

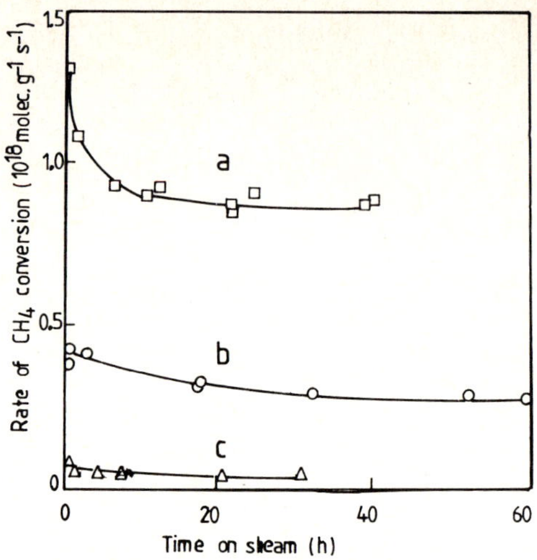

Fig. 2. Rate of CH_4 conversion vs time on stream at :
a - 907 K on fresh Li/MgO
b - 1023 K
c - 907 K after b.

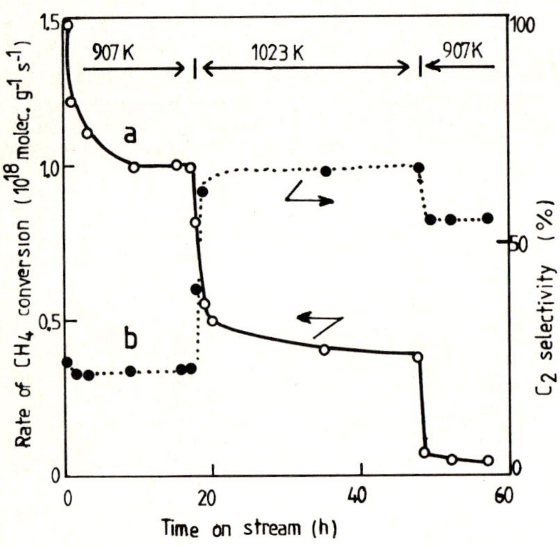

Fig. 3. Activity (a) and C_2 selectivity (b) vs time on stream and reaction temperature on Li/MgO.

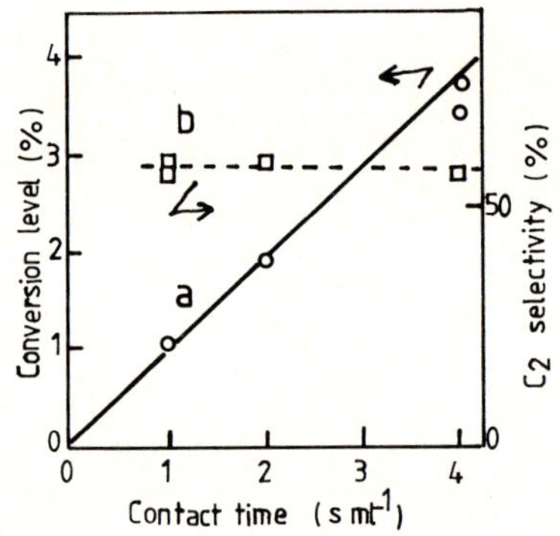

Fig. 4. Activity (a) and selectivity (b) vs contact time at 907 K on 1023 K - treated Li/MgO.

state of the active surface or could come from a kinetic effect pertaining to the decrease of conversion : Fig. 4 clearly indicates that increasing the level of conversion 4 times by decreasing the total flow-rate by 4 does not change significantly the C_2 selectivity, which rules out any kinetic effect on selectivity. Moreover this experiment confirms that the reaction proceeds without major diffusion limitation, as we could deduce from the nearly constant activity per gram of catalyst and this, irrespective of the sample weight.

Changes in texture and morphology

The significant decrease in the volume of a Li/MgO sample, before and after test at 1023 K suggests, as previously reported by Ito et al (ref.5) an important sintering. Consequently we studied more in details the evolution of texture and morphology during the different treatments by BET, BJH measurements, electron microscopy and DTA.

(i) O_2 treatments at low temperature (300-900 K) -Fig.5 shows the BET results obtained on MgO (curve a) and Li/MgO (curve b) heated under O_2 with the same procedure as in the catalytic reactor. A sharp increase of the surface area is noted after O_2 treatment at 723 K for the unpromoted magnesia while the surface area of the promoted sample, always lower whatever the temperature, increases smoothly in the 300-900 range.

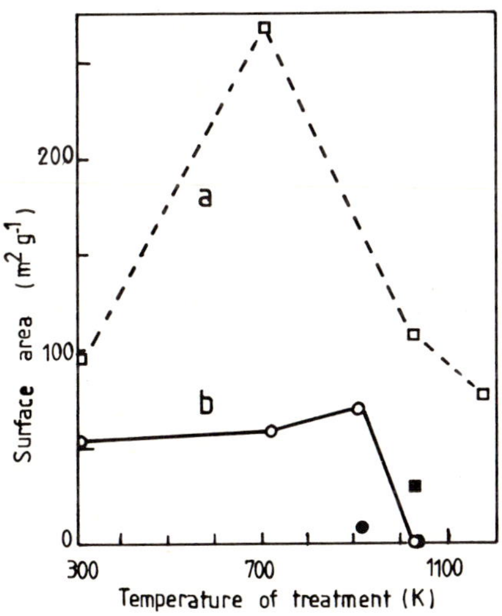

Fig.5. BET area vs O_2-treatment for MgO (a) and Li/MgO (b). Filled symbols : after 18 h reaction at the related temperature.

The corresponding porosity measurements are given in Table 1 for the Li/MgO solid. A porous system in the range 5-10 nm is observed for temperatures up to 903 K with a slight shift of the porosity towards higher pore sizes.

Changes in surface area and porosity are also revealed by electron microscopy (Fig.6. Table 1). The Li/MgO precursor is formed with nearly hexagonal flakes of $Mg(OH)_2$ (around 46 nm large with a thickness of 10 nm), more or less embedded in large crystals of Li_2CO_3 (the latter are dissolved in alcoholic preparations and visible only in dry preparations). After O_2 treatment at 723 K, the initial flakes of $Mg(OH)_2$ are more scattered, especially for the unpromoted magnesia (with numerous fragments of 5-6 nm) and a porosity, between 5-7 nm develops (Fig.6a).

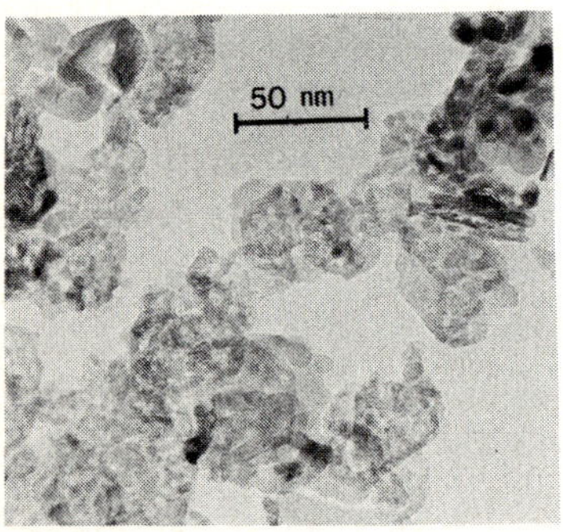

6 a

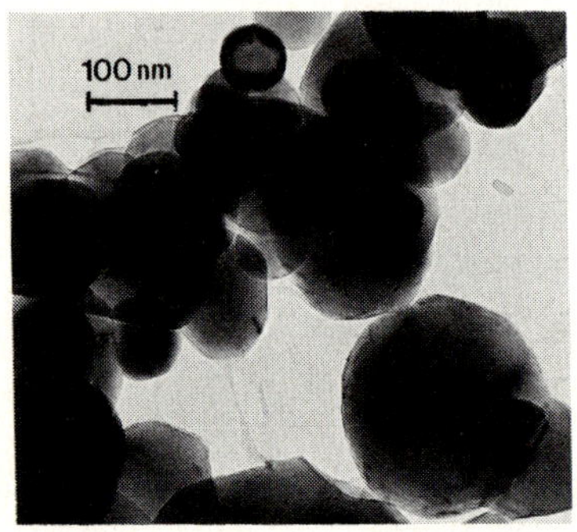

6 b

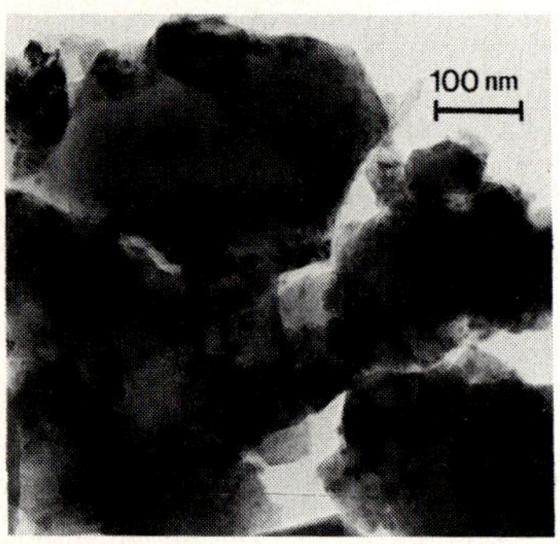

6 c

Fig.6. Electron micrographs of Li/MgO
a- after 723 K-O_2 treatment
b- after reaction at 907 K
c- after reaction at 1023 K.

These temperature changes probably correspond to the dehydroxylation of the initial $Mg(OH)_2$ phase into MgO, as confirmed by DTA analysis. For both unpromoted and promoted magnesia a large endothermic phenomenon is observed between 500 and 700 K in the DTA curves (Fig.7). The corresponding losses of weights are around 32 % in perfect accordance with the stoichiometric loss of weight of 31 % expected for : $Mg(OH)_2 \rightarrow MgO + H_2O$.

TABLE 1 : Characterization data of the Li/MgO catalyst after different thermal treatments.

T (K)	Thermal treatment gases	time on stream (mn)	S.BET (m^2g^{-1})	BJH pore size (nm)	particle size (nm)	Li/Mg (atomic)
333	vacuum	-	49.5	6.7 - 9.0	46	0.62
723	O_2	240	60.0	6.9 - 9.1	46	
903	"	1	64.1	7.7 - 10.3		0.63
1023	"	1	0.57	no porosity		0.59
907	CH_4+O_2	1080	4.3	"	90 - 350	0.57
1023	"	80	0.57	"		0.34
"	"	960	0.56	"		0.28
"	"	3600	0.44	"	250 - 600	0.18

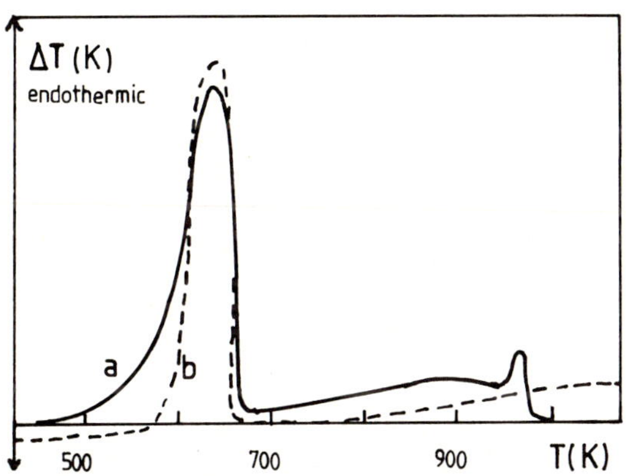

Fig.7. DTA curves of Li/MgO (a) and MgO (b) under flowing O_2-N_2 at 5 K mn^{-1}.

<u>(ii) Treatments at high temperature (> 900 K)</u> : upon heating, a sudden drop of the surface area from ca. 60 to 0.5 m^2g^{-1} is observed between 903 and 1023 K for the specific case of Li/MgO catalyst (see Fig. 5 and Table 1). It indicates a very fast sintering process since each sample was heated only 1 min at the cited temperature and it took only 60 min to heat from 903 to 1023 K. The unpromoted magnesia also underwent some sintering but still had a surface area

of 79 m^2g^{-1} at 1173 K. Clear evidence of a fast sintering process occuring specifically on the Li/MgO solid was also provided by DTA (Fig.7) : near 950 K, one or several endothermic events started with the promoted solid, followed by a sudden return to the base line. The latter was assigned to a loss of contact with the platinum cell due to a drastic shrinkage of the sample. By contrast, only a slow and regular endothermic drift was observed with the unpromoted magnesia, the sample remaining well in contact with the cell all along the experiment.

Together with the sintering phenomenon, a drastic change in porosity was deduced from BJH measurements (Table 1) since no mesoporosity was left after O_2-treatment at 1023 K.

(iii) Effect of the reaction at 907 and 1023 K : after 18 h of reaction at 907 K, the BET value of the Li/MgO catalyst has fallen from 64 to 4.3 m^2g^{-1}. (Fig.5 and Table 1). When the reaction was performed at 1023 K with a solid already extensively sintered (0.6 m^2g^{-1}) there was only a slight decrease of the surface area (0.4 m^2g^{-1} after 60 h on stream). For the case of pure magnesia, a catalytic run carried out at 1023 K for 15 h decreased the surface area from 108 to 31 m^2g^{-1}.

Supporting evidence was provided by electron microscopy : after reaction at 907 K, the promoted magnesia flakes have been transformed into large particles of regular shape from 90 to 350 nm, without any visible porosity (Fig.6b, Table 1). This trend to long distance cristallization was still much more marked after reaction at 1023 K where only very large agglomerates (250-600 nm) without specific shape were detected, suggesting a different sintering process by comparison with the previous case (Fig.6c).

Let us note that focussing the X-ray beam on most of the large particles or dark regions of the Li/MgO solid during the sample investigation made part of the solid disappear irreversibly. A similar effect, also observed with pure lithium carbonate but not with the unpromoted magnesia, is very likely related to liquefaction or decomposition of the Li_2CO_3 phase by the beam. This suggests that Li_2CO_3 is dispersed onto the magnesia phase after high temperature treatments.

Changes in chemical composition

The atomic ratios Li/Mg listed in Table 1 indicate that :

(i) after O_2 treatments, even at 1023 K, there was nearly no significant loss of lithium.

(ii) after dimerization runs, two cases were observed :

1. if the reaction was carried out at 907 K, the loss of lithium was very limited, the Li/Mg ratio decreasing from 0.63 to 0.57.

2. after reaction at 1023 K, a significant loss of lithium occurred during the first hour on stream, followed by a slower decrease of Li/Mg down to 0.18 after 60 h.

The chemical analysis of carbon for a sample treated at 1023 K under O_2 gives strictly the amount expected from the carbonate phase (5.34 %). After reaction for 60 h at 1023 K, the amount of carbon was somewhat lower than that expected from the carbonate phase, account being taken of the loss of lithium (1.33 % instead of 2,17 %). This indicates that i) part of the Li_2CO_3 has been decomposed during the reaction and ii) there is no evidence of carbon deposit at the catalytic surface, which excludes any hypothesis of deactivation by carbon poisoning.

The chemical and cristallographic composition of the Li/MgO solids deduced from XRD patterns are summarized in Table 2.

The changes from brucite $Mg(OH)_2$ to MgO structure after heat-treatment of the precursor are consistent with the previous characterization of the solids. Concerning the state of lithium, the XRD pattern of the Li_2CO_3 phase is still observed after O_2 treatment at 1023 K. After reaction at 1023 K for 60 h, the Li_2CO_3 bands are much less intense in agreement with the loss of lithium noted above. Traces of $Li(OH),H_2O$ were also observed, suggesting some decarbonatation of the Li_2CO_3 phase.

TABLE 2 : XRD composition of Li/MgO catalysts

Catalyst treatments	$Mg(OH)_2$	MgO	Li_2CO_3
precursor	*		*
O_2 at 1023 K		*	*
reaction at 1023 K		*	*

DISCUSSION

From the catalytic and the characterization results, one can draw the following conclusions.

(i) Catalytic activity appears to be more dependent on surface area than on lithium content. Thus, on Li/MgO catalyst, the fast and drastic deactivation which occurs around 1000 K coincides both with a large sintering of the solid and with a loss of lithium. However at 907 K on fresh catalyst, a significant deactivation coincides also with a surface decrease but not with a loss of lithium. With unpromoted magnesia, much more limited deactivation is observed, which is consistent with a rather stable surface area. No evidence of surface poisoning by carbon deposits has been found.

(ii) The stability of the surface is a function of :

- the temperature of treatment (collapse of the surface at 1023 K)

- the nature of the surrounding gases : at 907 K, the surface is stable under flowing O_2, whereas a sintering is observed after contact with the reaction mixture.

- the lithium promotion : whatever the surrounding atmosphere or temperature, the presence of lithium carbonate decreases significantly the stability of the magnesia surface area. This effect has been recently mentioned for magnesia promoted with various alkali salts (ref.7) and we observed it also with other supports such as silica and alumina (ref.11).

(iii) The addition of lithium carbonate to magnesia induces two promoting effects :

- increase of the total conversion per unit area,

- orientation of the reaction towards the methane coupling into C_2 hydrocarbons at the expense of the complete oxidation. This trend is as much marked as the catalyst has been heated at high temperature ($>$ 1000 K). For instance, the C_2 selectivity at 907 K increases from 23 to 56 % after intermediate run at 1023 K.

Before discussing these different points, some data should be provided concerning the possible physical and chemical states of lithium and magnesia throughout the various treatments.

The melting point of Li_2CO_3 is given between 970 and 1005 K in the literature. It forms with Li_2O and CO_2 equilibria which are reported in Fig.8. This figure reports also the possible equilibria between magnesia, basic magnesium carbonate and CO_2 pressure. From these data it may be deduced that the lithium carbonate i) is very likely liquid for samples treated or reacting at temperatures higher than 1000 K, ii) may be in equilibrium with the Li_2O phase (solid up to 1840 K) according to the surrounding P_{CO_2}. In regard to magnesia, its carbonatation into basic carbonate should not occur in the present T and P_{CO_2} conditions (see Fig.8). However, the formation of $MgCO_3$ is known to be enhanced in presence of water, which is actually the case in the dimerization reaction.

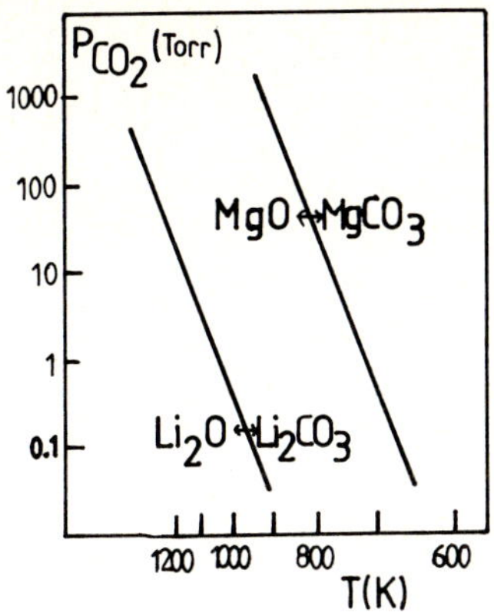

Fig.8 : Thermodynamic equilibrium diagrams.

Let us consider now the different steps of activation or reaction studied in this work.

Effect of treatment under oxygen

- At mild temperature, below the melting point of Li_2CO_3, the magnesia and lithium carbonate have been shown to form two distinct solid phases, the former remaining well dispersed. The initial effect of the alkali salt which is to reduce the surface area of the unpromoted magnesia (see Fig.5) cannot be assigned to some sintering process, the catalyst being far below the Tammann temperature of the support. Possibly, part of the lithium carbonate could act as a cement. The system could be represented as a conglomerate where Li_2CO_3 prevents the initial flakes of magnesia to scatter into smaller fragments.

- When Li/MgO is calcined at temperatures (above 1000 K), the drastic sintering which is observed has to be related to an effect of the Li_2CO_3 phase since the unpromoted magnesia remains well dispersed. Very probably fused at these temperatures, the Li_2CO_3 phase is assumed to spread over the magnesia (in accordance with the observation by electron microscopy), ensuring a tight contact between the two phases. It has been shown also (XRD, thermodynamic data) that the surrounding O_2 atmosphere could cause some decarbonatation in accordance with Kimble et al. (ref.10) who assume a complete decarbonatation into Li_2O at 1173 K under inert atmosphere. Accordingly, the actual process of magnesia sintering in the present conditions could come from a kind of dissolution of MgO into liquid lithium carbonate or possibly from a chemical effect of the CO_2 formed after Li_2CO_3 decomposition. The details of this latter process still have to be determined.

The resulting sample after being cooled is an agglomerate of MgO particles coated with Li_2CO_3, without any porosity left, as observed experimentally.

Effect of reacting atmosphere

(i) For reaction performed at mild temperature (e.g. 907 K), the fresh Li/MgO catalyst does not differ much from the unpromoted magnesia as for C_2 selectivity. This is consistent with the picture of two rather distinct solid phases (Li_2CO_3 and MgO), the whole reaction being still monitored by the magnesia activity. However, the surface will sinter in the reaction course under the specific action of the reacting atmosphere. Two gases are likely to participate to the process : H_2O and CO_2 (ca. 1 and 2 kPa as respective partial pressure). They would allow the formation of magnesium carbonate and/or magnesium hydroxide which could act as intermediate species in a recristallization process (leading to the well cristallized flakes of Fig.6b). As lithium carbonate remains in its solid state, no significant loss of material is expected, as observed even after long-term catalytic run.

This sintering of magnesia, different from the one proposed under O_2 atmosphere, would explain the deactivation of the catalyst reported in Fig.2 curve a.

(ii) For reaction performed at high temperature (e.g. 1023 K), the initial catalyst is already sintered and coated with Li_2CO_3, which limits any extra sintering of the magnesia in the course of the reaction. The loss of lithium during the reaction could be explained by a leakage of the fused carbonate not involved in the magnesia coating (only few percent of the Li_2CO_3 loading are required to form a layer on the magnesia surface). A reaction of the leaking carbonate with the reactor walls and porous disk is plausible since it was observed that used reactors displayed a higher residual activity than unused ones.

Let us add that this loss of lithium carbonate occurs specifically with the basic support-magnesia and not with neutral or acidic supports such as silica or alumina. The latter are shown to form ternary oxides as silicate or aluminate with the alkali salt, actual stabilizing agents of the alkali phase (ref.11).

At this stage of the discussion, we assume the tight contact between Li_2CO_3 and MgO to be the key point of the dimerization process.

Lunsford and coworkers (refs.3-5) have proposed that the active site for dimerization was O^- center created after substitution of Mg^{2+} by Li^+ ions in the magnesia lattice. The present picture of a mobile film of Li_2CO_3 coating the magnesia does not fit correctly with the static model of Li substitution. Moreover the dimerization also occurs with magnesia promoted by alkali ions such as Na^+ (ref.10) or K^+ (ref.7) too large to replace Mg^{2+}. Martin et al (ref.8) have recently proposed a mechanism which requires a first activation of methane on basic oxygens of magnesia and a second one on lithium species leading to carbene formation. This dual-site like scheme looks more consistent with the present picture of the catalytic surface.

CONCLUSIONS

This study of MgO and Li/MgO before and during methane dimerization has shown that :

(i) different modes of catalyst sintering have to be considered according to the temperature and the surrounding atmosphere :

- sintering via the liquid Li_2CO_3 phase at high temperature,
- sintering under the influence of H_2O and CO_2 in the course of the reaction.

(ii) two different types of catalytic deactivation can occur with respect to the two sintering processes,

(iii) the optimized catalytic performances are obtained when a tight interface between Li_2CO_3 and MgO phases is achieved, after a treatment allowing the liquefaction of the alkali salt.

These points which depend straightforwardly on the physical and chemical properties of the catalytic oxides should be considered when interpreting the behaviour and performances of the numerous formulas tested up to now and when developping new and still more efficient system for the coupling of methane.

ACKNOWLEDGMENTS : The authors thank Mrs. A. CHAMBOSSE, M.T. GIMENEZ, I. MUTIN and Mr. J. VARLOUD for valuable assistance and Dr. G.A. MARTIN for helpful discussions. This work has been supported by "Gaz de France".

REFERENCES

1 G.E. Keller and M.M. Bhasin, J. Catal., 73 (1982) 9.
2 W. Hinsen, W. Bytyn and M. Baerns, Proc. 8th Int. Congr. Catal., Dechema, Verlag Chemie, Berlin, 1984, pp. 581.
3 D.J. Driscoll, W. Martir, J.X. Wang and J.H. Lunsford, J. Am. Chem. Soc., 107 (1985) 58.
4 C.H. Lin, K.D. Campbell, J.X. Wang and J.H. Lunsford, J. Phys. Chem. 90 (1986) 534.
5 T. Ito, J.X. Wang, C.H. Lin and J.H. Lunsford, J. Am. Chem. Soc. 107 (1986) 5062.
6 K. Otsuka, K. Jinno and A. Morikawa, J. Catal., 100 (1986) 353.
7 E. Iwamatsu, T. Moriyama, N. Takasaki and K.I. Aika, J. Chem. Soc., Chem. Commun., (1987) 19.
8 G.A. Martin and C. Mirodatos, J. Chem. Soc., Chem. Comm., submitted for publication.
9 S.J. Gregg and K.S.W. Sing, in "Surface and Colloid Science", Vol 9, (Ed. E. Matijevic) J. Wiley and Sons, (1976) p. 231.
10 J.B. Kimble and J.H. Kolts, Energy Process, 6 (1986) 226.
11 M.C. Durupty and V. Perrichon, in preparation.

B. Delmon and G.F. Froment (Editors), *Catalyst Deactivation 1987*

PLATINUM REFORMING CATALYSTS: EFFECT OF CHLORINE CONTENT ON COKING AND CATALYST SELF-REGENERATION

A. PARMALIANA[1], F. FRUSTERI[1], G.A. NESTEROV[2], E.A. PAUKSHTIS[2] and N. GIORDANO[3]
[1]Istituto di Chimica Industriale, Università di Messina, 98100 Messina (Italy).
[2]Institute of Catalysis, 630090 Novosibirsk 90, USSR
[3]Istituto CNR/TAE, 98013 Pistunina, Messina (Italy).

ABSTRACT

The deactivation and subsequent self-regeneration of several Pt/γAl$_2$O$_3$/ honeycomb reforming catalysts have been investigated. Catalytic activity in the dehydrogenation of methylcyclohexane (MCH), taken as reaction model, has been evaluated at 400°C in a continuous flow microreactor. The determining role of surface chlorine during the deactivation and the H_2 self-regeneration is discussed. IR analysis of coked catalysts reveals different kinds of carbonaceous residues depending upon the chlorine presence on the catalyst surface. A catalyst with ca. 0.5% Cl shows complete self-regeneration. A regeneration mechanism, involving spillover of residual hydrogen, is proposed.

INTRODUCTION

Coking is the main cause of deactivation of bifunctional reforming catalysts. In spite of the practical importance of this phenomenon ("coking") and notwithstanding the fact that it has been the subject of intensive research for several decades, the formation and structure of the carbonaceous deposits on mono-or multimetallic reforming catalysts are still not well understood. According to some authors coke formation can be attributed to acid sites (refs. 1,2), others favour the metallic components (refs. 3-5) or a combination of both acidic and metallic sites (ref. 6). Cooper and Trimm (ref. 6) have pointed out that the extent of coke formation is controlled by the chemical stabilization of the hydrocarbon and that the rate of coking is associated with a polymerization reaction, most probably acid catalysed (Cl). The rate of deactivation of the catalyst depends mainly on the reaction temperature and partial pressure of hydrogen, but it is remarkable that the presence of hydrogen in the feed is not sufficient to avoid deactivation (coke formation) (ref. 7). Formation of unsaturated intermediates, which can condense or polymerize to coke, can be impeded by hydrogen either through a spillover (refs.4,8, 9) or a dynamic mechanism (ref. 10). Davis et al. (ref. 11) reported that the carbon deposit during reforming on platinum single crystal catalysts resulted from the activated nucleation and growth of unreactive polymeric species with an average hydrogen content of about 1.0-1.5 H atoms per surface C atom. Recently, it has been demonstrated that highly dispersed reforming catalysts are more resistant to deactivation from coke deposition. In fact it is claimed that the small platinum crystallites present an electron deficiency due to metal support interactions resulting into a lower stabilization of the intermediate adsorbed unsaturated hydrocarbons (ref. 12). Parera et al. (ref. 10) studied the influence of the chlorine content on deactivation of Pt/Al_2O_3 by coking and claimed that there is an optimum chlorine content which allows reduction of the coke deposit through a mechanism involving the activated spillover of superficial hydrogen. Cooper and Trimm claimed that coking can be connected with the catalyst acidity related to the presence of Cl (ref. 6).

Generally, catalyst regeneration is achieved by heating in an oxidizing atmosphere (refs. 13-14) or by appropriate chlorine treatments (ref. 15). These procedures may lead to further agglomeration of the metal and in some alloy catalysts they may alter the surface composition of metal particles or cause phase separation (ref.15). In previous work we have reported that coked reforming catalysts can be "fully" restored by a non-oxidizing H_2 treatment at 400°C (refs. 16,17). By this procedure metal sintering, encountered during oxidizing coke burning, can be avoided. The main goal of the present study was to gain further insight into the effect of the surface chlorine content on deactivation patterns of platinum honeycomb reforming catalysts during MCH dehydrogenation.

Furthermore, the fundamental role is discussed of surface chlorine on the catalyst self-regeneration step through a hydrogen spillover mechanism.

EXPERIMENTAL

Catalyst

Platinum supported catalysts were prepared from a ceramic honeycomb support of cordierite coated with a colloidal solution of γ-Al_2O_3 (Dispural

Condea Product, Hamburg, FDR), as described elsewhere (ref. 18). In order to differentiate the influence of the surface acidity of γ-Al_2O_3 and the chlorine content on the catalyst deactivation, three series of catalysts were prepared: Ser. B, Ser. P, Ser. C. All catalysts were obtained by wet impregnation using a recirculation system. The catalysts of Ser. B were prepared by impregnation of the support with an ammoniacal solution of $H_2Pt(OH)_6$ at different impregnation times. Catalysts of Ser. P were prepared by making use of a support preliminarly doped with 1.5% P to depress surface acidity of γ-Al_2O_3 (ref. 19). Afterwards the P-γ Al_2O_3/honeycomb support was impregnated with the ammoniacal solution of $H_2Pt(OH)_6$ at different impregnation times. Catalysts of Ser. C were prepared by impregnation with a H_2PtCl_6 solution with or without HCl (cat. C-2 and C-1, respectively). The catalysts were dried at 110°C for 24 h and then calcined in air at 500°C for 10 h.

Catalysts C-1A and C-1B were obtained from Cat. C-1 by dechlorination, based on water treatment at 500°C for 15 and 40 h respectively (ref. 20). Results are compared to a previously (ref. 16) investigated commercial 0.24% Pt/γ Al_2O_3/honeycomb reforming catalyst (PZM 4104, UOP, Des Plaines); the "as received" catalyst (here termed Z) was further subjected to dechlorination for 40 h (catalyst Z-B).

Surface areas of the support were measured by the BET method. The Pt content was determined photocolorimetrically using the stannous chloride method. The total amount of chlorine was determined by dissolution of the catalyst with sulfuric acid and titration of the distillate according to Volhard-Charpenter method (ref. 21).

Platinum particle size was determined by electron microscopy (JEOL 100 CX TEM, point-to-point resolution 5 Å) using finely ground and ultrasonically dispersed (in ethanol) catalyst samples, deposited on a thin carbon film supported on a standard copper grid. Prior to the TEM measurements the platinum samples were reduced at 400°C in flowing hydrogen for 2 h. To estimate the mean crystallite sizes, the normal statistical formulae were used (ref. 22). An average of 500 particles per sample was considered. Metal surface areas (MSA) and dispersion values have been evaluated according to Anderson (ref. 23).

The main physical and chemical characteristics of the catalysts used are given in table 1.

TABLE 1

Characterization of the catalysts.

Sample	B-1	P-1	C-1	C-1A	C-1B	Z	Z-B
γ-Al_2O_3/Honeycomb, wt/wt	0.15	0.15	0.15	0.15	0.15	n.d.	n.d.
BET S.A., $m^2 \cdot g^{-1}$	27	27	27	27	27	28	28
Pt content, wt%	0.19	0.23	0.26	0.26	0.26	0.24	0.24
Cl content, wt%	-	-	1.75	0.95	0.53	1.0	0.50
Mean crystallite size, Å	12	9	8	14	20	50	53
MSA, $m^2_{Pt} \cdot g^{-1}_{Pt}$	233	310	350	200	140	56	53

Apparatus and reaction methods

Tests of MCH dehydrogenation, including stability and regenerability of the catalysts, were carried out in a continuous flow fixed-bed microreactor operating at atmospheric pressure. Details concerning the apparatus and procedure have been described elsewhere (ref. 17).

Prior to reaction, the fresh catalyst (0.1 g, 40-70 mesh) was treated in a hydrogen flow at 400°C for 2 h. The reproducibility of the experimental data was established and found to be ± 2-3%.

All catalysts were tested at 400°C and WHSV= 48 h^{-1}. Runs were carried out at atmospheric pressure and with a molar ratio R = P_{H_2}/P_{MCH} of 2. Helium (350 cm^3 STP min^{-1}) was used as a carrier and N_2 (10 cm^3 STP min^{-1}) as an internal standard. On account of this, the molar ratio R'= $(P_{H_2}+P_{N_2}+P_{He})/P_{MCH}=20$. The performance of the catalysts was recorded over a period of 6 h. As besides toluene no byproducts were observed, the conversion to toluene was taken as a measure of the catalytic activity.

RESULTS

MCH dehydrogenation catalytic test

As it has been suggested that MCH dehydrogenation at 400°C is adequate for evaluation of coking on reforming catalysts (ref. 16), this reaction T was chosen as a reference. Before reaction, all catalysts were (pre)reduced in a hydrogen flow at 400°C for 2 h. Runs were made in the reaction conditions cited above. The values of the initial and final catalytic activity for all catalysts are summarized in Table 2.

TABLE 2

Catalytic MCH dehydrogenation activity of reforming catalysts at 400°C.

Cat.	% Pt	Ø Mean Crystallite Size, Å	Initial activity (% MCH conv.)	Final activity (% MCH conv.)
B-1	0.19	12	52.2	15.4
P-1	0.23	9	56.4	20.2
C-1	0.26	8	50.0	15.8
C-1A	0.26	14	35.0	10.8
C-1B	0.26	20	32.0	14.0
Z	0.24	50	27.0	12.0
Z-B	0.24	53	20.0	10.0

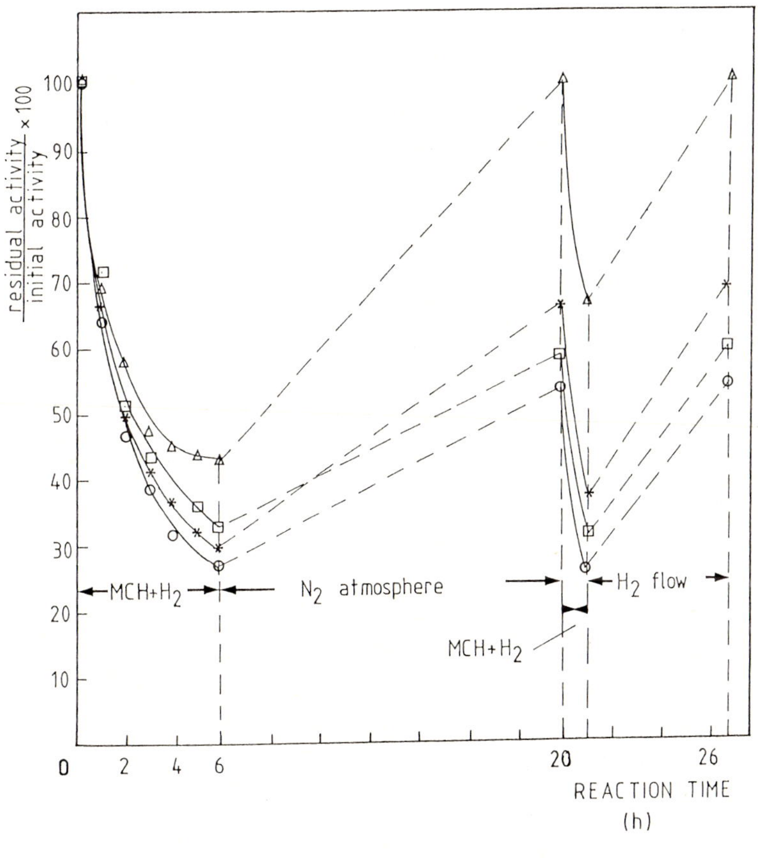

Fig. 1. Deactivation and subsequent regeneration test of reforming catalysts. T= 400°C, WHSV = 48 h^{-1}, R = P_{H_2}/P_{MCH} = 2 (O = cat. C-1; □ = cat. C-1A; Δ = cat. C-1B; ✱ = cat. B-1).

At first (up to about 2h) deactivation is very rapid, but then slows down until reaching almost constant conversion (see Figure 1).

Thermogravimetric analysis shows that the coke deposition on all catalysts during the 6 h run corresponds to about 2 wt%.

CATALYST REGENERATION TEST

H_2 static method

After 6 h run at T= 400°C the reaction mixture was vented and the "coked" catalyst was treated in a 500 cm^3 STP min^{-1} N_2 flow for 10 min, then the catalyst was kept at 400°C in an N_2 static atmosphere for 14 h.

H_2 dynamic method

After 6 h run at T= 400°C the reaction mixture was vented and the "coked" catalyst was treated in a 500 cm^3 STP min^{-1} N_2 flow for 6.5 h. During this regenerative process, the catalyst temperature was carefully monitored and found constant.

Products formed during the regeneration test by the H_2 static method have been analyzed by a gas-chromatograph unit. On cat. C-1B and Z-B the presence of CH_4, C_2H_6 has been revealed together with traces of C_2H_2. No such products have been noted on the other catalysts.

After regeneration, a MCH dehydrogenation catalytic test was duplicated (with the same procedure as for the initial run) in order to check whether the catalyst had regained its initial activity. All "coked" catalysts were subjected to both regeneration methods: most significant experimental results of these regeneration tests are summarized in Table 3.

TABLE 3

Regeneration tests of coked catalysts

Cat.	% Pt	% Cl	Initial Activity (% MCH Conv.)	Final Activity (% MCH Conv.)	Initial Activity after regeneration Test (% MCH conv.) H_2 Static Method	H_2 Dynamic Method
B-1	0.19	--	52.2	15.4	34.7	35.9
P-1	0.23	--	56.4	20.2	28.8	31.8
C-1	0.26	1.75	50.0	15.8	26.2	28.3
C-1A	0.26	0.95	35.0	10.8	20.4	20.5
C-1B	0.26	0.53	32.0	14.0	31.5	31.5
Z	0.24	1.0	27.0	12.0	18.3	18.8
Z-B	0.24	0.50	20.0	10.0	19.0	19.0

It was found that only catalysts C-1B and Z-B could be regenerated by both regeneration methods, with no substantial differences between the efficiencies of the two methods. The behaviour of cat. C-1, C-1B and B-1 during the catalyst deactivation-H_2 regeneration cycle are shown in Figure 1. In Figure 2 are summarized the results of the regeneration test of all coked catalysts with respect to their chlorine content.

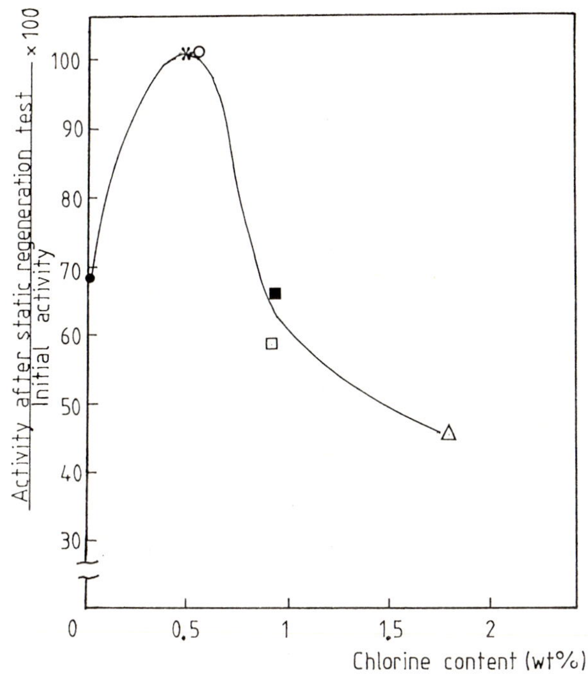

Fig. 2. Influence of catalyst chlorine content on the static regeneration test of coked reforming catalysts (● = cat. P-1; Δ = cat. C-1; □ = cat. C-1A; O = cat. C-1B; ■ = cat. Z; ✱ = cat. Z-B).

IR analysis of coke deposits

IR spectra of the coked catalysts were obtained, after heating in vacuum at 125°C, using UR-20 spectrometer within the range 1200-4000 cm^{-1}. The IR spectra, shown in Figure 3 revealed:

a) four absorption bands at : 1420-1470, 2860-2890, 2930-2940, 2960-2980 cm^{-1} characterizing stretchings of CH bands in CH_2 and CH_3 groups (refs.24,25). Coke type B.

b) two absorption bands at 1490 and 1590 cm^{-1} characterizing stretchings of aromatic rings (refs. 24,25). Coke type A.

c) one absorption band near 3020 cm^{-1} attributable to the stretchings of C-H bond in unsaturated aromatic compounds (refs. 24,25). Coke type A'.

It can be noted that coke on the catalysts C-1, C-1A and C-1B have a similar nature, attributable to the saturated hydrocarbon compounds. On the contrary on catalyst B-1 the coke is assigned mainly to aromatic compounds.

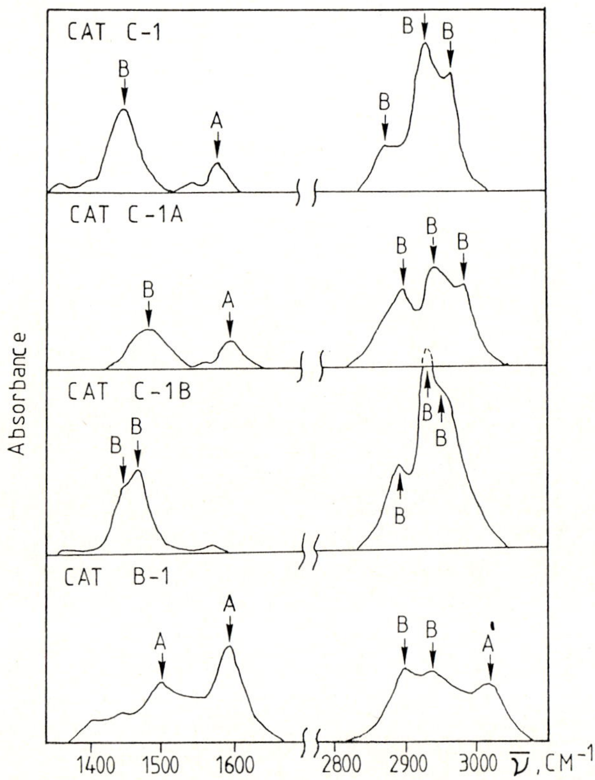

Fig. 3. Infrared spectra of coke deposits on reforming catalysts obtained by MCH dehydrogenation at 400°C.

DISCUSSION

Coking of Pt/Honeycomb Reforming Catalysts

Formation of coke over a Pt/Al_2O_3 catalyst is a very complex process. According to some authors (ref. 26), it starts on the metallic function of the catalyst and is initially characterized by rapid deactivation; afterwards, the process slows down in correspondence to coke deposition on the acidic function. Deposition of these carbonaceous residues is supposed to block the metallic sites causing severe deactivation of the catalyst (ref. 12). The results reported in Fig. 1 confirm this assumption and also indicate that the activity of catalysts of series C (C-1, C-1A, C-1B) decreases with reaction time depending on the chlorine content. Namely, the deactivation patterns (Fig. 1) show that the loss of initial activity for cat. C-1B (containing 0.53 wt% of Cl) is lower than for cat C-1 and C-1A with 1.75 and 0.95 wt% Cl, respectively. In his studies on the influence of chlorine content on coking, Parera et al. conclude that deactivation of re-reforming catalysts is minimum when the residual Cl content is 0.89% (refs. 9,21). This value optimizes hydrogen spillover (ref. 9) a factor which contributes to free the surface from carbonaceous residues , which are coke precursors.

The deactivation behaviour of the chlorine-free cat. B-1 (Fig. 1) clearly indicates that coking cannot be avoided by eliminating chlorine from the catalyst surface. Furthermore it must be noted that the results obtained with the chlorine free cat P-1, which has a support structure modified with P to block the γ-Al_2O_3 surface acidity, are similar to those obtained with cat. B-1 (Table 2).

On the basis of our results it is possible to rule out Cooper's assumption (ref. 6) that coking is a function of the catalyst acidity. Instead, we conclude that coking on a bifunctional catalyst involves the metallic sites possibly through steps involving dehydrogenation of chemisorbed species and consequent formation of unsaturated species which further condense over the acidic sites of the γ-Al_2O_3. These statements well agree with the views of Shum (ref. 4) according to whom the metallic function controls the long term decay of bifunctional reforming catalysts through formation of carbonaceous residues.

IR analysis of coked catalysts, reported in Fig. 3, shows that the presence of surface chlorine (cat C-1, C-1A and C-1B) leads to formation of linear saturated hydrocarbon residues. In our previous work aiming at the understanding of the reaction mechanism of MCH dehydrogenation and coke formation (refs. 16,17) it has been claimed that the chlorine content influences the nature and mechanisms of formation of carbonaceous residues contributing to coking.

It has been suggested that the main coke precursors, such as $MCH^{=}$ (methylcyclohexene) and methylcyclohexadiene, which are more prone to cracking, contribute to coking depending on the surface acidity (Cl) (ref.16). The coking mechanism involves desorption of the coke precursors from the metallic sites with subsequent adsorption on the acidic sites and ring opening. The hydrocarbon residues generated in the ring opening reaction can polymerize by an acid catalyzed process to form linear saturated hydrocarbons (refs.16,17). On chlorine free catalysts (e.g. cat. B-1) the ring opening reaction and subsequent polymerization of the hydrocarbon residues are not favoured and coking is due mainly to hydrocarbon residues having an aromatic structure originated by condensation process of coke precursors (ref. 17).

H_2 self-regeneration of coked reforming catalyst

It is well known that the presence of H_2 in the feed during reforming reduces the quantity of the carbonaceous deposits (refs. 27, 28). Moreover, it is generally agreed that H_2 exerts a hydrogenolytic activity on these deposits thus allowing their fast surface desorption (refs. 4,5,9,11,27). According to some authors the activity of H_2 has to be attributed to spillover of molecular H_2 followed by hydrogenolytic activity of atomic hydrogen (refs. 4,8,11,26), for which the determining role by the surface Cl has been indicated by Parera et al. (refs. 8-9). We have recently proposed regeneration of coked reforming catalysts, having an optimum chlorine content, by H_2 treatment at reaction temperature (ref. 16). The present study therefore aimed at better defining these statements and to attempt an interpretation of the influence of surface acidity on the H_2 spillover during catalyst self-regeneration. For this purpose the deactivated catalysts were treated with H_2 in the static and dynamic mode, with the latter probably being the more efficacious due to mass transfer effects. As experimental evidence (Tab. 3) clearly indicated that only catalysts C-1B and Z-B appear to be fully regenerable, it is suggested that the presence of chlorine is a prerequisite.

In the literature it is reported that the number of carbon atoms deposited per platinum surface site increases with the platinum particle size (ref. 12). This lead to think that the regenerability of big platinum crystallites could be more difficult than that of the small ones. Our results reported in

Table 3 show that catalyst C-1B, having bigger platinum crystallites than catalysts C-1 and C-1A, is fully regenerable. This indicates that the chlorine content constitutes the determining factor controlling the catalyst regenerability, as shown in Figure 2. Such an evidence is further supported by IR analysis of coked catalysts revealing that the coke on catalysts C-1, C-1A and C-1B has similar nature. Therefore the full regenerability of catalyst C-1B can neither be attributed to more easily removable carbonaceous residues.

On the basis of the mechanism postulated before (refs. 16,17) we suggest an interpretation based on the dissociative H_2 chemisorption and subsequent migration by a spillover mechanism. Hydrogenolysis of the unsaturated carbonaceous residues is postulated by means of atomic H via desorption of light hydrocarbons which free the active sites. The above hydrogen activity is confirmed by the presence of CH_4, C_2H_2, C_2H_6 in desorbed products for catalysts C-1B and Z-B. Some authors have found that the spillover is influenced by the Cl content of the catalyst (refs. 29-31). Benke (ref.31) suggested that the optimal concentration of Cl for the spillover on Al_2O_3 is of the order of $3x10^{13}$ atoms/cm^2 and that at the higher Cl concentrations the few Al ions left on the surface limit the proton migration because of the hindrance to the migration of hydride ions which are necessary to maintain electrical neutrality.

Tanaka et al. (ref. 32) found that the number of OH on Al_2O_3 heat treated at 500°C is $20x10^{13}$ cm^{-2}. Kramer et al. (ref.33) assume for Al_2O_3 (T= 400°C) $20x10^{14}$ OH cm^{-2}. Recently, some authors (ref. 34) have indicated a saturation value of the Cl atom on γ-Al_2O_3 of $10x10^{13}$ atoms/cm^2 which is of the same order of magnitude as the number of OH groups. In consideration of the above, we assume that on those samples characterized by 0.5 wt% Cl content (cat. C-1B and Z-B), OH groups are replaced half by Cl^- ions, and this give rise to maximum spillover. Under such conditions a quasi-neutrality in the surface electrical charges is assumed. In accordance with others (refs. 9,31), we claim that this constitutes a fundamental factor for high spillover, possibly through an ionic diffusion mechanism. The assumptions made above clearly explain the non regenerability of samples C-1 (1.75% Cl), C-1A (0.95% Cl) and Z (1% Cl) with $1.7x10^{14}$, $8.5x10^{13}$ and $9x10^{13}$ Cl atoms/cm^2 respectively. Such a high Cl coverage on the surface of those samples should prevent from conditions of electrical neutrality and therefore impede hydrogen spillover.

REFERENCES

1 B.C. Gates, J.R. Katzer and G.C.A. Schuit, Chemistry of Catalytic Processes, McGraw-Hill New York, 1979, ch. 3, p. 287.
2 T.M. John, R.A. Pachovsky and B.W. Wojciechowski, Adv. Chem. Series 133(1974) p. 422.
3 W.M.H. Sachtler and P. Biloen, Preprints, Div. Pet. Chem., ACS, Seattle (USA) March 20-25 (1983) p. 482.
4 V.K. Shum, J.B. Butt and W.M.H. Sachtler, Appl. Catal. 11 (1984) 151-154.
5 J. Volter and U. Kurschner, Appl. Catal. 8 (1983) 167-176.
6 B.J. Cooper and D.L. Trimm, in B. Delmon and G.F. Froment (Eds), Catalyst Deactivation, Elsevier, Amsterdam, 1980, p. 63.
7 L.W. Jossens and E.E. Petersen, J. Catal. 73 (1982) 377-386.
8 J.M. Parera, E.M. Traffano, J.C. Musso and C.L. Pieck, in G.M. Pajonk, S.J. Teichner and G.E. Germain (Eds),Spillover of adsorbed species, Elsevier, Amsterdam, 1983, p. 101.
9 J.M. Parera, N.S. Figoli, E.L. Jablonski, M.R. Sad and J.N. Beltramini, in B. Delmon and G.F. Froment (Eds), Catalyst Deactivation, Elsevier, Amsterdam, 1980, p. 571.
10 R.W. Coughlin, K. Kawakami and A. Hasan, J. Catal., 88 (1984) 150-162.
11 S.M. Davis, F. Zaera and G.A. Somorjai, J. Catal., 77 (1982) 439-459.
12 J. Barbier, G. Corro, Y. Zhang, J.B. Bournonville and J.P. Franck, Appl. Catal., 13 (1985) 245-255.
13 G.I. Straguzzi, H.R. Aduriz and C.E. Cigola, J. Catal., 66 (1980) 171-183.
14 J.P. Bournonville, J.P. Franck and G. Martino in G. Poncelet, P. Grange and P.A. Jacobs (Eds), Preparation of catalysts III, Elsevier Publ., B.V. Amsterdam, 1983, p. 81.
15 K. Foger and H. Jaeger, J. Catal. 92 (1985) 64-78.
16 F. Frusteri, V. Barcellona, G. Mento, A. Parmaliana and N. Giordano, Ann.Chim. (Rome) 75 (1985) 441-448.
17 A. Parmaliana, F. Frusteri, A. Mezzapica and N. Giordano, J. Catal. (1986), submitted for publication.
18 A. Parmaliana, M. El Sawi, G. Mento, U. Fedele and N. Giordano, Appl. Catal. 7 (1983) 221-232.
19 K. Gishti, A. Iannibello, S. Marengo, G. Morelli, P. Tittarelli, App. Catal. 12 (1984) 381-393.
20 A.A. Castro, O.A. Scelza, E.R. Benvenuto, G.T. Baronetti and J.M. Parera, J. Catal. 69 (1981) 222-226.
21 N.S. Figoli, M.R. Sad, J.N. Beltramini, E.L. Jablonski and J.M. Parera, Ind. Eng. Chem. Prod. Res. Dev. 19 (1980) 545-551.
22 D.J. Smith, D. White, J. Baird and J.R. Fryer, J. Catal. 81 (1983) 107-118.
23 J.R. Anderson, Structure of Metallic Catalysts, Academic Press, London 1975, p. 358.
24 L.J. Bellamy, The Infrared Spectra of Complex Molecules, Chapman and Hall, London, 1975, p. 13.
25 E.E. Wolf and F. Alfani, Catal. Rev. Sci Eng. 24(3)(1982) 329-371.
26 J.M. Parera, N.S. Figoli, E.M. Traffano, J.N. Beltramini and E.E. Martinelli, Appl. Catal. 5 (1983) 33-41.
27 E.E. Wolf and E.E. Petersen, J. Catal. 46 (1977) 190-203.
28 D.L. Trimm, Chem. Eng. Proces 18 (1984) 137-148.
29 J.L. Carter, P.J. Lucchesi, P. Corneil, D.C.J. Yates and J.H. Sinfelt, J. Phys. Chem. 69 (1965) 3070-3074.
30 G.C. Bond, J.M. Fuller and L.R. Molloy, Proc. Sixth Int. Congr. on Catalysis, London 1976, The Chemical Society 1977, p. 356.
31 A.H. Benke, Ph.D. Thesis, University of California, Berkeley, 1976.
32 M. Tanaka and S. Ogasowara, J. Catal. 16 (1970) 157-163.
33 R. Kramer and M. Andre, J. Catal. 58 (1979) 287-295.
34 G. Lietz, H. Lieske, H. Spindler, W. Hanke and J. Volter, J. Catal. 81 (1983) 17-25.

1987 Elsevier Science Publishers B.V., Amsterdam — Printed in The Netherlands

EFFECT OF RARE EARTH ON THE BEHAVIOR OF CARBON DEPOSITION ON NICKEL CATALYST

WU Xingya, ZHANG Jiyan and CHANG Liu
Department of Chemical Engineering, Tianjin University, Tianjin (P.R.China)

ABSTRACT
Two types of naphtha steam reforming catalyst have been compared. One is common Ni-Al-Mg catalyst, the other contains rare earth oxides. The coking rate curve of the common one is in "S" form, the other is in progressively decreasing form with high coking resistivity and decoking power and does not lose its activity at zero coking rate. The effect of RE oxides can only be displayed under close connection with Ni and in the presence of steam. A mechanism of improving coking resistivity is proposed. The RE content and preparation methods have also been investigated.

INTRODUCTION

Deactivation of Ni-catalyst by carbon-deposition is a general problem in hydrocarbon processing particularly in naphtha steam reforming process. Much work has been done in searching for high activity and high coking-resistivity catalysts [1]. In this paper we shall present our work of incorporating rare earth oxides into Ni-catalysts and their effect on coking suppression properties.

EXPERIMENTAL

Testings have been carried out in a flow system with a thermogravimetric balance reactor and with other techniques such as TPR (temperature programmed reduction), DTA (differential thermal analysis), TEM (transmission electromicroscopy) and XRD (X-ray diffraction).

The ID of the reactor is ca. 20 mm. The suspended basket is 10 mm in diameter and 2 mm high, in which 15-40 mg sample with 40-60 mesh are spread out in a single layer. The sensitivity of the balance is 0.01 mg. The heating rate is 13-16 °C/min.

The reactants n-heptane and n-octane are desulfurized to less than 0.12 ppm S. H_2 and N_2 are deoxygenized. The total gas-vapor flow rate of the reacting mixture is 350-600 ml/min. Catalyst is reduced by H_2-N_2 or H_2-H_2O-N_2 mixture at 800°C until constant weight is achieved, then the temperature is lowered to 550 °C and the gas stream is switched to hydrocarbon-steam-N_2 mixture.

Catalysts

Catalysts with different Ni and RE oxides content are prepared by coprecipitation or impregnation of incipient wetness. Catalyst A, B and C are obtained by impregnation and calcined at 800°C with carrier $MgAl_2O_4$ and a little Al_2O_3. Catalysts D, E and F are obtained by coprecipitation and calcined at 1000°C with carrier $MgAl_2O_4$ and some MgO.

Catalysts A and D contain Ni only. D_2 has a Ni-content twice as much as D_1.

Catalysts B and E contain both Ni and RE oxide. B and E have the same Ni content as A and D_1 respectively. B and E_1 are Ni-RE_1 oxide. E_2 is Ni-RE_2 oxide. E_1 and E_2 have the same weight percent of RE oxide.

Catalysts C and F contain RE oxide only. C and F_1 are RE_1 oxide. F_2 is RE_2 oxide.

The starting material of these catalysts are their corresponding nitrates. In copreicipitation the precipitant is Na_2CO_3-NaOH mixture.

RESULT

Reduction properties

TPR curves of caralysts A, B and C prepared by impregnation are transformed into the degree of reduction versus temperature, as shown in fig. 1. The initial reduction temperature of them are increased in the order of A<C<B. In the temperature range indicated, C is reduced in two stages with a total degree of reduction 67%, on the basis from higher valence state RE_1 to lower state RE_1 . A after a short interval of induction is reduced quickly, then slowly, till to completion. B is reduced in a rather even rate up to 100% reduction, including NiO to Ni and RE_1 to RE_1 . Here it is worthy to be noticed that the effect of RE_1 oxide on NiO only causes a delay of its reduction, while the effect of NiO on RE_1 oxide makes it completely reduced.

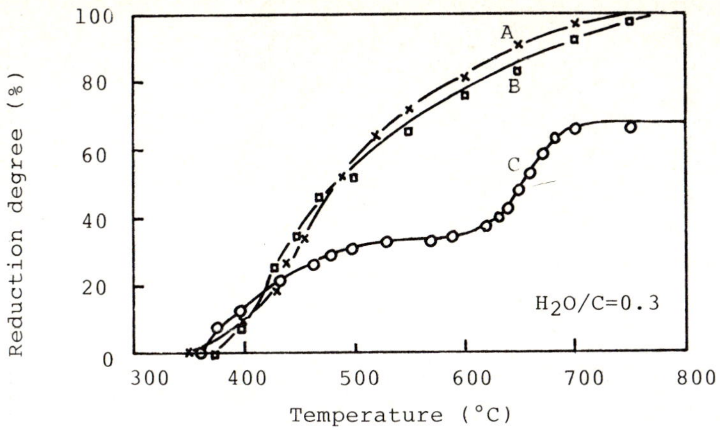

FIGURE 1. The temperature programmed reduction curves on catalysts.

TABLE 1
The XRD characteristics for RE_1 oxide in catalyst E_1 and F_1

RE oxide in catalyst	Angle of diffraction 2 ϑ (grad)	Height of diffraction peak Before red.* H_1 (mm)	After red.* H_2 (mm)	The ratio H_2/H_1
E_1	28.36	183	105	0.57
	32.90	56.65	32	0.56
	47.32	92	45	0.49
F_1	28.44	194	142	0.73
	32.90	55	40	0.73
	47.36	98.6	61	0.62

* Reduction with dry hydrogen

This fact suggests that in the mixture of NiO and RE_1 oxide, although there is no separate new compound can be detected by XRD, yet they are surely in intimate contact and have some strong influence on one another.

As for those catalysts prepared by coprecipitation, they have a rather lower degree of reduction, such as catalyst E_1 has its RE_1 oxide only partially reduced, as shown by XRD in table 1, in which F_1 is for comparison and is even lower. Such a trend is same as obtained from impregnation. Both F_1 and F_2 are reduced with changing color from their original light yellow and cream yellow to dark grey and pale grey respectively. The

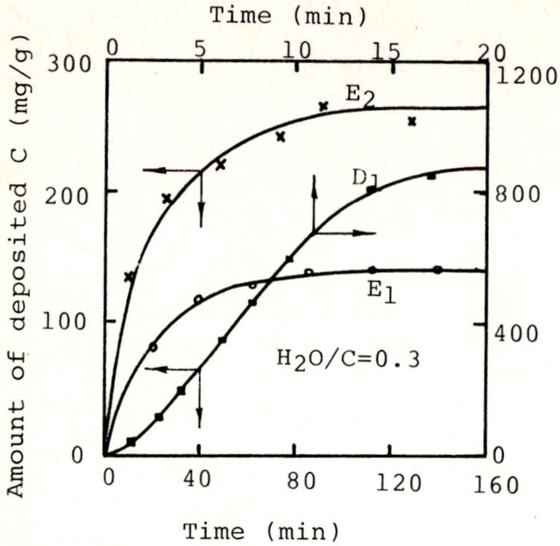

FIGURE 2. The carbon deposition curves on catalyst D_1, E_1 and E_2.

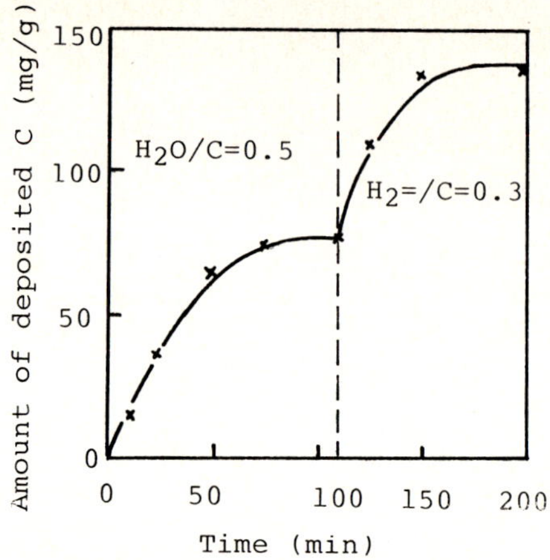

FIGURE 3. The carbon deposition curves on catalyst E_1 with diffrent H_2O/C.

degree of reduction of F_2 is somewhat lower than F_1. Their color and weight can be restored by reoxidation.

Coking behavior

When passing reactant 1 (heptane-steam-N_2) through catalysts D, E and F, there are filamentous carbon deposited on D and E with Ni-particles on the top, as usually happened[2,3], but there is none on F. The coking rate curve of D_1, E_1 and E_2 are shown in fig. 2.

Catalysts D and E have quite different profiles. D gives an "S" form curve, as normally exhibited [4,5], after a short induction period, the coking rate rises up and then turns to be constant, finally approaches to zero with complete loss of its catalytic activity. As for catalysts E_1 and E_2, their coking rate are high initially and comparable to that of catalyst D_1, but quickly decreases to zero and does not lose their catalytic activity at all. Here we call the zero rate point as zero coking rate. At that point, the rate of coking equals to that of decoking, i.e. coking and decoking are under dynamic equilibrium.

This fact is confirmed both by the tail gas chromatographic analysis and the immediate increase in carbon deposit, as H_2O/C is decreased after reaching zero coking rate, as shown in fig. 3. The average coking rate and total carbon deposit on E_1 and

E_2 are both much less than that on D_1. The difference between catalysts D and E is obviously due to the presence of RE oxide. The difference in E_1 and E_2 can be attributed to the oxides RE_1 and RE_2 having different oxidizing power [6,7,8]. RE_1 oxide is higher, so E_1 has a better coking resistance. But both RE_1 and RE_2 oxides after having been incorporated with Ni can enhance its despersity, its coking resistance and the mechanical strength of the final catalyst, which can be run at relatively low H_2O/C and high liquid space velocity [10].

In order to know the effect of RE oxide on depression of coking, an equal amount of catalyst D_2 and F_1 is mixed mechanically, with a Ni content same as E_1 and subjected to coking test. Its coking behavior is just like D_1 alone. It demostrates that mechanically incorporated RE oxide has no effect on coking mode.

When passing reactant II (heptane-N_2 without steam) through catalyst E_1, its coking curve is also in "S" form same as that of D_1. Such a phenomenon indicates that the effect of RE-oxide in RE-Ni catalyst can only be affected in the presence of steam and in the close connection with Ni.

Decoking behaviour

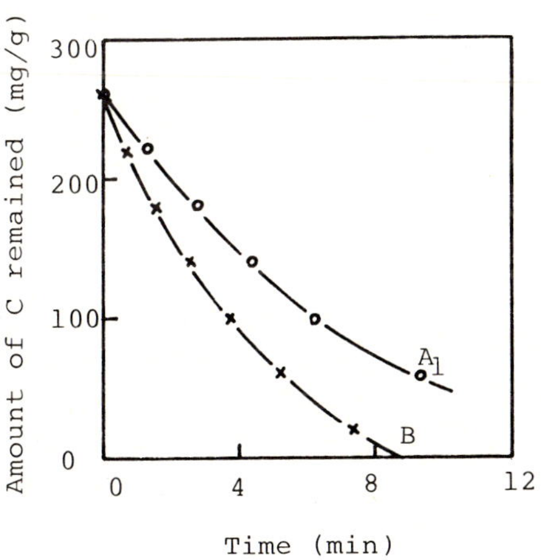

FIGURE 4. The carbon-elimination curves on catalyst A_1 and B.

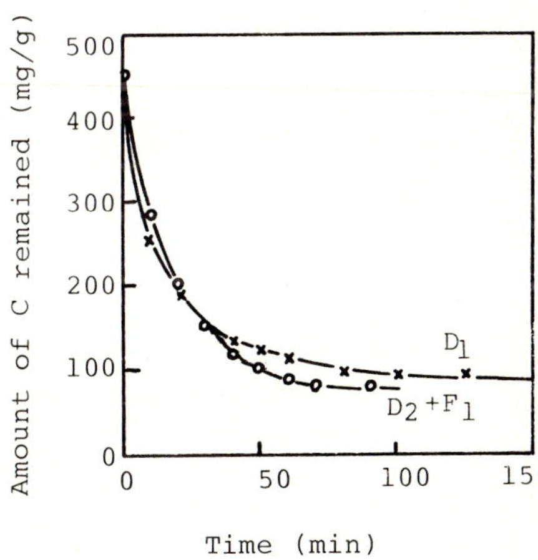

FIGURE 5. The carbon-elimination curves on catalyst D_1 and mechanically mixed catalyst of D_2 and F_1.

The decoking property of Ni and RE-Ni catallysts are investigated by passing reactant II through catalysts A_1 and B until the weight of carbon deposit is about 260 mg/g of catalyst, and then switching to steam-N_2 stream for carbon elimination. The decoking rate curve is shown in fig.4. Catalyst B has much higher rate of decoking. It is because there is RE_1 oxide in it, which adsorbs more steam than A_1 by our adsorption experiment and has greater oxidizing capacity.

A mechanically mixed catalyst D_2 and F_1 after having been deposited with about 450 mg carbon/g of catalyst is also tested for decoking by a mixture of H_2-steam-N_2. There are two decoking curves shown in fig.5, in which D_1 is for comparison. They have nearly the same manner of decoking. Here it is proved again that uncombined RE oxide has no effect on Ni.

Besides, when filamentous carbon without any contamination of Ni is mechanically well mixed with equal weight of pre-reduced catalysts D_1, E_1 and F_1 in same proportion separately and put into the reactor, heated to 550°C in the stream of deoxygenized pure nitrogen and then switched to H_2O-H_2-N_2 mixture, there is no weight change observed from any of the three samples. Such a result tells that Ni only chemically bonded with the

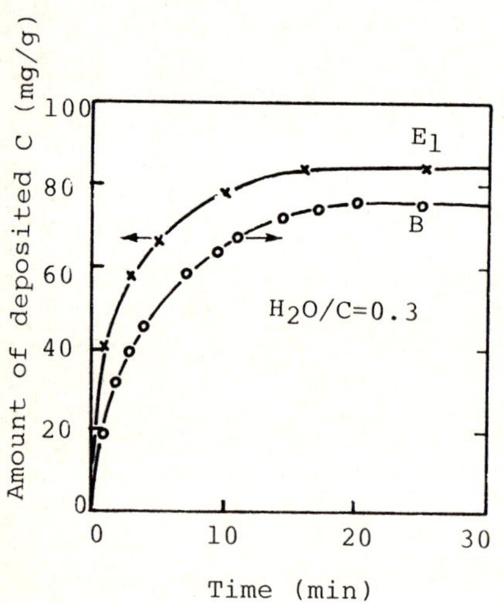

FIGURE 6. The carbon-deposition curves on catalyst B and E_1.
Cat. E_1 - coprecipitated RE-Ni cat.
Cat. B - impregnated RE-Ni cat.

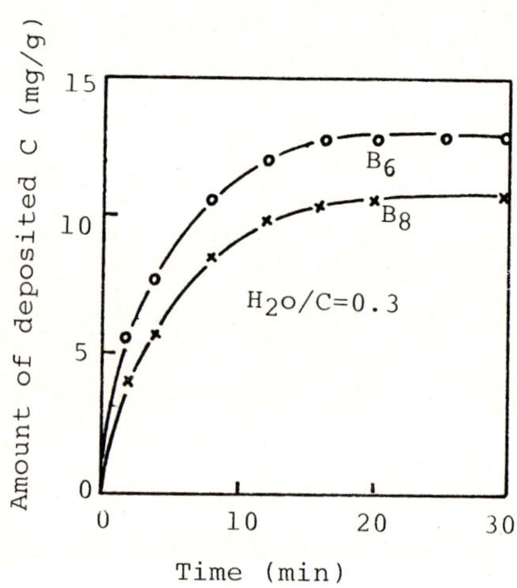

FIGURE 7. Effect of calcination temperature on amount of carbon deposited.
Cat. B_6- B_1 calcined at 600°C
Cat. B_8 - B_1 calcined at 800°C.

deposited carbon is the active site for carbon-elimination.

Methods of preparation [9]

When passing the reactant III (octane-steam-N_2) through catalysts E_1 (made by coprecipitation) and B (by impregnation), E_1 and B have same form of coking rate curve, as shown in fig.6. But B has better coking resistivity. It can be explained by that on the surface of impregnated catalyst the concentration of the active components is higher.

The precursor of catalyst B containing 6% NiO and 1% RE oxide is treated at different calcination temperature 600°C and 800°C to get catalyst B_6 and B_8. Their coking rate curves are shown in fig.7. Catalyst with higher calcination temperature behaves higher coking resistance. Because at higher heat treating temperature the mutual dispersion and interaction between RE_1 oxide and NiO are greater. As our experiment on DTA of B, its peak temperature is at 735°C and on TG the constant weight temperature is at 675°C, which are both higher than 600°C, thus calcination temperature of 600°C is somewhat too low to make the involved solid-solid reaction complete.

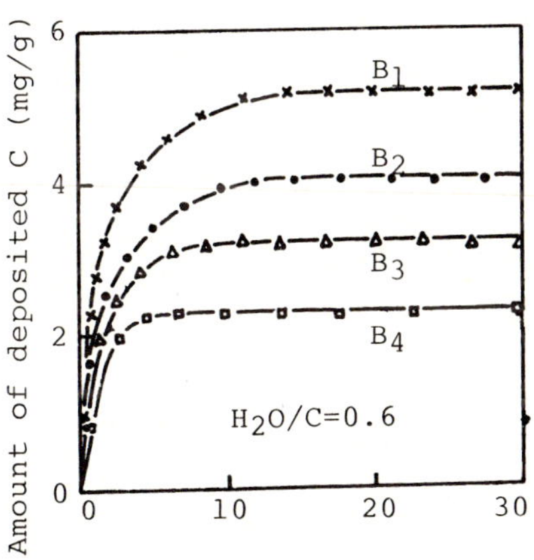

FIGURE 8. Effect of RE content in catalyst E on carbon deposiion.
Cat. B_1(6% Nio, 1% CeO_2)
Cat. B_2(6% Nio, 2% CeO_2)
Cat. B_3(6% Nio, 3% CeO_2)
Cat, B_4(6% Nio, 4% CeO_2)
Calcined at 800°C, $H_2O/C=0.6$.

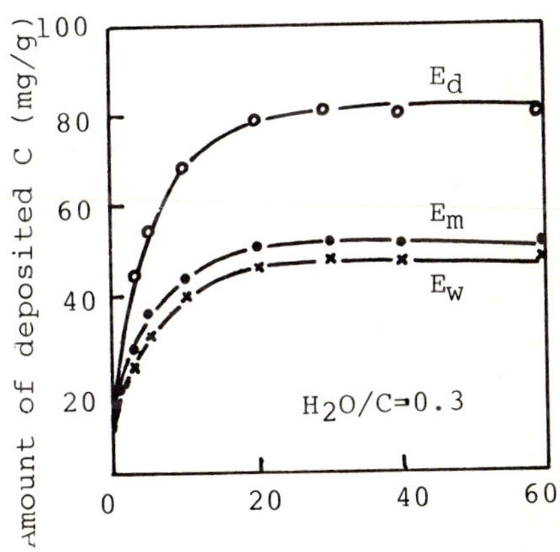

FIGURE 9. Effect of reduction conditions on carbon deposition.
Cat. E_d - reducted with dry H_2
Cat. E_m - reducted with dry H_2 first, then treated with steam for 10 min
Cat. E_w - reducted with mixture of H_2 and steam.

Four different catalysts of B each containing 1, 2, 3 and 4% of RE_1 oxide are prepared and indexed as B_1, B_2, B_3 and B_4. They gave the same form of coking rate curve as shown in fig.8. The catalyst with more RE_1 oxide has higher coking resistance and shorter time to reach zero rate point. Basically, naphtha steam-reforming reaction is an oxidative dehydrogenation reaction, naphtha is oxidized by steam to form CO and CO_2, and gives up H_2 simultaneously. RE_1 oxide is an oxidizing agent which can accelerate the above reaction, hence when more RE_1 oxide is present, the carbon deposit is less and the time of reaching equilibrium is shorter. But the optimal quantity of RE oxide in the catalyst should be carefully determined, too much will cause phase separation or formation of undesired compound.

When catalyst E_1 is reduced under different atmosphere, the resulted catalysts have different coking resistivity, as shown in fig.9. Curve E_d, E_w and E_m represent catalyt E_1 being reduced by dry hydrogen, wet hydrogen (containing 10% H_2O) and by dry hydrogen first then switched to steam for 10 min. After reduction by hydrogen with or without steam, the degree of reduction can be calculated by the weight change from their original quantity of NiO and RE^{n+} oxide present. In this experiment, NiO in E_d is 100% reduced, RE oxide is partially reduced. If assuming in the presence of steam, RE^{n+} oxide is unchanged, even having been prereduced to RE^{m+} oxide in dry hydrogen atmosphere, it can be reoxidized back to RE^{n+} oxide, then here the degree of reduction of E_w and E_m referring to NiO only are 92% and 90.7% respectively. E_w has the highest coking resistivity. E_m is a litter less, yet very close to it. Since they have nearly the same degree of reduction, but it still shows the difference due to different treatments. The idea of incomplete reduction by wet hydrogen is pratically used in industry for obtaining better coking resistance.

DISCUSSION AND CONCLUSION

Active site

For RE-Ni catalyst, the active site is Ni together with its intimately contacted RE oxides, even in the case when Ni particles is positioned on the top of filamentous carbon, otherwise the RE-Ni catalyst will not show both better coking resistance and decoking ability than catalyst containing Ni alone. RE oxides itself does not have any substantial catalytic activity both in coking and decoking, except in some sort of interaction with Ni. So Ni and RE compound must be calcined at high enough temperature such as 800-1000°C to ensure the requirement satisfied, but the optimum temperature has to be found by the overall optimation of the system.

Role of RE oxide

In RE-Ni catalyst, RE oxide is a valuable promoter, but its promoting action can only be fully displayed under the condition of the presence of steam. the combined action of RE oxide with Ni and H_2O can be visualized from the following scheme.

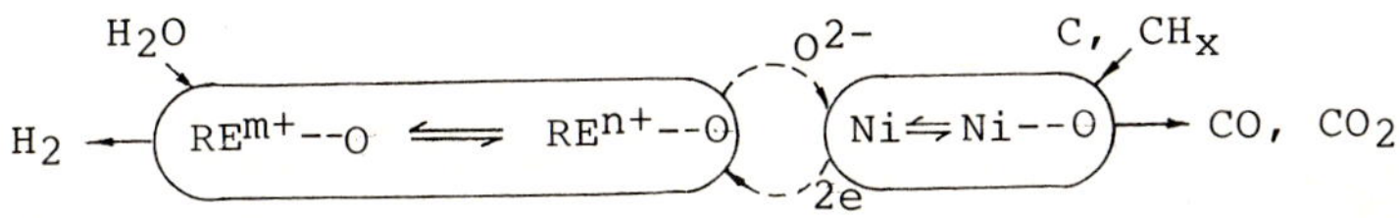

Water dissociatively adsorbs on lower valence state RE^{m+} oxide resulting in formation of $2H^+$ and O^{2-}. RE^{m+} gives up 2 e to $2H^+$ which are then reduced to H_2 and RE^{m+} itself is oxidized to RE^{n+}. O^{2-} combines with RE^{n+} to form a part of the activated lattice O^{2-} in its higher valence state oxide, and then migrates to the nearest Ni atom to form metastable surface compound Ni-O, which in subsequence, reacts with the adsorbed carbon and its precursors to form CO, CO_2 and H_2, at the same time Ni atom gives up 2e back to RE^{n+} to restore its lower valence stste RE^{m+}, thus completes the oxidation-reduction cycles, In the absence of RE oxide, H_2O should be directly adsorbed on Ni to accomplish the above redox cycle. But it is carried out in a much slower rate. In the presence of RE oxide, it accelerates the rate. In this sense, it can be said that the rate determing step of CO and CO_2 formation in the naphtha steam-reforming reaction is dissociative adsorption of steam on the active site and RE oxide is actually an oxygen-quick-transfer station.

Zero-coking rate

For a well made RE-Ni catalyst, during the naphtha steam reforming reaction the coking rate curve appears to be a progressively decreasing form. The rate of decreasing depends on RE oxide content in the catalyst and the reduction condition, the H_2O/C ratio etc. But at last a zero-coking rate point is reached. At that point no net carbon will be deposited and no activity loss will happen. We say such a state is in dynamic equilibrium estabished between coking and decoking at the definite operating condition. If, for example, H_2O/C is changed, the original equilibrium will be destroyed at once and be followed by a new equilibrium.

Dry and wet hydrogen reduction

In the dry hydrogen stream NiO and RE^{n+} oxide in the coprecipitated catalyst can be reduced completely to Ni and partly to RE^{m+} oxide which can be reoxidized by steam in the naphtha steam reforming process to form RE^{n+} oxide and H_2, yet its coking resisting property is no good. It is because as above mentioned, one of the main point of depressing coking is the active lattice oxygen quickly transferred from RE^{n+} oxide to Ni, while in the rather deeply reduced RE-Ni catalyst which contains comparatively less amount of lattice oxygen to migrate. Therefore, it will take quite a long time to build up RE^{n+} oxide before the zero coking rate is reached. During such a long period large quantity of carbon has already been deposited. In the steam RE^{m+} oxide-Ni system, there exists a dynamic equilibrium between the rate of oxygen coming from steam to form RE^{n+} oxide and that of lattice oxygen migrating from RE^{n+} oxide to Ni. In the case of wet hydrogen reduction, the reduced catalyst contains a significant amount of RE^{n+} oxide which will soon estabish equilibrium with steam and reach the zero-coking rate point and thus appears to be a very good catalyst. Hence the content of RE^{n+} oxide in the catalyst affects its coking behaviour considerably.

REFERENCES

1 J.R. Rostrup-Nielsen, Caralytic Steaming Reforming, Teknisk Forlag A/S, Copenhagen, 1984
2 L.S. Lobo and D.L. Trimm, Nature (London), 234 (1971) 15
3 S.D. Jackson, S.T. Thomson and G. Webb, J. Catal. 70 (1981) 249
4 J.R. Rostrup-Nielsen, J. Catal, 33 (1974) 184
5 C.H. Bartholomew, Catal. Rev.- Sci. Eng., 24 (1982) 67
6 A.W. Peters and G. Kim, in K.A.G. Schneider Jr. (Ed.), Industrial Applications of Rare Earth Elements, American Chemical Society, Washington, D.C., 1981, ch. 7, pp. 117-131.

7 G.V. Samsonov (Ed.), The Oxide Handbook, 2nd ed., IFI/Plenum Data Company, New York, N.Y.

8 K. Otsuka, M.Hatano and A. Morikawa, J. Catal., 79 (1983) 493

9 T. Borowiecki, Appl. Catal., 10 (1984) 273

10 X.Y. Wu, Q.L. Liao, Z.C. Liang, Y.D. Ding, Y.N. Qin and L. Chang, in G.X. Xu and J.M. Xiao (Ed.),New Frontiers In Rare Earth Science And Applications, Proc. Int. Conf. Rare Earth Development and Applications, Beijing, P.R. China, Sep. 10-14, 1985, Science Press, Beijing, 1985, Vol. 1, pp.672-674.

B. Delmon and G.F. Froment (Editors), *Catalyst Deactivation 1987*

PREVENTION OF GROWTH OF FILAMENTARY CARBON IN SUPPORTED IRON AND NICKEL CATALYSTS.

E.T.C. Vogt, A.J. van Dillen, and J.W. Geus,

Department of Inorganic Chemistry, University of Utrecht,

Croesestraat 77A, 3522 AD Utrecht, Netherlands.

ABSTRACT

Two different lines of approach in the prevention of filamentary carbon growth on supported Fe and Ni catalysts are discussed. Suppression of intermediate carbide formation by alloying the active metal leads to a decrease of carbon whisker growth, although at a considerable loss of Fischer-tropsch activity. On the one hand introduction of the SMSI-like interaction between active metal and support leads to interesting changes in the selectivity, but does not succeed in prevention of filamentary carbon growth. On the other hand, enhancement of the interaction due to the formation of a layer of nickel hydrosilicate between the nickel particles and silica support prevents whisker growth without activity loss.

INTRODUCTION.

A major problem in processing carbon-containing feeds, such as used in Fischer-Tropsch synthesis, methanation, and steam-reforming, is extensive carbon deposition. Whereas dissociation to adsorbed carbon atoms is considered to be a prerequisite and thus carbon atoms an important intermediate in the above processes, growth of the carbon atoms to larger moieties can lead to deliterious catalyst poisons.

On transition metal catalysts, the carbon moieties can exhibit a variety of properties and morphologies [1,2,3]. McCarthy et al. [4], for instance, distinguished seven different types of carbon on nickel catalysts. Using ethylene as a carbiding agent, he observed formation of long carbon filaments at temperatures between 625 and 1050 K. In this paper we will focus on the prevention of the growth of this filamentary carbon in supported catalysts. Firstly since this carbon species grows mainly at temperatures at which the processes referred to above are carried out. Secondly filamentary carbon turns out to be the most detrimental form of carbon. The high mechanical strength of the carbon fibers brings about disintegration of the catalyst bodies and leads to plugging of the reactor. Removal of a catalyst thus deactivated from the reactor is fairly difficult and regeneration of the catalyst by oxidation of the carbon can not be done readily either.

A representative picture of the carbon filaments is shown in figure 1. This figure contains a scanning and a transmission electronmicrograph of a nickel-on-silica catalyst prepared by impregnation of the support with a nickel nitrate solution. After being exposed

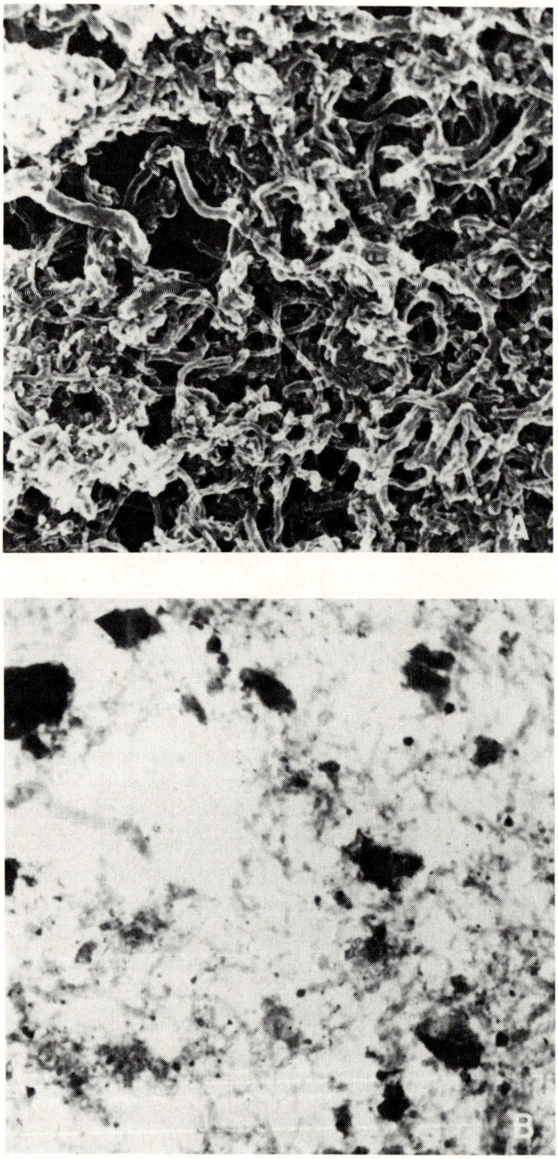

Figure 1. a. SEM image of carbided nickel catalyst prepared by impregnation of $Ni(NO)_3$ onto silica. b. STEM image of area shown in the SEM image. Magnification : 30000 x.

to carbon monoxide-hydrogen at about 700 K, the catalyst has the structure of figure 1. It can be seen that numerous carbon filaments are present within the catalyst, many of which having a nickel particle on top as has been reported earlier [3,4].

Though many investigations devoted to the prevention of the growth of filamentary carbon in catalysts have been published [1-9], the problem is still not resolved. To develop catalysts that are less liable to the growth of filamentary carbon, we will first survey the mechanism of the formation of carbon filaments. From the mechanism it will appear that either alloying with a metal not capable of forming a carbide, or strongly enhancing the interaction with the support can prevent the growth of filamentary carbon. Results with nickel and iron alloys, as well as with supports strongly interacting with iron or nickel particles will be presented.

Mechanism of Growth of Filamentary Carbon.

Several authors reporting on the growth of carbon filaments have proposed different mechanisms [5,6,7,8]. Most workers agree on a metal carbide being an intermediate. To evaluate the possibility of the formation of a metal carbide out of carbon monoxide and the decomposition of the carbide into the metal and graphite, we will first consider the thermodynamics.

Carbon monoxide contacting nickel or iron catalysts can react according to the following reactions :

Reaction	ΔH_r kJ/mol	ΔS_r J/mol.K	
$2\ CO + 2\ Fe \rightarrow Fe_2C + CO_2$	-152.7	-167.4	(1)
$2\ CO + 3\ Ni \rightarrow Ni_3C + CO_2$	-126	-129	(2)
$2\ CO \rightarrow C + CO_2$	-172.4	-177.4	(3)

The above data show that the decomposition of carbon monoxide according to reaction (3) is always thermodynamically favored. Graphite can result either from reaction (3) or from reaction (1) or (2) followed by

$$Fe_2C \rightarrow 2\ Fe + C \qquad (4)$$
$$Ni_3C \rightarrow 3\ Ni + C \qquad (5)$$

Dissociation of carbon monoxide on graphite will not proceed readily, whereas this reaction proceeds rapidly on iron and slightly less easily on most nickel surfaces. Accordingly, carbon monoxide will dissociate onto iron and most nickel surfaces and the adsorbed oxygen atoms thus formed will react with another carbon monoxide molecule to carbon dioxide. The carbon atoms thus set free will convert the metal into metal carbide, which subsequently excretes the thermodynamically more stable graphite.

It is very interesting to note that no growth of filamentary carbon has been reported under conditions where reactions (1) or (2) are thermodynamically not favorable [8]. It has, moreover, been demonstrated that the thermodynamic equilibrium with the gas phase involves the metal carbides in an extensive range of temperatures [8]. We therefore conclude that formation of a metal carbide is a prerequisite for growth of carbon filaments.

The carbon filaments grow with nickel on one side and with iron mostly on one, but also on two sides of the metal particles. Therefore the carbon taken up at the free surfaces of a metal particle must migrate through the metal towards the growing carbon filament(s). It has been proposed that a temperature gradient over the metal particle is providing the driving force for the migration of carbon atoms through the metal particles [5]. According to this theory, no carbide is formed, but carbon atoms dissolved into the metal migrate to the growing filament. The temperature gradient causes a different solubility of carbon atoms and thus provides the concentration gradient. However, a substantial temperature gradient over a metal particle of about 40 nm calls for a very high flow rate of thermal energy. It can be questioned whether such a flow rate of thermal energy can be established continuously. A concentration gradient brought about by different carbon species dissolved in the metal with a different solubility has also been proposed [6], as well as a non-stoichiometric carbide able to exhibit a concentration gradient [7].

Using magnetic measurements de Bokx et al [8] found evidence for the presence of a carbide intermediate during interaction of supported iron and nickel catalysts with carbon containing gases. The authors therefore reject transport of carbon interstitially dissolved , since the solubility of interstitial carbon is too low to account for the magnetic effects. A combination of magnetic measurements and temperature-programmed hydrogenation indicated that the intermediate carbide with silica-supported iron is the ε/ε'-carbide ($Fe_{2+x}C$), while silica-supported nickel reacts to a non-stoichiometric carbide [9]. The magnetization passing through a maximum during exposure to a carbiding gas mixture points to an induction period before the growth of carbon filaments starts. Apparently nucleation of graphite does not proceed immediately.

High-resolution electronmicroscopy and electron diffraction have shown [10] that the carbon filaments consist of small graphite platelets. The platelets are excreted parallel to the surfaces of the metal particles that are excreting the carbon atoms. The growth can be explained by the fact that on nickel (111) surfaces graphite layers are fitting almost perfectly, while on iron (110) surfaces the fit is also good. Since for the nucleation of a graphite layer interaction with the metal surface is required, the graphite is growing only on the above crystallographic surfaces. Nickel particles assume a morphology in which two (111) surfaces are excreting carbon atoms, and the remaining surfaces have a different crystallographic orientation. As a result graphite layers enclosing the angle that is enclosed also by the two (111) surfaces are growing. With iron particles, a morphology exhibiting four closely packed (110) surfaces is sometimes established. As a result a particle exhibiting growth of a carbon filament on two sides can be seen (fig.2).

Extensive evidence on monocrystalline nickel surfaces can guide the development of a more detailed mechanism. Though the structure of nickel carbide slightly differs from that of pure nickel, the characteristics of the different crystallographic nickel surfaces will not be strongly modified.

Blakely and coworkers [11] investigated the equilibrium segregation of carbon on

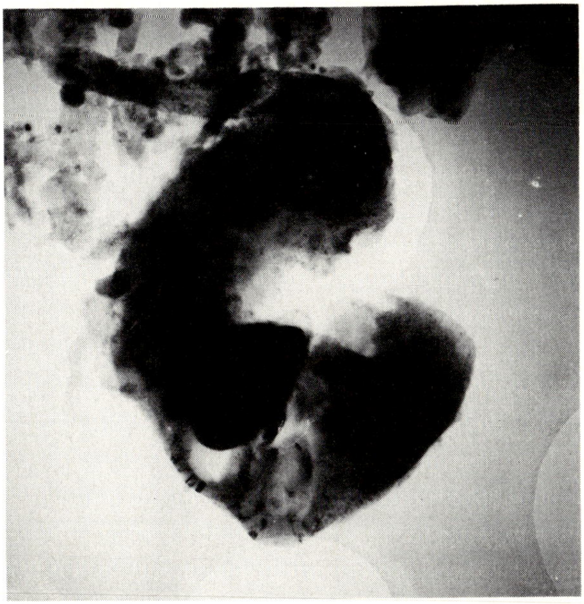

Figure 2. TEM image of carbon filaments formed on a silica supported iron catalyst. Clearly, the formation of the so-called octopus carbon can be observed. Magnification : 162000 x.

different crystallographic surfaces of nickel starting from carbon dissolved in the bulk. On Ni(111) surfaces the authors observed segregation of multilayers of graphite. The carbon atoms in the graphite layer contacting the Ni surface atoms were found to be slightly more stable than carbon atoms in bulk graphite. Segregation of graphite layers onto Ni(111) surfaces, where an almost perfect epitaxial fit is present, has therefore been firmly established.

Depending on the temperature and the bulk carbon concentration, graphite can locally segregate on the Ni(100) surface. At temperatures higher than that at which graphite segregates, Blakely and coworkers [11] found two stable structures of adsorbed carbon atoms covering the surface completely. From the experimental carbon coverages at different temperatures, the authors calculated the heat of segregation. Above 652 K a structure saturating at a Ni(s)/C ratio of four was observed exhibiting a heat of segregation of about 46 kJ/mol. Below 652 K a structure saturating at a Ni(s)/C ratio of 2 and a heat of segregation of 21 kJ/mol was found. A stepped Ni (100) surface showed a much higher heat of segregation, viz. about 84 kJ/mol. Remarkably, a Ni (110) surface did not exhibit segregation of carbon.

The above experimental data show that segregation of graphite layers preferably proceeds on Ni (111) surfaces. The Ni (110) surface does not display carbon segregation and the (stepped) Ni (100) surface exhibits segregation of carbon atoms in stable structures not related to the graphite structure. The mechanism based on segregation of graphite layers from a carbide phase preferably on Ni (111) planes also involves migration of carbon atoms from Ni surfaces into the bulk.

Schouten et al. [12] have investigated migration of carbon atoms deposited from methane onto Ni (100) and Ni (110) surfaces into the bulk. Methane does not decompose on Ni (111) surfaces. It was observed that carbon deposited onto Ni (110) is completely taken up into the bulk. Carbon atoms deposited onto Ni (100) appeared to be much more stable. As in the above segregation experiments two stable coverages were found, again of Ni(s)/C ratios of four and two. The coverage of the higher Ni(s)/C ratio was also the most stable.

The segregation and dissolution experiments hence agree very well. However, the values for the heats of segregation determined in both types of experiments are different. The dissolution experiments led to higher values. Schouten et al observed surface segregated carbon atoms to be less stable at higher bulk concentrations of carbon [12]. They therefore ascribe the quantitative differences to the different bulk concentrations of carbon in both types of experiments.

We now will consider the relative rates at which carbon atoms will be made available on different nickel surfaces from molecules as CO or CH_4. Using ellipsometry, which does not affect adsorbed CO, Labohm et al. [13] established that dissociation of CO does not proceed on Ni (111). On the Ni (110) and (100) surfaces adsorbed CO dissociates at temperatures above about 150°C. Interaction of Ni surfaces with CH_4 and CO is therefore highly structure-sensitive. Carbon atoms are deposited onto Ni (100) and (110) surfaces in contrast to Ni (111) surfaces. Labohm et al. [13] also found that carbon deposited onto the Ni (100) surface suppresses the adsorption of CO. At a carbon coverage of about 0.5 the adsorption of CO at low pressures is completely absent. Since adsorbed carbon atoms at this coverage are stable against dissolution into the bulk, dissolution of carbon atoms from CO from Ni (100) surfaces is not likely to be important. Dissociation of CH_4 and CO on Ni (110) and subsequent dissolution, on the other hand, will proceed relatively rapidly.

The above experimental data suggest formation and dissolution of adsorbed carbon mainly on surfaces such as the Ni (110) of a Ni crystallite. The carbon atoms are excreted as graphite layers on the (111) surfaces, where rapid nucleation of graphite is possible. From magnetic measurements on nickel crystallites exposing crystallographic planes of different dimensions, it could be established that hydrogen atoms can penetrate into the nickel surface yielding a nickel surface hydride, provided the crystallographic planes are small. With small planes a sidewards shift of the metal surface atoms is relatively easy. We thus assume that Ni (111) surfaces of a small dimension will accommodate carbon atoms in between the metal surface atoms and thus behave analogously to Ni (100) planes. The structure of the closely packed surfaces is hence distorted, and graphite layers do not fit on the modified surface. Excretion of graphite therefore calls for relatively large (111) planes and thus for relatively large metal particles.

Prevention of Growth of Filamentary Carbon.

The growth of filamentary carbon can thus be suppressed by preventing either the formation of a metastable metal carbide or relatively large carbided metal particles assuming a morphology with at least two extended (111) planes with nickel and (110) planes with iron. Formation of an intermediate, metastable metal carbide can be avoided by alloying of the active metal with a metal not forming a carbide of a significant stability. Since the alloying metal cannot form a carbide, dissociative adsorption of carbon monoxide will only proceed on sufficiently large ensembles of the active metal at the alloy surface. The dilution of the surface with inactive metal atoms can be expected to cause a significant decrease in the activity. In our laboratory copper and platinum, metals not forming bulk carbides, have been used to alloy nickel and iron. The results on these alloy catalysts will be reviewed. Since a relatively small number of supported metal particles of pure iron or nickel, or containing a small amount of the inactive metal can produce a large amount of carbon, it is essential that the alloy particles have a uniform composition. Special preparation procedures were used to produce supported alloy catalysts containing alloy particles of a very small variation in chemical composition.

The second of the above approaches calls for relatively small metal particles strongly adhering to the support. Carbon can also be segregated at the interface with the support. With large particles the morphology at the interface will change due to the excreted carbon atoms so as to display two closely packed planes enclosing a small angle at the interface with the support. Another possibility to prevent growth of filamentary carbon can therefore be the establishment of a strong interaction of the metal particle with the support. Experimental results for nickel supported on silica, titania, and silica covered by a thin layer of vanadia will be reviewed.

Prevention of Filamentary Carbon Growth by Suppression of Carbide Formation.

Van Stiphout et al. [14] reported on the activity and stability of silica-supported Ni/Pt catalysts. The catalysts containing alloy particles of a uniform composition were prepared by consecutive deposition-precipitation of nickel and platinum onto silica. It was observed that alloying with platinum indeed suppresses the growth of filamentary carbon provided the platinum content is above about 10 at.%. At platinum contents above 10 at.%, the methanation activity of the catalyst is significantly lower than that of pure nickel. Though the activity with methanation is not a problem in view of the high exothermicity of the reaction, the cost of platinum is a drawback.

Copper is much less expensive and, hence, more favorable to alloy with nickel or iron.

The tendency of copper to react to a carbide is very small indeed, as is evidenced by the use of copper containing catalyst in the methanol synthesis. The selectivity is highly elevated and no marked amounts of hydrocarbons are being produced. Mesters [15] , van Stiphout et al. [16] and Ponec [17] have studied the activity and stability of nickel-copper alloy catalysts. Particles of a very homogeneous chemical composition were produced by the decomposition of nickel carbonyl into a fluidized bed of a supported copper catalyst. The copper catalyst was produced by precipitation of copper(II) onto suspended silica from a homogeneous solution using the hydrolysis of urea. The resulting catalyst contains small copper particles that are very thermostable. It was established that alloying with copper suppresses the growth of filamentary carbon. To suppress the growth of carbon almost completely a copper content of about 30 at.% is required. Though copper-nickel catalysts of a copper content of 30 at.% or more exhibit a lower activity, the drop in activity is less severe than the suppression of the growth of carbon. Coprecipitation of copper(II) and nickel(II) also leads to particles of a fairly uniform chemical composition. It was observed that a small fraction of relatively large pure nickel particles brings about a rapid growth of filamentary carbon. A simultaneous deposition-precipitation of copper and nickel did not lead to the formation of large pure nickel particles.

In view of the more favorable selectivity of iron for Fischer-Tropsch synthesis, it seemed to be more interesting to produce copper-iron than copper-nickel catalysts. Wielers et al. [18,19] produced copper-iron catalysts both by the afore mentioned decomposition of iron carbonyl and by simultaneous deposition-precipitation of copper and iron. With the latter catalysts the iron was reduced in two steps, first to iron(II) and subsequently to metallic iron. The high solubility of iron(II) in silica brought about a selective removal of iron(II) out of the mixed copper-iron moieties deposited onto the silica. Reduction at more elevated temperatures led to formation of pure iron particles out of a fraction of the iron ions taken up intermediately by the silica. The iron particles were found to exhibit a rapid growth of very long carbon fibers during Fischer-Tropsch synthesis.Dissolution into the silica and subsequent formation of pure metallic iron was assessed by Mössbauer spectroscopy. The growth of long carbon fibers was observed in TEM investigations.

Mössbauer experiments also indicated that a large fraction of the iron in the reduced catalysts was present in copper-iron alloy particles. Infrared spectra of carbon monoxide adsorbed on the alloy catalysts indicated no substantial surface enrichment of one of the constituents of the alloy. However, as with copper-nickel catalysts, a considerable enrichment of the surface with iron was found on prolonged interaction with carbon monoxide.

Iron-copper alloys are endothermic and thus liable to decomposition into a copper- and an iron-rich phase. Experiments on single crystals have indicated that decomposition into two phases indeed proceeds easily with copper-iron alloy surfaces. Van Pruissen et al. [20] have observed that a surface alloy prepared by decomposition of iron carbonyl on a copper single crystal initially leads to a copper-rich surface. The iron is present virtually completely below the first atomic layer. However, interaction with oxygen leads to separation of iron oxide at the surface of the oxidized copper. Wielers [19] analogously found that interaction of a copper-iron catalyst with a carbon monoxide hydrogen flow leads to separation of an iron carbide on the surface of the remaining copper particles. At the interface between the iron and the copper very thin carbon filaments of a low mechanical strength were growing.

Prevention of Filamentary Carbon by Enhanced Interaction with the Support.

In the literature a strong interaction between metal particles and the support has been reported for titania and vanadia supports [20–27]. After reduction of the catalysts at elevated temperatures some peculiar phenomena such as a low extent of adsorption of hydrogen and carbon monoxide can be observed. The extent of adsorption corresponding to the size of the metal particles as determined by electronmicroscopy can be re-established by oxidation and reduction at a lower temperature. After much debate the above strong metal support interaction (SMSI) has appeared to be due to reduced moieties of the support covering the metal particles. Oxidation of the reduced moieties decreases the interaction and the surface of the metal particles is again (partly) denuded. With nickel migration of reduced species of the support on top of the metal particles can be explained readily. It has been shown that calcination of titania-supported nickel oxide leads to formation of some nickel titanate. Subsequent reduction leaves some reduced titanium oxide on the nickel particles.

The above strong interaction between metal particles and supports that can be reduced to a lower valence state may be utilized to suppress the growth of filamentary carbon. Since hydrogenation of CO leads to formation of water that can oxidize the reduced support and thus strongly diminish the interaction with the metal, we want to assess the degree of reduction of the support contacting the metal particles during the catalytic reaction. The assessment can be made from the selectivity of the hydrogenation. The presence of strong metal support interaction during the catalytic reaction is apparent from a higher selectivity for higher hydrocarbons.

Balkenende et al. [22] investigated the hydrogenation of carbon monoxide and the deposition of carbon on nickel-on-titania catalysts. De Bokx et al.[21] prepared these nickel

TABLE 1.
Ethane to Methane ratios at different temperatures at methanol pressure of 8 kPa.

catalyst	C_2H_6 / CH_4 ratio 476 K	497 K
20% Ni / SiO_2 [1]	<0.01	<0.01
10% Ni / Al_2O_3 [2]	0.16	0.08
5% Ni / TiO_2	0.40	0.16

[1] prepared by HDP using urea decomposition
[2] prepared by HDP using alkali injection

catalysts by deposition-precipitation on nickel ions onto titania (Degussa FRG P25, 80% anatase 20% rutile). The catalysts reduced at 723 K exhibited SMSI behaviour during the catalytic reaction as is evident from the data of table 1. In this table selectivities measured for a nickel-on-silica and a nickel-on-alumina catalyst are compared with the selectivity of the titania-supported catalyst. The much higher production of C_2 hydrocarbons is apparent.

The results of table 1 agree well with observation of other authors (Bartholomew et al. [23], Burch and Flambard [24], and Vannice [25,26]). These authors also observed a shift in the selectivity towards higher hydrocarbons, which is acribed to the presence of special sites at the boundaries between the reduced moieties of the support and the metal (Burch and Flambard [24]). However, the above authors all reported deactivation of the catalysts during prolonged use. The deactivation was acribed to carbon deposition, though the nature of the deposited carbon has not been described. Apparently, SMSI during the catalytic reaction does not prevent formation of carbon.

To investigate the possibly beneficial effect of SMSI on the prevention of growth of carbon fibers more closely, we used vanadia as a support. SMSI effects for vanadia have been published in the literature. To assess the effect of SMSI on the growth of carbon accurately, we will compare the results of a vanadia-supported nickel catalyst with those of silica-supported nickel catalysts. Silica has not been reported to exhibit SMSI effects. Two different nickel-on-silica catalysts were investigated, a catalyst in which the nickel particles are bonded weakly to the support and one in which the interaction with the support is much stronger. The first nickel catalyst is prepared by impregnation of silica with a solution of nickel formiate and drying. The second nickel catalyst, in which the nickel particles are anchored to the silica, will be dealt with in detail later on.

To enable us to arrive at a reliable comparison, we used a newly developed procedure to cover supports, such as silica, with a layer of vanadia. This procedure involves deposition-precipitation of vanadium(III) onto suspended silica (Vogt et al. [28,29]). In a recent paper Vogt et al. [30] described the use of this technique for the preparation of a catalyst in which nickel has been applied onto a silica support covered by vanadia. The data of table 2 show the selectivities of the three nickel catalysts. The low selectivity for higher hydrocarbons of the silica-supported nickel catalysts shows the absence of SMSI effects, whereas the high production of higher hydrocarbons demonstrates SMSI to be exhibited by the vanadia-silica supported catalyst. The higher hydrocarbons produced by the vanadia containing catalyst ranged up to C_4 and are mainly olefinic. With the catalysts supported on pure silica, the formation of higher hydrocarbons was limited to ethane.

Though the presence of SMSI has been demonstrated unambiguously for the vanadia-containing catalyst, it is still liable to deactivation by carbon deposition. During a typical run of 15 h, the activity dropped to about 15% of the initial value. Model carburisation experiments have been performed in a flow of 3.0% of CO and 0.6% of H_2 at 550°C and a total pressure of 1 bar. With the vanadia containing catalyst and the nickel catalyst

TABLE 2.
C_2 to CH_4 ratios of catalysts at 570 K, CO 5%, H_2 15%, total pressure 1 bar, s.v = 8000 h^{-1}.

catalyst	C_2-CH_4 ratio
15% Ni-SiO_2[1]	0.018
17% Ni-SiO_2[2]	0.003
4% Ni-28%V_2O_3/SiO_2	0.31

[1] prepared by impregnation of nickelformate
[2] prepared by HDP using urea decomposition

prepared by impregnation, Ni/C ratios of 0.1 or less were determined. This indicates a take up of carbon far in excess of Ni_3C and thus the growth of carbon filaments.

Investigation of the carbided samples in the electronmicroscope showed that the large amount of carbon in the vanadia containing catalyst was due to a relatively small number of large nickel particles. The large nickel particles had produced a very large amount carbon, that was present as very long carbon fibers. The much more numerous, very small nickel particles had not grown carbon fibers. Evidently, a small fraction of the nickel had not properly been deposited onto the vanadia-covered silica. As a result, some large nickel particles resulted during the thermal pretreatment, that led to an extensive growth of carbon. To prevent growth of carbon, it is therefore essential to avoid formation of even a small number of metal particles, not being attached properly to the support. Due to the small interaction with the support or to an improper application onto the support, some larger nickel particles result that give rise to a large amount of carbon.

We assume that the activity of the small nickel particles in the catalyst is not affected during the reaction. The drop in activity is therefore attributed to the diffusion limitation brought about by the dense carbon fibers. That small particles are not deactivated is indicated by the fact that the nickel-silica catalyst produced by deposition-precipitation did not show growth of carbon fibers and did not loose activity. We now will discuss the origin of the absence of carbon growth in this catalyst.

Hermans and Geus [31] reported on the preparation of nickel-on-silica catalysts by deposition-precipitation from homogeneous solution. It was established, that the use of the hydrolysis of urea at 363 K results in surface reaction of the silica support with nickel ions to form nickel hydrosilicate. Upon reduction with hydrogen, only up to 70% of this hydrosilicate will be reduced to metallic nickel, as was determined thermogravimetrically and magnetically by Kuijpers et al. [32]. Catalysts of this type were tested by several authors [22,30,32,33].

In the previously mentioned carburisation experiments performed by Vogt et al. [30]), a sample with a loading of 17 wt% was tested. It was found, that upon prolonged exposure to reaction mixture of a 5/1 ratio of CO/H_2 at 550°C, virtually no carbon uptake occurred. A Ni/C ratio of 10 was reported indicating mere partial formation of nickel carbide. As mentioned before, under these conditions, samples prepared by impregnation extensively formed carbon filaments. Kuijpers and Geus [33] reported on carbon deposition from CO and CH_4 at several temperatures. Using CH_4 up to 350°C only surface carbide formation is reported, whereas CO-decomposition resulted in and remained restricted to bulk carbide formation. Kuijpers et al [32] described the use of the catalyst under more severe process conditions. H_2/CO ratios below unity at a total pressure of 600 kPa required steam addition to maintain activity. At higher ratios, addition of steam was not necessary, and the catalysts activity remained constant over periods of up to 1000 h.

Van Stiphout [34] recently described a preparation technique utilising electrochemical deposition of the nickel onto the silica. Using this technique, a number of disadvantages of the preparation by urea decomposition, such as waste problems and the preparation time can be resolved without changing the catalyst characteristics.

Concluding remarks.

Three techniques for the prevention of filamentary carbon growth have been described. The prevention of the formation of an intermediate carbide by alloying seems to be able to prevent carbon whisker growth, however, at a loss of activity with Ni/Cu and Ni/Pt catalysts. Alloying Fe with Cu leads to an alloy that is not sufficiently stable against segregation of iron carbide. Moreover, the iron is liable to be separated from the copper by intermediate dissolution into the silica support, which leads to some pure iron particles. Carbon fibers can grow from these pure iron particles.

The enhancement of metal support interaction by SMSI effects seems to be able to prevent carbon whisker growth. However, virtually all the metal particles must be strongly bonded to the reducible support. Even a small fraction of metal particles not being attached strongly to the support can produce rapidly a large amount of carbon and thus can deactivate the catalyst.

A reducible support exhibiting the selectivity characteristic of SMSI is not required to suppress the growth of carbon. A strong chemical interaction of metallic nickel with an intermediate partially reduced hydrosilicate layer has appeared to provide the best stability against the growth of carbon up till now. However, total reduction of the hydrosilicate remains thermodynamically possible in the reducing atmospheres and at temperatures usually present in important processes, which could give rise to possible filamentary carbon.

REFERENCES

1 *C.H. Bartholomew, Catal.Rev.-Sci.Eng 24 (1982) 67.*

2 *D.L. Trimm, Catal.Rev.-Sci.Eng 16 (1977) 155.*

3 *J.G. McCarty, H. Wise, J. Catal 57 (1979) 64.*

4 *J.G. McCarty, P.Y. Hou, D. Sheridan, H. Wise, in "Coke Formation on Metal Surfaces" (L.F. Albright, R.T.K. Baker, eds.), ACS Symposium Series 202, p.253, Amer. Chem. Soc., Washington D.C., 1982.*

5 *R.T.K. Baker, M. Barber, M. Harris, F. Feates, R. Waite, J. Catal 26 (1972) 51.*

6 *J.R. Rostrup-Nielsen, D.L. Trimm, J. Catal 48 (1977) 155*

7 *R.A. Buyanov, V.V Chesnokov, A.D Afasen'ev, V.S. Babenko, Kinet.Katal. 18 (1977) 839; R.A. Buyanov, V.V Chesnokov, A. Afasen'ev, Kinet. Katal. 20 (1979) 166.; R.A. Buyanov, Kinet.Katal 21 (1980) 189.*

8 P.K. de Bokx, A.J.H.M. Kock, E. Boellaard, W. Klop, J.W. Geus, J. Catal. 96 (1986) 454-467.
9 A.J.H.M. Kock, P.K. de Bokx, E. Boellaard, W. Klop, J.W. Geus, J. Catal. 96 (1986) 468-480.
10 E. Boellaard, P.K. de Bokx, A.J.H.M. Kock, J.W. Geus, J. Catal. 96 (1986) 481.
11 J.C. Shelton, H.R. Patil, and J.M. Blakely, Surf. Sci. 43 (1974) 493-520; L.C. Isset and J.M. Blakely, Surf. Sci. 47 (1975) 645-649 and Surf. Sci. 58 (9176) 397-414; M. Eizenberg and J.M. Blakely, Surf. Sci. 82 (1979) 228-236.
12 F.C. Schouten, O.L.J. Gijzeman and G.A. Bootsma, Bull. Soc. Chem. Belg., 88 (1979) 541.
13 F. Labohm, C.W.R. Engelen, O.L.J. Gijzeman, J.W. Geus and G.A. Bootsma, J. Chem. Soc., Farad. Trans. I, 78 (1982) 2435.
14 P.C.M. van Stiphout, J.W. Geus, Appl. Catal., 25 (1986) 19.
15 C.M.A.M. Mesters, On the Preparation and Reactivity of Copper-Nickel Alloys, Ph.D. Thesis, University of Utrecht, 1984
16 P.C.M. van Stiphout, in publication.
17 V. Ponec, Int. J. Quant. Chem. Suppl. 2, 12 (1977) 1.
18 A.F.H. Wielers., C.E.C.A. Hop, J. van Beynum, A.M. van der Kraan, J.W. Geus, J. Catal, submitted.
19 A.F.H. Wielers, G.W. Koebrugge, J.W. Geus, J. Catal., submitted.
20 O.P. van Pruissen, M.M.M. Dings, E. Boellaard, O.L.J. Gijzeman and J.W. Geus, Appl. Surf. Sci. 27 (1986) 24-51.
21 P.K. de Bokx, R.L.C. Bonné, J.W. Geus, J. Catal., accepted.
22 A.R. Balkenende, P.K. de Bokx, J.W. Geus, Appl. Catal., accepted.
23 C.H. Bartholomew, R.B. Pannell, J.L. Butler, J. Catal. 65 (1980) 335.
24 R. Burch, A.R. Flambard, J. Catal. 78 (1982) 389.
25 M.A. Vannice, Proc. Pan-pacific synfuels conference, vol 1, p.208, Japan Petroleum Institute, 1982.
26 M.A. Vannice, R.L. Garten, J. Catal. 56 (1979) 236.
27 S.J. Tauster, S.C. Fung, J. Catal. 55 (1978) 29.
28 E.T.C. Vogt, M. de Boer, A.J. van Dillen, J.W. Geus, Appl. Catal, submitted.
29 H. Barten, R. Leferink, F.J.J.G. Janssen, F.M.G. van der Kerkhof, E.T.C. Vogt, A.J. van Dillen, J.W. Geus, in Proceedings 4th International Symposium on Heterogeneous Catalysts, Louvain la Neuve, 1986.
30 E.T.C. Vogt, A.Q.M. Boon, A.J. van Dillen, J.W. Geus, Ind. Eng. Chem. Prod. Res. Dev., submitted.
31 L.A.M. Hermans, J.W. Geus, in Studies of Surface Science and Catalysis, vol 3, Elsevier, Amsterdam, 1979, p 113.
32 E.G.M. Kuijpers, R.B. Tjepkema, J.W. Geus, J. Molec. Catal. 25 (1984) 241.
33 E.G.M. Kuijpers, J.W. Geus, Fuel 62 (1983) 158.
34 P.C.M. van Stiphout, in ref 25.

B. Delmon and G.F. Froment (Editors), *Catalyst Deactivation 1987*

COPPER CATALYSTS FOR THE HYDROLYSIS OF ACRYLONITRILE TO ACRYLAMIDE: DEACTIVATION AND CURE

J.C. LEE, D.L. TRIMM, M.S. WAINWRIGHT, N.W. CANT[1], M.A. KOHLER and N.I. ONUOHA

School of Chemical Engineering and Industrial Chemistry, The University of New South Wales, P.O. Box 1 Kensington N.S.W. 2033, Australia.

[1]School of Chemistry, Macquarie University, North Ryde N.S.W. 2109, Australia.

ABSTRACT

The deactivation of copper based catalysts for the hydrolysis of acrylonitrile to acrylamide has been studied using Raney copper and supported copper on silica catalysts. Initial rapid deactivation is due to the fouling of the surface by polymer produced from acrylamide. At least part of the polymer is formed by a process involving the catalysts. A second deactivation process caused by the interaction of the catalyst with oxygen is observed. This deactivation can be very significant with supported catalysts where small copper particles oxidise more easily. The activity of the catalyst after the initial deactivation is found to depend on the size of the pores in the catalyst.

INTRODUCTION

The hydrolysis of acrylonitrile to acrylamide over heterogeneous catalysts is an important industrial process [1]. The reaction

$$CH_2{=}CHCN \ + \ H_2O \ \rightarrow \ CH_2{=}CHCONH_2 \qquad (1)$$

is catalysed by a variety of metals and metal oxides [2-8], with copper based catalysts being preferred on an industrial scale [9].

All catalysts for the reaction deactivate during use. At least part of the deactivation appears to result from the accumulation of acrylamide polymers on the surface [10,11]. Raney copper is the preferred industrial catalysts not only because it is selective for the hydrolysis but also because removal of polymer deactivant can be achieved without significant degradation of the solid by exposing the spent catalyst to sodium hydroxide solutions similar to those used to activate the Raney copper alloy.

There is also preliminary evidence that deactivation caused by oxygen dissolved in the feed may be important [10]. This deactivation is reported to be slower than that caused by polymer deposition.

Hirai et al [12] have reported that deactivation is significantly reduced by the use of supported copper catalysts containing copper particles of less than 10 nm diameter. If the formation of polymer is related to copper, such supported catalysts should have a lower density of surface copper atoms, a smaller initiation surface for polymerisation and less deactivation. As a result, the present studies were initiated to compare deactivation on Raney and supported copper catalysts, to study the causes of deactivation and to attempt to minimise deactivation by control of catalysts and operating conditions.

EXPERIMENTAL

The Raney copper catalysts were prepared by the selective leaching of aluminium from a copper alloy (50 wt% Cu : 50 wt% Al) using the procedure described by Onuoha and Wainwright [13] and Tomsett et al [14]. Supported copper on silica was prepared by ion exchange following the technique described by Kobayashi et al [15] and developed by Kohler et al [16]. All catalysts were fully characterised and the principal results are summarised in Table 1.

The apparatus and analytical procedure for measuring the activity of catalysts for the hydrolysis of acrylonitrile have been previously described [13,17]. Approximately 1.5 g of Cu/SiO_2 or 0.4 g of Raney copper were placed in a 6 mm i.d. stainless steel U tube reactor and were reduced in a flowing 5% H_2/N_2 mixture at 523 K. The temperature was then raised to 573 K and reduction in pure H_2 was performed for a further 16 hours. The reactor was then cooled and placed in a vigorously stirred oil bath so that the catalyst bed was maintained at 323 ± 1 K. The feed stream (7 wt% acrylonitrile in distilled water) was passed through the reactor and the product stream was analysed for acrylamide by HPLC (Gow-Mac Series 80-600) using a U.V. detector operating at fixed wavelength (254 nm). Separation was achieved by on line sampling to a 250 x 4.6 mm column packed with 10 μ Bondapak C_{18} silica gel using methanol/water (30/70 vol %) as the mobile phase. Where necessary, the oxygen content of the feed stream was measured using a E.I.L. Model 1520 portable dissolved oxygen meter.

Fractional conversion was always kept below 0.03 to ensure differential rate measurements. Several samples were taken to establish rate (r) at particular times. Activities were reported as $a = r/r_0$.

RESULTS AND DISCUSSION

Initial studies were carried out using Raney copper catalysts (samples A to D) which had previously been used to establish the kinetics of the hydrolysis reaction [13]. The catalysts were prepared by leaching the parent alloy to different extents, the characteristics of the resulting solids being summarised in Table 1.

The catalysts were then used to promote the hydrolysis of acrylonitrile and showed evidence of two types of deactivation. These initial experiments were

TABLE 1

Characteristics of fresh catalysts

Sample	Designation	Time of leaching (min)	Copper (wt%)	S_{BET} (m^2/g.cat)	Pore Volume (cm^3/g.cat)	Average Pore radius (nm)
Raney Cu	A	40	55.7	4.54	.029	12.8
Raney Cu	B	140	72.8	12.6	.117	21.4
Raney Cu	C	180	79.1	13.9	.159	22.8
Raney Cu	D	1440	98.8	15.3	.238	32.0
Raney Cu	E	2880	98.9	14.2	.107	13.0
Cu/SiO_2	F	-	3.9	190	1.041	10.6
Cu/SiO_2	G	-	7.2	190	1.247	9.5

S_{BET} : Catalyst surface area

Catalysts A-D were leached at 313 K, catalyst E was leached at 274 K.

conducted using feed mixtures prepared from distilled water without attempt to control oxygen levels. An initial rapid deactivation was followed by a period of slower deactivation (Figure 1), with the most leached catalyst deactivating least.

Rapid deactivation has been suggested to result from the deposition of polymerised acrylamide on the surface [10]. If this is so, then the polymer should foul the surface and block pores. Samples of catalyst were removed from the reactor after various times on line, dried and characterised. Available pore volume and average pore radius were both found to decrease with time on line (Table 2).

TABLE 2

Catalyst morphology at various stages of deactivation of Raney copper.

Time on stream t (h)	Total surface area S_{BET} (m^2/g.cat)	Pore volume (cm^3/g)	Average pore radius (nm)	Relative activity r/r_o
0	13.9	.159	22.8	1.0
29	14.9	.108	14.5	0.49
72	13.9	.084	12.0	0.21
169	13.4	.060	9.0	0.13

Given the structure of the catalysts, most of the available copper surface area is within the pore system. Deactivation would then be expected to result from polymer nucleating on the surface and growing to close off pores, thus restricting access to the interior of the catalyst particles. In this case the extent of pore closure and catalyst deactivation would be expected to depend on the square of the radius of the pores. As seen from Figure 2, this is found to be the case.

Initial rapid deactivation is known to occur on Raney copper catalysts [10, 11] and it has been suggested that a thermal polymerisation produces the foulant. However, if copper is associated with the polymerisation, there should be a dependence of rate of deactivation on copper surface area. As a result, comparisons were made between deactivation on a Raney copper catalyst with two supported copper catalysts of very different copper surface area [13,16] (Figure 3). These comparisons showed that the initial deactivation differs markedly between the catalysts and that the second deactivation (obvious after ca 10 h on line) also differs

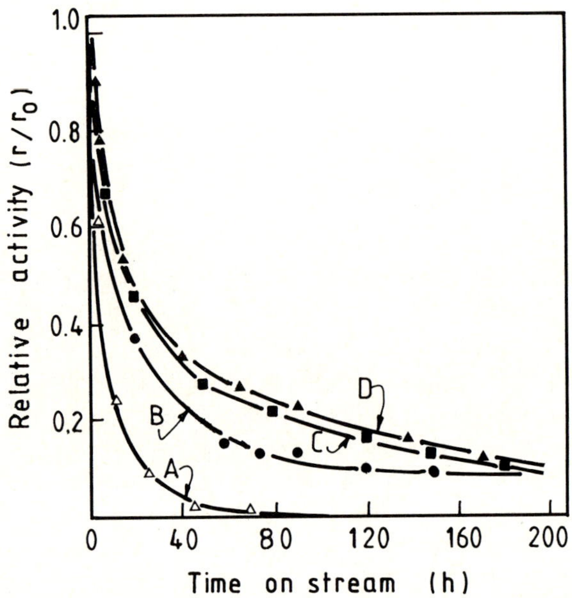

Fig. 1. Catalyst deactivation with time on stream for alloys of different structure. A,B,C,D refer to catalysts reported in Table 1.

Since this second deactivation may be interfering with the initial deactivation, attention was focused on establishing the magnitude of the former effect. Long term deactivation has been suggested to be caused by oxygen in the feed [10]. Distilled water was boiled and cooled under an atmosphere of helium, air or oxygen and then used to prepare standard feed. This feed was passed over the catalyst with the conversion and oxygen level in the feed being measured. The results, summarised in Figure 4, show clearly that the second deactivation step is dependent on oxygen concentration. It is also

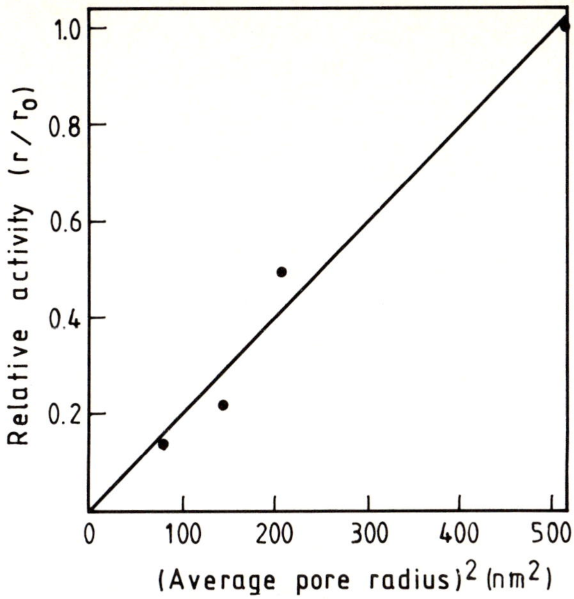

Fig. 2. Relative activity as a function of (average pore radius)^2 of Raney copper during the course of reaction. Data plotted here were obtained from Table 2.

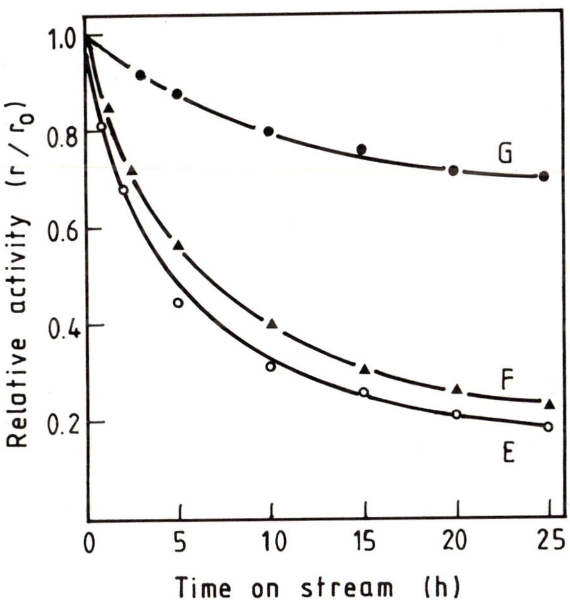

Fig. 3. Relative activities of different catalysts as a function of time on stream. E, F and G refer to catalysts reported in Table 1.

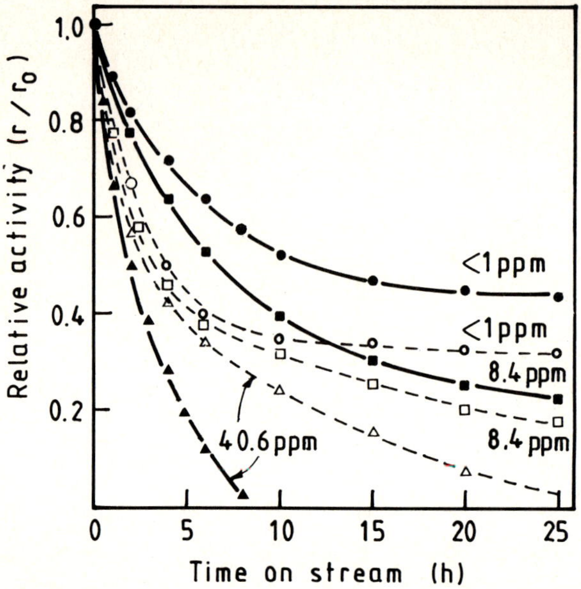

Fig. 4. Catalyst deactivation with time on stream as a function of dissolved oxygen for Cu/SiO_2 (Sample F, solid line) and Raney copper (Sample E, dashed line). Oxygen levels in solution shown on graph.

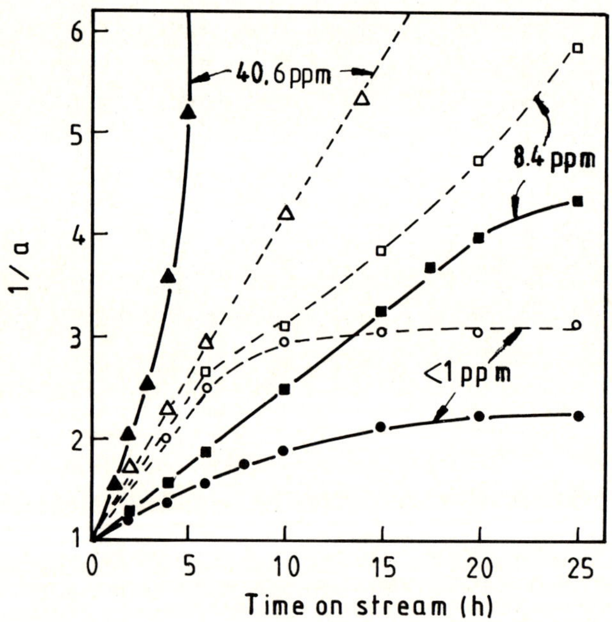

Fig. 5. Plots of 1/a vs time on stream for Cu/SiO_2 (Sample F, solid line) and Raney copper (Sample E, dashed line) based on the data from Figure 4.

obvious that, at least in the case of Cu/SiO_2 converting feed containing oxygen, the second deactivation step is large enough to compete with deactivation by polymer fouling.

Loss of activity (-da/dt) can be expressed generally in terms of the equation [18]

$$\frac{-da}{dt} = k_d\, a^d C^m(A/D/P) \tag{2}$$

where the subscripts to the concentration, C,(i.e. A, D or P) refer to reactant, product or poison respectively and are applied singly or in combination depending on the source(s) of deactivation. If, as has been suggested for polymer fouling [10], deactivation is second order, this equation reduces to

$$\frac{-da}{dt} = k_d\, a^2 (C_{A/D/P} \text{ constant or negligible}) \tag{3}$$

where k_d is the rate constant for deactivation caused by polymers. If activities (a) are calculated in terms of $a = r/r_0$, then this equation becomes [10]

$$a = \frac{1}{1+k_d t} \tag{4}$$

Plots of 1/a vs t can then be used to establish if the deactivation is second order and, if so, to determine values of k_d. Plots based on the data from Figure 4 are shown in Figure 5, from which it is seen that deactivation is second order in all cases up to at least 4 h on line. Values of k_d are summarised in Table 3. From this table, it is clear that k_d values on Raney copper are quite insensitive to oxygen but corresponding values on Cu/SiO_2 increase significantly with oxygen in the feed. It would not be unreasonable to expect that small copper particles oxidise more readily than bulk copper and, as a result, the sensitivity of Cu/SiO_2 to oxygen is not unexpected.

TABLE 3.
Values of k_d (h^{-1}), the deactivation rate parameter for catalyst fouling at 323K.

Catalyst	Oxygen level (ppm)		
	<1.0	8.4	40.6
Raney copper sample E	2.52×10^{-1}	2.68×10^{-1}	3.15×10^{-1}
Cu/SiO_2 sample F	9.20×10^{-2}	1.52×10^{-1}	5.12×10^{-1}

On an industrial scale, the level of near steady state activity that can be achieved after the initial deactivation is of considerable importance. Inspection of the characteristics of the catalysts and their near-steady state activities suggested that pore size was the main determinant of final performance. As seen from Figure 6, this is found to be the case with the

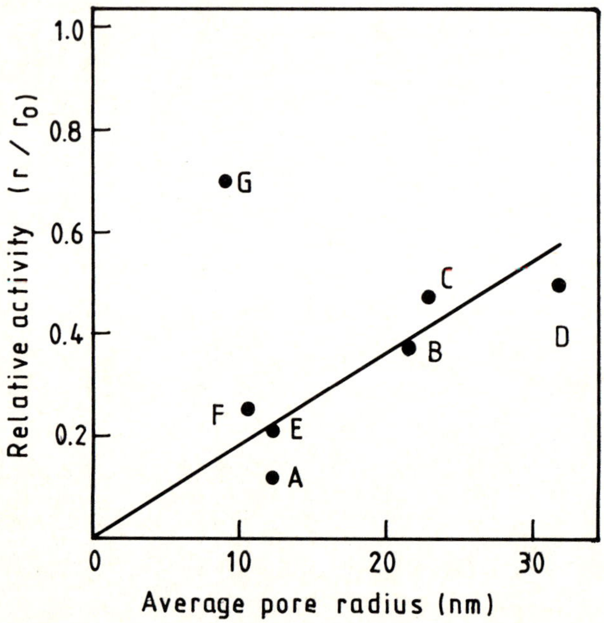

Fig. 6. Plot of activity after 20h on line vs average pore radius. A to G refer to catalysts reported in Table 1.

exception of 7 wt% Cu/SiO_2. If polymer nucleates on the surface and grows to obstruct the pores (see Fig. 2) then the permeability of the polymer gel can be expected to increase as the pore radius increases. As a result, access to copper within wide pores should be restricted but should still be possible. The near steady state rate should then be higher, the wider the pore and the more permeable the polymer foulant. These predictions agree with the main trend observed in Figure 6.

The reproducible result observed with 7 wt% Cu/SiO_2 does show, however, that other factors may influence the near equilibrium activity of the catalyst. These factors, of obvious industrial importance, are currently under study.

ACKNOWLEDGEMENTS

Funding of this research by the Australian Research Grants Scheme is gratefully acknowledged.

REFERENCES

1 F. Matsuda, Chemtech., 7 (1977) 306.
2 F. Nozaki, T. Sodesawa and T. Yamamoto, J. Catal., 84 (1983) 267.
3 L.R. Haefele and H.J. Young, Ind. Eng. Chem. Prod. Res. Dev., 11 (1972) 364.
4 H. Miura, K. Sugiyama, S. Kawakami, T. Aoyama and T. Matsuda, Chem. Lett., (1982) 183.
5 I.O. Mikhailishin, O.J. Amankona and T.M. Mokrivskii, through Chem. Abstr., 99 (1983) 71190s.
6 V.A. Lifanova and O.N. Temkin, Kinetika i Kataliz, 23 (1982) 868.
7 V.I. Trachenko, Zh. Prikl. Khim., 52 (1979) 1570.
8 H. Hayashi, H. Nishi, Y. Watanabe and T. Okazaki, J. Catal. 69 (1981) 44.
9 D.L. Werges and L.A. Goretta, US Patent 3,894,084 (8 July 1975).
10 N.I. Onuoha and M.S. Wainwright, Chem. Eng. Commun., 29 (1984) 13.
11 N.I. Onuoha and M.S. Wainwright, Appl. Catal., 14 (1985) 361.
12 H. Hirai, H. Wakabayashi and M. Komiyama, Chem. Lett., (1983) 1047.
13 N.I. Onuoha and M.S. Wainwright, Chem. Eng. Commun., 29 (1984) 1.
14 A.D. Tomsett, M.S. Wainwright and D.J. Young, Appl. Catal. 12 (1984) 13.
15 H. Kobayashi, N. Takezawa, C. Minochi and K. Takahashi, Chem. Lett., (1980) 1197.
16 M.A. Kohler, J.C. Lee, D.L. Trimm, N.W. Cant and M.S. Wainwright, Appl. Catal. (in press).
17 N.I. Onuoha, R.P. Chaplin and M.S. Wainwright, Chromatographia, 12 (1979) 703.
18 O. Levenspiel, J. Catal. 25 (1972) 265.

B. Delmon and G.F. Froment (Editors), *Catalyst Deactivation 1987*

DEACTIVATION OF ALUMINAS AND PHOSPHATES CATALYSTS IN 1-BUTANOL DEHYDRATION

M. RUWET, P. BERTEAU, S. CECKIEWICZ[1] and B. DELMON

Unité de Catalyse et Chimie des Matériaux Divisés, U.C.L.,
Place Croix du Sud, 1, B-1348 Louvain-la-Neuve (Belgium).

[1] On leave from the Institute of Chemistry, Jagiellonian University,
Karasia 3, 30-060 Krakow, Poland.

ABSTRACT

The resistance to deactivation of aluminas(γ-Al_2O_3 pure or modified with F^-, Zn^{++}, Na^+) and phosphates(B-PO_4, Al-PO_4, Ca-Ni-PO_4) catalysts was investigated with pure 1-butanol under various reaction conditions. In the corresponding laboratory tests, our catalysts are not subject to deactivation. An activity decrease and selectivity changes were observed after a run with synthetic acetonobutylic mixtures containing, in addition to 1-butanol, acetone, ethanol, acetic acid and water. After the catalytic tests, the coke content was low. The combined role of the presence of water and organic molecules other than 1-butanol (especially acetic acid) in the feed explains the catalytic activity decrease.

INTRODUCTION

Potentially, acetonobutylic (ABE) fermentation, which gives 1-butanol, together with acetone, could be the source of valuable chemical products. The present paper concerns the results of part of a programme we have conducted with the purpose of transforming 1-butanol to produce butenes and/or butyraldehyde. It describes the results obtained using aluminas (γ-Al_2O_3 either pure, or modified with F^-, Zn^{++} or Na^+) and phosphates (B-PO_4, Al-PO_4, Ca-Ni-PO_4) as catalysts for the dehydration of 1-butanol, either pure or in synthetic mixtures corresponding to the product of ABE fermentation, namely containing also acetone, ethanol, water, acetic and butyric acids.

Aluminas and phosphates are active in many catalytic reactions, such as alkylation, olefins isomerization, oxidation, polymerization, dehydrogenation (phosphates only) and alcohol dehydration (1,2). The acid-base properties of these solids play the central role and determines selectivity.

1-Butanol dehydration yields water, 1-butene and dibutylether (DBE). In addition, isomerization of 1-butene occurs alongside 1-butanol dehydration and gives 2-butenes (cis and trans).

Butyraldehyde can also be produced by dehydrogenation which occurs on some catalysts (oxides containing P, Ca and Ni, or P and Bi, or P, Bi and Mo, generally in the presence of a small quantity of oxygen) (3,4).

When the more complex ABE mixtures were used as reactants, the products were ethylene, propylene, butylacetate and mesityloxide, in addition to those formed from pure 1-butanol. Ethylene is formed from ethanol, propylene and mesityloxide from acetone, and butylacetate results from the esterification of 1-butanol with acetic acid.

In the work reported here, we investigated the resistance of the catalysts to deactivation with pure 1-butanol under our standard as well as under "tougher" reaction conditions. We also studied the influence of impurities coming from the ABE fermentation liquor, under the standard reaction conditions. With pure 1-butanol, our catalyst did not seem to be subject to deactivation. However, after a run with ABE mixtures, an activity decrease and selectivity changes were observed.

The coke content of the used catalysts was low, coke alone is therefore, not the factor explaining the catalytic activity decrease. We suggest that deactivation is an indirect consequence of the combined presence of water and organic molecules other than 1-butanol (especially acetic acid) in the feed.

EXPERIMENTAL

Catalysts

The starting alumina was a commercial Rhône-Poulenc G.F.S.C. γ-Al_2O_3. The modified catalyst were prepared by impregnation with aqueous solutions of HF, $Zn(CH_3COO)_2.2H_2O$ or NaOH, respectively. The concentrations of these solutions were adjusted to obtain 1% by weight of F^- and Zn^{++}, and Na^+. The volume of solution employed was exactly equal to the total pore volume of the starting alumina (0.70 $cm^3.g^{-1}$). After standing overnight, the samples were dried for 24 hours at 100°C and calcined in air during 4 hours at 823 K (5,6,7). The samples will be referred to as γ-Al_2O_3, γ-Al_2O_3/F^-, γ-Al_2O_3/Zn^{++}, γ-Al_2O_3/Na^+.

Boron phosphate was obtained (8) by heating mixtures of triethyl-borate and 85% H_3PO_4 taken in the adequate proportion (B/P = 1) with continuous stirring at 353 K for 45 minutes. The resulting preparation product was dried for 2 h at 393 K (under low pressure) and then calcined in air for 18 h at 873 K. In the text it will be noted B-PO_4.

Aluminium phosphate was prepared (9) by the slow neutralization (0.1 cm^3/min) of a mixture composed of $Al(NO_3)_3.9H_2O$ and H_3PO_4 by NH_{3aq} until pH = 6. The precipitate was washed with distilled water until traces of NO_3^- ions disappeared, dried for 20 h at 373 K and then calcined at 673 K during 3 h. In the text it will be referred to as Al-PO_4.

Calcium-nickel phosphate was precipitated (10) from a solution containing ammonium phosphate, calcium chloride and nickel chloride ($NiCl_2.6H_2O$). After adding the ingredients, the stirring was continued for 0.5 hour. The supernatent liquor was removed by decantation and the residue washed with distilled water until total elimination of chlorides and soluble nickel salts. The slurry of calcium-nickel phosphate was then filtered, dried for 12 h at 333 K and finally for 24 h at 403 K. The product was calcined 8 h at 673 K. In the next it will be noted Ca-Ni-PO_4.

The investigated samples are listed in Table 1. We verified by X-ray diffraction that the correct structure was obtained. The X-ray patterns were recorded on a Siemens Kristalloflex 805 diffractometer using nickel-filtered CuK_α radiation (40kV, 40 mA).

TABLE 1
Catalysts and some of their characteristics

catalytic system	crystallographic system	BET specific surface area ($m^2.g^{-1}$)	NH_3TPD ($mmol.g^{-1}$)	CO_2TPD ($mmol.g^{-1}$)
γ-Al_2O_3	cubic	222	0.56	0.11
γ-Al_2O_3/F^-	cubic	221	0.49	0.04
γ-Al_2O_3/Na^+	cubic	232	0.35	0.33
γ-Al_2O_3/Zn^{++}	cubic	237	0.38	0.28
B-PO_4	tetragonal	43.6	0.32	0.27
B-PO_4 after ABE mixture dehydration	-	38.2	-	-
Al-PO_4	amorphous	126	5.52	0.04
Ca-Ni-PO_4	amorphous	144	1.70	0.06

The specific surface areas are also reported in Table I. They were determined by adsorption of nitrogen at 77 K in a conventional volumetric (aluminas) or gravimetric (phosphates) B.E.T. apparatus.

The acid-base properties of the catalysts were studied by NH_3 or CO_2 TPD measurements combined with IR spectroscopy of probe molecules (ammonia, pyridine,. or pyrrole). Those results have been reported and discussed in other publications (11,13). We only reported, in Table 1, the total acidity and basicity of the catalysts in terms of the total amount of NH_3 or CO_2, desorbed from the samples during TPD measurements.

Reactants

In the catalytic tests, the reactants used were : 1-butanol (>99.5%, Merck), acetone (>99.7%, Janssen chemica), ethanol (>99.8%, Merck), acetic acid (>99.8%, Merck), butyric acid (>98%, UCB) and helium (99.995%, l'Air Liquide Belge).

Catalytic test

The activity of catalysts was measured in an all-glass flow reactor (int. diameter of 4 mm). The samples were the 100-200 μm fraction obtained by sieving. A catalyst of ca. 40 mg was placed in the reactor (with a fixed bed height of 6-10 mm) and was heated under a stream of helium (65 $cm^3.min^{-1}$) at 573 K during 2 h. Then a helium stream saturated with 1-butanol vapour (partial pressure of 1-butanol being equal to 3.7 kPa and Liquid Hourly Space Velocity (LHSV) being equal to 4.4 to 7.4 h^{-1}) was passed through the catalytic bed and the products were analyzed by a HP 5880 A chromatograph equipped with a 2.5 m Porapak Q column and a microthermal conductivity detector. These reaction conditions are hereafter referred to as the "standard" ones. In the case of the ABE mixture, the saturator system was replaced by an automatic dosing system (B. Braun-Melsungen) with a syringe of 10 cm^3 and a rate of pumping of ca. 0.0166 $cm^3.min^{-1}$. To prevent any condensation of reactants and reaction products in the apparatus, all connections from the saturator to the chromatograph were heated by a wired resistance.

The catalytic test results were expressed as percentage conversion, defined as the total percentage of 1-butanol transformed. Selectivities were defined as the percentage of converted 1-butanol transformed into a given product. The activity of a catalyst was defined as the number of 1-butanol mmoles transformed in one hour per g of catalyst.

Carbon analyses

Carbon analyses were performed following the method described by Jones et al. (14). The sample was exposed to a pure O_2 stream at 1250°C. The CO_2 formed (during the combustion of carbonaceous species) was adsorbed in an N-N-dimethylformamide solution and then titrated with 0.02 M tetra-n-butylammonium hydroxide solution.

RESULTS

Catalytic tests

1. Experiments with pure 1-butanol

The results of 1-butanol dehydration on the studied catalysts are presented in Table 2. The alumina, pure or modified by F^- and Zn^{++}, showed higher conversions than the phosphates. The Na^+ modified alumina did not transform

1-butanol.

The best catalytic properties among the phosphates were exhibited by B-PO_4. For all these samples, no deactivation was observed during a minimum of 3 hours of time on stream.

The analysis of product distribution revealed great differences between the catalysts. Pure γ-Al_2O_3 and γ-Al_2O_3 /Zn^{++} were highly selective to butenes (1-butene >> 2-butene), whereas γ-Al_2O_3/F^-, also selective to butenes, presented a higher ability for isomerization of 1-butene to 2-butenes. BPO_4 transformed 1-butanol to butene isomers (2-butene > 1-butene), Al-PO_4, in addition, yielded dibutylether, whereas Ca-Ni-PO_4 produced only butyraldehyde.

Moreover, as we previously reported, aluminas present very good resistance to deactivation in our working conditions (12) :

- γ-Al_2O_3 tested at a temperature reaction of 603K, a LHSV equal to 13.4 h^{-1}, a butanol partial pressure of 22 kPa, did not present any variation of the catalytic activity and product distribution during 6 hours;
- after 16 hours of operation at very high temperatures, namely 748K, and LHSV equal to 13.4 h^{-1}, the γ-Al_2O_3 catalytic activity measured in the standard conditions was the same as the initial one.

TABLE 2
The results for pure 1-butanol after 0.3 h/3 h of reaction under standard conditions

catalyst	conversion (%)		selectivity (%) 1-butene		2-butene		dibutylether		butyraldehyde	
	0.3h	**3h**	0.3h	**3h**	0.3h	**3h**	0.3h	**3h**	0.3h	**3h**
γ-Al_2O_3	100	**100**	95.0	**95.0**	5.0	**5.0**	-	-	-	-
γ-Al_2O_3/F^-	100	**100**	60.0	**60.0**	40.0	**40.0**	-	-	-	-
γ-Al_2O_3/Na^+	0	**0**	-	-	-	-	-	-	-	-
γ-Al_2O_3/Zn^{++}	100	**100**	95.0	**95.0**	5.0	**5.0**	-	-	-	-
B-PO_4	97.8	**97.9**	21.6	**23.5**	78.4	**76.5**	-	-	-	-
Al-PO_4	46.7	**48.8**	17.5	**18.1**	5.8	**5.6**	76.7	**76.3**	-	-
Ca-Ni-PO_4	8.2	**8.0**	-	-	-	-	-	-	100	**100**

2. <u>Experiments with the ABE mixtures</u>

The composition of the ABE mixtures used is presented in Table 3. Table 4 shows the results of the catalytic tests with the ABE mixtures in terms of conversion and selectivity in the various products derived from 1-butanol after 0.3 and 3 hours of reaction.

In addition to the typical products of 1-butanol conversion, namely butenes, dibutylether and butyraldehyde, ethylene, propylene, butylacetate and mesityloxide were identified. Considering only the products derived from 1-butanol, more side products were formed with the ABE mixtures than with pure 1-butanol (table 2). The catalytic activity of the various samples in the reaction of pure 1-butanol and ABE mixtures nr 8 and 9 are compared in Table 5. For all studied samples, the catalytic activity with respect to 1-butanol is much depressed with the ABE mixtures. B-PO_4 exhibited the highest activity among the various studied catalysts, but an important deactivation (20%) was observed after 3 hours of time on stream. Nevertheless the BPO_4 activity after 3 hours of reaction was still higher (by 14 to 97%) than that of the other catalysts.

TABLE 3

ABE mixtures composition

ABE mixture	components (wt %)					
	butanol	acetone	water	ethanol	acetic acid	butyric acid
1	-	20.0	80.0	–	-	-
2	77.0	22.0	1.0	–	-	-
3	57.0	20.0	23.0	–	-	-
4	95.0	-	3.5	–	1.5	-
5	78.0	19.5	1.0	–	1.5	-
6	57.0	20.0	21.5	–	1.5	-
7	58.0	19.5	21.5	1.0	-	-
8	57.0	20.0	20.5	1.0	1.5	–
9	45.3	12.9	30.5	3.2	7.1	1.0

3. Experiments with pure 1-butanol after contact with ABE mixtures

After the run with the ABE mixtures, we returned to pure 1-butanol and measured the catalytic properties with γ-Al_2O_3 and BPO_4. The results are presented in table 6. If we compare the results of pure 1-butanol reaction with fresh catalysts and catalysts having worked with ABE mixtures, we observe a decrease of conversion (except after a run with ABE mixtures nr 1 and 7, used with γ-Al_2O_3). Selectivity is also impaired, and dibutylether is formed in several cases. We notice that, with γ-Al_2O_3, larger losses of conversion are observed with ABE mixtures containing acetic acid and ca. 20% of water. Particularly conspicuous changes are observed with γ-Al_2O_3 after the run with ABE mixtures nr 6 and 8, and with BPO_4. It is also interesting to compare those results (table 6) with the ones of 1-butanol conversion during the run with the ABE mixtures (table 4). The γ -Al_2O_3 catalyst regained part of the activity loss observed in the ABE run. But the loss observed with BPO_4 (value after 3h in table 4 and value in table 6) was irreversible. This corresponds to a diminution of about 28% of the activity.

Table 4

Test results of ABE mixtures after 0.3h and 3h of reaction.

Catalyst	ABE mixture	Butanol conversion (%)		Selectivity (%)									
				1-butene		2-butene		dibutylether		butyraldehyde		Butylacetate	
		0.3h	3h	0.3h	3h	0.3h	3h	0.3h	3h	0.3h	3h	0.3h	3h
γ-Al_2O_3	1	0	0	0	0	0	0	0	0	0	0	0	0
	2	73.0	72.6	30.2	30.1	1.0	1.0	49.0	49.2	19.8	19.7	-	-
	3	65.0	65.2	30.1	30.2	0.5	0.5	54.4	54.5	15.0	14.8	-	-
	4	46.0	45.4	17.1	17.2	0.3	0.4	81.1	79.9	0.3	0.3	1.2	1.2
	5	58.0	57.8	16.7	16.8	0.5	0.5	76.7	76.6	5.2	5.2	0.9	0.9
	6	43.2	43.0	15.4	15.2	0.3	0.3	75.4	75.5	7.3	7.4	1.6	1.6
	7	73.4	73.1	36.1	35.8	1.7	1.6	43.3	43.8	18.9	18.8	-	-
	8	39.0	38.0	13.7	13.1	2.6	2.5	73.5	74.6	7.7	7.5	2.5	2.3
	9	17.2	18.3	7.3	6.3	2.5	3.1	29.2	41.8	9.8	7.3	51.2	41.5
γ-Al_2O_3/F^-	8	56.0	58.0	16.1	20.3	6.0	8.1	66.2	59.0	9.4	10.9	2.3	1.6
	9	30.5	29.8	9.8	6.8	6.9	7.4	24.5	36.8	10.3	9.4	48.5	39.6
γ-Al_2O_3/Zn^{++}	8	40.0	38.6	14.2	13.9	2.7	2.3	73.4	74.6	7.3	7.1	2.4	2.1
	9	16.9	17.5	6.9	7.2	2.5	3.4	31.3	39.8	9.7	7.3	49.6	42.3
B-PO_4	8	84.9	67.6	29.9	39.9	67.8	55.0	1.1	3.4	-	-	1.2	1.7
	9	85.9	71.5	25.1	36.8	62.5	50.1	-	-	3.7	2.9	8.7	10.2
Al-PO_4	8	17.0	15.6	11.1	8.9	3.2	3.4	68.2	72.9	12.5	9.6	5.0	5.2
	9	9.2	8.5	9.5	8.4	2.5	2.3	65.5	67.2	14.4	13.9	8.3	8.2
Ca-Ni-PO_4	8	2.0	2.0	-	-	-	-	-	-	36.4	36.4	63.6	63.6
	9	0	0	-	-	-	-	-	-	-	-	-	-

TABLE 5

Compared catalytic activities of the various studied catalyts

catalyst	catalytic activity (mmol BuOH $g^{-1}.h^{-1}$)					
	pure 1-butanol		ABE mixture 8		ABE mixture 9	
	0.3 h	**3h**	0.3h	**3h**	0.3h	**3h**
γ-Al_2O_3	152	**152**	59	**58**	25	**27**
γ-Al_2O_3/F^-	152	**152**	85	**88**	45	**44**
γ-Al_2O_3/Zn^{++}	152	**152**	61	**59**	25	**26**
B-PO_4	148	**148**	129	**102**	130	**198**
Al-PO_4	71	**74**	26	**24**	14	**13**
Ca-Ni-PO_4	12	**12**	3	**3**	0	**0**

TABLE 6

Test results for pure 1-butanol dehydration of γ-Al_2O_3 and B PO_4 fresh and after 3 hours of run with ABE mixtures

catalyst	butanol conversion %	selectivity 1-butene	selectivity 2-butene	dibutylether	catalytic activity mmol BuOH $g^{-1}h^{-1}$
γ-Al_2O_3 fresh	100	95.0	5.0	-	152
γ-Al_2O_3 after mixture 1	100	95.0	5.0	-	152
2	98.0	97.0	3.0	-	149
3	98.0	97.0	3.0	-	149
4	97.0	97.0	3.0	-	147
5	95.2	97.0	3.0	-	145
6	81.0	83.0	1.0	16.0	123
7	100	97.0	3.0	-	152
8	84.1	90.0	2.0	8.0	128
BPO_4 fresh	97.9	23.5	76.5	-	148
BPO_4 after mixture 8	69.2	29.8	68.2	2.0	105

Coke content

After pure 1-butanol dehydration under the standard conditions, the aluminas and the phosphates did not exhibit any change of colour. Under tougher conditions, the aluminas became grey/black.

After the dehydration of ABE mixtures, the catalysts exhibited no or only slight changes of colour.

Table 7 presents the coke content of the various studied catalysts after catalytic tests with pure 1-butanol under standard and "tougher" reaction conditions, and with ABE mixture 8.

TABLE 7
Coke analyses results

catalyst	catalytic reaction conditions reactant	temp. (K)	LHSV (h^{-1})	duration (h)	% coke after catalytic test
γ-Al_2O_3	1-butanol	573	7.4	3	0
	1-butanol	603	13.4	6	0
	1-butanol	748	13.4	16	1
	ABE mixture 8	573	7.4	3	2.6
γ-Al_2O_3/F^-	1-butanol	573	7.4	3	0
	1-butanol	623	13.4	72	4
	ABE mixture 8	573	7.4	3	3.1
γ-Al_2O_3/Na^+	1-butanol	573	7.4	3	0
	1-butanol	623	13.4	24	3.7
γ-Al_2O_3/Zn^{++}	1-butanol	573	7.4	3	0
	ABE mixture 8	573	7.4	3	2.3
B-PO_4	1-butanol	573	6.8	3	0
	ABE mixture 8	573	6.8	3	1.3
$AlPO_4$	1-butanol	573	4.4	3	1.2
	ABE mixture 8	573	4.4	3	2.6
Ca-$NiPO_4$	1-butanol	573	6.5	3	1.8
	ABE mixture 8	573	6.5	3	2.9

DISCUSSION

With respect to deactivation processes, three striking features are to be pointed out in our results. The first one is that coke, deposited in small quantities during pure 1-butanol dehydration, does not modify the catalytic activity of phosphates or pure or modified γ-Al_2O_3 (even under "tough" reaction conditions). The two other features concern the observed deactivation in pure 1-butanol dehydration after a run with ABE mixtures containing acetic acid and water. These are :

- a permanent depression of the catalytic activity of γ-Al_2O_3 and B-PO_4
- a permanent change of the selectivity.

However, the behaviour of γ-Al_2O_3 and BPO_4 is different in that BPO_4 practically does not regain activity when returning to pure 1-butanol after the ABE run, whereas part of the activity depression observed with γ-Al_2O_3 is recovered.

The results have to be discussed in the general context of the mechanism of the dehydration.

It is known that the dehydration of alcohols requires the simultaneous presence of acidic and basic centres in adequate proportions, on the catalyst surface (11,13,15). The strength of the acid sites is crucial. A certain acidity level is required in order to have a great dehydration activity : if acidity is too weak, the dehydration activity lessens and if the acidity is too strong, cracking may occur. We have previously shown that the strength of the acid sites determines the reaction product distribution (11).

The fact that coke is deposited only in small quantities leads us to think that, if deposited carbon has a role in deactivation, this is as a poison, and not as a fouling agent (mechanical blocking of pores and mechanical limitation to the access of molecules to the surface). One important question arises, namely : is the deactivation effect due to poisoning by deposits formed during catalysis, or by a change in the strength of the catalytic (acidic) centres ?

In the case of the aluminas and phosphates used with pure 1-butanol, there is no poisoning by coke deposition. But water or foreign organic molecules present in the feed could bring about modifications explaining the activity changes with pure 1-butanol after the ABE mixture runs. We shall thus focus our discussion on the possible effect of the presence of water and foreign organic molecules.

The presence of water in the feed can bring about changes in the equilibrium between Lewis and Brönsted acidic sites; the following hydroxylation equilibrium is shifted to the right, in the presence of large amounts of water :

$$\text{Lewis acid site} + H_2O \rightleftharpoons \text{Brönsted acid site}$$

In principle, an interconversion leading to a decrease of the Lewis acidity could explain the diminution of the activity in alcohol dehydration (11,13,15,16). In addition, the interconversion should affect preferably the strong Lewis sites. The role of the weak Lewis acid sites would be enhanced in comparison to that of the strong ones. As the weak sites play a predominant role in the formation of DBE (11,20), this could also explain an increase in the formation of this product.

Concerning the other molecules present in the ABE mixtures, there is little information on acetone, but the role of acetic acid is better known. Various authors have shown that, in the case of zeolites, this substance interacts with both basic and vicinal acid sites according to the scheme presented below :

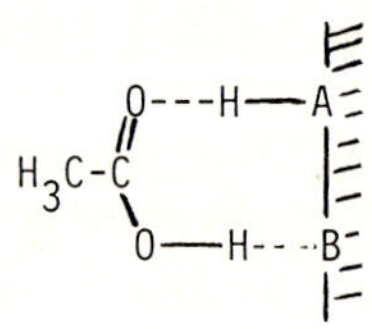

Acetic acid is irreversibly retained on those sites leading to a dramatic lowering of the catalytic activity (17,18). Moreover, Przystajko et al. have shown that the basic centres of aluminas are more reactive with acetic acid than those of zeolites (19).

With these data in mind, we shall examine, in succession, the case of the aluminas and that of the phosphates and more particularly that of BPO_4.

1. Aluminas

All the studied aluminas presented lower dehydration activities in the ABE mixtures than in the case of the pure 1-butanol (table 5). As one conspicuous feature of deactivation after a run with the ABE mixture is the change of selectivity (formation of dibutylether in several cases) accompanied by a loss of activity, it is worthwhile to examine, in the first place, the results obtained **during the ABE run.** We shall thus discuss the catalytic properties of pure γ-Al_2O_3 with the different ABE mixtures (table 4). In a second section we shall examine the results obtained with pure 1-butanol **after runs with ABE mixtures** (table 6).

1.1 Catalytic properties of pure γ-Al_2O_3 with ABE mixtures

The comparison of butanol **conversions** of γ-Al_2O_3 with the different ABE mixtures (1 to 9) indicates that the presence of acetone, water or acetic acid in the feed, even in small quantities, causes a decrease of activity. The lowest values are obtained with the combined presence of acetic acid and large amounts of water.

We explain these changes by the simultaneous occurrence of two effects.

Although the water produced by dehydration at the reactor outlet is in quantities comparable (ca. 30%) to those added in the ABE mixtures, the interconversion phenomenon can be substantially more intense in the case of the ABE mixtures' dehydration. Indeed, in the case of pure 1-butanol, the water content increases as conversion increases, from the top (0% water) to the bottom (30%) of the catalytic bed. In the ABE mixtures nr 3, 6, 7 and 8, containing about 20% water, the water contents vary from 20% at the top to 30% at the bottom. As a whole, the water content is higher in the latter case.

The interconversion of the sites could thus partially explain the activity decrease observed in the ABE mixtures' dehydration. In addition, this could explain, at least partially, the formation of DBE. But this does not appear to constitute the whole explanation, as DBE is also produced when returning to pure 1-butanol after a run with the ABE mixtures nr 6 and 8.

The second effect is indicated by the increased formation of DBE in the presence of acetic acid. DBE formation is favoured because the role of the weak Lewis sites becomes proportionally more important. Two reasons could be proposed. The first one is, as we have seen above, a preferable interconversion of the strong Lewis sites to Brönsted sites. The second one should be found in the influence of acetic acid on active centres. This weak acid would preferably interact with the strong acid sites vicinal to basic sites.

All these phenomena would lead to a modification in the acidic/basic centres ratio and in the site density, and thus DBE/butene selectivity changes would occur (12).

1.2 Pure γ-Al_2O_3 with 1-butanol after run with ABE mixtures

The contact of -Al_2O_3 with some mixtures (particularly nr 6 and 8) leads to a permanent depression of the catalytic activity (table 6). Three components are present in the corresponding mixtures, namely acetone, acetic acid and water. The results indicate that neither acetone alone (mixture 1) nor water alone (mixtures 2, 3, 7) lead to such an effect. But acetic acid, acetone and large quantities of water (ca. 20%) lead to a permanent depression.

The fact that the catalytic activity of γ-Al_2O_3 (depressed after the runs with ABE mixtures) is partially restored when the catalyst is contacted with pure 1-butanol, indicates that the moderate quantities of coke deposited (table 7), and the presence of more water leading to an interconversion of Lewis to Brönsted acid sites, cannot be the only factor explaining deactivation.

The explanation of the permanent deactivation is thus the inhibition of the active centres by acetic acid. This inhibition would change the acid/base centres ratio and thus explain the activity decrease and the selectivity change. It remains to be explained why a large water vapor pressure makes this inhibition stronger.

2. Phosphates

As was also observed for the aluminas, the catalytic properties of phosphates are depressed in the ABE mixtures' dehydration. We shall examine the particular case of B-PO_4. Among all our catalysts, BPO_4 had the highest catalytic activity in the presence of the ABE mixtures. Its catalytic activity was only 13% lower than that with pure 1-butanol after 0.3h of reaction whereas the catalytic activity decrease of the aluminas and the other phosphates varied between 44 to 75% (ABE mixture 8) and 70 to 100% (ABE mixture 9) (table 5). But BPO_4 in contact with the ABE mixture deactivated with time. After 3 hours of reaction, its catalytic activity had further decreased by 20%, whereas that of all the other samples remained equal to that observed after 0.3 hour. The phenomenon is thus more complex. Moreover, in contrast with γ-Al_2O_3, the catalytic activity of BPO_4 in pure 1-butanol dehydration after the run with ABE mixture 8, remained as low as during that run.

Although there are many common features between BPO_4 and aluminas, a special deactivation process occurs which should explain these differences. The formation of coke during the ABE run is small (table 7); it is therefore unlikely that coke alone could explain deactivation. Part of the origin of deactivation could be explained by an additional effect of the presence of large quantities of water. Indeed, it is shown that water, when in large quantities, affects drastically the surface area of BPO_4. This effect increases in intensity upon prolonged contact (2). The decrease (by 12.4%) of the BET specific surface area (table 1) of BPO_4 after catalytic test with ABE mixture 8 shows that this phenomenon takes place in our case. This loss of surface area (sintering or recrystallization) corresponds to a loss of active sites. But this explains only a part of the activity depression, namely ca. 12.5% compared to the overall loss of 28% observed.

It must be noted that a selectivity change is observed. This indicates that, in addition to the loss of active sites, an inhibition of the active centres by acetic acid occurs, as in the case of γ-Al_2O_3.

CONCLUSION

Aluminas and phosphates catalysts are resistant to deactivation at the time scale of laboratory tests, with pure 1-butanol as reactant. However, the contact with ABE mixtures containing acetic acid and large quantities of water leads to deactivation, as detected by measurements with pure 1-butanol after a run with the ABE mixtures.

Part of the effect is reversible due to the interconversion of Lewis to Brönsted centres. Another part is irreversible. It is explained by a poisoning effect of acetic acid on active centres.

In the case of BPO_4, an additional irreversible effect is due to a textural change of this catalyst.

ACKNOWLEDGEMENTS

We acknowledge the "Services de la Programmation de la Politique Scientifique" in Belgium for their financial support. The text has been elaborated within the framework of the Belgian National Energy R&D Program. The authors assume all scientific responsibility.

REFERENCES

1. F.S. Wagner, in B.E. Leach (Editor), Applied Industrial Catalysis, Vol 2, Academic Press, New York, 1983, pp 27-108
2. J.B. Moffat, Catal. Rev. Sci. Eng. 18 (1978) 199-257
3. C.L. Kibby and W.K. Hall, J. Catal. 20 (1973) 144
4. M. Ruwet, S. Ceckiewicz and B. Delmon, Ing. Eng. Chem. Prod. Res. Dev., submitted for publication

5. K. Jiratova, L. Beranek, Appl. Catal. 2 (1982) 125
6. P.O. Scokart, S.A. Selim, J.P. Damon, P.G. Rouxhet, J. Coll. Int. Sci. 70 (1979) 209
7. J.P. Damon, J.M. Bonnier and B. Delmon, J. Coll. Int. Sci. 55 (1976) 381
8. J.B. Moffat and L.H. Goltz, Can. J. Chem. 43 (1965) 1680-1688
9. M.G. Mitichenko, A.A. Kubasov, V.V. Yuschenko, K.V. Topchieva, I.V. Arkhangel'skii, L.V. Kubasova, S.L. Vol'fkovitch, USSR, SU, 910 (1982) 187
10. E.C. Britton, A.J. Dietzler and C.R. Noddings, Ind. Eng. Chem. 43(12) (1951) 2871-2874
11. P. Berteau, S. Ceckiewicz and B. Delmon, Appl. Catal., accepted for publication
12. P. Berteau, M. Ruwet and B. Delmon, Bull. Soc. Chim. Belg. 94(11-12) (1985) 859-868
13. M. Ruwet, P. Berteau and S. Ceckiewicz, Bull. Soc. Chim. Belg. 96(4) (1987)
14. R.F. Jones, P. Gale, P. Hopkins and L.N. Powell, Analyst 90 (1965) 623
15. H. Knözinger in B. Imelik et al. (Editors), Catalysis by Acids and Bases, Elsevier Science Publishers, Amsterdam, 1985, 111-125
16. A. Corma, V. Fornes and E. Ortega, J. Catal. 92 (1985) 284-290
17. A. Bielanski and J. Datka, J. Catal. 32 (1974) 183
18. E. Santacesaria, D. Gelosa, E. Giorgi and S. Carra, J. Catal. 90 (1984) 1-9
19. W. Przystajko, R. Fiedorow and I.G. Dalla Lana, Appl. Catal. 15 (1985) 265-275
20. E.A. Paukshtis, K. Jiratova, R.I. Soltanov, E.N. Yurchenko and L. Beranek, Collect. Czech. Chem. Commun. 50 (1985) 497-508
21. E. Garbowski and M. Primet, J. Chem. Soc. Faraday Trans. I, 81 (1985) 497-508

B. Delmon and G.F. Froment (Editors), *Catalyst Deactivation 1987*
1987 Elsevier Science Publishers B.V., Amsterdam — Printed in The Netherlands

THE ROLE OF COBALT AND NICKEL ADDED TO MOLYBDENUM-ALUMINA IN HYDROTREATING CATALYSTS

T. Hisamitsu, K. Komori and H.Ozaki

Central Research Laboratories, Nippon Mining Co., Ltd., 3-17-35, Niizo-Minami, Toda, Saitama, 335 (Japan)

ABSTRACT

Studies have been made on the role of promoter metals, cobalt and nickel, added to MoO_3-Al_2O_3 catalysts for hydrodemetalation(HDM), hydrodesulfurization (HDS) and hydrodenitrogenation(HDN) of heavy residual oils. The addition of nickel or cobalt has been confirmed to promote initial activities for both reactions of HDM and HDS. However, it has also been observed that deactivation rates are accelerated at the same time. It has been demonstrated in a hydrotreating test for 4,600 hours that the unpromoted MoO_3-Al_2O_3 catalyst achieved better HDM and HDS performance than the promoted catalyst when they were used in a guard reactor of HDS units processing heavy residual oils.

INTRODUCTION

Molybdenum-based catalysts have been extensively used industrially for hydrorefining petroleum for many years. In addition, it is well established that activities of molybdenum based catalysts for HDS, HDN, hydrogenation(HY) and hydrocracking(HC) reactions are promoted by the addition of cobalt or nickel.

Although a large amount of research has been directed towards elucidating the promoting effect of cobalt and nickel, the role of promoter in these catalysts is not fully understood. Various promoting effects have been recognized and summarized by Massoth: 1)increases Mo area; 2)increases Mo reduction; 3)increases H_2 mobility; 4)due to Co intercalation of MoS_2; 5)due to MoS_2/Co_9S_8 synergism; 6)due to specific kinetic effects; 7)prevents catalyst deactivation; 8)enhances surface segregation; 9)prevents MoS_2 crystallization (ref. 1).

Although feedstocks for industrial hydrorefining processes are usually very complex, fundamental research on the role of promoter metals has been performed for the most part using pure compounds for reactants, such as thiophene (ref. 2,3), benzothiophene (ref. 4,5), dibenzothiophene (ref. 6), o-xylene (ref. 7) and cyclohexene (ref. 8). There are several literatures available, in which residual oils have been used as feedstocks for studies on the relationship between HDM, HDS and HDN activities and atomic ratio of promoter metals to molybdenum supported on alumina (refs. 9-11). It should be stressed, however, that all results, in contrast to industrial practice, have been derived from short-run experiments.

Here the effects of cobalt and nickel added to MoO_3-Al_2O_3catalysts on HDM, HDS and HY performance has been studied, based on results obtained in three series of experiments which have been carried out for 76 to 4,600 hours using feedstocks of heavy residual oils.

In the first series of experiments the effect of nickel added to 4% molybdenum-alumina catalyst on the initial activities and the deactivation rates during 76 hours have been evaluated. In the second series of experiments, the initial activities and the deactivation rates during 250 hours have been compared between unpromoted and promoted catalysts containing 4 or 8% molybdenum. In the third series of experiments, which have been carried out for 4,600 hours, the performance of a catalyst containing 4% molybdenum has been evaluated for use in a guard reactor, in comparison with catalysts containing a similar amount of molybdenum and promoter metals to typical HDS catalysts.

EXPERIMENTALS

Catalysts

A γ-alumina extruded into a quadrulobe of 1.2 mmø has been used for a support. Its surface area, pore volume, and mean pore diameter are 190 m^2/g, 0.71 ml/g and 150 Å, respectively. Metals have been supported in the following order by the pore filling method. First, the alumina support was impregnated with ammonium heptamolybdate solution and dried at 130°C for 4 hours. One part of the dried MoO_3-Al_2O_3 was then calcined at 500°C for 2 hours and defined as unpromoted catalysts. Promoted catalysts were prepared by impregnating the other part of the dried MoO_3-Al_2O_3 with cobalt and/or nickel nitrate solution, drying and calcining. The unpromoted catalysts were designated as XMo, while the promoted catalysts were termed as XMo-YCo, XMo-YNi and XMo-YCoNi, with X giving molybdenum content and Y giving the content of cobalt, nickel or cobalt plus nickel as a percentage. In the third series of experiments, a commercial nickel-molybdenum-alumina catalyst for HDS of heavy residual oils(HOP-802 supplied by Orient Catalyst Co., Ltd. Tokyo, Japan) was used in the second reactor. All catalysts were presulfided in-situ with gas oil containing 1% carbon disulfide prior to use.

Hydrotreating

The experiments have been carried out using continuous flow high-pressure units equipped with two down-flow reactors. The dimensions of reactors are 25 mm in inner diameter and 1,200 mm in length. One reactor loaded with 100 ml of catalyst was used for each unit in the first and second series of experiments, while two reactors connected in series and loaded with 60 and 140 ml of catalysts, respectively, were used for each unit in the third series of experiments. Reaction conditions are summarized in Table 1.

TABLE 1

Reaction Conditions

	First Series of Experiments	Second Series of Experiments	Third Series of Experiments
L.H.S.V. (hr^{-1})	1.0	1.0	0.3
Reaction Pressure (kg/cm^2)	120	120	140
H_2 Feed Rate (l-H_2/l-oil)	1000	1000	670
Reaction Temperature (°C)	Base + 30	Base + 40	0-300hr:Base after 300hr:81%HDS

Two lots of a mixture of equal amount of atmospheric and vacuum residues derived from Arabian heavy crude oil were used for feedstock in the first and second series of experiments. The feedstock used in the third series of experiments was a mixture of equal amount of atmospheric and vacuum residues derived from a half and half blend of Maya and Middle Eastern crude oils. Inspection data for these feedstocks are summarized in Table 2.

TABLE 2

Feedstock Properties

	Feed-I	Feed-II	Feed-III
Specific Gravity (15/4°C)	1.0131	1.0141	1.0217
Sulfur (wt.%)	4.80	4.85	4.19
Nitrogen (wt.%)	0.36	0.39	0.50
Vanadium (ppm)	130	139	343
Nickel (ppm)	36	44	74
Hydrogen/Carbon Atomic Ratio	1.52	1.50	1.48
Conradson Carbon Residue (wt.%)	18.2	20.3	20.5

Analysis

Sulfur content was measured by burning samples with oxygen in a ceramic tube according to Japan Industrial Standard K-2541. Nitrogen content was measured by chemiluminescence with a Dhoman model DN-10. Hydrogen and carbon contents were determined with a CHN-analyzer using a Perkin-Elmer model 240-C. Some of the used catalysts taken from the reactors were subjected to X-ray microanalysis (XMA) for internal metal deposition profiles. XMA was carried out using a Hitachi model X-560 after oil absorbed in used catalysts was removed using a Soxhlet extractor with toluene.

RESULTS AND DISCUSSION

The promoting effect of nickel added to 4Mo has been evaluated in the first series of experiments. In this hydrotreating experiment the HDM and HDS activities and the deactivation rates during 76 hours have been compared between 4Mo-0.5Ni, 4Mo-1Ni, and 4Mo. Sulfur and metals(V+Ni) removal is plotted as a function of time on stream in Figures 1(a) and (b).

The addition of 0.5% nickel increased the initial HDM activity by 5% in metals removal; the deactivation rate, however, was simulteniously accelerated. On the other hand, there was no decline observed in metals removal with the unpromoted catalyst, although the initial HDM activity of 4Mo was the lowest among the three catalysts. Consequently, the advantage of initial activity gained by the addition of nickel has already disappeared at 60 hours. The addition of 1% nickel resulted in a small gain of the initial activity and the same deactivation rate when compared with the addition of 0.5% nickel.

As for the HDS reaction, the addition of 0.5 and 1% nickel had a similar influence to each other. The initial sulfur removal of 58% with 4Mo has increased to 76% by the addition of nickel. This increase in activity corresponds to the more than double increase in the rate constant for the second order reaction rate equation. Although the deactivation rate increased at the same time with the addition of nickel, the promoted catalysts still maintained higher sulfur removal than the unpromoted catalysts by 8% at the end of the experiments.

The results of this series of experiments can be summarized as follows: addition of nickel to 4Mo adversely affects HDM activity. Although it significantly promotes the initial HDS activity, this advantage decreases with increasing time on stream.

In the next series of experiments studies have been made with the objective of investigating the effect of cobalt added to 4Mo in the place of nickel and also the effect of promoter metals added to MoO_3-Al_2O_3 which contains a similar amount of molybdenum to typical HDS catalysts. The initial activities and the deactivation rates during 250 hours have been compared between 4Mo-1Co and 4Mo and between 8Mo-2CoNi and 8Mo. The experimental results are shown in Figures 1(c), (d), and (e).

Although the data can not be directly compared between the two series of experiments since the reactions in this series have been conducted at a temperature 10°C higher than in the previous series, it can be said that the advantage of initial HDM activity gained by adding cobalt to 4Mo lasts longer than in the case of adding nickel; the advantage, however, disappears at 250 hours. Cobalt also seems to promote initial HDS activity and to accelerate the deactivation rate to a greater extent than nickel. Sulfur removal with 4Mo-1Co and 4Mo crossed each other at about 150 hours. Consequently, the

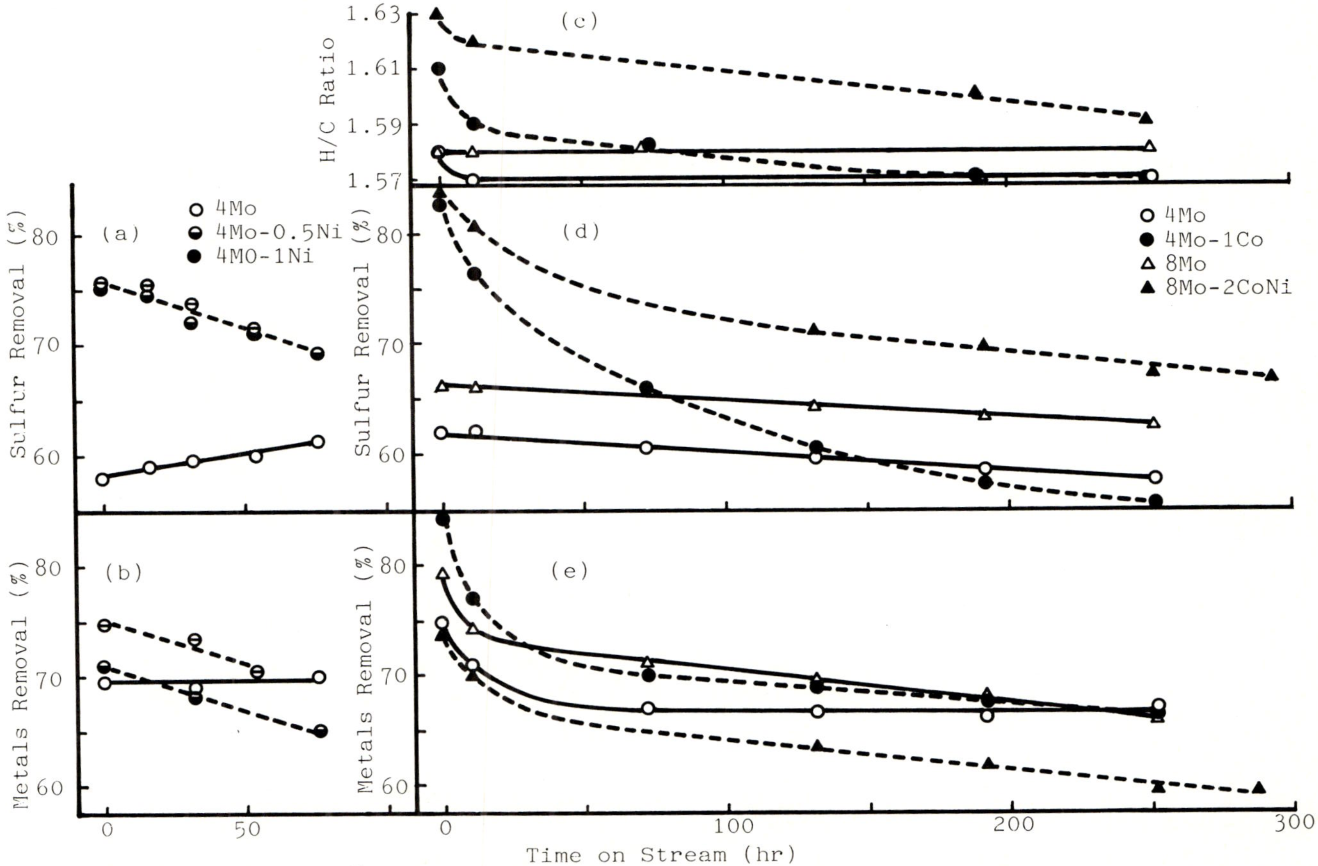

Figure 1 The First and Second Series Experimental Results. (a),(b) 1st Series. (c),(d),(e) 2nd Series.

addition of nickel or cobalt to 4Mo seems to be disadvantageous from the standpoint of total catalyst performance, although it promotes initial activities for both HDM and HDS reactions.

In the case of MoO_3-Al_2O_3 containing 8% molybdenum, the addition of 1% cobalt and 1% nickel adversely affected not only the deactivation rate but also initial activity for HDM reaction, in contrast to the results mentioned above where the addition of 1% cobalt to 4Mo promoted the initial activity. 8Mo-2CoNi had almost the same initial HDS activity as 4Mo-1Co, which was significantly higher than that of the unpromoted catalysts. It is interesting to note that although the deactivation rate of 8Mo-2CoNi was also higher than that of 8Mo, it was significantly reduced in comparison with 4Mo-1Co, so that 8Mo-2CoNi was able to maintain higher sulfur removal than 8Mo by 5% even after 250 hours. It agrees with a generally accepted concept that 8Mo-2CoNi, which contains an amount of metals similar to that of typical HDS catalysts, gives the best performance among the catalysts tested here as far as HDS reaction is concerned. With respect to the HDM reaction, however, it is interesting to note that 8Mo-2CoNi gives the poorest results and that 4Mo seems to be a promising catalyst.

Hydrogen/carbon atomic ratio of product oils, which may correspond to the catalyst activity for HY reaction, seems to vary in a similar way to HDS activity.

The used catalysts were subjected to X-ray microanalysis. Figure 2 illustrates vanadium distribution profiles in the catalyst pellet cross-section taken from the upper position of the catalyst bed. It is obvious that the addition of promoter metals and the increase of molybdenum content enhance the preferencial deposition of vanadium on the exterior of catalyst pellets.

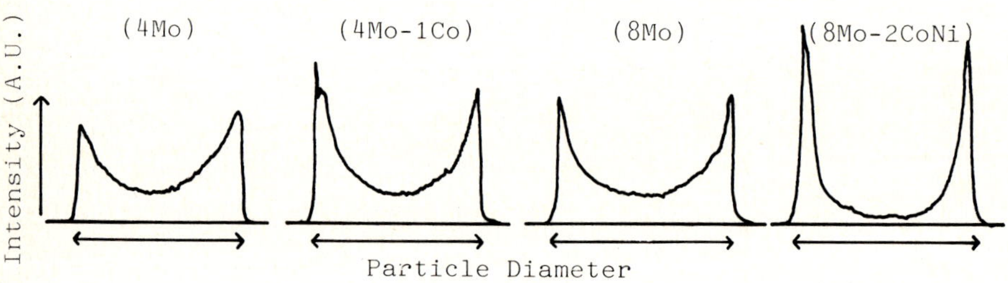

Figure 2 Vanadium Distribution Profiles in The Cross-Section of Used Catalysts.

Thus, an unpromoted MoO_3-Al_2O_3 catalyst indicates the possibility of giving better performance than a promoted one when it is used in a guard reactor of HDS units processing heavy residual oils, where better HDM ability is required rather than HDS ability. In order to evaluate the performance of unpromoted catalysts in such a use, a couple of long life tests with different catalyst combinations have been conducted for 3,700 and 4,600 hours with a feedstock containing vanadium and nickel in relatively high concentrations. A 60 ml of unpromoted catalyst(3Mo) or promoted catalyst(8Mo-2CoNi) was loaded in the first reactor of each unit. And a 140 ml of commercial HDS catalyst was loaded in each second reactor.

During the first 300 hours after the tests began, reaction temperature was held at the base temperature in order to make sure that activity changes coincided with the results obtained in the previous experiments. Reaction temperature was then raised at rates required to maintaining the sulfur content of the second reactor effluent at 0.8%, up to a predetermined maximum temperature. In Figure 3, reaction temperature and sulfur, metals and nitrogen contents of the first and second reactor effluents are plotted as a function of time on stream.

Metals contents of the first and second reactor effluents decreased gradually as reaction temperature began to increase after 300 hours. Metals content of the effluents from 3Mo was lower than that from 8Mo-2CoNi during the first 1,500 hours where the reaction temperature was kept the same with each other. Although the reaction temperature for 8Mo-2CoNi was raised at a higher rate than that for 3Mo after 1,500 hours, metals content stayed at the same level with each other. The slightly lower metals content observed after 3,000 hours with 8Mo-2CoNi may be due to its higher reaction temperature. Reaction temperature for the combination between 8Mo-2CoNi and the HDS catalyst attained the predetermined maximum temperature at 3,700 hours, whereas the combination between 3Mo and the HDS catalyst has lasted up to 4,500 hours. During that times the amount of metals deposited on catalysts in the first reactors, which was calculated based on the difference of metals content between the feedstock and the first reactor effluents, had reached 1.88 and 1.29 g/g-fresh catalyst for 3Mo and 8Mo-2CoNi, respectively. Thus, it has been demonstrated that 3Mo has a better HDM performance than 8Mo-2CoNi when they are used in a guard reactor.

Sulfur content of the first reactor effluent from 8Mo-2CoNi was lower than that from 3Mo by about 0.4% just after the tests were started, as expected from previous results. Accordingly, sulfur content of the second reactor effluent from the combination between 8Mo-2CoNi and the HDS catalyst was lower than that from the combination between 3Mo and the HDS catalyst by about 0.03%. The difference of 0.03% in sulfur content of the second reactor effluents corresponds well to the difference of about 0.4% in sulfur content of the first reactor effluents on the assumption that the HDS reaction rate is a function of the second order with respect to sulfur concentration in feedstock. Sulfur content of the first reactor effluents rapidly got nearer and crossed each other at around 300 hours. As for the HDN reaction, no difference was observed between the two catalyst combinations.

Vanadium and nickel distribution in the cross-section of the used catalyst

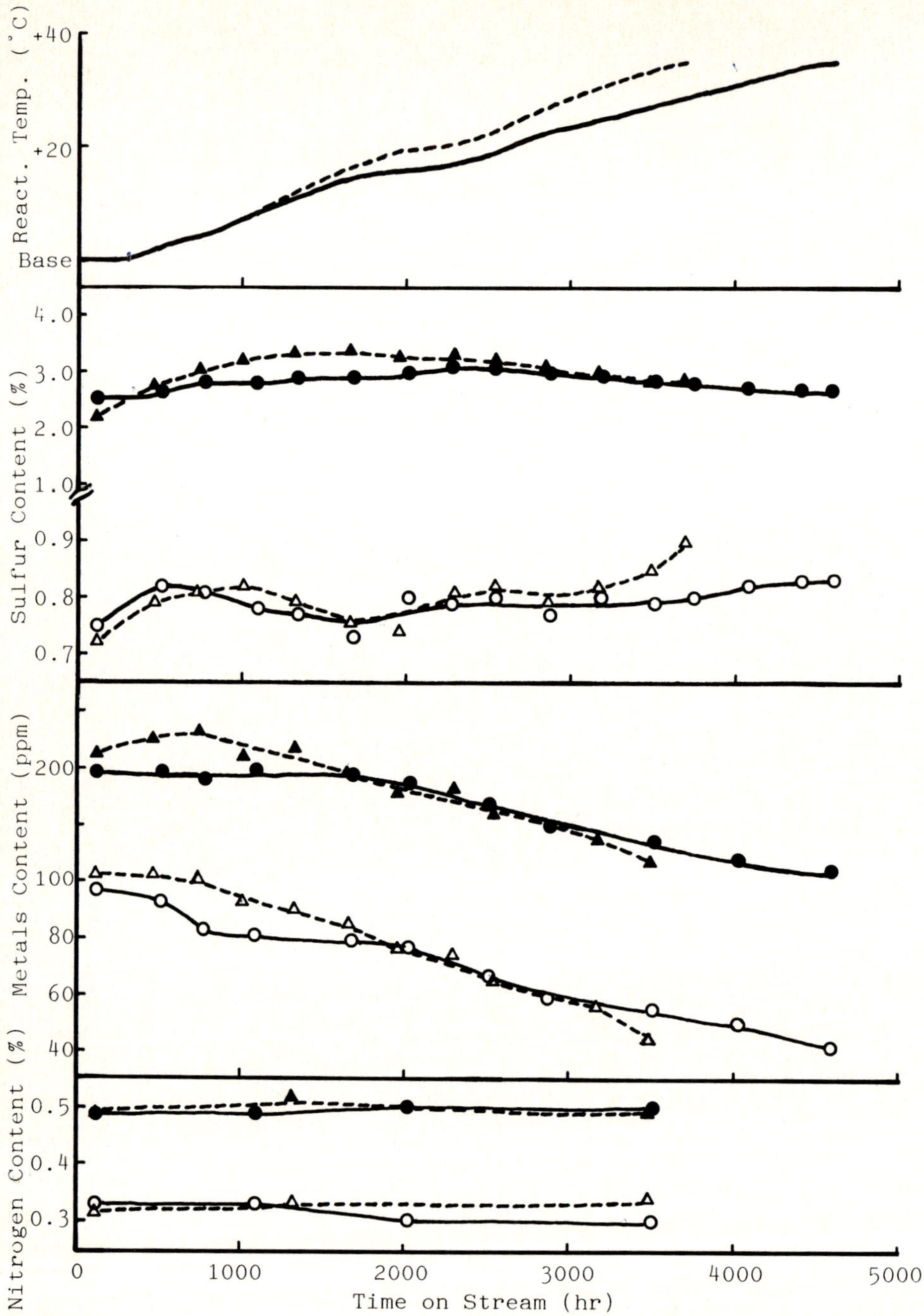

Figure 3 The Third Series Experimental Results. Effluents of 1st(●) and 2nd(○) reactors from 3Mo/HDS-catalust combination(——). Effluents of 1st(▲) and 2nd(△) reactors from 8Mo-2CoNi/HDS catalyst combination(---).

pellets taken from the first reactors are illustrated in Figure 4. It is clearly shown that the interior of the catalyst pellets of 3Mo has been utilized for removal of vanadium and nickel to a greater extent than that of 8Mo-2CoNi.

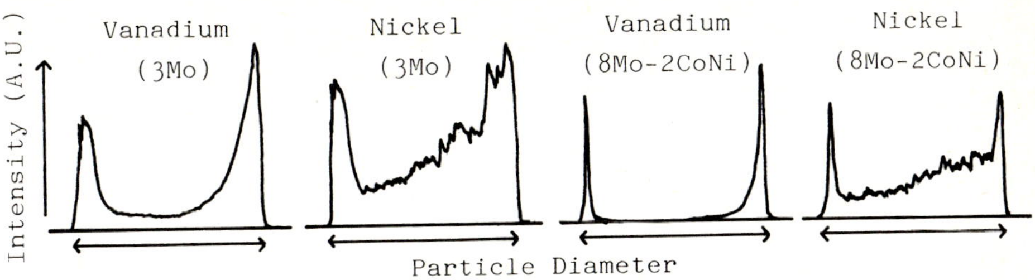

Figure 4 Vanadium and Nickel Distribution Profiles in The Cross-Section of Used Catalysts.

CONCLUSIONS

The effects of promoter metals added to MoO_3-Al_2O_3 have been studied using heavy fuel oils as feedstocks under reaction conditions employed in industrial hydrotreating processes. The results lead to the following conclusions:

1) The addition of cobalt or nickel to MoO_3-Al_2O_3 resulted in only a small gain in initial HDM activity and a significant acceleration of the deactivation rate. Consequently, the addition of such metals is considered to be disadvantageous as far as HDM reaction is concerned.

2) With respect to the HDS reaction, the addition of promoter metals increased the initial activity significantly; however, it also accelerated the deactivation rate. In addition, the deactivation rate is higher with lower molybdenum content. Therefore, improvement of HDS performance by the addition of promoter metals is anticipated only when molybdenum content is as high as that of typical HDS catalysts.

3) It has been demonstrated in a hydrotreating test for 4,600 hours that MoO_3-Al_2O_3 containing only 3% molybdenum achieves better performance than a catalyst containing a similar amount of molybdenum and promoter metals to typical HDS catalysts when they are used in a guard reactor of HDS units, where effective removal of vanadium and nickel is required for catalysts.

REFERENCES

1 F.E. Massoth, Adv. Catal. 27 (1978) 265-310.

2 P. Canesson, B. Delmon, G. Delvaux, P. Grange and J.M. Zabala, Proc. 6th Internat. Congr. Catalysis (1976) 927-936.

3 J. Laine, J. Brito, J. Gallardo and F. Severino, J. Catal., 91 (1985) 64-68.

4 V.H.J. De Beer, J.G.J. Dahlmans and J.G.M. Smeets, J. Catal., 42 (1976) 467-470.

5 D.S. Thakur and B. Delmon, J. Catal., 91 (1985) 308-317.

6 M.L. Vrinat and L. De Mourgues, Appl. Catal., 5 (1983) 43-57.

7 E.D. Radchenko, M.V. Landau, B.K. Nefedov, L.I. Nikulina, G.D. Chukin, P.A. Zhdan, D.A. Agrivsky and A.A. Slinkin, Proc. 8th Internat. Congr. Catalysis, (1984) II 399-410.

8 D.S. Thakur, P. Grange and B. Delmon, J. Catal., 91 (1985) 318-326.

9 M. Kurita, T. Watanabe and N. Takayama, Kogyokagaku Zasshi, 74 (1971) 2264-2268.

10 N. Todo, K. Muramatsu, M. Kurita, K. Ogawa and Y. Kotera, Bull. Japan Petrol. Inst., 14 (1972) 89-93.

11 S. Kushiyama, Y. Koinuma, R. Hizawa, S. Kobayashi, H. Mishikata, K. Inoue, Y. Shimizu and K. Egi, Sekiyu Gakkaishi, 19 (1976) 1016-1021.

B. Delmon and G.F. Froment (Editors), *Catalyst Deactivation 1987*

POISONING OF HYDRODESULFURIZATION CATALYSTS BY VANADIUM.

M.J. LEDOUX, O. MICHAUX and S. HANTZER

Laboratoire de Catalyse et Chimie des Surfaces, UA423-CNRS, Université L. Pasteur, 4 rue Blaise Pascal, 67000 Strasbourg (France).

ABSTRACT

The HDS activity of a commercial NiMo catalyst has been followed versus the amount of vanadium added to it, either by an oxidic procedure or by a sulfided route, using a highly soluble vanadyl porphyrin, simulating the industrial process. At the same time, Metal Solid NMR and EPR spectroscopies have been used to characterize the nature of the vanadium deposit.

INTRODUCTION

Several authors have studied the deactivation of molybdenum-based hydrotreatment catalysts for the HDM reaction. They used either vanadium and/or nickel poisonous compounds (ref. 1-3) and they observed a very rapid deactivation at low coverage of poison, followed by a much slower monotonous deactivation. The deactivation for HDS or HDN reactions by these poisons has not been published, except HDS tests made by Mitchell et al. (ref. 4) on phtalocyanine poisoned $CoMo/Al_2O_3$. Their poisoning procedure was not however really adequate for observing a difference between the poisoning effect by the ring of the phtalocyanine or by the metal itself contained in the ring. Finally, none of these authors has tried to characterize the poison deposit.

A tentative characterization of the vanadium deposit either by EPR or by non-pulsed solid NMR, has been successfully accomplished by Silbernagel (ref. 5) on industrial catalysts, but without the corresponding catalytic tests. He showed that at low loading vanadium is mainly under the vanadyl form; then, between 1% and 10%, most of the vanadium is contained in an uncharacterized phase which become V_2S_3 above 10% loading.

Because of the important deactivation for HDS or HDN reactions of CoMo or NiMo catalysts due to the vanadium content of crude oil, we have analyzed simultaneously the catalytic reaction and the nature of the metallic deposit by EPR and by Metal Solid NMR (ref. 6). The purpose of this article is to discuss the structural interaction between vanadium and a $NiMo/Al_2O_3$ catalyst in the sulfided state, and its consequences on the activity and the regeneration of the catalyst.

EXPERIMENTAL

The entire study was performed on the NiMo HR346 from PROCATALYSE. Two methods of vanadium deposition have been followed.

- For the oxidic method, the oxidic precursor of the catalyst was impregnated with a water solution of ammonium vanadate, dried at 120°C for 12h and calcinated at 500°C for 2h in air. The normal procedure of in situ sulfidation, described later, was then followed before catalytic test or spectroscopic analyses.

- For the sulfided method, the presulfided catalyst (normal procedure) was transferred under argon in a batch reactor containing a toluene-thiophene-0.5% solution of the required amount of a highly soluble vanadyl porphyrin (vanadyl meso-tetra-(p-n-hexyloxipheryl) porphyrin) (ref. 6,7). The mixture was stirred and left under reflux for 2 hours; the solvent was distilled to dryness and the catalyst transferred back to the reactor, under argon, to be re-treated by H_2S/H_2 for 2h at 450°C. The same procedure was followed to impregnate pure alumina without the NiMo active phase.

The catalytic tests (thiophene HDS under normal pressure : 20 torr thiophene, 740 torr H_2) were performed under differential conditions, on a fixed-bed reactor. The rate of the reaction was calculated, assuming a first order reaction, at very low conversion (below 2%), obtained by varying the space velocity (ref. 8,9). This rate of reaction will hereafter be called "activity". These tests were always made after a sulfidation step which was called "normal procedure" above : Purge of the reactor at room temperature, 30 min. under pure H_2; switch to H_2S/H_2-2% mixture; increase of temperature to 450°C at 13°/min.; left 2h at this temperature; rapid cooling (less than 2 min.) to 227°C for catalytic test or to room temperature before transfer under argon for EPR or NMR analyses in sealed cells.

The EPR and metal solid NMR experimental conditions have already been described (ref. 6,10).

RESULTS

HDS Activity.

The activity of the different poisoned catalysts versus the vanadium concentration is illustrated in Figure 1. Blank reactions on catalysts without vanadium but which had been treated either by water and calcination for the oxidic method of poisoning, or by H_2-porphyrin for the sulfidic method, showed no decrease in activity.

The deactivation due to the vanadium on the first series of catalysts (oxidic method) is slower than the deactivation observed on the second series (sulfidic method by porphyrin). But both of them are linear with the logarithm of the vanadium concentration, which is consistent with a statistical distribu-

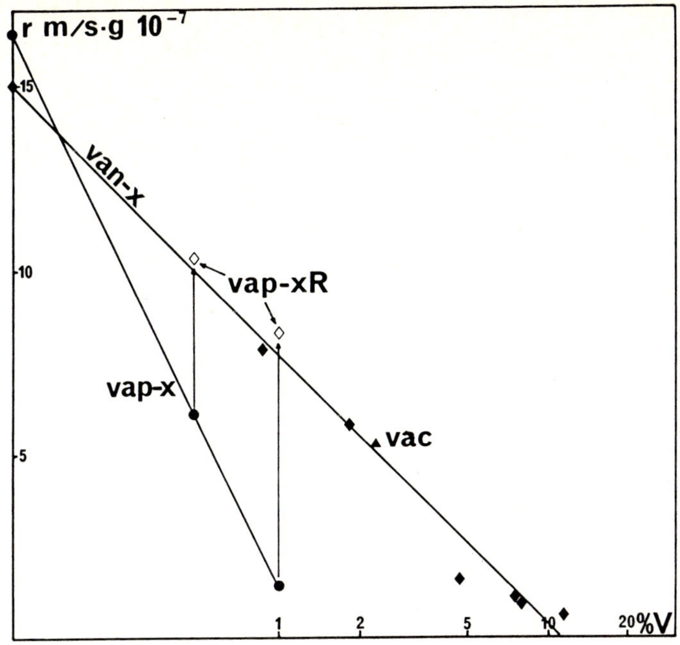

Figure 1 : HDS activity of $NiMo/Al_2O_3$. Van-x: first series of catalysts (oxidic method) from ammonium vanadate; vac: from vanadyl acetylacetonate. vap-x: second series of catalysts (sulfidic method) from vanadyl porphyrin; vap-xR: "regenerated" vap-x.

tion of the vanadium on the surface of the catalyst.

Finally, when the catalysts of the second series are "regenerated" in air at 500°C and resulfided, their activity increases at the level of the first series' activity.

EPR-Analyses.

Table 1 shows the main physical parameters measured from the EPR spectra.

Bulk sulfides (V_3S_5 and V_5S_8), like the first series of catalysts (oxidic method), do not show any signal as long as they are kept under oxygen-free atmosphere.

Standard spectra are obtained from solid vanadyl porphyrins (VOTPP and VOMTHPP) and from vanadyl acetylacetonate, where the vanadyl ion is surrounded either by four nitrogen or four oxygen atoms.

The EPR spectra of the second series of catalysts (sulfided method) (Figure 2) or of vanadyl porphyrin impregnated on the pure alumina (without the NiMo active phase) are identical after the second sulfidation step.

Table 1 : Physical constants obtained from the EPR analysis of the samples.

samples	T °K	a// (Gauss)	a⊥ (Gauss)	g//	g⊥	$\bar{a}_0$* (G)
(VO)TPP	300					
solid	120	173	60	1.972	1.987	98
(VO)MTHOPP	300	170	60	1.971	2.006	97
solid	120	173	60	1.958	1.999	97
VO-acac	300	ΔH = 340G				
solid	120	ΔH = 310G		g = 2.008		
VAP-0.5** 1)	300	168	55	1.978	1.991	92
and VAP-1 3)	300	152	55	1.978	1.991	87
1)	120	168	56	1.970	1.988	93
VAPAL-1 1)	300	171	56	1.966	1.984	94
3)	300	154	56	1.966	1.984	89
1)	120	171	56	1.971	1.986	94

* $\bar{a}_0 = (2a_\perp + a_{/\!/})/3$ mean value of the hyperfine coupling constant which must be theoretically equal to a_0 in solution. ** species 1) and 3), see text. Spectra at 300 °K and 120 °K identical. VAPAL-1 = porphyrin on pure alumina after sulfidic treatment.

Three different species of vanadyl environment are detected, one with four nitrogen atoms (as for the solid porphyrin), a second, probably with four sulfur atoms, which disappears to the benefit of the third when air is admitted to the sample, and a third with four oxygen atoms (as for the $VO(acac)_2$) .

A quantitative measurement made by double integration shows that all the vanadium is present under the vanadyl form and that the four nitrogen atoms' environments represent 20% of the total, the four sulfur atoms' environment also represents 20%, and the four oxygen atoms' environment 60%.

Finally, after "regeneration" the EPR signal disappears completely (Figure 3).

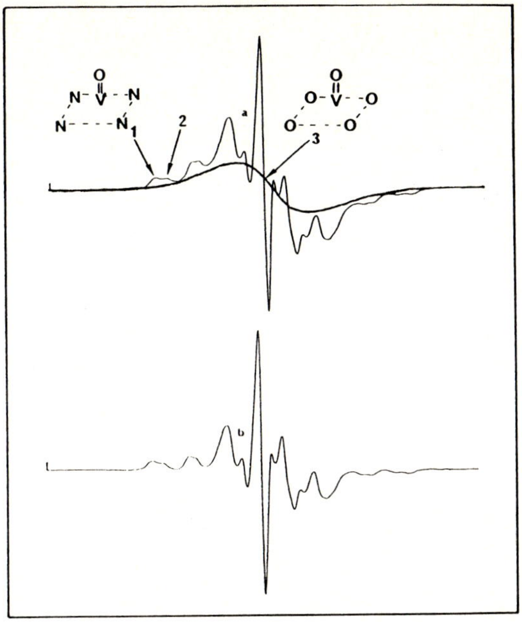

Figure 2: a) EPR spectrum of vap-1% showing the three environment of the vanadyl ion. b) Same spectrum after substraction of the species 3.

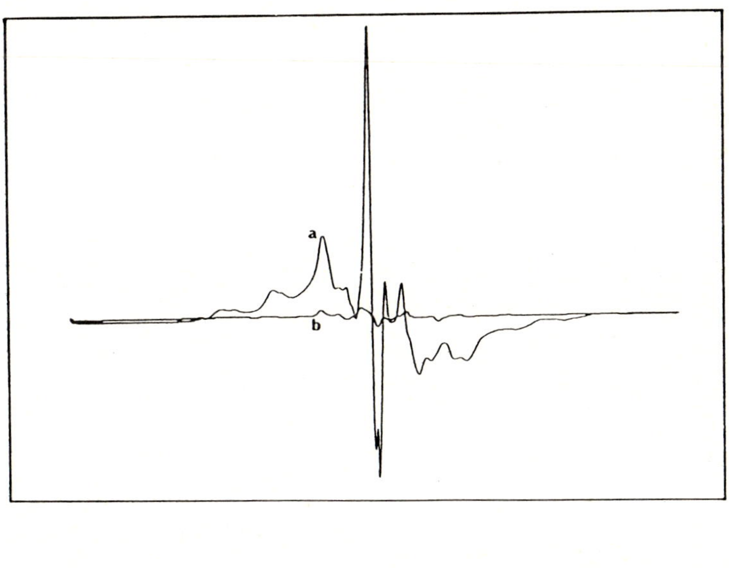

Figure 3: a)EPR spectrum of vap-0.5%. b) vap-0.5%, after "regeneration".

NMR Measurements.

The pure solid porphyrins, like the second series of catalysts (sulfidic method), have no NMR signal.

However, one has been able to show that, either on silica or on alumina, the first series of catalysts (oxidic method) has a spectrum similar to the bulk V_3S_5 or V_5S_8 in terms of Knight Shift and longitudinal relaxation time T_1 (Figure 4a and 4b).

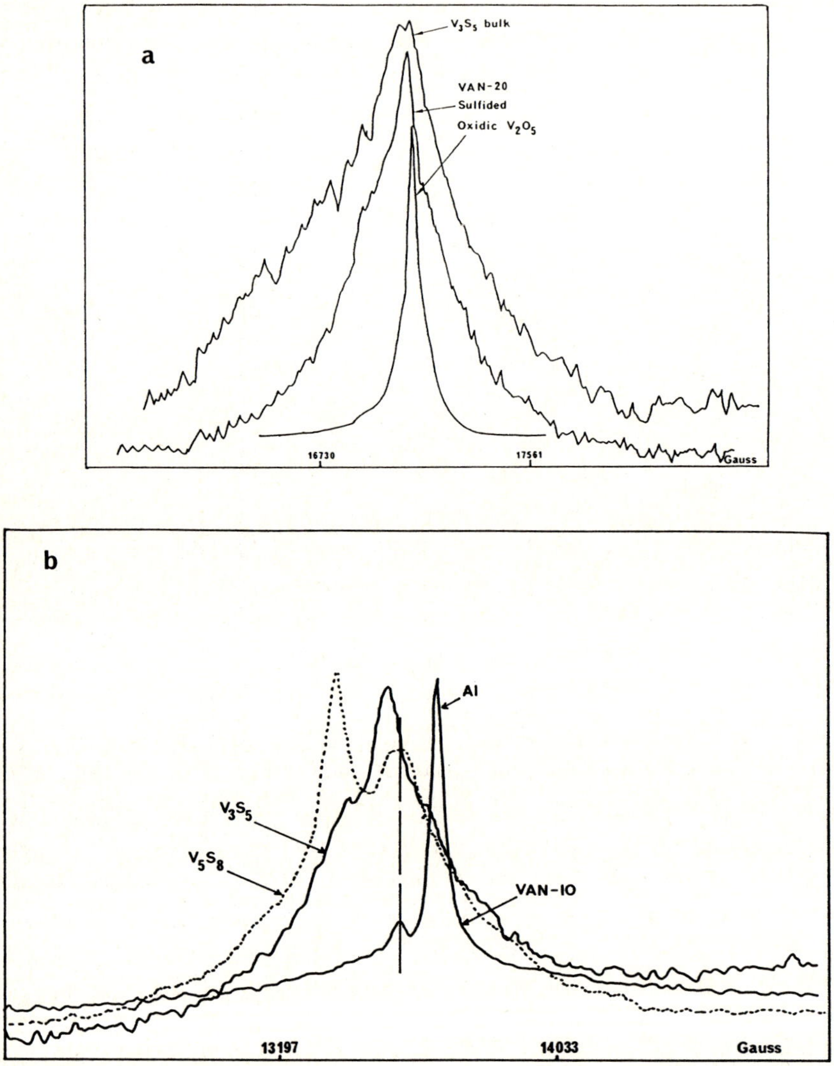

Figure 4: Metal solid NMR. a) At 4.2°K; van-20 = 20% of vanadium on $NiMo/SiO_2$. Time Interval: 10 ms for the sulfides and 2 s for the oxide. b) At 80°K; van-10 = 10% of vanadium on $NiMo/Al_2O_3$. Time Interval: 0.5 ms.

DISCUSSION

In preceding works (ref. 8-10), our group has proposed a description of the active sulfided CoMo or NiMo catalysts which takes into account both our NMR and activities measurements and the Harris and Chianelli theory (ref. 12) on the electronic transfer from Co or Ni to the molybdenum. In this model three sites are active for HDS, sulfur vacancies on molybdenum atoms with molybdenum neighbours (indice of activity: ≃1), sulfur vacancies on distorted tetrahedral cobalt sulfide, a phase which is stabilized by the presence of the molybdenum, (indice of activity: ≃1), and sulfur vacancies shared by a "rapid octahedral cobalt atom" and a molybdenum atom (indice of activity: ≃15) (Scheme 1). These "rapid cobalt atoms" (rapid because of their short relaxation time) behave like a glue, stabilizing the distorted tetrahedral cobalt phase on the molybdenum sulfide. In such a structure, Harris and Chianelli have shown that the cobalt atom can transfer electrons towards the molybdenum atom and thus strongly increase the activity of the molybdenum.

Two other effects must be taken into account in explaining the synergy between Co or Ni and Mo, an increase of the dispersion of the active phase and a stabilization of the degree of sulfidation, but these two effects are also due to this specific bond between "rapid octahedral cobalt" atoms and molybdenum atoms.

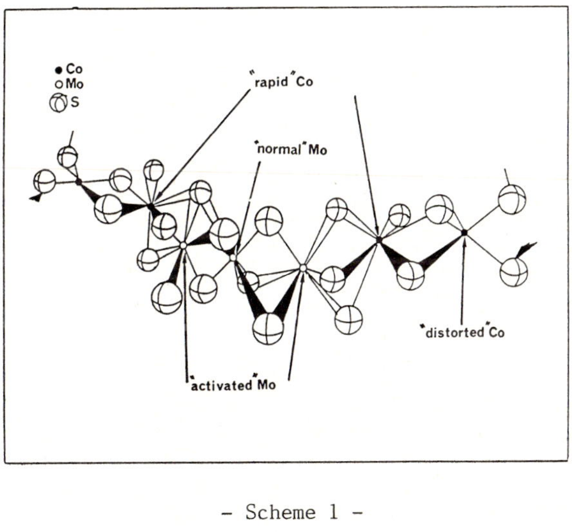

- Scheme 1 -

The NMR analysis has given, for the maximum of synergy (Co/Mo ≃ 0.5), one "rapid octahedral cobalt" for eight to ten distorted tetrahedral cobalt; thus only one molybdenum atom among twenty is bound to a "rapid cobalt" and is a very active site for HDS. A very selective poison can completely destroy the apparent synergy between Co or Ni and Mo with only a small number of atoms, if these atoms choose these very active sites.

It has been shown above that 60% of the vanadyl poison (ex. porphyrin) is surrounded by four oxygen atoms and therefore certainly lies on the support, as no oxygen atoms can possibly be found on the sulfided active phase under our conditions of measurement. In addition, the surface distribution of 20% of instable vanadyl surrounded by the four sulfur atoms, or of 20% of vanadyl surrounded by four nitrogen atoms, cannot be totally assigned either to the support or to the active phase; as there is no difference between the pure alumina and the catalyst, one can be reasonably confident of a statistical distribution. Thus, if one estimates that half of the surface is covered with the active phase, only 20% of the total vanadyl poison lies on this active phase.

20% of 1% in weight of vanadium on the NiMo catalyst corresponds to one atom of vanadium for twenty atoms of molybdenum, which is enough to poison the very active sites responsible for the synergy. Such a catalyst must have the same activity as a non-promoted Mo catalyst, which is observed (see Figure 1). This description means that the vanadyl species choose preferentially the very active site on the sulfided active phase; this is not in contradiction with the fact that these species are rich in electrons while the site of desulfurization is very electrophile.

For the other family of catalyst (oxidic method) or for "regenerated" porphyrin poisoned catalysts, the vanadyl ion is oxidized to V_2O_5 and then sulfided to a vanadium sulfide of the non stoechiometric phase VS-VS_2 as shown by the EPR and NMR analyses. Two explanations can be given for the poisoning effect of the vanadium.

At low concentration, during the sulfidation step, the vanadium can compete with the nickel (or cobalt) to bind the molybdenum atoms and prevent the formation of the pair : "rapid Ni(Co)" - Mo.

Silbernagel et al. (13) have shown that the non-stoechiometric phase VS-VS_2 can be described as a classical sandwich structure, as in MoS_2 for instance, with sulfur-metal-sulfur layers of VS_2 stochiometry, and additional vanadium atoms filling the plan between two sulfur layers. In this structure V_5S_8 can be written $V_{1/4}VS_2$, where one site on four is occupied, and VS can be written VVS_2 where all the sites are occupied.

The NMR spectrum shows that the poisonous vanadium (oxidic method) is very close to V_5S_8 at high loading (~10% of vanadium). At lower loading, one can propose that the MoS_2 layers are used as a basal plan to develop a $V_{1/4}MoS_2$ stable structure, as in V_5S_8 ($V_{1/4}VS_2$), preventing the formation of most of the very active CoMo or NiMo sites. Thus one atom of vanadium for four atoms of molybdenum will be sufficient to destroy the apparent synergy, a value which corresponds to about 3% of vanadium in weight statistically distributed between the support and the active phase. This is observed in Figure 1.

At higher coverage, the vanadium sulfide develops its structure to V_5S_8 or V_2S_3 by adding more layers of metal and sulfur atoms and progressively blocks the accessibility of the remaining active sites to reach the activity of a poorly dispersed pure vanadium sulfide catalyst.

CONCLUSION

It has been shown that the vanadium, contained as vanadyl ion in a porphyrin structure, maintained its vanadyl configuration under HDS conditions, even at high temperature, on an industrial NiMo catalysts. This vanadium is a powerful poison for the HDS reaction because it neutralizes selectively the very active sites responsible for the apparent synergy observed between Ni and Mo. Only 1% in weight of metal is sufficient to totally destroy the synergy.

After an oxidic regeneration, followed by resulfurization, the vanadium is present on the surface in a sulfided dispersed phase similar to V_5S_8. Its poisoning effect is less dramatic because it does not choose selectively the very active site to cover the surface.

In both case, the vanadium is statistically dispersed on the full surface of the catalyst, support and active phase.

ACKNOWLEDGMENT

The DRRT Alsace has supported this work financially (83.j.0365); P.Petit and J.J. André are gratefully acknowledged for the EPR analysis, P. Panissod for the NMR analysis, H.J. Callot for the porphyrin synthesis and R.R. Chianelli for supplying bulk vanadium sulfides.

REFERENCES

1 C. Takeuchi, S. Asoaka, S. Nakata and Y. Shiroto, Preprints, Am. Chem. Soc., Division of Petroleum Chemistry, 30 (1985) 96.
2 J. Weitkamp, W. Gerhardt and D. Scholl, Proceedings of the 8th Inter. Congr. Catal., Berlin, Verlag Chemie Ed., (1985) p.II 269.
3 J.C. Plumail and H. Toulhouat, Proceedings of the 2nd Franco-venezuelian Colloque on Catalysis, IFP, Rueil Malmaison, (1985) p.E.
4 P.C.H. Mitchell and J.A. Valero, React. Kinet. Catal. Lett., 20 (1982) 219.
5 B.G. Silbernagel, J. Catal., 56 (1979) 315.
6 M.J. Ledoux, O. Michaux, S. Hantzer, P. Panissod, P. Petit, J.J. André and H.J. Callot, J. Catal., In press.
7 M.J. Ledoux, O. Michaux and H.J. Callot, To be patented.
8 M.J. Ledoux, O. Michaux, G. Agostini and P. Panissod, J. Catal., 102 (1986) 275.
9 O. Michaux, Thesis, Université L. Pasteur, Strasbourg (1986).
10 M.J. Ledoux, O. Michaux, G. Agostini and P. Panissod, J. Catal., 96 (1985) 189.
11 M.J. Ledoux, O. Michaux, S. Hantzer, 9th Int. Congress. Catal., Calgary 1988, submitted.
12 S. Harris and R.R. Chianelli, J. Catal., 98(1986) 17.
13 B.G. Silbernagel, J. Catal., 56 (1979) 315.

B. Delmon and G.F. Froment (Editors), *Catalyst Deactivation 1987*

MILD HYDROCRACKING: COPING WITH CATALYST DEACTIVATION

J.W. Gosselink, W.H.J. Stork, A.F. de Vries and C.H. Smit

Koninklijke/Shell-Laboratorium, Amsterdam (Shell Research B.V.), Badhuisweg 3, 1031 CM Amsterdam (The Netherlands)

ABSTRACT

The mild hydrocracking process imparts extra cracking capacity to a vacuum gas oil desulfurization unit simply by the increase in temperature. With conventional hydrotreating catalysts, the resulting exponential increase in catalyst deactivation by coke formation limits the conversion levels achievable. If a catalyst more resistant to coke deactivation is used, higher operating temperatures/conversion levels are feasible. A direct increase in conversion can be achieved by means of multiple catalyst systems in which dedicated cracking catalysts are included. As dedicated cracking catalysts are susceptible to poisoning by organic nitrogen compounds, the deactivation behaviour of systems containing them is very complex.

INTRODUCTION

The rapid increase in oil prices during the late seventies brought about a marked reduction in the consumption of oil products, especially of heavy fuel. The resulting shift in the balance of demand towards higher-grade products could only be met by increased conversion. Additional "conventional" conversion units such as cat. crackers, hydrocrackers and thermal crackers have certainly been installed. Since such units generally require major investments and have long lead times, though, efforts were also made to bring on stream more quickly alternative conversion facilities that were cheap but possibly had only limited conversion capabilities. A prime example of this approach is "mild hydrocracking" (MHC) (refs. 1-4), whereby the catalysts and mode of operation of existing vacuum gas oil (VGO) desulfurization units are adapted so that, apart from the product sulfur specification being met, some 15-40 % of VGO is converted into, in particular, valuable middle distillates of acceptable quality.

In the MHC process, conditions such as pressure (35-90 bar) and gas rate (200-500 $Nl.kg^{-1}$) are fixed and, apart from the use of dedicated catalysts, the only variations possible are in the operating temperature (360-420 °C) and, in some cases, space velocity (0.4-1.5 $m^3.m^{-3}.h^{-1}$). The hydrogen consumption in MHC is higher than in conventional HDS but beyond a given level (0.5-1.0 %(m/m) on feed) it decreases again with increasing conversion/temperature. Heteroatom removal is deep in any case, and hydrogen consumption by additional cracking is (over)compensated by lower hydrogenation, connected with the increased aromatics content of the product.

Furthermore, on progression to higher temperatures at the low prevailing hydrogen partial pressures, catalyst deactivation also increases, presumably due to increased coke lay-down on the catalyst. As a result, the optimum operating regime for a MHC unit reflects a balance between the higher conversion and the shorter catalyst life. It is thus evident that the study and control of catalyst deactivation are crucial to progress in MHC. Some of the ways in which stability can be increased are obvious (such as maximization of hydrogen partial pressures within the unit constraints). This paper focusses on the progress that can be made by optimizing the design of catalyst systems.

EXPERIMENTAL

A number of catalysts were tested for different cases (1-4), i.e. different combinations of operating conditions (Table 1) and feedstocks (Table 2).

TABLE 1

Operating conditions

Case		1	2	3	4
P (total)	(bar)	40	40	40	62.5
WHSV	($kg.l^{-1}.h^{-1}$)	0.9	0.3	0.4	0.8
T	(°C)	390-400	370-390	400	380-425
H_2/feed	($Nl.kg^{-1}$)	250	300	300	330

The experiments were performed in once-through trickle-flow reactors with a catalyst inventory of about 100 ml except for the experiments in which the effect of nitrogen poisoning was investigated, where two separate microflow reactors, catalyst inventory 5-15 g, were used. The details of the test equipment and procedures have been reported earlier (refs. 1-3). It has to be stressed that >370 °C conversion (i.e. conversion to bp >370 °C products) has been used as the measure of the cracking activity and is defined as:

$$>370\ ^{\circ}C\ \text{conversion} = 1 - \frac{>370\ ^{\circ}C\ \text{content of total product}}{>370\ ^{\circ}C\ \text{content of feedstock}}$$

CATALYST DEACTIVATION UNDER MHC CONDITIONS

In normal VGO desulfurizers conventional hydrotreating (HT) catalysts are generally used. Shell HT catalysts are S-344 and S-444 $Co/Mo/Al_2O_3$ catalysts, the more active in hydrodesulfurization (HDS) and S-324 and S-424 $Ni/Mo/P/Al_2O_3$

TABLE 2

Feedstock characteristics

Case		1	2	3	4
C	(%(m/m))	83.68	85.25	85.63	86.02
H	(%(m/m))	11.83	11.78	11.98	12.30
S	(%(m/m))	3.22	3.04	2.65	1.94
N	(%(m/m))	0.10	0.14	0.11	0.14
Ni	($mg.kg^{-1}$)	0.5	0.8	0.7	0.6
V	($mg.kg^{-1}$)	0.2	1.1	0.5	1.0
density 70/4	(g/ml)	0.898	0.899	0.897	0.878
TBP-GLC Initial boiling point	(°C)	344	216	340	228
10 % recovered at	(°C)	398	329	405	331
20 % recovered at	(°C)	420	369	431	366
30 % recovered at	(°C)	437	398	451	393
40 % recovered at	(°C)	454	423	468	416
50 % recovered at	(°C)	471	446	486	436
60 % recovered at	(°C)	489	470	501	455
70 % recovered at	(°C)	510	495	520	475
80 % recovered at	(°C)	536	526	539	498
90 % recovered at	(°C)	553		564	532
Final boiling point	(°C)	614			

catalysts, the more active in hydrodenitrogenation (HDN) and hydrocracking (HC). As a start to our research on MHC these conventional catalysts were investigated extensively under MHC conditions.

When a VGO HDS unit is being operated with a conventional catalyst in the MHC mode, significant catalyst deactivation can be encountered as a result of the low hydrogen pressure (compared with HC) and high-temperature operation (compared with HDS). Under first-stage HC conditions (e.g. 100 bar H_2 pressure or higher), the decline in the HDS activity of, for instance, S-424 is about 1-2 °C per 1000 run hours. Under MHC conditions (case 1 at 40 bar, accelerated life test) and >370 °C conversion level of 18 % a deactivation rate of 17 °C per 1000 run hours is found. The deactivation of the HDS reaction under MHC conditions is generally more pronounced than that of HDN and cracking, for reasons not completely understood. However, the HDS reaction is of prime importance, because the total cycle length is often determined by the sulfur specification of the liquid product.

Coke deposition is generally accepted to be the main cause of catalyst deactivation under these conditions (ref. 5). By analyses of the carbon content of samples of S-324 after 600 run hours operation at mean >370 °C conversion level of 27 % (case 1) we have investigated the coke profile over the catalyst bed. The carbon, coke, content of the catalyst gradually increases with depth in the catalyst bed, as illustrated in Fig. 1.

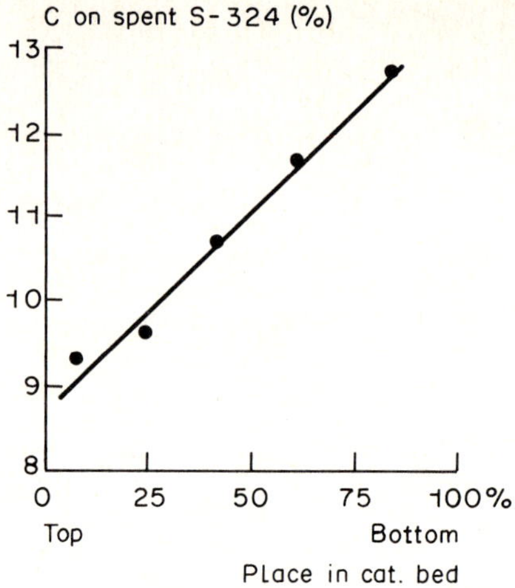

Fig. 1. C profile over spent S-324 after 600 run hours at a mean >370 °C conversion level of about 27 % (values not corrected for the relative increase in catalyst density).

Conversion in a MHC unit over a conventional HT catalyst can be augmented by further increasing the temperature (refs. 1-3,6,7), leading, however, to faster deactivation of the catalyst. The extent of this penalty has been investigated in bench-scale experiments with S-344 at 40 bar (case 2). Figure 2 shows clearly that the gradual increase in the conversion level is accompanied by an exponential increase in the catalyst deactivation.

For the same case S-324 was also tested. As stated earlier this catalyst is somewhat more active in cracking. Therefore the same conversion level of 27.6 % (S-344 at 388 °C) can be reached at a lower temperature, i.e. 383 °C. Figure 3 shows that, at equal conversion levels, the deactivation rates of S-324 and S-344 are about the same.

The complete description of the deactivation by coke formation is very complicated. Coke precursors responsible for this type of deactivation are presumably resins, asphaltenes, polycyclic aromatics, and nitrogen, oxygen and sulfur heterocyclic compounds. They adsorb on the catalyst surface and compete with, in particular, sulfur compounds for active (HDS) sites. H_2 addition will saturate these intermediates, eliminating them as coke-making compounds. But H_2 removal will lower their H/C ratios, with coke formation as a result (ref. 5). Obviously, high temperature and low H_2 partial pressure (compare MHC with HDS and HC) favour the H_2 removal reaction and thus the coke formation. Both the (HDS, HDN and cracking) reactions and the formation of more volatile products will lower the hydrogen partial pressure (low H_2/feed ratios in MHC) and

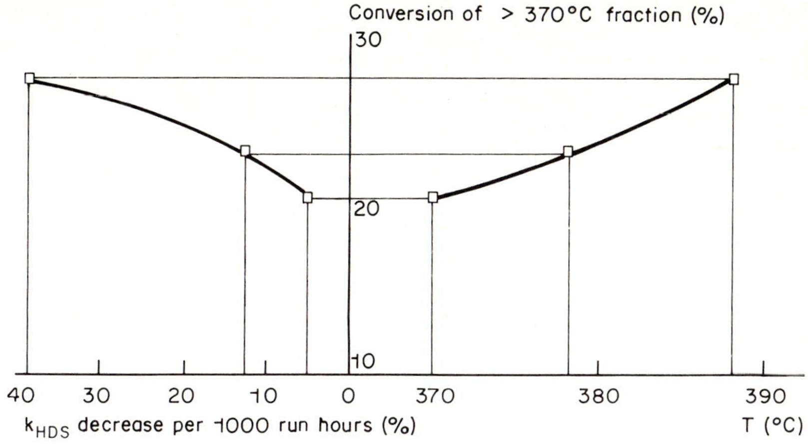

Fig. 2. Effect of temperature on MHC of VGO (case 2) over S-344. Conversion and catalyst deactivation.

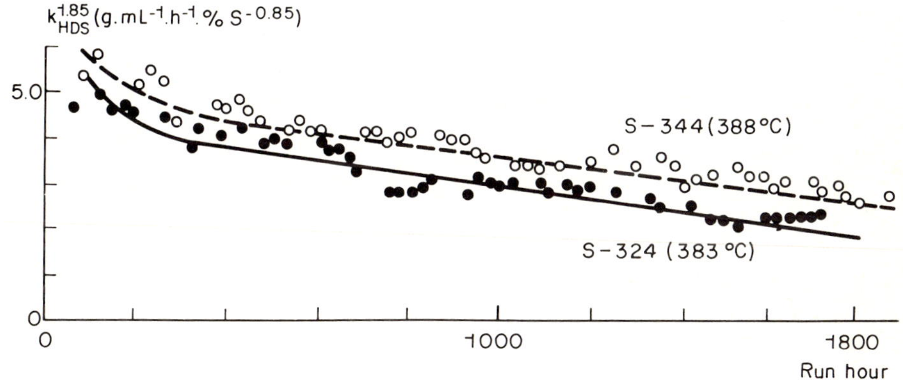

Fig. 3. Comparison of HDS deactivation of S-344 and S-324 at 27.6 % conversion level (case 2).

consequently increase coke formation on progression down the reactor (see Fig. 1). The fact that catalyst deactivation seems to be primarily a function of the conversion level suggests that coke precursors formed in the cracking reaction play an important role and that coke precursors present in the feedstocks studied might be less harmful.

CATALYSTS MORE RESISTANT TO COKE DEACTIVATION

Operating with a catalyst with enhanced stability allows a further increase of temperature/conversion. To this end we have studied existing and experimental catalysts in dedicated MHC bench-scale accelerated life tests.

Figure 4 shows the higher stability of a new MHC catalyst (0.8 mm cylinders) under low-pressure MHC conditions (case 1: 16 % conversion and case 3: 28 % conversion) in the HDS reaction compared with conventional HT catalysts.

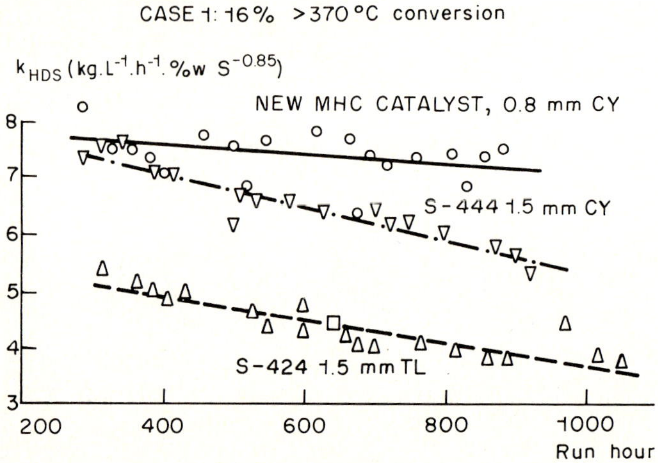

Fig. 4. Improved stability of the new MHC catalyst (0.8 mm cylinders).
CY - cylinders; TL - trilobes.

It is possible that the combination of porous texture and metals loading has a beneficial effect on the resistance to coke formation.

Another approach to increasing the stability of HT catalysts is the use of Ni/Mo over Co/Mo stacked beds, which show increased stability under Cat. Feed Hydrotreating conditions in the processing of heavier feedstocks (ref. 5). In particular, the Ni/Mo catalyst at the top will hydrogenate coke precursors, which would otherwise poison the intrinsically more active Co/Mo HDS catalyst.

COMPLEX DEACTIVATION IN MULTIPLE CATALYST SYSTEMS

A direct increase in cracking activity can be achieved by means of dedicated cracking (HC) catalysts. Such catalysts are generally sensitive to organic nitrogen compounds. Stacked beds with S-424 (having a high HDN activity) on top of an HC catalyst have therefore been studied. Figure 5 shows the performance of such a stacked bed (68/32 v/v) under typical conditions for a high-pressure (60 bar) MHC unit (case 4), compared with that of a S-424 single bed in bench-scale equipment. The advantage of the stacked bed with respect to the >370 °C conversion increases with increasing temperature. The yield of extra distillates in this case is concentrated in the naphtha range. By replacement of the second catalyst by HC catalysts more tailored to middle-distillates make the product palette can be shifted in the direction of the gas oil and kerosine ranges.

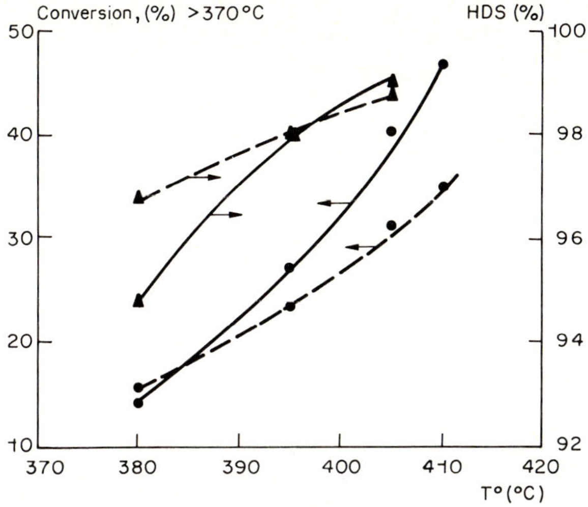

Fig. 5. Comparison of MHC performance of S-424/HC cat. (——) and S-424 (---), case 4.

The fact that the HC catalysts are much more susceptible than the HT catalysts to poisoning by nitrogen compounds makes deactivation of these dedicated multiple catalyst systems very complicated. A simplified scheme for the deactivation network is given in Fig. 6.

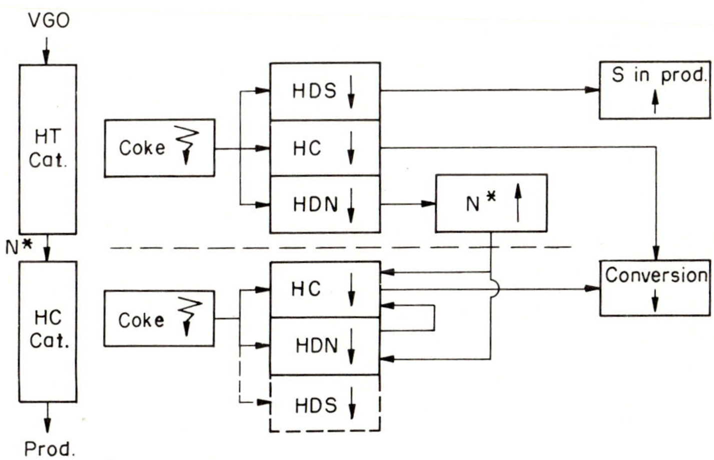

Fig. 6. Simplified scheme for deactivation of multiple catalyst systems.

The influence of the decline in the HDN activity of the HT catalyst on the performance of the HC catalyst has been investigated in microflow equipment by decreasing the temperature of the HT bed while keeping that of the HC bed constant (case 4). Figure 7 shows the dramatic effect of the increasing nitrogen level of the HT bed effluent on the conversion level reached over the HC bed. A comparable effect on the HDN activity of the HC bed is found.

Computer models have been developed to describe the effect of this N poisoning on the overall stacked-bed activity and are currently been used to design optimal stacked-bed systems.

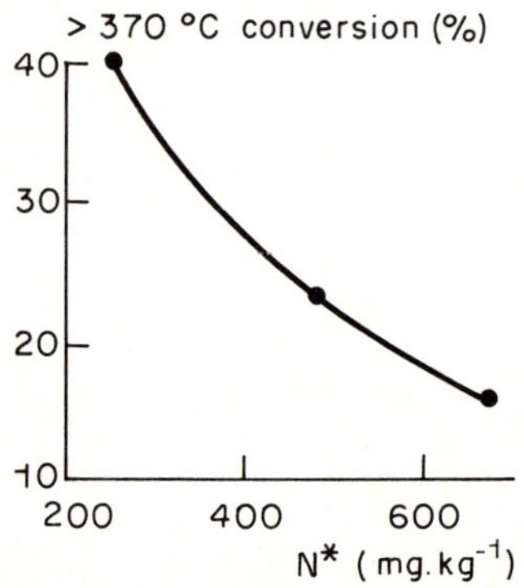

Fig. 7. Effect of N poisoning on HC catalyst of multiple catalyst system (case 4, T(HC bed) = 405 °C).

In addition to direct deactivation the coke lay-down on the catalyst of the multiple systems also enhances the N poisoning of the HC catalyst. Fortunately, recent experiments (case 4) have shown that stable operation with such systems is possible under conditions where they perform better in terms of conversion than the conventional systems. Moreover, deactivation of these multiple systems is more easily compensated for by temperature increase, common practice in refinery units, because of their higher apparent activation energies. This phenomenon is illustrated in Fig. 5. Increase of temperature results in higher rates of desorption of N compounds from the surface of the HC catalyst.

CONCLUSIONS

1. In MHC the high temperature and the low H_2 pressure (compare HDS and HC) lead to enhanced coke make and subsequently catalyst deactivation.
2. Coke formation is most pronounced in the lower reactor parts because of the local lower H_2 pressures.
3. Coke deactivation seems to be primarily a function of the conversion level applied.

4. Increase of the conversion level in a MHC unit with a conventional HT catalyst by increasing the operating temperature is limited by the resulting exponential increase of coke deactivation.
5. Catalysts more resistant to coke deactivation permit a temperature/conversion increase beyond these limits.
6. In multiple catalyst systems, such as S-424/HC cat., which enable a direct increase of cracking activity/conversion level, coke deactivation potentially also results in an increase in poisoning of the dedicated cracking catalyst by organic nitrogen molecules.

ACKNOWLEDGEMENT

The authors wish to thank Mr. P. Slaman, Mr. B.L. van Liemt, Mr. A. van de Paverd and Ms. C.M. Heijs for valuable contributions to this paper.

REFERENCES

1. I.E. Maxwell, W.H.J. Stork, B. Schaper, L. Lundqvist and M. Yoguchi, Petrotech, 5 (1982) 816-817.
2. W.H.J. Stork, I.E. Maxwell, A.F. de Vries, C.H. Smit, L. Lundqvist and B. Schaper, Paper presented at the Shell Catalyst Seminar, Tokyo, Japan, November 9, 1983.
3. J.W. Gosselink, W.H.J. Stork and A.F. de Vries, Paper presented at the Shell Catalyst Seminar, Tokyo, Japan, May 27-29, 1986.
4. M.M. van Kessel and R.H. van Dongen, Paper presented at the Institute of Petroleum Economics and Refining Seminar, November 11, 1986.
5. C.T. Adams, D.N. Washecheck, R.H. Slade and W.J. Daniels, Paper AM-86-26 presented at the 1986 USA National Petroleum Refiners Association (NPRA) Annual Meeting, March 23-25, 1986, Los Angeles, USA.
6. J.W.M. Sonnemans, F.L. Plantenga, P.H. Desai, V.J.D'Amico and P.H. Dixon, Paper AM-84-60 presented at the 1984 NPRA Meeting, March 25-27, 1984, San Antonio, USA.
7. J.W. Ward, J.W. Miller, J.D. Probst and G.E. Dolbear, Paper presented at the Japan Petroleum Institute, October 23-24, 1984, Tokyo, Japan.

B. Delmon and G.F. Froment (Editors), *Catalyst Deactivation 1987*

COKING OF IRON SULFIDE CATALYSTS DURING HYDROLIQUEFACTION OF COAL

R. BACAUD[1] , M. BESSON[1] , M. OBERSON[1] , D. BRODZKI[2] , P. BUSSIERE[1] , H. CHARCOSSET[1] , G. DJEGA-MARIADASSOU[2] and B. NICKEL[3]

[1]Institut de Recherches sur la Catalyse, CNRS, Conventionné avec l'Université Claude Bernard, Lyon I, 2 Avenue A. Einstein, 69626 Villeurbanne Cedex (France)

[2]Université P. & M. Curie, Laboratoire de Réactivité de Surface et Structure, UA 1106, CNRS, 4 Place Jussieu, 75252 Paris Cedex 05, France

[3]USM Grenoble, LEDSS (LA 332), Bât. 52, Chimie Recherche, BP 68, 38402 Saint Martin d'Hères

ABSTRACT

Catalysis of coal hydroliquefaction (HL) was studied over highly dispersed and non porous iron sulfide catalysts (non stoichiometric pyrrhotites). The active interface between the bulk catalyst and the reactional mixture was built during liquefaction and a coke layer was deposited on the $Fe_{1-x}S$ surface. During HL the first role of this coke was to prevent the sintering of the catalyst particles. Two kinds of coke were identified according to the mode of sulfidation and introduction of the catalyst into the autoclave. The catalytic roles of the interface were discussed in terms of solvent rehydrogenation, pool of active hydrogen(spillover effect) and stabilization of radicals.

INTRODUCTION

Hydroliquefaction (HL) of coal can be carried out using iron-based catalysts like red-muds, pyrite, iron oxides in the presence of an excess of sulfur (1). During the catalytic process, what may be the initial iron-based precursor, the active phase has been shown to be a non stoichiometric pyrrhotite $Fe_{1-x}S$ (2-6). For sake of comparison between different experiments and in order to study the activity of the catalytic phase, surface composition and specific surface areas must be more particularly defined.

We used aerosol iron oxides prepared by a flame method (7). These precursors generally presented a well defined morphology which could be preserved, during their evolution into pyrrhotite, during HL. The catalysts were non porous materials.

Liquefactions were carried out in an autoclave (Sotelem, France) and the reaction products extracted by different solvents. The extraction by tetrahydrofurane (THF) solubilized most of the organic products and permitted studies of the catalyst particles in the final solid residue by X-ray diffraction and transmission electron microscopy (TEM) associated with an X-ray emission microanalyser.

The evolution of the "catalyst-coal" interface and its role in the reaction solvent rehydrogenation and in the stabilization of radicals, are the main objectives of this paper. The THF washed surface of the catalyst was shown to vary according to the experimental conditions. Assumptions could be made to correlate the nature of the catalytic surface with liquid phase composition and hydrogen consumption. Coke deposition appeared to be one of the major component of the catalytic surface.

II EXPERIMENTAL

Different Fe_2O_3 aerosols (with various specific surface areas, Table 1, Fig. 1) were used as catalyst precursors. In standard conditions, HL process

TABLE 1
Main characteristics of two iron oxide precursors.
Every precursor have been shown to transform into pyrrhotite (2, 3).

Samples	$S_{BET} m^2 g^{-1}$	d_{BET}(nm)	d_{XRD}(nm)	d_{TEM}(nm)	Phases
SFEC	18	65	50	20 –	α , γ ,
				110	, β
THV3	44	30	22	15	Fe_2O_3

was conducted in a stirred autoclave (0.3 l) with a highly volatile bituminous coal (40 g, Freyming, France), in suspension in tetralin (hydrogenating solvent, 95 g); 2 wt % iron oxide (related to coal) and elemental sulfur were added in order to obtain a 1 % H_2S partial pressure and to sulfide the precursor. Initial hydrogen pressure, at room temperature, was 15 MPa.

Blank experiments without any catalyst or coal were also carried out in order to determine the sulfidation state and activity of the internal surface of the autoclave. The autoclave was heated to the reaction temperature (673K) at 3K/min. and held at this temperature for one hour. A total pressure of 22 MPa was generally maintained constant at 673K.

Introduction of the catalyst at high temperature could also be made. Some catalysts were pre-sulfided in the autoclave, in suspension in tetralin, with elemental sulfur, but without coal. The influence of temperature has already been studied in a previous work (2).

At the end of each run, the value of conversion, based on solubilities of HL products in hexane (HEX), toluene (TOL) and THF, was determined using the

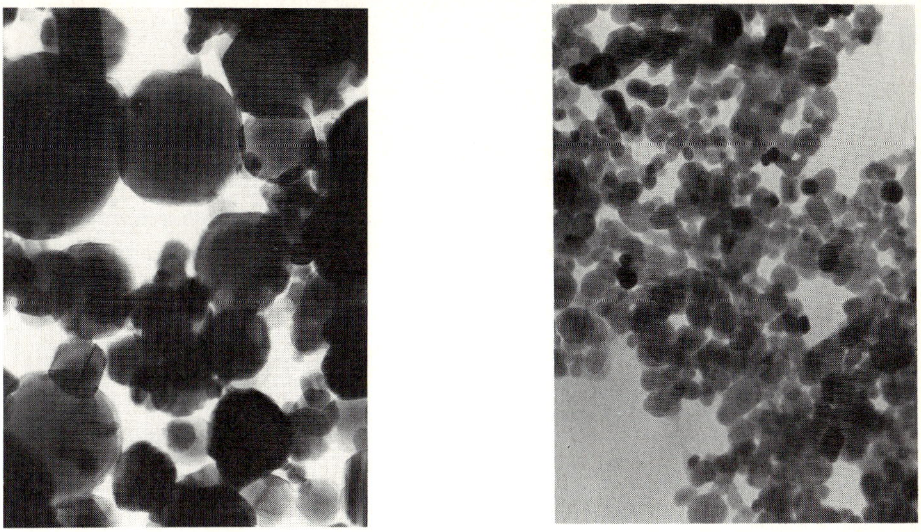

Fig. 1. Iron oxide precursors (Fe_2O_3) : 18 and 44 m^2g^{-1} respectively.

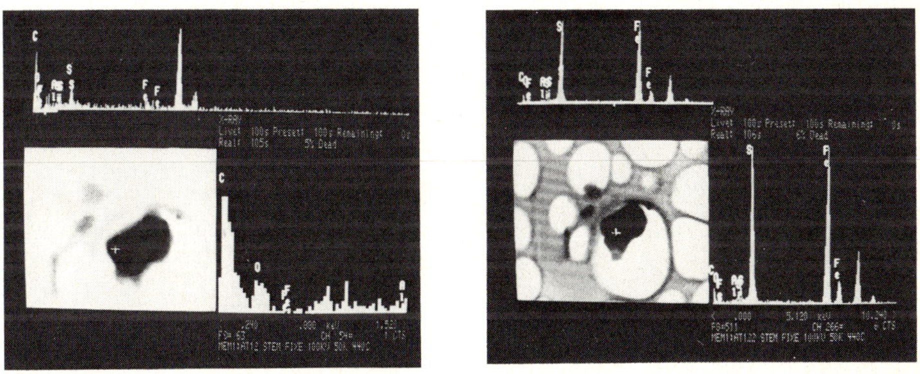

Fig. 2. THF washed catalyst : coke deposited on the surface of pyrrhotite particles.

pressure microfiltration procedure described by Tischer and Utz (8). The total hydrogen consumption was obtained from the decrease of total pressure in the autoclave plus the hydrogen quantity transferred from the solvent to coal fragments. Evaluation of the percentage of dehydrogenated tetralin (into naphtalene was made using the Naphtalene/(Naphtalene + Tetralin) ratio (N/N + T) as measured by gas chromatography.

The solid residues remaining from THF extractions were separated by centrifugation (5200 rpm). X-ray diffraction patterns (XRD) were performed using an internal reference (quartz). A Seeman-Bolhin device was used, with a FeKα radiation.

The stoichiometry of $Fe_{1-x}S$ was determined by plotting the d_{102} X-ray spacing versus x (3,9). XRD also allowed the determination of the particle sizes of pyrrhotites (using the Scherrer equation).

Total surface areas of the initial iron oxide precursors were made using the BET method, at 77K.

Ultra-high resolution electron microscopy using a JEM 100 CX II apparatus was associated to a LINK AN 10000 system for X-ray emission microanalysis (Energy Dispersive Spectroscopy). Small areas, as low as 15 nm, could be analyzed. The X-ray detector was a LZ5 analyzer (ultra fine window, equiped with a 30 mm^2 SiLi single crystal). Automatic correction of the baseline at low energies gave good peak to noise ratios for C, O and N elements.

Mössbauer spectrometry (conventional constant acceleration spectrometer) was used to control the composition of iron compounds after HL. In order to avoid any oxidation, the solid HL residue was immediately transferred, after filtration, into a polypropylene cup which was then sealed. Isomer Shifts (IS) referred to sodium nitroprusside with a 0.03 mm s^{-1} precision. Accuracies for quadrupole Splitting (QS) and line widths (W) were 0.05 and 0.02 mm s^{-1} respectively. The accuracy for effective fields H_{eff} was 2 kOe.

TABLE 2
Analytical data for the Freyming coal.

Ultimate analysis (wt % MAF basis)	
C = 85	H = 5.35
S = 0.85	pyritic S = 0.3
N = 1.1	O = 7.7
Petrographic composition (vol %)	
Vitrinite = 67	Exinite = 15
Inertinite = 13	Mineral matter = 4

As can be seen on Table 2, coal already contained pyritic sulfur. Pyrite grains have been previously shown to present rather large particle sizes and, consequently, low specific surface area contributions (2).

III RESULTS

Bulk sulfidation of the catalyst was already detected at 523K after 1 hour and was rapid enough to be complete when the autoclave attained the temperature of HL (673K). In these conditions, sulfidation was homogeneous, as observed by EDS, TEM (Figs 2, 4) and XRD measurements. Sulfide stoichiometry (1 - x) varied between 0.870 and 0.995, but the most frequent composition was $Fe_{0.915}S$. The pyrrhotite stoichiometry deduced from Mössbauer spectrometry, was found to be $Fe_{0.905}S$ which is not far from the XRD data. The value was calculated as described by Montano and Granoff (10).

A textural promotor effect of the reactional mixture avoided sintering of the catalyst particles (3); isolated particles could be easily observed in the residue (Fig. 4). On the contrary, at 720K, in the standard conditions, but without coal, a drastic sintering of pyrrhotite particles was observed. Presulfidations of iron oxide precursors in autoclave at lower temperatures attenuated this phenomenon.

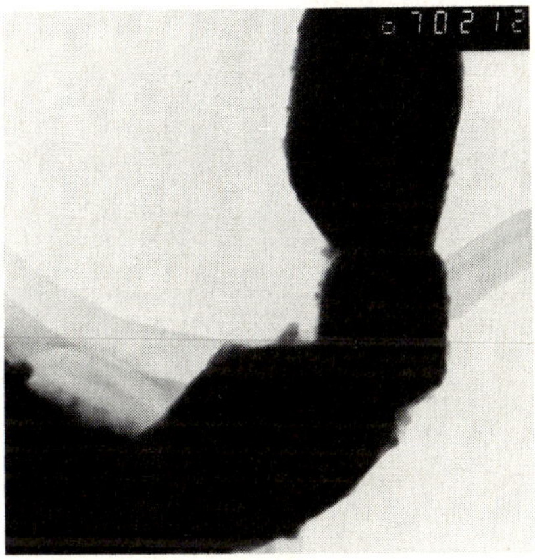

Fig. 3. Coking and sintering without coal.

Coking of the surface of the pyrrhotite particles was always observed. Figure 2a clearly shows, using EDS technics, the formation of a coke layer where only C element could be detected (beam size : about 20 nm). As soon as the electron beam attained the pyrrhotite cristallite, Fe and S peaks were observed with approximately a 1 : 1 ratio, in good agreement with the pyrrhotite composition (Fig. 2b).

"Hard" coke was rather observed in the case of presulfidation of iron oxides in the autoclave (Fig. 3). Morphology of this deposit was quite irregular. In contrast, "smooth" surface coke seemed to be the rule when HL was conducted in standard conditions with coal.

The interface "pyrrhotite-coke" is clearly defined on Figure 4 where lattice fringes of pyrrhotite are observed, showing the total sulfidation of the cristallite. Lattice fringes of the coke deposit are also clearly evidenced. We

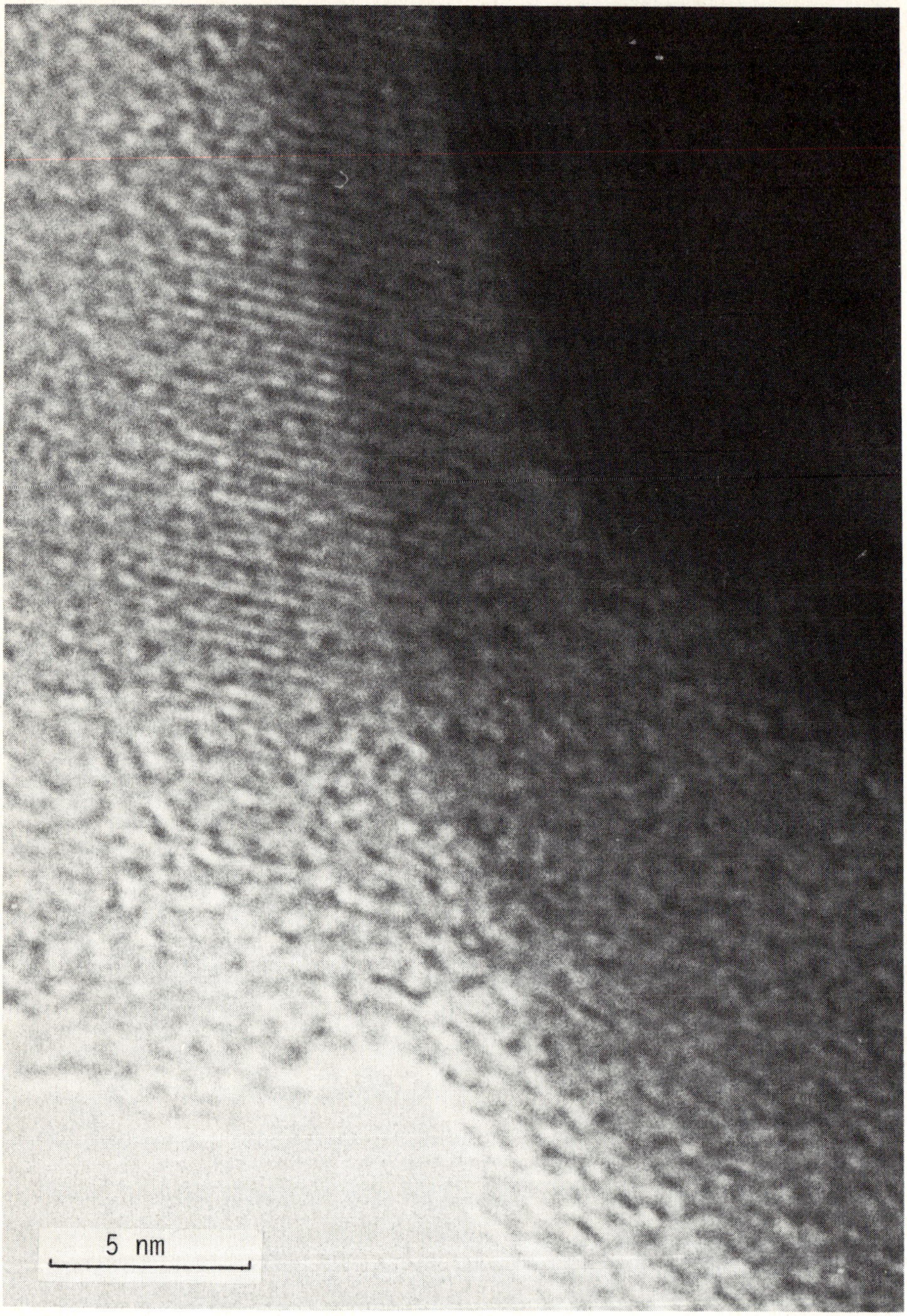

Fig. 4. Pyrrhotite-coke interface after HL (THF washed residue). Lattice fringes of both compounds can be seen.

have to remember that these TEM micrographies (ultra high resolution) were obtained after a THF extraction of the liquid products of HL. THF is considered as producing a total extraction of the heavier carbonaceous species. The carbonaceous "print" observed in TEM micrographies can be considered as really present in the HL conditions.

Looking at the solid residues obtained after toluene or hexane extractions, thickness of the carbonaceous layer was growing as shown by TEM.

Two other modes of treatment of the iron oxide precursor were made. The first one concerned a presulfidation in gas phase. This kind of sulfidation have been shown to produce a drastic sintering. The second mode consisted in introducing the iron precursor at high temperature into the autoclave, once the HL process was already initiated. Coking of the catalyst in this case was heavier and TEM observations rather difficult.

The results of the catalytic activities measurements are reported in Table 3 for different modes of utilisation of the Fe_2O_3 aerosol.

The results are expressed on a daf basis : N/N + T measures the degree of the tetralin dehydrogenation after hydroliquefaction; wt % H_2 is the overall hydrogen consumption from H_2 gas plus H_2 from tetralin dehydrogenation. Comparison of Expt 2 (standard mode of Fe_2O_3 utilisation) with the blank experiment shows a clear effect of the catalyst on the conversion of coal into toluene solubles (oils + asphaltenes) as well as on the overall H_2 consumption . The N/N + T ratio is further lower in expt 2 than in Expt 1 (blank).

Experiments 3 to 5, are related to different modes of utilisation of the Fe_2O_3 aerosol catalyst, and mainly show that none of these experimental procedures gave rise to better results than the standard one (Expt 2). At these low % conversions of coal into oils, the more accurate evaluation of any experiment was the % coal conversion into toluene solubles. It should be noticed that : i) the variation of temperature in this series of experiments is as large as 13K, which makes a very detailed comparison of the results somewhat difficult, because the hydroliquefaction of coal is very sensitive to temperature. ii) the N/N + T ratio varies very much from 0.02 to 0.13.

DISCUSSION

The inhibition of commercial catalysts such as $NiMo/Al_2O_3$ for the direct liquefaction of coal has already been studied (1). "Coke" deposits as well as metallic deposits cause a gradual loss of catalyst performance. On the other hand, little is known about the effects of "coke" in the case of iron catalysts. The lack of studies in this case is obviously related to the much lower cost of the iron catalysts. However, BOMANAVAR and MONTANO (11) reported that an additional catalyst $Fe_{1-x}S$-H_2S present during hydroliquefaction allowed the initial iron sulfides of coal to be activated; they should be

TABLE 3

Hydroliquefaction of coal at about 673K with iron catalyst, in solvent tetralin

Expt	Fe_2O_3 catalyst precursor (S_{BET},m²/g)	Sulfidation mode	Temperature (K)	% Conversion of coal in Products soluble in			$\frac{N}{N+T}$	wt % H_2 consumption
				THF	TOL	HEX		
1	No (blank)		676	85	41	8	0.13	1.41
2	59	In Situ sulfidation, by H_2S from S added to tetralin (standard)	678	87	55	16	0.08	2.33
3	44	Presulfidation in 15% H_2S-H_2 at 523K (no solvent)	676	86	42	10	0.03	1.48
4	44	Presulfidation of Fe_2O_3 suspended in Tetralin + S (T = 593K)	681	85	49	9	0.13	2.25
5	59	Fe_2O_3 suspended in Tetralin + S introduced into the autoclave at about 673K	673	87	53	17	0.14	2.16

otherwise inhibited by adsorbed organic compounds.

A first and main point in the present study lies in the textural promoter effect of heavy carbonaceous products from coal against the sintering of the small $Fe_{1-x}S$ particles which arise from in situ sulfidation of the Fe_2O_3 aerosol. This is very important for the very fine granulometry of the present Fe_2O_3 catalyst precursor (Ø < 0.05 μm). It gives a proof that very finely dispersed iron sulfides catalysts may be kept in such a favourable state of dispersion because they are prevented from sintering by undissolved coal products or by heavy dissolved and possibly adsorbed compounds or still by repolymerisation of coal liquid products. The inertinite of the coal is presumed to belong to the concerned heavy carbonaceous materials, but it is probably not the unique involved species. As regard to inertinite, it is nevertheless of interest to note that the percentage of THF insoluble is close to the % inertinite in coal, in every case (Expts 1 to 5, Table 3).

It was further shown that in the standard mode of the Fe_2O_3 catalyst utilisations, it does exist a very close contact between the iron sulfide surface and the carbonaceous deposits. These last ones are named "smooth coke" in the following : they represent a print of the reactional interface created during hydroliquefaction. Everything occurs as if all or at least most of the iron sulfide surface would be covered by a layer of carbonaceous material.

Assuming that those deposits would only deactivate the $Fe_{1-x}S$, H_2S active surface, the Fe_2O_3 aerosol used in standard conditions (Expt 2, Table 3) should be inactive. That is definitely not the case (comparison of Expts 2 and 1) since the % conversions in toluene or hexane solubles are increased, as well as the hydrogen consumption, while the N/N + T ratio is decreased.

It has then to be considered that the catalytically active surface is not merely composed of the $Fe_{1-x}S$ (plus adsorbed H_2S) surface, but is more complex and include a surface layer of carbonaceous heavy deposits named "smooth coke". Nevertheless it cannot be stated that at least a small part of the iron sulfide surface is not free of any carbonaceous deposits. The effective surface of the catalyst should then rather combine only a small percent area of a bare $Fe_{1-x}S$, H_2S surface, with large patches of a "smooth coke"-$Fe_{1-x}S$, H_2S interface. What about the role of those carbonaceous deposits ? It should be recalled that metallic catalysts like Pt when supported on carbon give easily rise to the so-called hydrogen spillover effect, that is to migration of active hydrogen, generally presumed to be more or less alike atomic hydrogen, from the Pt particles to the carbon support (12). It was further shown that hydrogen spillover takes place in a Pt black/Ce-Y zeolite/perylene system. Large quantities of hydrogen are adsorbed in fact at room temperature by cerium-Y zeolite after small amount of perylene are deposited on physical mixtures of Pt black and Ce-Y sieve (13). The hydrogen spillover phenomenon over metallic sulfides deposited on active carbon was shown by Fujimoto et al (14). It works alike the hydrogen spillover over noble metal supported catalysts apart that higher hydrogen pressure and higher temperatures are needed to activate the hydrogen molecule. In our actual standard conditions of coal hydroliquefaction, $Fe_{1-x}S$, H_2S may well act as a source of active hydrogen which migrates into and through the "smooth coke" layer and gives then rise to a pool of highly mobile and reactive hydrogen. The spillover effect and how it is affected by carbonaceous deposits has been recently reviewed (15).An active form of hydrogen is very likely able to play a role in the stabilization of free radicals arising from thermolysis of coal, in the naphtalene to tetralin rehydrogenation, or in the breaking of relatively stable bonds like Ø-O-Ø (ether bridged) or (and) Ø-CH_2-Ø (methylene bridges) in coal structure. This last function of the catalyst interface will be discussed in more detail in another paper (16). The active form of hydrogen included within the "smooth coke" layer, should present at least an intermediate reactivity between molecular hydrogen and atomic hydrogen. Atomic hydrogen is well known to be highly reactive towards the coal itself (17), as well as towards model compounds simulating the chemical bridges between the polyaromatic units in coal structure (18, 19).

Related phenomena described in detail elsewhere (20) strongly support the hypothesis of the occurence of hydrogen spillover phenomenon under the present standard conditions of hydroliquefaction (in situ sulfidation of the catalyst). It was shown in fact that the Fe_2O_3 aerosol allowed the stabilization of a very high percentage of fossile radicals in the coal inertinite to take place at a temperature as low as 623K. These fossile radicals should not be accessible to the larger tetralin molecules under these conditions, but more available to react with the mobile atomic form of hydrogen due to spillover.

Expt 3 also corresponds to "smooth coke" formation whilst, Expts 4 and 5 showed "hard coke" formation. Hard coke has clearly greater rugosity factor than smooth coke. Table 4 summarizes the state of coke ("smooth" or "hard") the apparent degree of sintering of $Fe_{1-x}S$ and the catalyst activity evaluated by the % toluene solubles, and by the tetralin dehydrogenation ratio. It may be considered from most of our observations : 1) that any divided solid, even when chemically inert, like SiO_2 aerosol, gives rise to an increase in the % toluene solubles but remains without any effect on the N/N + T ratio (20). This is explained by physical adsorption of the free radicals from coal by SiO_2. Free radicals repolymerization is then slowed down and % toluene solu-

TABLE 4

Different catalyst sulfidations and the corresponding kinds of coke

Exp.	Sulfidation mode	Catalytical* activity (soluble TOL)	$\frac{N}{N+T}$ *	Sintering	kind of "coke"
2	standard (in Situ)	high	↘	small	smooth
3	Presulfidation in H_2S-H_2 at 523K (no solvent)	low	↘↘	high	smooth
4	Presulfidation of Fe_2O_3 suspended in tetralin + S (T =593K)	medium	→	high	hard
5	Fe_2O_3 suspended in tetralin + S injected into the autoclave at about 673K	high	→	high	hard

* Compared to the blank (without catalyst).

bles consequently increased. Such an explanation for the role of the catalyst in hydroliquefaction has also been assumed by other authors (21);
2) that "hard coke" at the difference of "smooth coke" should be inactive towards the hydrogen spillover effect. "Hard coke" should only be acting as an inert solid.

As a matter of fact the global tetralin dehydrogenation ratio is only (and strongly) decreased in the presence of "smooth coke".

As regard to the catalytic activity evaluated by the % toluene solubles it is of the same level in three cases (Expts 2, 4, 5) of which two correspond to "hard coke" and one to "smooth coke". Some compensation effects are possible between a higher specific activity of "smooth coke" and a higher area (increased rugosity) of "hard coke". The last case (Expt 3, presulfidation by H_2S, H_2), where almost no change of % toluene soluble arises from the added catalyst, is accounted for by a higher sintering of $Fe_{1-x}S$ than in Expt 2 (in situ sulfidation). The extent of the "smooth coke" area is then decreased accordingly.

In conclusion, catalysis of coal hydroliquefaction by highly dispersed iron sulfide catalysts has to take into account strong effects of the "coke" deposited on the $Fe_{1-x}S$, H_2S surface.

1) This "coke" is responsible for the increased resistance of the catalytically active phase, against sintering.

2) At least two kinds of "coke" have been identified, named "smooth coke" (formed during in situ sulfidation or after dry presulfidation by H_2, H_2S) and "hard coke" formed during some more specific modes of utilisation of the highly dispersed Fe_2O_3 aerosol.

3) "hard coke" merely acts as a physical adsorbent for the free radicals produced by the thermolysis of coal. It stabilizes those radicals against repolymerization, and gives rise, provided that its available surface area is sufficient, to an increased conversion in toluene solubles compounds.

4) "Smooth coke" is like to operate with this same mechanism but with a lower efficiency due to a lower rugosity factor (smaller available area). But "smooth coke" by contrast with hard coke is strongly presumed to further have a chemical function, which lies in its ability to give a pool of active hydrogen, due to the hydrogen spillover effects.

Finally the catalytically active reaction interface is created by the conditions of liquefaction themselves; the properties of the coal could be another factor.

REFERENCES

1 M. Andres-Besson and H. Charcosset, Rev. Inst. Fr. Petr., 39 (1984) 209 - 233 ; 365 - 382.
2 G. Djega-Mariadassou, M. Besson, D. Brodzki, H. Charcosset, Tran Vinh Huu and J. Varloud, Fuel Process. Techn., 12 (1986), 143 - 153.
3 G. Djega-Mariadassou, D. Brodzki, M. Besson, H. Charcosset, Tran Vinh Huu and J. Varloud, Intern. Conf. on Coal Science, (1985), pp. 177 - 180.
4 P.A. Montano and V.I. Stenberg, Ibid., p. 788.
5 V.I. Stenberg, Ibid., p. 103
6 B.O. Strobel and F. Friedrich, Ibid., p. 7.
7 P.G. Vergnon and H. Batis Landousli, Ind. & Eng. Chem., Prod. Res. Dev., 19 (1971) 147 - 151.
8 R.E. Tischer and B.R. Utz, "A standard batch screening test for coal liquefaction catalysts. A preliminary report", Report DOE / PET C/TR–83/2, March, 1983.
9 G. Bugli, Thèse de Doctorat d'Etat, Université P & M Curie, 1971.
10 P.A. Montano and B. Granoff, Fuel, 59 (1980) 214.
11 A. Bommanavar and P.A. Montano, Fuel, 62 (1983) 932.
12 A.J. Robell, E.V. Ballou and M. Boudart, J. Phys. Chem., 68 (1964) 2748.
13 W.C. Neikam and M.A. Vannice, J. Catal., 27 (1972) 207.
14 K. Fujimoto, A. Ohno and T. Kunugi, Studies in Surface Science and Catalysis 17 - Spillover of Adsorbed species, G.M. Pajonk, S.J. Teichner and J.E. Germain Ed., Elsevier (1983) p. 241.
15 B.K. Hodnett and B. Delmon, Studies in Surface Science and Catalysis 27 - Catalytic Hydrogenation, L. Cerveny, Elsevier (1986) Ch. 2, p. 53.
16 V.L. Cebola, R. Bacaud, M. Besson, D. Cagniant, H. Charcosset, J.L. Lemberton and D. Sambanis, to be published.

17 A. Amano, M. Yamada, T. Shindo and T.A. Akalura, Fuel, 63 (1984) 718.
18 L.W. Vernon, Fuel, 59 (1980) 102.
19 B.C. Bockrath, K.T. Schroeder and G.L. Keldsen, "Proceedings of 1985 International Conference on Coal Science", 28 - 31 october 1985, Sydney, Australia, 1985, p. 83.
20 H. Charcosset, R. Bacaud, M. Besson, A. Jeunet, B. Nickel and M. Oberson, Fuel Process. Technol., 12 (1986) 189.
21 P.J. Cassidy, Chemtech., (1983) 562.

B. Delmon and G.F. Froment (Editors), *Catalyst Deactivation 1987*

DEACTIVATION OF CLAUS TAIL-GAS TREATING CATALYSTS

P.H.BERBEN, A.SCHOLTEN, M.K.TITULAER, N.BRAHMA, W.J.J.van der WAL[o] and J.W.GEUS

Department of Inorganic Chemistry, University of Utrecht, Croesestraat 77[a], 3522 AD Utrecht (The Netherlands)

[o]VEG Gasinstituut n.v., P.O. Box 137, 7300 AC Apeldoorn (The Netherlands)

ABSTRACT

The selective oxidation of hydrogen sulfide in Claus tail gas is catalyzed by iron oxide and iron oxide/chromium oxide on α-alumina catalysts. These catalysts deactivate either by sulfation or by sulfiding of the iron oxide. The effect of deactivation on the aforementioned catalysts is studied. It has been found that the initially existing epitaxial relation between iron oxide and α-alumina, present after preparation of the catalyst, is broken up during use. The denuded α-alumina surface establishes the Claus equilibrium. Therefore, the activity and selectivity of the catalyst after deactivation is decreased. The development of a catalyst which does not deactivate during the oxidation of hydrogen sulfide is dealt with. Furthermore, the mechanism of sulfation of a Claus catalyst is discussed.

INTRODUCTION

The conversion of hydrogen sulfide from hydrodesulfurization processes or sour natural gas into elemental sulfur is carried out in the Claus process. In this process hydrogen sulfide reacts with sulfur dioxide to elemental sulfur and water. Since at the temperature required for the catalytic reaction the thermodynamic equilibrium is not completely at the right-hand side, the off-gas of Claus plants contains appreciable amounts of sulfur dioxide and hydrogen sulfide. Since a slight increase of the hydrogen sulfide/sulfur dioxide ratio of the gas flow entering the first catalytic Claus reactor decreases substantially the SO_2 content of the tail gas, selective oxidation of the hydrogen sulfide in the tail gas with molecular oxygen to elemental sulfur can abate air-pollution due to emission of incinerated tail gas.

In a previous paper (ref. 11) we showed that iron oxide/chromium oxide supported by alfa-alumina is a selective catalyst in the oxidation of hydrogen sulfide. However, this catalyst is susceptible to deactivation under certain circumstances.

The deactivation of Claus catalysts has already been studied by Quet et al.

(ref. 1). Furthermore, several authors attempted to elucidate the mechanism of the Claus reaction and of the sulfation of the alumina catalysts studying the adsorption of hydrogen sulfide and sulfur dioxide on different catalysts by infrared spectroscopy (ref. 2-8, 19).

This paper deals with the deactivation of the iron oxide and iron oxide/chromium oxide on α-alumina catalyst. Both catalysts can oxidize Claus tail gas. We established the reaction conditions leading to deactivation of the catalysts, the change in catalyst structure during deactivation and the performance of the catalyst after deactivation. Also the mechanism of sulfation of Claus catalysts will be discussed.

EXPERIMENTAL

catalyst preparation

All catalysts were prepared by means of the incipient wetness impregnation method. In this technique the previously evacuated pores of the carrier material are just filled with a solution in which a precursor of the active compound has been dissolved. Keeping the thus carefully impregnated support at moderate temperatures (373-393 K) leads to evaporation of the solvent. Finally, the precursor is converted into the active oxide by calcination in air at 773 K.

In this study α-alumina (Fluka puriss.) was used as the support material. X-ray diffraction patterns of the carrier material were recorded. The diffraction maxima could be attributed to α-alumina only. The diffraction pattern did not show other forms of alumina. The BET surface area was 6.5 m^2 per g. Mercury porosimetry showed that this support material mainly contains macropores. From the penetrated amount of mercury the pore volume was calculated to be 0.50 ml. per g.

TABLE 1

Amount of active oxides present in the catalysts

catalyst	total loading[a]	percent Fe_2O_3	percent Cr_2O_3
A	1	100	0
B	1	90	10
C	5	90	10

[a] the loading of the catalyst was calculated on the basis of

$$\frac{\text{wt. } Fe_2O_3\ (+\ Cr_2O_3)}{\text{wt. } Fe_2O_3\ (+\ Cr_2O_3) + \text{wt. } Al_2O_3} * 100\%$$

The impregnation solution consisted of a Fe complex of an organic chelating agent, viz. EDTA (ethylene diamino tetra-acetic acid). The pH of the solution was brought at 6.

After calcination in air the catalyst was pressed into tablets at a pressure of 160 MPa. These tablets were crushed into a sieve fraction between 850 μm and 1000 μm.

In table 1 the loading of the catalysts used in this study is given.

apparatus and procedures

The activity and selectivity of the catalysts have been measured in a conventional atmospheric flow apparatus. The reactants, hydrogen sulfide and oxygen, balance helium, were passed downstream through the reactor (i.d. 18 mm). The product sulfur condenses in the lower part of the reactor, which is kept at 403 K. Next, the effluent gasflow passes through a vessel in which Sicapent (fosfor pentoxide on silica) is used as a drying agent. The dried gas flow, which contains sulfur dioxide, helium, and possibly hydrogen sulfide and oxygen, is quantitatively analyzed. No condensation of water can proceed in the equipment between the catalyst and the vessel containing the Sicapent drying agent. This is important, because liquid water is able to catalyze reactions between the components to be analyzed, e.g. hydrogen sulfide and sulfur dioxide react to sulfur and water in the so called Claus reaction. When condensation of water occurs, a reliable detection of the products of the oxidation of hydrogen sulfide is therefore not possible.

Temperature-programmed reduction experiments were performed also in an atmospheric flow reactor (i.d. 8 mm). The hydrogen consumption was monitored by measurement of the difference in thermal conductivity of the incoming and effluent gas. The sample weight was approximately 250 μg. A physical mixture was made by grinding of the different components. A detailed description is given elsewhere (ref. 10).

The surface morphology was studied in a Philips EM 420 transmission electronmicroscope.

Differential Thermal Gravimetric (DTG) patterns were recorded on a Perkin Elmer TGS2 apparatus. The sample weight was approximately 10 mg. The sample was heated in an oxygen gas flow at a rate of 10 K per min.

RESULTS

catalyst A

In fig. 1 the activity of the 1 wt.% iron oxide on alfa-alumina (catalyst A) is given as a function of time at three different temperatures. We have defined the activity as the conversion of hydrogen sulfide. The selectivity of the

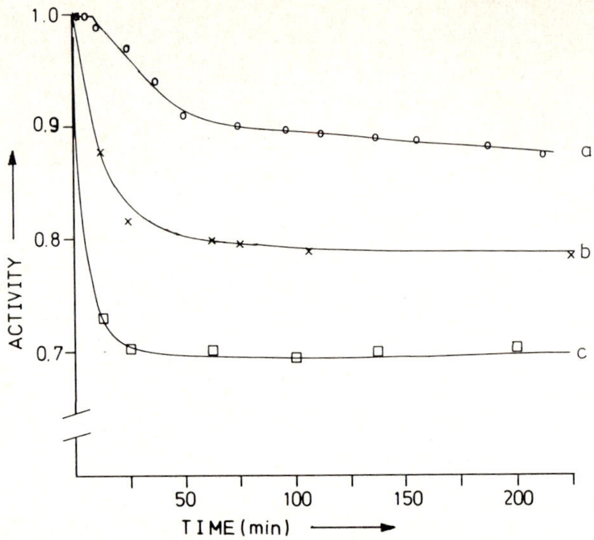

fig.1. activity as a function of time for catalyst A during the oxidation of hydrogen sulfide at different temperatures. a. 548 K b. 523 K c. 493 K reaction conditions: H_2S= 3 vol.% ; O_2= 2.4 vol.% ; S.V.= 5000 per hr.

reaction, that is the fraction of the converted hydrogen sulfide that reacts to elemental sulfur, is a function of the temperature at which the reactor is operated. The amount of catalyst in the reactor was adjusted in such a way that the initial activity was about 1.0.

It can be seen that after a period of initial deactivation the activity assumes a stable level. The time during which this initial deactivation proceeds can be shortened by lowering the reactor temperature. The level of conversion increases with the reactor temperature. It should be emphasized that the experiments shown in fig. 1 were carried out at a space velocity of 5000 hr^{-1}.

To investigate the possibility that the effluent gas of the hydrogen sulfide oxidation reaction reached thermodynamic equilibrium, the space velocity was decreased until no further change in composition of the outcoming gas was observed. From the composition of the gas leaving the reactor at a space velocity of 1000 hr^{-1}, the equilibrium constant of the Claus reaction was calculated. In table 2 the result of this calculation is given. The reaction conditions, except for the space velocity, are similar to those mentioned in fig. 1. The thus calculated equilibrium constant is equal to the theoretical constant within the experimental error. This implies that after the initial deactivation of the catalyst, the catalyst can establish the Claus equilibrium.

To investigate whether the initial deactivation is caused by formation of iron sulfate, the deactivated catalyst is characterized by means of X-ray diffraction and temperature-programmed reduction (TPR) experiments. In the X-ray

TABLE 2

Equilibrium constant for the reaction

$3/n\ S_n + 2\ H_2O \leftrightarrow 2\ H_2S + SO_2$

temperature (K)	activity	selectivity	ln K (calculated)	ln K (theoretical)
523	0.975	0.870	-10.74	-10.38

diffraction pattern no maxima could be observed due to a solid phase containing iron ions, probably because of the low amount of iron oxide present in the freshly prepared catalyst. In fig. 2 the TPR patterns of both the deactivated catalyst and a physical mixture of 1 wt.% iron(III) sulfate and α-alumina are represented. The three peak pattern observed for a freshly prepared catalyst (not given) has drastically changed. The profile for the deactivated catalyst is in part characteristic of iron sulfate shown in fig. 2b.

Furthermore, the deactivated catalyst was heated both in a helium and an oxygen flow at temperatures stepwise increased. The temperature of the reactor was raised in each experiment by 25 K, starting at 373 K. A constant temperature was maintained for 15 min during which the outcoming gas was analyzed for the presence of sulfur dioxide. As oxygen and helium are both inert gases towards iron sulfate, production of sulfur dioxide starts as the decomposition temperature of the sulfate is reached. If iron sulfide would be present in the catalyst, the production of sulfur dioxide should begin at a lower temperature only in the flow of oxygen. Helium does not produce sulfur dioxide out of iron sulfide. The formation of sulfur dioxide out of the deactivated catalyst started at 548 K in helium as well as in oxygen. Iron oxide thus reacts exclusively to iron sulfate during the catalytic reaction of hydrogen sulfide with oxygen at moderate temperatures.

Catalyst B

In order to investigate whether addition of chromium oxide to the catalyst could prevent formation of iron sulfate, the activity of catalysts both with and without chromium oxide was measured in the oxidation of hydrogen sulfide (fig.

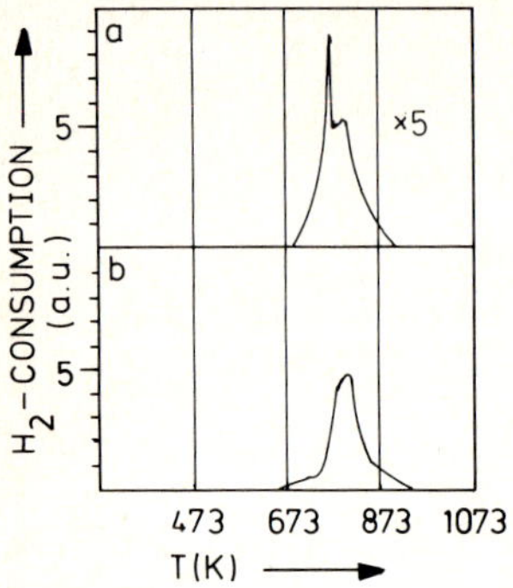

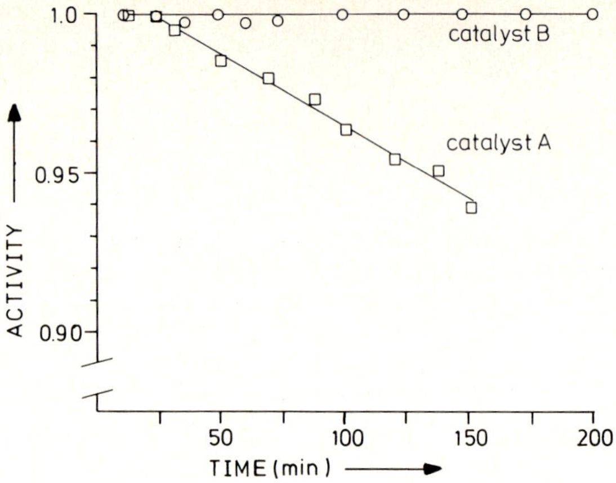

left: fig.2. Temperature programmed reduction profiles.
a. catalyst A after deactivation
b. physical mixture of Fe(III)-sulfate and alfa-alumina

right: fig.3. activity as a function of time for catalyst A and B during the hydrogen sulfide oxidation reaction.
reaction conditions: H_2S= 3 vol.% ; O_2= 2.4 vol.% ; S.V.= 1700 per hr. ; temperature= 523 K

3). The amount of catalyst was adjusted so as to adjust the initial activity at about 1.0. No deactivation could be observed with catalyst B, whereas catalyst A showed the same performance as described in the previous section.

Catalyst C

As catalyst B catalyst C appeared to be not susceptible to formation of iron sulfate. Initial deactivation as observed with catalyst A can thus be prevented. In fig. 4 an electronmicrograph, which is indicative for the texture of catalyst C, is shown. In the micrograph Moire patterns are visible indicating the presence of epitaxial layers of iron oxide on the α-alumina. Characterization of catalyst C with complementary techniques confirmed the presence of a layer of iron oxide without any micropores.

In fig. 5 the performance of catalyst C as a function of the reactor temperature is shown. Below approximately 573 K the activity is 1.0, while the selectivity slightly decreases with increasing temperature. Above a temperature of 573 K, the colour of the catalyst changes from brown into black. This change in colour starts in the lower part of the reactor. At this temperature the oxygen is exhausted due to the formation of sulfur dioxide. The hydrogen sulfide therefore can not be totally converted. The resulting gas flow is reducing. The

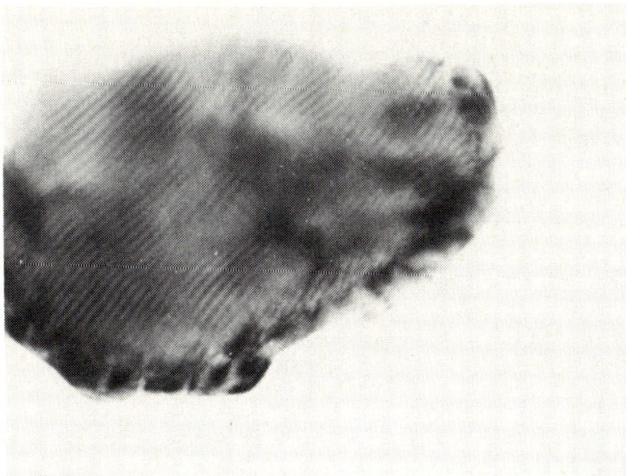

fig.4. representive electron micrograph of catalyst C before the reactor experiments.

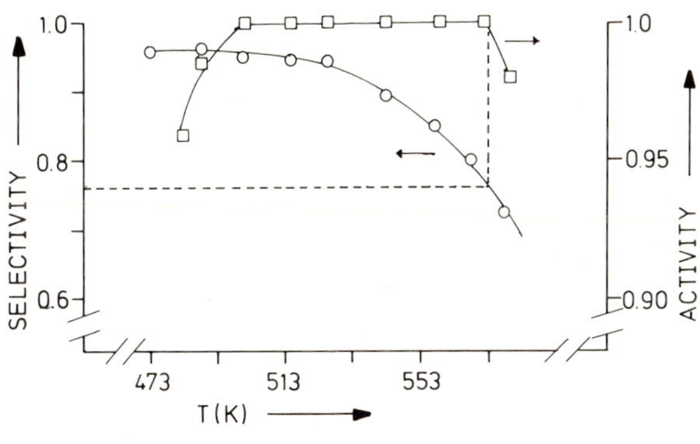

fig.5. activity and selectivity as a function of temperature for the hydrogen sulfide oxidation reaction over catalyst C. reaction conditions: H_2S= 1 vol.% ; O_2= 0.75 vol.% ; S.V.= 1000 per hr.

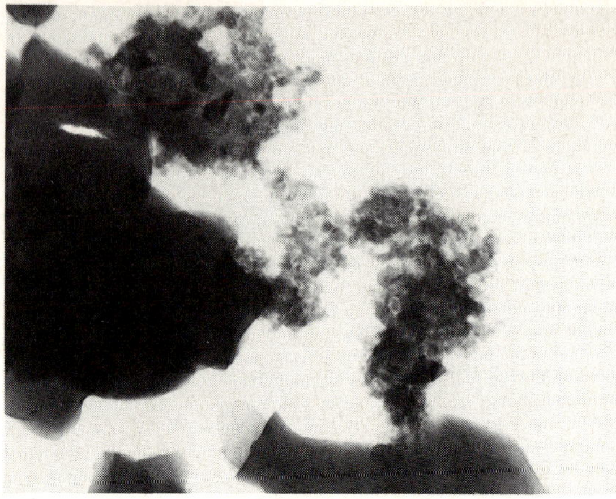

fig.6. representive electron micrograph of catalyst C after deactivation.

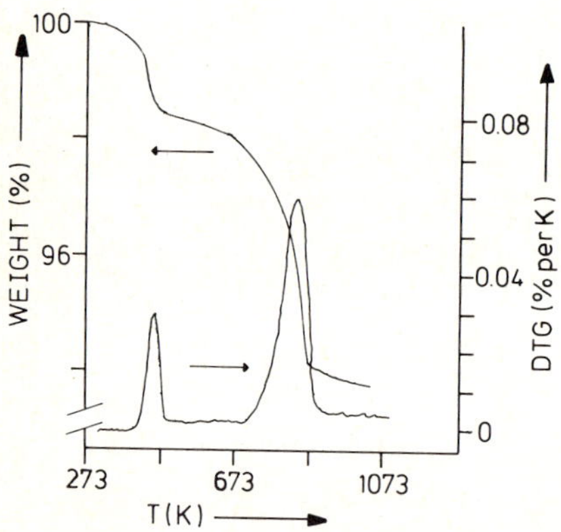

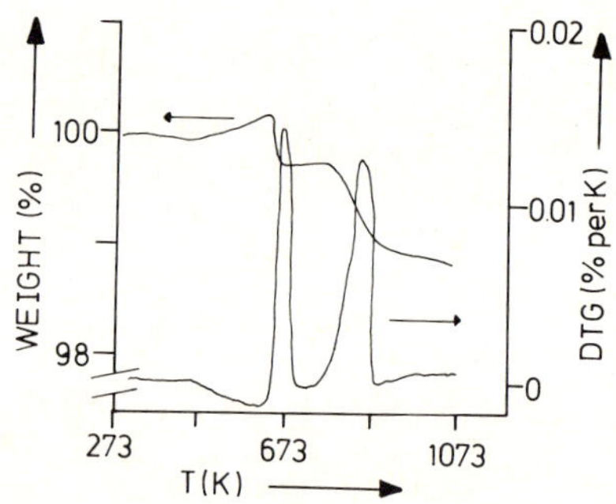

left: fig.7. Differential Thermal Gravimetric (DTG) plot for catalyst C after deactivation.
conditions: heating in 20 % O_2 in N_2 by 10 K per min

right: fig.8. Differential Thermal Gravimetric (DTG) plot for catalyst C after sulfiding in a 1 vol.% H_2S in He flow.
conditions: heating in 20 % O_2 in N_2 by 10 K per min

temperature at which this phenomenon starts, is indicated in fig. 5 by the dotted line.

Characterization of the catalyst after being exposed to a reducing atmosphere was performed with several complementary techniques, such as electronmicroscopy, X-ray diffraction, differential thermogravimetry, temperature-programmed reduction, and wet chemical analysis. X-ray diffraction patterns of the deactivated catalyst revealed no maxima that could be attributed to an iron phase. The iron oxide originally covering the alumina surface epitaxially is not longer contacting the carrier as can be seen from the electronmicrograph shown in fig. 6. It appears that the iron oxide is torn from the alumina. The DTG pattern (fig. 7) shows two distinct peaks with maxima at temperatures of 453 K and 853 K. The low-temperature peak is attributed to iron sulfide, which is converted to iron oxide in an oxygen gas flow. The formation of (black) iron sulfide causes the change in the colour of the catalyst. The decomposition of aluminium sulfate results in the high-temperature peak in the DTG profile. This aluminium sulfate can be formed from a denuded aluminium oxide surface that is kept in a reducing, hydrogen sulfide containing atmosphere as mentioned afore. The experimental decrease in weight points to pyrite being the iron sulfide phase which has been formed (the conversion of pyrite into iron oxide gives rise to a theoretical loss in weight of about 2%). Furthermore, α-alumina is not very reactive towards SO_2. This is apparent from the weight loss at 853 K shown in fig. 7. The 4% loss in weight points to at most 2% of the aluminium oxide having reacted to aluminium sulfate during the deactivation.

Fig. 8 shows a DTG pattern of catalyst C after deliberate sulfidization in a 1% H_2S-helium flow at 573 K. During the DTG experiment the weight of the catalyst initially increases. Two distinct weight loss peaks at about 663 K and 853 K can be distinguished. At these temperatures iron sulfate and aluminium sulfate, respectively, are decomposed. The sulfur dioxide, required for the formation of sulfates, is originating from the regeneration of iron sulfide. It is known that the regeneration of iron sulfide with air to iron oxide, sulfur, and sulfur dioxide already proceeds at ambient temperature (ref. 9). The sulfates can thus be formed either during keeping the sulfided catalyst at room temperature and/or during the initial phase of the DTG experiment. The fact that this weight loss can be hardly discerned is illustrative for the very low amounts of sulfates formed during the regeneration of iron sulfide. The DTG pattern of catalyst C, which was treated in air for 20 hr. at 598 K after being sulfided in the same way as the catalyst shown in fig. 8, can be seen in fig. 9. It is obvious that treatment in air at this temperature removes the iron sulphate almost completely. The peak at 853 K, indicative for aluminium sulphate, is slightly increased in comparison with fig. 8.

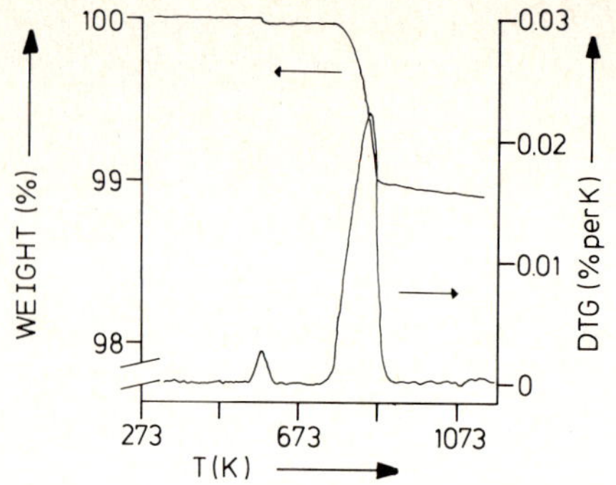

fig.9. Differential Thermal Gravimetric (DTG) plot for catalyst C after sulfiding in a 1 vol.% H_2S in He flow and subsequent heating in air at 598 K for 20 hr.
conditions: heating in 20 % O_2 in N_2 by 10 K per min

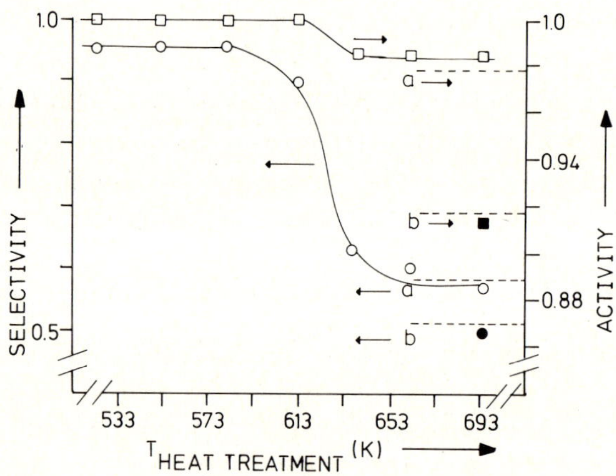

fig.10. Activity and selectivity measured at 523 K as a function of temperature of thermal treatment. The dotted lines correspond with Claus equilibrium levels.
conditions: H_2S= 1 vol.% ; O_2= 0.9 vol.% ; S.V.= 1000 per hr.
□ and ○: without H_2O in the feed gas
■ and ●: with 2.6 vol.% H_2O in the feed gas

A temperature-programmed reduction profile (not shown) of a freshly prepared catalyst C shows three reduction peaks. After deactivation of this catalyst as described in this section, the profile has drastically changed. The original pattern could be restored only by heat treatment in an oxygen containing gas flow at a temperature of 1073 K or higher.

By means of wet chemical analysis of a deactivated catalyst C both sulphate and aluminium ions were determined. No iron(III)-ion could be extracted from catalyst C. All three ions could be extracted from catalyst A after deactivation in a reducing atmosphere containing hydrogen sulfide.

In fig. 10 the activity and selectivity measured in the oxidation of hydrogen sulfide at 523 K are given as a function of the temperature of thermal treatment. The treatment involves a procedure in which the hydrogen sulfide oxidation reaction is carried out over catalyst C at the temperatures indicated in the figure. After keeping the catralyst at the temperature of the thermal treatment for 1 hr, the temperature is decreased to 523 K at which temperature the activity and selectivity are measured. It is obvious that above a temperature of about 613 K the catalyst is subjected to an irreversible deactivation. Both the activity and selectivity of the catalyst are diminished untill a constant level is reached. The dotted lines, marked a in fig. 10, are the theoretical activity and selectivity that correspond to an effluent gas that has reached the Claus equilibrium. It can be seen that after a heat treatment of about 693 K, this equilibrium is established. After a heat treatment at 693 K the catalyst is cooled down to 523 K. At this temperature, 2.6 vol.% water was brought into the incoming gas flow. Both the activity and selectivity levels are decreased to their corresponding theoretical Claus equilibrium levels corrected for the extra amount of water present in the feed gas (dotted lines b in fig. 10).

DISCUSSION

To avoid capillary condensation of sulfur in the catalyst, the oxidation of hydrogen sulfide has been carried out at temperatures above the dewpoint of sulfur (approximately 450 K). At these temperatures, a low active surface area suffices to oxidize the hydrogen sulfide virtually completely. In an earlier study the selectivity to elemental sulfur of catalysts supported on either α-alumina, or γ-alumina, and a commercial catalyst (CRS-31, Rhone Poulenc) was compared (ref. 11). It was concluded that a high selectivity to elemental sulfur could be achieved with a catalyst in which the active component had been applied onto a support of a low surface area (e.g. iron oxide on α-alumina). Furthermore, the catalyst should not catalyze the equilibrium reaction between hydrogen sulfide and sulfur dioxide, known as the Claus reaction. The huge amount of water (about 30 vol.%), present in Claus tailgas, shifts the equilibrium to the hydrogen sulfide side. As a result, the activity and selectivity of the oxidation of hydrogen sulfide are decreased.

From Moire patterns apparent in electron-micrographs taken from catalyst C, it was established that α-alumina is covered by a thin, continuous layer of iron oxide (ref. 12). The interaction between these oxides is based on an epitaxial relation. We revealed that this special texture of the catalyst can prevent the establishment of the Claus equilibrium. However, this equilibrium could be established when hydrogen sulfide and sulfur dioxide are passed over the uncovered α-alumina (ref. 11). The epitaxial layer is broken up when iron oxide is subjected to a solid state transformation. As a result, the iron phase is torn from the alumina. As can be seen from table 2 and fig. 10, the effluent gas has reached Claus equilibrium after the catalyst was deactivated. The α-alumina surface therefore has been denuded during the deactivation. Although X-ray diffraction did only exhibit maxima that could be attributed to α-alumina, the presence of other (surface)phases of alumina may not be excluded. Treatment of the α-alumina, used in this study, at temperatures above 1023 K led to a decrease of the BET surface area due to sintering. The presence of some metastable, highly porous alumina phases formed before the final complete conversion to α-alumina in the sintering process (ref. 13) may be responsible for the fact that the Claus equilibrium is established after deactivation of the catalyst.

The characterization of the deactivated samples was mainly performed by temperature-programmed techniques, such as TPR and DTG. These techniques are very sensitive, which is essential with loadings of 1 to 5 wt.% of the active components. Moreover, they can distinguish between different sulfur containing compounds.

In this study the iron oxide is subjected to two different phase transformations. Catalyst A is sulfated as hydrogen sulfide is oxidized over the catalyst at moderate temperatures. Saussey et al. (ref. 14) compared the sulfation of an alumina of a moderate BET surface area during the oxidation of hydrogen sulfide and of sulfur dioxide. Sulfation during sulfur dioxide oxidation was more difficult, as it proceeds at higher temperatures than the oxidation of hydrogen sulfide. Moreover, it is known that the presence of oxygen is a prerequisite for sulfation (ref. 1). Formation of iron sulfate at reaction temperatures of 473 - 573 K during oxidation of hydrogen sulfide is thus well possible. It is remarkable that the iron sulfate could be again transformed into iron oxide already at 600 K, as determined with several techniques. According to Ostroff and Sanderson iron sulfate is thermally decomposed at 810 K (ref. 15). The decomposition temperature of surface and bulk sulfates of the same cation may differ. The denuded α-alumina surface is not very susceptible to sulfate formation. As the α-alumina has less hydroxyl groups on its surface than γ-alumina, this agrees with the study of Saussey et al. (ref. 14). These authors concluded that sulfation during the oxidation of sulfur dioxide is promoted by the hydroxyl groups on the alumina surface.

The addition of chromium oxide to iron oxide (catalyst B) could prevent formation of iron sulfate. The French company Elf Aquitaine has developed a Claus catalyst that forms less sulfates (ref. 1). Unfortunately, the nature of this modified alumina has not been published. Kung (ref. 16) explained the catalytic behavior of a cation in a solid solution by the difference in the electrostatic potential, as the cation is placed into different oxidic solid solutions of the same crystal structure. We did not study the change in surface properties when chromium oxide is added to the catalyst.

The α-alumina surface of catalyst C is denuded by another iron oxide phase transformation as mentioned afore. As the temperature of the reactor is raised, the formation of sulfur dioxide becomes a faster reaction than the oxidation of hydrogen sulfide. The gas atmosphere in the reactor hence becomes reducing. As a result, the iron oxide is transformed into pyrite (FeS_2) and the α-alumina surface is uncovered. Because sudden rises in the hydrogen sulfide content of Claus tailgas can happen regularly, this kind of deactivation is a severe problem. The formation of pyrite agrees the observations by van der Wal (ref. 17). He concluded that the final product of the desulfurization reaction is FeS_2, if the process gas does not contain any reducing compound, such as hydrogen or carbon monoxide. Pyrhotite (FeS) is formed when these reducing compounds are present. Some of the denuded α-alumina surface reacts to aluminium sulfate. It must be stated that no iron sulfate formation was observed.

Two catalysts not deactivating on exposure to an increased hydrogen sulfide content were developed. In the first, the amount of the active oxide was decreased. The amount of sulfur dioxide per catalyst charge at temperatures around 573 K is thus lowered. The temperature where the formation of sulfur dioxide exhausts the oxygen is consequently raised. The second catalyst consists of an active oxide on an α-alumina, which exhibits a surface area of about 0.5 m^2 per g. This support can not catalyze the Claus equilibrium reaction.

Finally, we will make some remarks about the mechanism of sulfating. Quet et al. showed the existence of non-deactivating and deactivating sulfates on alumina (ref. 1). Chang (ref. 18) and recently Datta et al. (ref. 4) studied the adsorption of sulfur dioxide using infrared spectroscopy. The species which could only be removed after a severe thermal treatment was assigned to a sulfite-like species. This species reacts with oxygen to a sulfate. The sulfite-like species exhibits a low frequency band in the infrared spectrum. Various authors discuss the possibility that this sulfite-like species plays a role as an intermediate in the Claus equilibrium reaction (e.g. ref. 2, 19). Very recently, a hydrogen sulfite species was observed on different catalysts (ref. 3, 7, 20). It is believed that this hydrogen sulfite species is the intermediate in the Claus equilibrium reaction. As the sulfite-like species reacts with oxygen to sulfate, the Claus equilibrium is not affected. When the hydrogen sulfite species reacts with oxygen to sulfate (ref. 14), the alumina can not catalyze the Claus reaction anymore. So, the sulfite-thiosulfate mechanism proposed by Quet et al. (ref. 1) is in part probably correct, although the authors did not publish any spectrometric evidence for this mechanism.

ACKNOWLEDGEMENT

The authors express their gratitude to the VEG Gasinstituut n.v. in Netherlands for financially supporting these investigations.

REFERENCES

1 C.Quet, J.Tellier and R.Voirin, in B.Delmon and G.F.Froment (Eds.), Stud. Surf. Sci. Catal. (Catal. Deact.), 6 (1980) 323-329
2 H.G.Karge and J.C.Dalla Lana, J. Phys. Chem., 88 (1984) 1538-1543
3 J.C.Lavalley, J.Lamotte, O.Saur, A.B. Mohammed Saad, C.Tripp and B.A.Morrow, in J.G.Grasselli and D.G.Cameron (Eds.), proc. Int. Conf. on Fourier and Computerized Infrared Spectroscopy, Ottawa, June 24-28, 1985, 486-487
4 A.Datta, R.G.Cavell, R.W.Tower and Z.M.George, J. Phys. Chem., 89 (1985) 443-449
5 A.Datta and R.G.Cavell, J. Phys. Chem., 89 (1985) 450-454
6 A.Datta and R.G.Cavell, J. Phys. Chem., 89 (1985) 454-457
7 M.Laniecki, M.Ziolek and H.G.Karge, J. Phys. Chem., 91 (1987) 4-6
8 H.G.Karge, R.W.Tower, Z.Dudzik and Z.M.George, in T.Seiyama and K.Tanabe (Eds.), Proc. 7th Int. Symp. Catal., Tokyo, June 30- July 4, 1980, pp. 643-652
9 J.W.Geus and W.J.J. van der Wal, Proc. 8th Int. Symp. Catal., Berlin, July 2-6, 1984, pp. II 245-256
10 A.J.H.M.Kock, H.M.Fortuin and J.W.Geus, J. Catal., 96 (1985) 261
11 P.H.Berben, N.Brahma, M.K.Titulaer and J.W.Geus, to be published
12 D.W.Pashley, in B.M.Siegel (Ed.), Modern Developments in Electron Microscopy, Academic Press Inc., New York, 1967, ch.5.
13 S.J.Wilson and J.D.C.Mc Connell, J. Solid State Chem., 34 (1980) 315-322
14 H.Saussey, A.Vallet and J.C.Lavalley, Mater. Chem. Phys., 9 (1983) 457-466
15 A.G.Ostroff and R.T.Sanderson, J. Inorg. Nucl. Chem., 9 (1959) 45-50
16 H.H.Kung, J. Catal., 53 (1982) 387-395
17 W.J.J. van der Wal, Thesis, Utrecht, 1987, ch.6.
18 C.C.Chang, J. Catal., 53 (1978) 374-385
19 H.G.Karge, J.G.Dalla Lana, S.Trevizan de Suarez and Y.Zhang, Proc. 8th Int. Symp. Catal., Berlin, July 2-6, 1984, pp. III 453-463
20 P.H.Berben, M.J.Kappers and J.W.Geus, to be published

B. Delmon and G.F. Froment (Editors), *Catalyst Deactivation 1987*

NEW TECHNIQUE FOR THE CHARACTERIZATION OF CARBONACEOUS COMPOUNDS RESPONSIBLE FOR ZEOLITE DEACTIVATION

P. MAGNOUX, P. ROGER, C.CANAFF, V. FOUCHE, N.S. GNEP and M. GUISNET

Unité Associée au CNRS 350, Catalyse en Chimie Organique, Université de Poitiers, 40, avenue du Recteur Pineau, 86022 Poitiers Cedex, France

ABSTRACT

A new technique has been developed for characterizing the carbonaceous compounds deposited in zeolites, responsible for their deactivation ("coke"). The technique consists in treating the coked samples at room temperature by a solution of hydrofluoric acid at 40 % in order to dissolve the zeolite and to liberate the internal "coke". This treatment does not cause any transformation of the carbonaceous compounds as shown by the tests carried out with two reactive hydrocarbons : 1-tetradecene and 9-methylphenanthrene impregnated on an inert solid. The soluble components of "coke" extracted by an organic solvent (CH_2Cl_2) are analyzed by classical techniques : G.C., H.P.L.C., H-N.M.R., M.S... Two examples are given here to show the interest of this technique. The first concerns the effect of the reaction temperature (120-450°C) on the composition of the "coke" formed during propene transformation on a USHY zeolite ; the reactional steps involved in "coke" formation were able to be defined. In the second example, the mode of deactivation of three protonic zeolites : USHY, H mordenite and HZSM5, during dimethylether conversion into hydrocarbons, was specified by using results obtained from adsorption measurements on the "coked" zeolites and from analysis of the carbonaceous compounds.

INTRODUCTION

Deactivation of acid catalysts which occurs during the transformations of organic compounds is mainly due to the formation of carbonaceous compounds ("coke"). Characterization of "coke" is limited most often to the measurement of its atomic H/C ratio [1-5] .With classical catalysts, the values of H/C are between 0.4 and 0.7 [1], which proves that "coke" is polyaromatic. In the case of zeolites, values greater than 1 were found [4,6,7]. This can be explained by the possibility that "coke" can be formed not only on the outer surface but also in the zeolite pores. Internal "coke" in zeolites can be non-polyaromatic [8-11] because of steric constraints exerted by the porous structure on the formation of large molecules through bimolecular reactions and because of limitations for the desorption of not very bulky compounds. Internal and external "cokes" can coexist on a same zeolite [8,11], their relative significance depending on the zeolite and on operating conditions : temperature, reaction time... The characteristics concerning the coke considered globally give therefore little information. For instance the H/C ratio of a coke which is the mean value of the H/C ratio of its internal and external parts give no information at all on its composition.

The method presented in this work allows to separate the carbonaceous compounds deposited on zeolites into two fractions, one soluble in methylene chloride, the other non-soluble. The non-soluble fraction constituted by highly polyaromatic compounds, generally too bulky to be situated in the zeolite pores can be characterized chemically (atomic H/C ratio) and physically (Electron microscopy, Electron Energy Loss Spectroscopy...[12]). The soluble fraction, polyaromatic with less than 7 rings or non polyaromatic, situated in the zeolite pores [11] can be characterized by conventional analysis : G.C., H.P.L.C., N.M.R., M.S.... These carbonaceous compounds cannot be solubilized by treating the "coked" samples with methylene chloride [10]. The first step of the method consists therefore in liberating the coke components blocked in the zeolite porosity by dissolving the zeolite in a hydrofluoric acid solution. Internal coke could also be liberated by destruction of the zeolite structure by ball milling for a significant period of time [6], the inconvenience of this technique being that it modifies probably the characteristics of the external "coke", in particular its shape.

After having shown that the coke does not undergo any transformation during its recovery and that therefore the information concerning the composition is exact, two examples illustrating the interest of the method will be given. The first example concerns the effect of the reaction temperature on the composition of the carbonaceous compounds deposited on an ultrastabilized protonic Y zeolite (USHY) during propene transformation. The detailed analysis allows in particular to define the reactional steps involved in their formation and their relative significance as a function of the temperature. The second example shows that the mode of deactivation of three protonic zeolites (USHY, H mordenite, HZSM5) can be defined thanks to coke analysis and to adsorption measurements on the coked samples.

RESULTS AND DISCUSSION

1. Determination of the coke composition ; discussion of the method

In the first step, the aim of which is to liberate the coke components blocked in the zeolite porosity, the zeolite is dissolved at room temperature in a hydrofluoric acid solution at 40 % [10]. The soluble components are then extracted by a solvent (CH_2Cl_2) and analyzed by the conventional methods : GC, HPLC, H-NMR, MS... No significant change in the coke composition must occur before analysis, in particular because of the use of acid solutions. Indeed the carbonaceous compounds formed in the zeolites can be constituted not only of non-reactive polyaromatic compounds but also of olefinic or of alkyl aromatic products (and even of components with heteroatoms) which can evidently undergo numerous transformations by acid catalysis.

It has been shown elsewhere that no isomerization occurs during the recovery by this method of n-alcanes included in 5A molecular sieves [13]. Saturated and unsaturated fatty acids (stearic and oleic) adsorbed on alumina or on magnesium oxide are recovered pure [14]. We show here that with this method there is no transformation of very reactive hydrocarbons impregnated on an inert solid (SiO_2). The hydrocarbons chosen were an olefin : 1-tetradecene and an alkylaromatic : 9-methylphenanthrene. Figure 1 shows that the GC of the compounds recovered in CH_2Cl_2 (Fig. 1b) are identical to the GC of the starting compounds (Fig. 1a). These GC can be compared to those of the transformation products of 1-tetradecene and of 9-methylphenanthrene on acid catalysts (Fig. 1c). The contact of 1-tetradecene with the hydrofluoric acid solution which occurs during the dissolution of SiO_2 is therefore insufficient to cause a double bond shift, a reaction which however does not require strong acid sites [15]. Likewise hydrofluoric acid does not catalyze the isomerization and the disproportionation of 9-methylphenanthrene either since these reactions require stronger acid sites [16].

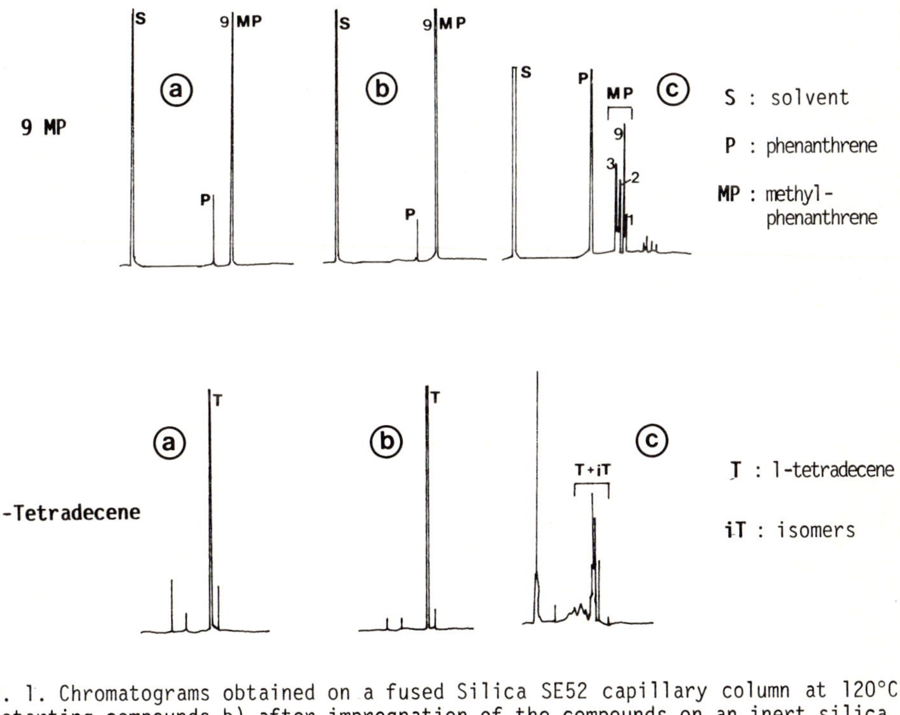

Fig. 1. Chromatograms obtained on a fused Silica SE52 capillary column at 120°C a) starting compounds b) after impregnation of the compounds on an inert silica, dissolution of silica in a 40 % hydrofluoric acid solution, extraction by methylene chloride c) after reaction of 9-methylphenanthrene on USHY and of 1-tetradecene on alumina at 300°C.

We can thus conclude that the method used for the recovery of the carbonaceous compounds blocked in the porosity of the zeolites will not cause any significant change of their nature. This is not surprising since the temperature is low and the coke and the acid molecules are in two different phases.

2. Effect of the reaction temperature on the composition of the carbonaceous residues formed during propene transformation on an USHY zeolite

Olefins are often produced during the transformations of organic compounds on acid catalysts (e.g. methanol conversion, alkane cracking...). Highly reactive, they can undergo numerous secondary reactions and in particular can lead to carbonaceous compounds responsible for catalyst deactivation ("coke"). We shall show how the reaction temperature affects the composition of the carbonaceous compounds deposited in a USHY zeolite during propene conversion. The mechanism of their formation will be discussed.

The operating conditions were the following : flow reactor, p-propene = 0.1 bar, pN_2 = 0.9 bar, weight of propene injected per weight of catalyst and per hour close to 1, reaction time 15 min, temperature equal to 120°C, 200°C, 350°C or 450°C. For all these temperatures the coke content was between 4 and 6 %.

2.1. Composition of the carbonaceous compounds ; effect of the reaction temperature

The "coke" composition depends strongly on the reaction temperature. Thus the atomic H/C ratio decreases when the reaction temperature θ increases : it is equal to 1.8 at 120°C, 1.2 at 200°C, 1.0 at 350°C and 0.8 at 450°C. For the first three temperatures, the coke is completely soluble in CH_2Cl_2 whereas for θ = 450°C, only 30 % of the coke is soluble ; the non-soluble part, remaining as small black particles on the surface of the solution of hydrofluoric acid, is constituted of highly condensed polyaromatic compounds. After elimination of the solvent, the soluble "coke" for θ = 120°C is a viscous yellow liquid whereas for the other values of θ it is a brown solid, all the darker than θ is higher.

The soluble "cokes" were analyzed by GC, HPLC, H-NMR, MS. The GC analysis shows that the soluble "cokes" are always very complex mixtures, whose compositions are very different : the higher the reaction temperature, the more difficult is the elution of the components. However for θ = 450°C, part of the products is easily eluted. HPLC analysis shows that for θ = 120°C, the products are non aromatic ; for θ = 200°C, they have 2 or 3 aromatic rings, for θ = 350°C 2 to 4 and for θ = 450°C 3 to 5 (Fig. 2). This aromaticity increase is confirmed by H-NMR at least up to 350°C (Fig. 3) : the percentages of aromatic and of alkylaromatic protons (from groups carried by aromatic rings) increase at the

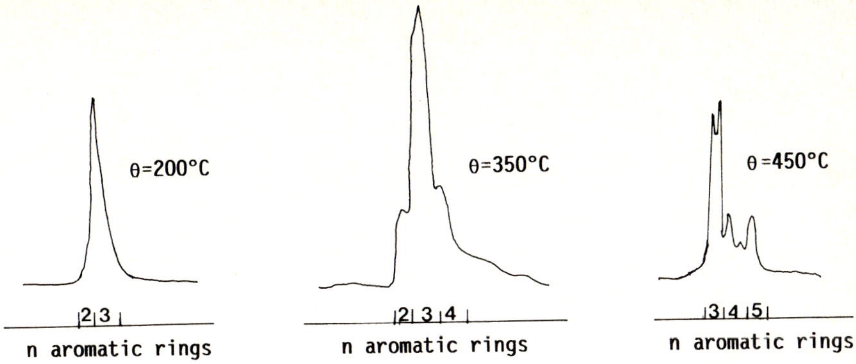

Fig. 2. HPLC analysis of the soluble coke obtained for different reaction temperatures θ. 250 mm Column packed with ultrasil NH_2 ; solvent : n-heptane ; UV detection.

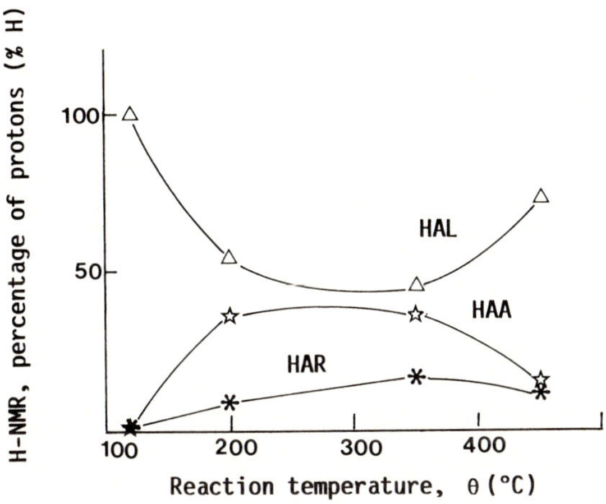

Fig. 3. Analysis of the soluble coke by H-NMR. Change of the percentages of aromatic protons (H_{AR}) of alkylaromatic protons (H_{AA}) and of aliphatic protons H_{AL}) as functions of the reaction temperature θ.

expense of the percentage of aliphatic protons. The contrary occurs between 350°C and 450°C : in the soluble coke for θ = 450°C, a large proportion of aliphatic and cyclic protons is found (73 %) and the percentage of aromatic protons and above all of alkylaromatic protons is very low. This shows that either the polyaromatic compounds existing in the soluble fraction have large alkyl (or naphtenic) groups or the soluble coke is a mixture of polyaromatic and of aliphatic compounds. The latter hypothesis, in agreement with GC analysis, is more probable. It allows to understand why the global H/C ratio of the coke is high when 70 % of this coke is constituted by highly polyaromatic (since non-soluble) compounds. If a value of 0.4 is taken for the atomic H/C ratio of this non-soluble coke [12], the atomic H/C of the soluble coke is indeed close to 1.4. The MS analysis is carried out at low ionisation energy (10eV) after solvent evaporation ; this evaporation can cause the elimination of the more volatile "coke" components. For θ = 120°C, the main components found by MS are heavy (386 < molecular weight M < 470) which corresponds, since they are non aromatic, to compounds having 28-34 carbon atoms and C_nH_{2n-4} or C_nH_{2n-6} as general formulas (therefore with 3 or 4 cycles plus unsaturations). For the highest values of θ, M and n of the main components are lower :

θ = 200°C	198 < M < 328	15 < n < 25
θ = 350°C	258 < M < 324	20 < n < 25
θ = 450°C	254 < M < 296	20 < n < 23

and the general formulas correspond to polyaromatic compounds (2 to 5 aromatic rings).

2.2. Detailed composition of the carbonaceous compounds. Modes of formation

For θ = 120°C, the main products have as formulas C_nH_{2n-4} or C_nH_{2n-6} with n between 28 and 34 and are consequently naphtenic or/and olefinic (Table 1). H-NMR shows the existence of some olefinic protons (small signals for δ between 5.6 and 6.5 ppm corresponding to less than 1 % of all the protons) and of CH_2 groups in α of a double bond (δ = 2.15 ppm corresponding to less than 5 % of the protons). This presence of double bonds is confirmed by IR. The percentage of protons of saturated cycles (1.5 ppm < δ < 1.7 ppm) is also very low (< 1 %). On the other hand, as found by other authors [9], the number of protons of CH_3 aliphatic groups is at least 1.5 greater than those of the CH_2 and of the CH groups. The carbonaceous compounds are therefore mainly aliphatic, highly branched with probably one or two double bonds and one or two saturated cycles. Most of the compounds have a carbon number which is not a multiple of 3. These compounds cannot therefore result directly from propene polymerization. They are probably formed through the following reactional steps : 1) formation of oligomers and polymers of propene 2) rearrangement and scission of the products of step 1 (C_2-C_6, mainly branched, are the principal products desorbed from the zeolite) 3) formation of other polymers from propene and from the products of step 2 ; 4) cyclization in one or two positions of the polymers ; 5) hydrogen transfer from the polymer to the olefinic products of the reaction 2 (most of the C_2-C_6 products desorbed from the zeolite are saturated). Since only very few cycles and double bonds are formed, steps 4 and 5 are slow.

It can be noted that the kinetic diameter of these compounds is significantly smaller than the pore size. They are not very basic and consequently not strongly adsorbed on the acid sites. They are therefore blocked in the zeolite porosity only because of their low volatility : their boiling point is indeed higher than 400°C.

For $\theta = 200°C$, the main components of the "coke" have 2 or 3 aromatic rings. However most of the protons (92 %) are aliphatic or carried by groups situated in α of the aromatic rings. The protons of the CH_2 or of the CH aliphatic groups are about twice more numerous than the protons of the CH_3 groups. No olefinic protons and practically no protons of saturated cycles are observed. The compounds are therefore bi or triaromatic with numerous branched alkyl groups, the branching of these groups being however less significant than for $\theta = 120°C$. Three main families of compounds can be distinguished by mass spectrometry (Table 1) :

- A C_nH_{2n-12} family, i.e. with 7 unsaturations or cycles. The main compounds have 15 to 17 carbon atoms (M = 198, 212, 226).
- A C_nH_{2n-18} family, i.e. with 10 unsaturations or cycles. The main compounds have 19 to 21 carbon atoms (M = 248, 262, 276).
- A C_nH_{2n-22} family, i.e. with 12 unsaturations or cycles. The main compounds have 22 to 24 carbon atoms (M = 286, 300, 314).

The mass spectrum of the main compounds of each family was obtained by GS-MS coupling. Figures 4 show on the example of the compounds with M = 226 and M = 262 how it is possible to deduce from the scissions the developed formula. The lighter compounds (family 1) are alkyl naphtalenes, the alkyl groups having 5 to 7 carbon atoms. The compounds of families 2 and 3 have probably 2 or 3 aromatic cycles, one unsaturated C_5 cycle plus alkyl groups (3 to 8 carbon atoms).

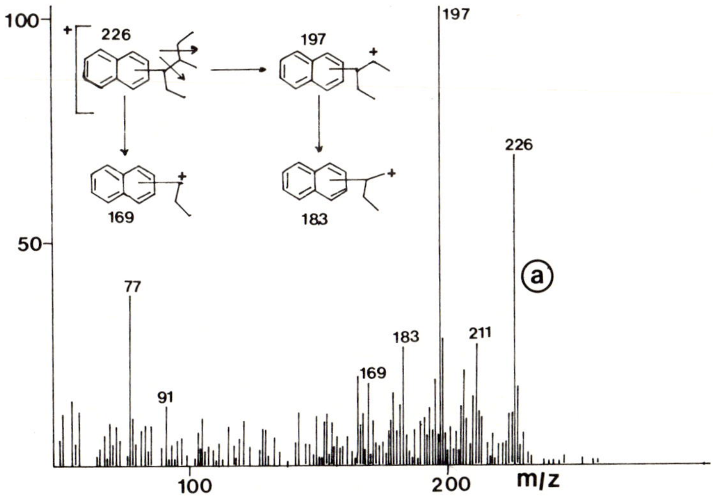

Fig. 4a. Mass spectrum of a main component of the soluble coke (M=226) for a reaction temperature $\theta = 200°C$, obtained by GC-MS coupling. Ionisation energy = 40 eV.

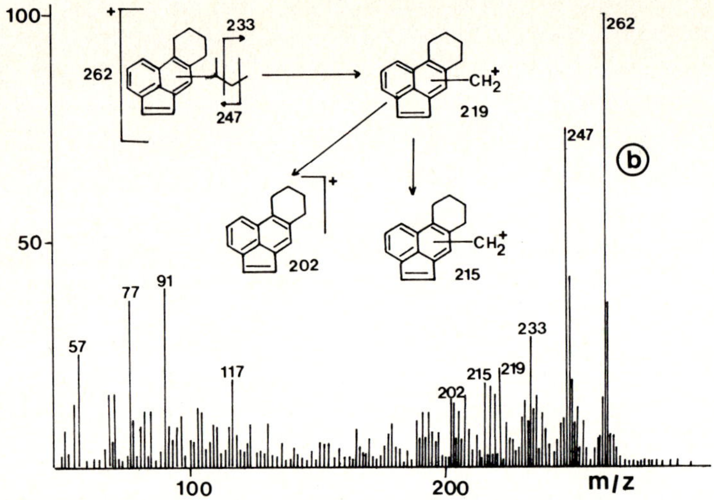

Fig. 4b. Mass spectrum of a main component of the soluble coke (M=262) for a reaction temperature θ = 200°C, obtained by GC-MS coupling. Ionisation energy = 40 eV.

The reactional steps involved at θ = 120°C can explain the formation of all these compounds. The number of their carbon atoms is smaller because an increase in temperature favors thermodynamically scission reactions at the expense of oligomerization and of polymerization reactions. Aromatic rings are formed at 200°C because hydrogen transfer reactions (step 5) from naphtenes to olefins become rapid.

The naphtalenic compounds (family 1) are not very bulky and could circulate in the porosity of the zeolite if they were more volatile. A significant desorption of these compounds is moreover observed if the coked sample is rapidly heated (in order to avoid "coke" transformations) at higher temperature under nitrogen flow. The other compounds, bulkier, are probably blocked in the supercages of the Y zeolite.

For θ = 350°C, the main products have 3 or 4 aromatic rings. Most of the protons (83 %) are either alkylaromatic or aliphatic. The protons of the CH or of the CH_2 aliphatic groups are three times more numerous than those of the CH_3 groups. The number of protons in saturated cycles is very small. The compounds are therefore tri or tetra aromatic with numerous alkyl groups. Two main families of compounds can be distinguished by mass spectrometry (Table 1) :

- The first family is the one already observed for θ = 200°C having as general formula C_nH_{2n-22}, n being however smaller : the main compounds have 20 to 22 carbon atoms (M = 258, 272, 286).

- The second family has a C_nH_{2n-26} general formula (14 unsaturations or cycles). The main components have 22 to 24 carbon atoms (M = 282, 296, 310). From their analysis through GC-MS coupling we can deduce the formula given in table 1. All these compounds, too bulky to circulate in the porosity of the Y zeolite, would be blocked in its supercages. The reactions 1-5 allow to explain their formation, the significance of the cyclization and of the hydrogen transfer reactions increasing once again when θ increases from 200°C to 350°C.

TABLE 1
Nature of the carbonaceous compounds formed during propene conversion on a USHY zeolite at different temperatures.

Reaction temperature	Compound series formula	Main components
120°C	C_nH_{2n-4}, C_nH_{2n-6} 1 or 2 double bonds and 2 or 3 cycles	$C_{30}H_{56}$, $C_{31}H_{58}$, $C_{32}H_{60}$
200°C	C_nH_{2n-12} 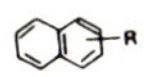	$C_{15}H_{18}$, $C_{16}H_{20}$, $C_{17}H_{22}$
	C_nH_{2n-18} 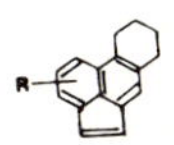	$C_{19}H_{20}$, $C_{20}H_{22}$, $C_{21}H_{24}$
	C_nH_{2n-22} 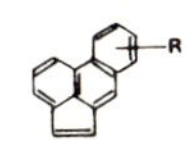	$C_{22}H_{22}$, $C_{23}H_{24}$, $C_{24}H_{26}$
350°C	C_nH_{2n-22} 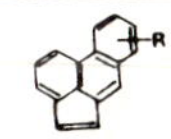	$C_{20}H_{18}$, $C_{21}H_{20}$, $C_{22}H_{22}$
	C_nH_{2n-26} 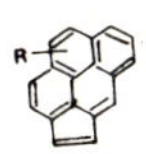	$C_{22}H_{18}$, $C_{13}H_{20}$, $C_{24}H_{22}$

For θ = 450°C only 30 % of the coke is soluble ; the non-soluble part comprises highly polyaromatic compounds. H-NMR shows that the soluble compounds have only a small number of aromatic and alkyl of aromatic protons. Most of the protons are probably in saturated cycles (28 % with δ = 1.5 ppm) and small signals corresponding to olefinic protons can be observed. On the other hand, MS (after evaporation of the solvent) and HPLC analysis show the existence of alkyl polyaromatic compounds with 3 to 5 rings. Thus the soluble coke comprises probably two parts : the first composed of polyaromatic compounds C_nH_{2n-26} like for θ = 350°C, the second of olefinic, aliphatic or cyclic compounds, highly volatile since eliminated during solvent evaporation. These latter compounds result probably from propene transformation somewhere in the zeolite porosity, coke deposits allowing the entry of the linear molecules of propene and preventing the exit of the branched or cyclic transformation products. Similar phenomenona were already observed with H mordenite during n-heptane cracking [10].

2.3. Conclusion

The carbonaceous compounds formed from propene in the porosity of an USHY zeolite and responsible for its deactivation were recovered after dissolution of the zeolite in a hydrofluoric acid solution and their composition determined by GC, HPLC, H-NMR and MS. At low temperature (120°C) the main compounds had over 28 carbons. They were formed through polymerization of propene and of olefins resulting from propene transformation. These compounds not being very basic nor very bulky were blocked in the zeolite porosity only because of their low volatility. When the reaction temperature was increased, scission reactions in comparison to the polymerization reactions became more and more favored. The number of carbons of the polymers became smaller and these compounds being more volatile could be desorbed from the zeolite. This increase in the rates of desorption with the temperature explains why the coking rate did not increase significantly with reaction temperature. The rates of cyclization and of hydrogen transfer were also increased and aromatic rings formed. The polyaromatic compounds obtained (2 to 5 rings) being very bulky, remained blocked in the supercages of the zeolite. Heavier polyaromatic compounds, therefore non-soluble in organic solvent could also be formed probably through growth of the lighter polyaromatics situated in the supercages near the outer surface.

3. Composition of "coke" ; effect on the adsorption properties of zeolites. Mode of deactivation

Three protonic zeolites : two with large pores (USHY and H mordenite (HM)) and one with intermediate pore-size (HZSM5) were used. Their characteristics were given in ref. [17]. Their deactivation was studied in a flow reactor during dimethylether conversion at 400°C with p_{DME} = 0.2 bar and p_{N_2} = 0.8 bar. The soluble carbonaceous compounds were analyzed by GC, HPLC, H-NMR and MS. The adsorption capacities of the coked samples were measured for nitrogen at - 196°C and for n-hexane at 0°C [17].

3.1. Coking and aging of the zeolites

The initial activity (after 5 minutes' reaction) of HZSM5 is about 60 times greater than for USHY and 80 times than for HM. The deactivation of HZSM5 is very low ; on the contrary USHY and above all HM loses rapidly nearly all its activity. This more rapid deactivation of the large pore-size zeolites is partly due to a more rapid coking rate : indeed the initial rate of coking is at least 20 times greater on USHY and on HM than on HZSM5. The low coking rate on HZSM5 is due to the steric constraints exerted by the narrow pore structure of this zeolite on the numerous bimolecular reactions involved in the formation of coke and also to the low density of its acid sites [5]. On the other hand, the fast deactivation of HM can also be attributed to a greater coke "toxicity". Initially, one gram of carbonaceous deposit eliminates the activity of at least 100 g for HM against only 5-10 g for HZSM5 and 10-20 g for USHY. This greater effect of coke on the HM activity can be related to the monodimensional framework of this zeolite [10].

3.2. Number of coke molecules and of acid sites

As in the case of n-heptane cracking [10] , the composition of the carbonaceous compounds depends on the zeolite and on the reaction time (Table 2). From H-NMR, HPLC and MS analysis it is possible to deduce formulas for the main components of the soluble part of coke. The number of molecules in the soluble coke can then be estimated from the amount of this coke (total amount of coke x yield of solubilization) and from the mean molecular weight of the components (Table 2). An approximate value of the number of molecules in the non-soluble coke was also calculated by admitting for these molecules a mean number of carbon atoms equal to 40. This number corresponds to a polyaromatic with about 12 aromatic rings and an atomic H/C ratio equal to 0.4 which is the value found for H/C of the non-soluble coke of the most coked sample of USHY.

The total number of coke molecules n_k is always much more smaller than the total number of the zeolite acid sites, n_{A1} obtained from their chemical formula (Table 2). It is also smaller than the number of strong acid sites (n_{A2}), A_2 representing the sites on which the NH_3 adsorption heat is greater than 100 kjoule mole^{-1}, [17]. Thus for 17 % coke on USHY, n_k is equal to about 2/3 of n_{A2} and yet the zeolite is practically inactive. With 7 % coke, HM is completely inactive while n_k is equal to only 10 % of n_{A2}. On HZSM5 with 2.5 % coke n_k is equal to about 35 % of n_{A2} and the decrease in activity to about 25 %. We can therefore conclude that on HZSM5, aging occurs probably through site coverage (one molecule of coke deactivating one active site) while on USHY and above all on HM it occurs through pore blockage.

TABLE 2

Characteristics of the zeolites and of the carbonaceous compounds. n_{A1} is the theoretical number of acid sites drawn from the chemical formulas of the zeolites and n_{A2} the number of acid sites for which the NH_3 adsorption heat was greater than 100 kjoule $mole^{-1}$. n_k : number of coke molecules ; ρ : coke density ; H-NMR : H_{AR} : aromatic protons ; H_{AA} : alkylaromatic protons ; H_{AL} : aliphatic protons.

		USHY		HM		HZSM5	
Zeolites	n_{A1} (10^{20} sites/g)	25		11		2.2	
	n_{A2} (10^{20} sites/g)	3.4		7.5		1.6	
Total "coke"	coking time (hrs)	0.5	6	0.17	0.5	0.5	24
	coke (wt%)	7	17	1.3	7	0.6	2.5
	atomic H/C	0.65	0.55	≃ 2	0.6	≃2.5	1
	solubilization (wt%)	75	5	100	20	100	100
	ρ(g/cm^3)	1.5	2.15	1.1	1.95	0.8	1
	n_k(10^{20}molecules/g)	1.2	2.2	0.35	1	0.1	0.6
Soluble "coke"	H-NMR (%)						
	HAR	5	5	20	ε	ε	20
	HAA	30	20	45	ε	ε	30
	HAL	65	75	35	100	100	40
	HPLC n aromatic rings	3-5	4-5	3-4	-	-	2-3
	MS n carbon atoms	18-26	18-26	14-18	15-44	26-35	16-22
	Main components	C_nH_{2n-26}	C_nH_{2n-26}	C_nH_{2n-18} C_nH_{2n-24}	C_nH_{2n-4} C_nH_{2n-12}	C_nH_{2n-6}	C_nH_{2n-16}
	ρ(g/cm^3)	1.3	1.3	1.1	0.9	0.8	1
	n_k(10^{20}molecules/g)	1	0.2	0.35	0.2	0.1	0.6

3.3 Real and apparent volumes occupied by "coke"

The density of coke ρ_R can be estimated from its composition. For this, we have given to the density of the insoluble part of the coke that of graphite (2.2 g/cm^3) and estimated that of the soluble part from the densities of its main components (Table 2). The volume V_R really occupied by coke (cm^3/g) is equal to ρ_R^{-1}. The volume V_A apparently occupied by coke was deduced from adsorption experiments on the coked samples : $(V_A)_H$ and $(V_A)_{N_2}$ are respectively the porous volumes made inaccessible to n-hexane and to nitrogen. On USHY, V_R is always smaller than $(V_A)_H$ and $(V_A)_{N_2}$, the differences in values increasing with the coke content (Fig. 5a). This means that coke causes a blockage of the zeolite porosity. At low coke content, the blockage is more pronounced for n-hexane (kinetic diameter 4.9 A) than for nitrogen (3.6 A). On HM even at low coke content, coke deposits block the access of n-hexane to a large part of the porous volume : for 1.3 % coke, $(V_A)_H$ is 5 times greater than V_R. This is quite characteristic of a channel blockage. At low coke content, the volume made inaccessible to nitrogen $(V_A)_{N_2}$ is equal to the volume really occupied by coke (Fig. 5b) This difference between n-hexane and nitrogen is due to the fact that the circulation of nitrogen occurs in all the directions whereas that of n-hexane is monodimensional [17]. At high coke content, $(V_A)_{N_2}$ is greater than $(V_A)_H$, coke preventing the access of nitrogen both to the large and to the narrow channels. On HZSM5 (Fig. 5c) blockage of the porous volume is also observed, at least for coke contents higher than 2 %. However this blockage is much more limited here than with the other zeolites.

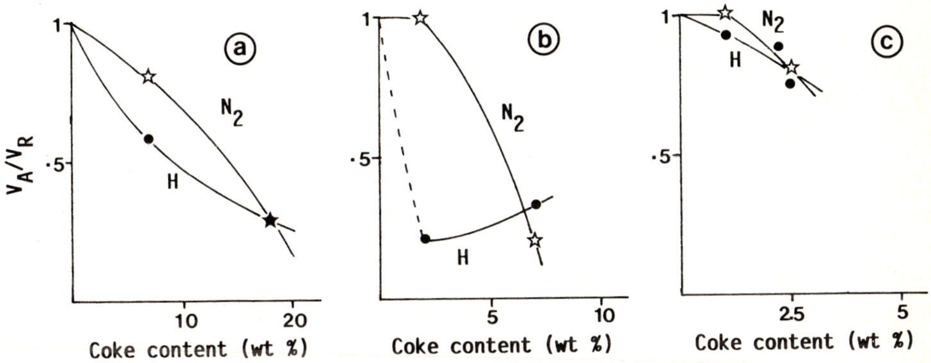

Fig. 5. Change of the ratio V_A/V_R as a function of the coke content (wt %). V_A apparent volume occupied by coke determined by nitrogen adsorption (N_2) or by n-hexane adsorption (H) ; V_R real volume occupied by coke.

In conclusion : by considering both the adsorption measurements on the coked samples and the information obtained on coke composition the mode of zeolite deactivation can be specified. Thus for USHY, for HM and probably for HZSM5 at high coke content the deactivation observed during the conversion of dimethylether into hydrocarbons at 400°C was shown to be due to pore blockage.

REFERENCES

1 E.E. Wolf and F. Alfani, Catal. Rev. Sci. Eng., 24 (1982) 329-371.
2 W.G. Appleby, J.W. Gibson and G.M. Good, Ind. Eng. Chem., Process, Des. Dev., 1 (1962) 102-110.
3 R.C. Haldeman and M.C. Botty, J. Phys. Chem., 63 (1959) 489-496.

4 L.D. Rollmann and D.E. Walsh, in J.L. Figueiredo (Ed.), NATO Asi Series E, 54, Progress in Catalyst Deactivation, Martinus Nijhoff Publishers, The Hague, Boston, London, 1982, pp. 81-91.
5 E.G Derouane, in B. Imelik et al (Eds.), Studies in Surface Science and Catalysis Vol. 20, Catalysis by Acids and Bases, Elsevier, Amsterdam, Oxford, New-York, 1985, pp. 221-240.
6 B.E. Langner, Ind. Eng. Chem. Process Des. Dev., 20 (1981) 326-331.
7 P.B. Venuto, L.A Hamilton, Ind. Eng. Chem. Prod. Res. Dev., 6 (1967) 190-192.
8 D.M. Bibby, N.B. Milestone, J.E. Patterson and L.P. Aldridge, J. Catal., 97 (1986) 493-502.
9 A.K. Ghosh and R.A. Kydd, J. Catal., 100 (1986) 185-195.
10 M. Guisnet, P. Magnoux and C. Canaff, in R. Setton (Ed.), NATO Series C, 165, Chemical Reactions in Organic and Inorganic Constrained Systems, D. Reidel Publishing Company, Dordrecht, Boston, Lancaster, Tokyo, 1986, pp. 131-140.
11 M. Guisnet, P. Magnoux and C. Canaff, in Y. Murakami et al. (Eds.), Proceeding of the 7th International Zeolite Conference, New developments in Zeolite Science Technology, Elsevier, Tokyo, 1986, pp. 701-707.
12 P. Gallezot, S. Leclercq, P. Magnoux and M. Guisnet, in preparation.
13 G. Eglinton, P.M. Scott, T. Belsky, A.L. Burlingame and M. Calvin, in Advances in Organic Geochemistry, Pergamon Press, London, 1964, p. 162.
14 C. Bearez, Thesis Poitiers 1985.
15 H. Pines, The Chemistry of Catalytic Hydrocarbon Conversions, Academic Press, 1981, p. 7.
16 M. Guisnet, in B. Imelik et al. (Eds.), Studies in Surface Science and Catalysis, Vol. 20, Catalysis by Acids and Bases, Elsevier, Amsterdam, Oxford, New-York, Tokyo, 1985, pp. 283-297.
17 P. Magnoux, P. Cartraud, S. Mignard and M. Guisnet, submitted for publication.

B. Delmon and G.F. Froment (Editors), *Catalyst Deactivation 1987*

DEACTIVATION OF PLATINUM CATALYSTS STUDIED BY ELECTROCHEMICAL METHODS

E. LAMY-PITARA, L. BENCHARIF, L. LGHOUZOUANI, Y. TAINON and J. BARBIER
Laboratoire de Catalyse en Chimie Organique, UA CNRS 350
40, Avenue du Recteur Pineau
86022 POITIERS CEDEX

Abstract
Transient electrochemical methods can be used for the characterization of the adsorbed species on the surface of metal catalysts.

In the case of poisons adsorbed on platinum catalysts and studied by cyclic voltammetry, several informations can be obtained such as the stoichiometry and the mean valency of the adsorbed poisons and their effects on the adsorption of organic compounds.

Competitive reactions of substituted maleic acids have been used for the investigation of the electronic effects of sulfur and copper poisons. The obtained changes of the selectivities are compared with the changes of the free energy of adsorption of the organic compounds for $\Theta \rightarrow 0, \Delta Go$, which are determined directly by electrochemical methods.

INTRODUCTION

The characterization of the surface state and of the chemisorbed species on metal catalysts is a common feature in heterogeneous catalysis, surface science and interfacial electrochemistry. The important development of high-vacuum techniques has been profitable to these three fields but there is not yet quite a communication between catalysis and electrochemistry.

However, as it has been proved for many reactions, the adsorbed species and the mechanisms can be the same in heterogeneous catalysis and in electrocatalysis. A typical example concerns the nature of adsorbed hydrogen on a transition metal surface. It has been shown by thermodesorption and electrochemical desorption (Ref. 1) that the obtained curves have both two maxima, indicating two energeticaly different adsorbed hydrogen species, and more advanced studies on single crystal faces establish correlations between electrochemical and high vacuum techniques (Ref. 1-5). Moreover, the rate of H_2-D_2 equilibration in gas-phase and the rate of the electrochemical oxidation of hydrogen on Pt are the same and this fact proves that the rate determining step is the same (Ref. 6), i.e. the dissociative adsorption-desorption of hydrogen on the Pt surface : $H_2 \rightleftarrows 2\ H_{ads}$. Another example is related to the reactions of liquid phase hydrogenation of olefin and electrochemical reduction (Ref. 7,8). In this case the same determining step in both reactions is the interaction between adsorbed organic species and adsorbed hydrogen.

This close correlation suggests that neither the electrolyte nor the electrolyte-metal interface significantly affects the chemisorption process and this can be explained by the magnitude of the chemical forces involved in these processes compared with the electrostatic double layer forces and the solvatation energy (Ref. 6).

In such conditions, it can be allowed to make use of the electrochemical methods to study the adsorbed species involved in the catalytic processes and this approach is not quite developped. These methods are based on the measurement of the exchanged quantities of electricity, q, during the formation or the destruction of superficial layers. The relation between the exchanged quantity of electricity and the potential of the electrode-catalyst, gives informations on the surface process, as a function of free energy changes.

In order to study the surface processes, which are limited by the quantity of adsorbed species, transient methods must be used. A transient electrochemical method, largely employed, is the linear potential sweep cyclic voltammetry (L.P.S.C.V.) or potentiodynamic technique, that allows a direct evaluation of charge and coverage, with a resolution of 115-230 cal. and a very good sensitivity and precision in the scales of energy and charge.

So, in this paper, transient electrochemical methods are used in order to study the adsorption of different poisons (Cu, S) on platinum and their effects on the adsorption of olefinic diacids and on the competitive interaction of these compounds with hydrogen (Ref. 9-11). It must be noticed that the characterization of the catalytic system and the test-reaction are carried out in the same conditions (in situ).

The use of these transient electrochemical methods allows :

- the determination of the initial metallic area of the catalyst,
- the control of the poison deposition so as to obtain adatoms in fractions of a monolayer
- the measurement of the area occupied by the deposited poison
- the determination of the quantity of adsorbed poison,
- the evaluation of the adsorption stoichiometry and of the electronic charge of the adatom,
- the measurement of the equilibrium coverage by the adsorbed organic species in absence or in presence of adatoms, which allows to obtain the adsorption isotherms .

EXPERIMENTAL

1) Cyclic voltammetry

The linear potential sweep cyclic voltammetry is a perturbation technique, using a linear potential variation, analogous to the flash desorption spectroscopy when a thermal variation is used.

This technique gives a means of evaluating the quantity of electricity associated with an adsorbed monolayer of hydrogen or oxygen on the catalyst surface. Through integration of the anodic or cathodic part relative to the hydrogen zone of the voltammogram (I, in fig 1) it is possible to obtain the quantity of electricity, Q_H^o, associated with a hydrogen monolayer and to calculate the initial number, N_H^o, of the surface platinum atom (Ref. 12) :

$N_H^o = Q_H^o$ (μC)/1.6 x 10^{-13} (1),

or the initial surface area (assuming that a platinum atom occupies an average area close to 7.6 $Å^2$).

2) Experimental conditions

The apparatus and the measuring cell used for the voltammetric study are described in Ref. 9-11.

The platinized platinum catalyst (which constitutes the working electrode) is prepared by electrolytic deposition, at a potential of - 0.05 V/SCE (versus a saturated calomel electrode), in a solution of 2 to 4% of chloroplatinic acid in 1 M HCl. The roughness factor of the platinum surface, defined as the ratio of the actual area to the geometric area, $r = S_r/S_g$, is kept equal to 50-100.

The supporting electrolyte is a solution of Merck "Suprapur" 0.5 M H_2SO_4, diluted in very pure water of a resistivity equal to 17-18 MΩ . cm. The products used to modify the surface of the platinum catalyst are pro analysi Merck $Cu(SO_4)_2$ $5H_2O$ and purum Carlo Erba Na_2S 38 % H_2O. Maleic acid and citraconic acid are pro analysi Fluka.

3) Operating mode

Before each experiment the surface of the catalyst is thoroughly cleaned by several successive cycles between 0.05 and 1.5 V/R.H.E. (versus a reversible hydrogen electrode). The cleanliness of the cell-solution-electrode system can be checked by recording a voltammogram, the shape of which changes in the presence of minute quantities of impurities.

After the measurement of the initial area, the catalyst surface is modified by adsorption of copper, or sulfur adatoms. This modification is achieved at controlled potential, in the double layer region, where no electrochemical reaction occurs in the sulphuric medium (II, in fig 1). This treatment can be carried out in a nearby cell, in the case of sulfur only, because the sulfur adatoms are not oxidized during the transfer of the electrode from one cell to the other, conversely to copper adatoms, which are kept in the same cell under nitrogen flow during the evacuation of the copper containing solution and the refilling of the cell by clean acidic solution. The modified catalysts can be used either for the study of the adsorbed species, or for the study of the adsorption of the organic compounds or for the hydrogenation experiments. In the second case the equilibrium coverage of organic species is measured, for different concentrations in solution, in absence and in presence of poison adatoms on the surface. In the last case the simple or competitive hydrogenations are followed by HPLC analysis.

RESULTS AND DISCUSSION

I Characterization of copper and sulfur adatoms deposited on platinized platinum catalysts

The adatoms deposition is carried out by electrolysis of the corresponding mineral salt, at a potential that is fixed in the double layer region where no undesirable adsorption occurs. Furthermore in the case of copper in this region of potential it is possible to cover only a fraction of the surface by adatoms without any bulk deposition, the potential being more positive than the thermodynamic potential of bulk deposition ("under potential deposition") (Ref. 9,13).

During the deposition of copper a negative transient current occurs, which is due to the reduction of Cu^{++} to Cu adatoms. In the case of sulfur, a positive transient current occurs, which indicates that the added sulfide (H_2S an acidic medium), is oxidized during its adsorption at a degree of oxidation higher than - 2 (Ref. 10). The observed curves $i = f(t)$ can be integrated and the obtained quantity of electricity, Q_{ads}, is proportional to the number of exchanged electrons and also to the number of adsorbed adatom molecules.

The adatoms deposited on platinized platinum modify the cyclic voltammetry curves characteristic of this metal.

In the adsorption region of hydrogen, the observed decrease of the height of the adsorption or desorption peaks shows that a fraction of the surface area has been occupied by the adatom, thus inhibiting the adsorption of hydrogen. In fig 1, the change of the platinum voltammogram by copper adatoms is illustrated as an example. The difference between the curves (2) and (1), corresponding to the desorption (or adsorption) of hydrogen in the absence and in the presence of copper adatoms, allows the measurement of the fraction, Θ_{Cu}, of the platinum surface which is occupied by the copper :

$$\Theta_{Cu} = \frac{Q_H^o - Q_H^{Cu}}{Q_H^o} = \frac{N_{Cu}^H}{N_H^o} \qquad (2)$$

with Q_H^{Cu} = the quantity of electricity associated with the oxidation of adsorbed hydrogen in presence of copper adatoms.
and N_{Cu}^H = the number of hydrogen adatoms displaced by the copper adatoms.

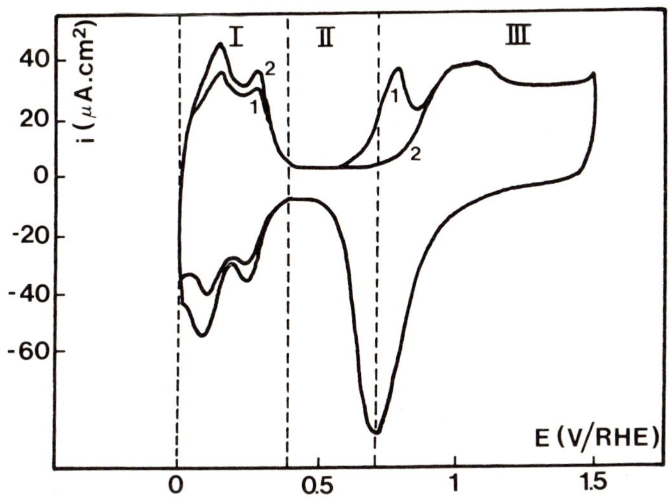

Figure 1 : Voltammogram of a platinum electrode modified by adsorption of copper.

(1) in presence of adsorbed copper

(2) in absence of adsorbed copper

The adsorbed copper is oxidized at potentials higher than 0.5 V/RHE (before the platinum oxidation), as it is shown in Fig 1, and it is desorbed : $Cu_{ads} \rightarrow Cu^{2+} + 2e^-$. The quantity of electricity, associated with the copper oxidation, Q_{ox}^{Cu}, leads to the total number of adsorbed copper atoms,

$$N_{Cu} = \frac{Q_{ox}^{Cu}\ (\mu C)}{2 \times 1.6.10^{-13}} \qquad (3)$$

The degree of the surface coverage by copper, Θ_{Cu}, varies linearly with N_{Cu}/N_H^o (fig 2), and the slope, $n_{Cu/Pt} = N_{Cu}/N_{Cu}^H = 1$ (4) , expresses the adsorption stoichiometry of copper on platinum. Thus, it has been confirmed that one copper adatom occupies one platinum atom on the surface of platinized platinum, as on the surface of smooth platinum (Ref. 14,15).

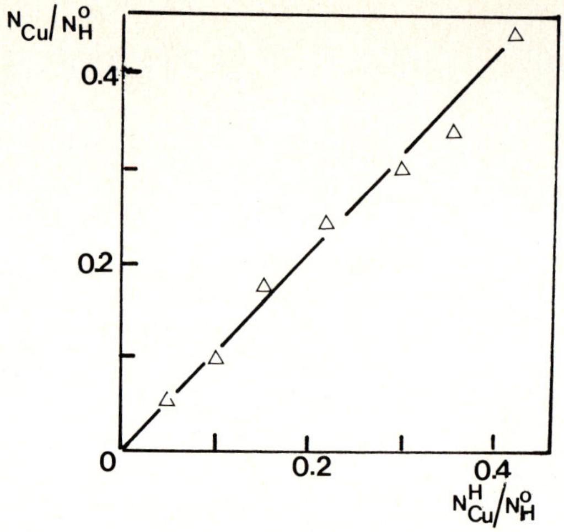

Fig 2 : Number of adsorbed copper adatoms versus the number of displaced hydrogen adatoms on platinum.

The adsorption of sulfur on platinum, has been extensively studied (Ref. 10,11). As the sulfide species are oxidized during their adsorption at a degree of oxidation higher than - 2, and then they are desorbed as sulfate in more positive potentials, it is possible to calculate the charge of the sulfur adatoms by comparison of the exchanged quantities of electricity, respectively Q_{ads}^S and Q_{ox}^S.

It has been found, that the mean valency of the adsorbed sulfur species, x_S, varies with the degree of coverage Θ_S, and also with the coefficient of roughness, r (Ref. 10) (fig 3).

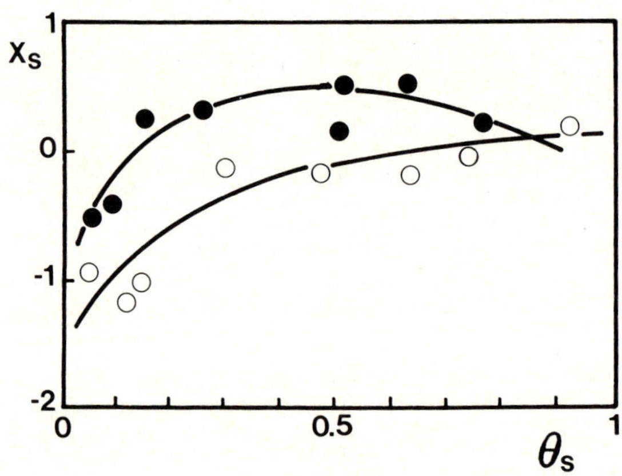

Figure 3 : Mean valency of the sulfur adatoms on platinum as a function of the degree of sulfur coverage ● r = 100 o r = 20

The mean stoichiometry also, $n_{Pt/S}$, varies with the degree of coverage from $n_{Pt/S}$ = 2-3, for a low value of Θ_S, to n = 1, for Θ_S near the monolayer (fig 4).

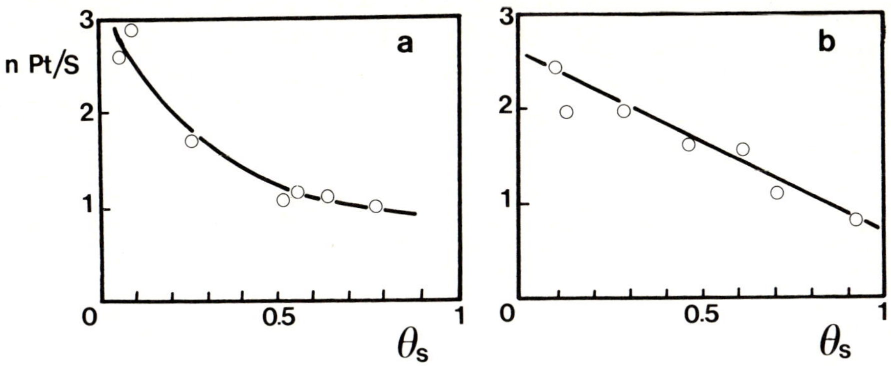

Figure 4 : Mean stoichiometry of sulfur adatoms on platinum in function of the degree of sulfur coverage
a) r = 100 b) r = 20

This can be explained by the occurence of two (or more) different adsorbed sulfur species of variable proportion in function of Θ_S and of the surface structure. Other electrochemical or radiotracer results relative to the system S/Pt (Ref. 16,17), or the S/Au system (Ref. 18,19) and XPS results (Ref. 19, 20), corroborate this statement.

II - Effect of copper and sulfur adatoms on the adsorption of maleic and methylmaleic acids

The mechanism of catalytic hydrogenation of olefinic compounds involves a chemisorption step (Ref. 11). Fig 5 gives as an example the adsorption isotherms for methylmaleic acid in absence and in presence of copper adatoms. In presence of copper on the platinum surface, the equilibrium coverages decrease, for all concentrations, pointing out that the adatoms inhibit, by a geometrical effect, the adsorption of the organic compounds.

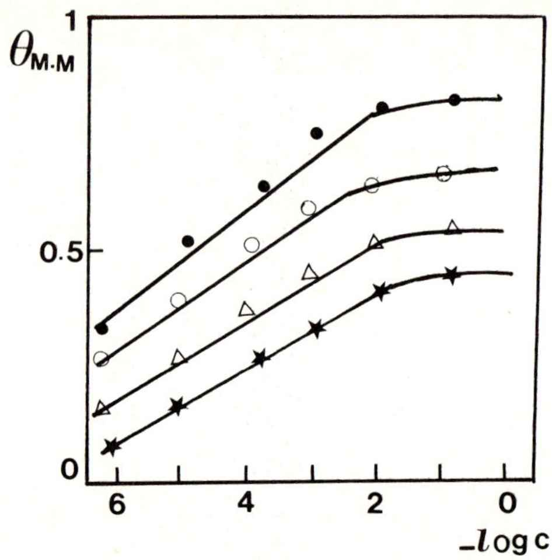

Figure 5 : Adsorption of the methylmaleic acid on platinum modified by copper adatoms.

● Θ_{Cu} = 0, ○ Θ_{Cu} = 0.07 △ Θ_{Cu} = 0.17 ✱ Θ_{Cu} = 0.25.

The obtained isotherms can be described by two straight lines in function of log C, so they follow a Temkin type law : $\Theta = a + 1/f \log C$, with f, the heterogeneity coefficient, which represents the variation of the free energy of adsorption as a function of the degree of coverage : $\Delta G = \Delta Go + f\ RT\Theta$, and "a", the adsorbability : $a = 1/f \log Ko$ (Ref 21), ΔGo and Ko being ΔG and K when $\Theta \rightarrow 0$.

In a general way, the adsorption isotherms of these compounds, determined experimentaly can fit in with a Langmuir or a Temkin equation, which are approximations of the more general Frumkin model : $e^{f\Theta}\Theta/(1-\Theta) = KC$ (Ref. 14).

During a catalytic hydrogenation, in the zone of low olefin concentration (order 1 in respect to the olefin), a competition between the adsorption of the olefin and the adsorption of hydrogen occurs. So the Θ_{olef} is very low ($\Theta_{ol} \rightarrow 0$), as it is shown by radiotracer methods (Ref.22). Moreover, when $\Theta \rightarrow 0$, the interactions between adsorbed organic species can be neglected, and ΔGo, which represents the affinity between the substrate and the first adsorbate molecules, will be sensitive to the change of the electronic properties of the catalyst. Furthermore by comparison of the affinity of modified platinum catalyst for two "probe" molecules, like maleic acid and methylmaleic acid, it is possible to define the direction of the electronic transfer induced by the adatoms deposition. Indeed, the methyl group, as an electrodonor one, is able to increase the electronic density of the double bond, and the adsorption of methylmaleic acid, in comparison with maleic acid, will be favoured on electron deficient metals.

The results relative to the adsorption of maleic and methylmaleic acids, in absence and in presence of copper and sulfur adatoms are summarized in fig 6.

Copper adatoms (fig 6a) cause a decrease of Δ Go for these two olefinic compounds. This result can be explained by an enrichment in electrons of the platinum atoms, caused by an electronic transfer from copper adatoms towards platinum atoms :

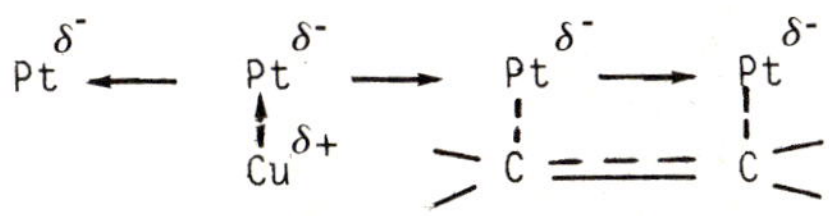

This long-range electronic effect should weaken the strength of the bond olefin-platinum. Indeed it is known that metal adatoms can be partialy positively charged (Ref. 13,23), and the copper adatoms on platinum have a small charge (about equal to + 0.20) depending on Θ_{Cu}.

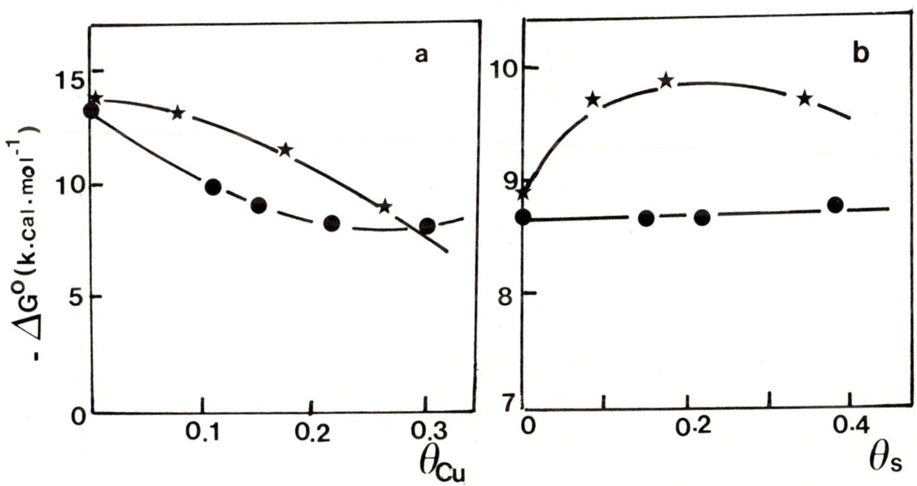

Figure 6 : Variation of the free energy of adsorption of maleic acid, ●, and methylmaleic acid, ★, on platinum
a) in function of the degree of copper coverage
b) in function of the degree of sulfur coverage.

The adsorbed sulfur species cause different effects on the adsorption of these two organic compounds. In fact ΔGo increases in presence of sulfur for the methylmaleic acid, while it remains quite constant in the case of maleic acid (Fig 6b)

According to an electronic transfer from platinum to sulfur, the increase of ΔGo can be explained by the electron donnor effect of the methyl group, which induces an increase of the electronic density of the double bond, and so favours the adsorption of the methylated compound on the electron deficient platinum atoms :

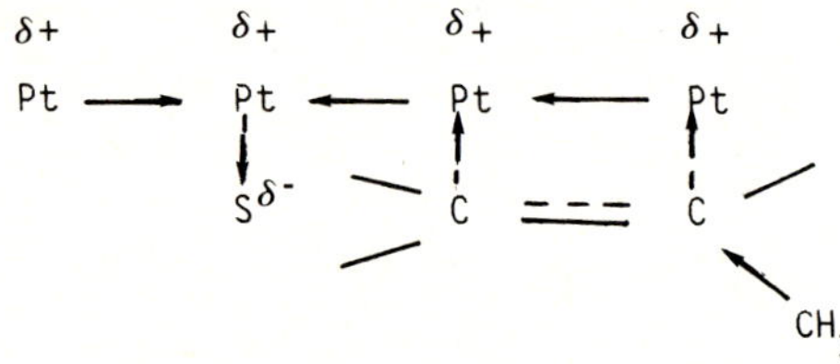

III - Effect of adsorbed copper or sulfur on the competitive hydrogenation of maleic and methylmaleic acids

The hydrogenation of maleic acid in an aqueous solution at 25°C, catalyzed by a platinized platinum unsupported catalyst, follows a Horiuti-Polanyi mechanism, which for low hydrogen pressures and low concentrations leads to the rate equation :

$$v = k.K_H.K_M.pH_2.C_M = k'pH_2C_M \quad (4)$$

with : k' the apparent rate constant, which is the product of the pure kinetic constant k (that is the constant of the rate determining step), by the constant of equilibrium of hydrogen adsorption K_H, and by the constant of equilibrium of the maleic acid adsorption K_M, pH_2 and C_M being the hydrogen pressure and the maleic acid concentration.

The competitive hydrogenation of two compounds A and B, for $C_A = C_B$, (in the region of low concentrations) can be defined by another parameter, the selectivity, R :

$$R_{A/B} = \frac{v_A}{v_B} = \frac{k'_A}{k'_B} = \frac{k_A K_A}{k_B K_B} = \text{Log } (Co/C)_A / \text{ Log } (Co/C)_B \quad (5)$$

It is evident from equation (5) that a variation of the selectivity for a pair of olefins having a similar structure, as for example the maleic acid and the methylmaleic acid, means that the ratio of the r.d.s. constants k_A/k_B, or the ratio of the constants of equilibrium K_A/K_B, can vary. This parameter, R, has been studied in the literature, for different substituted olefins, in function of the number of methyl substituents (Ref. 24) or in function of additives that modify the behaviour of the catalysts (Ref. 28-29)).

In many cases, it has been found that the changes of selectivities are due to changes of the equilibrium constants (Ref. 24,26,28,29) which are sensitive to the electronic change of the surface. So, the measure of selectivities can also be used to evaluate the electronic effects of adatoms (or poisons).

Table 1 shows that the selectivity for the hydrogenations of maleic and methylmaleic acids, $R_{M/MM}$, decreases in function of Θ_S, indicating that the methylated olefins are less deactivated by the sulfur than the simple olefin. Indeed, this result can be explained by the variation of the ratio K_{oM}/K_{oMM} or $\Delta G_{oM}/\Delta G_{oMM}$ (figure 6b).

TABLE 1 :
Selectivities for the competitive hydrogenations of maleic acid and methylmaleic acid, at different platinum catalysts modified by sulfur and copper poisons

Θ_S	$R_{M/MM}$	Θ_{Cu}	$R_{M/MM}$
0	3.05	0	3
0.07	1.92	0.09	1.82
0.12	1.72	0.16	2.00
0.19	1.28	0.31	2.33

In the same way the selectivity increases with an increasing copper coverage in the range $0.1<\Theta_{Cu}<0.3$ (Table 1). Such a result is in good agreement with an electronic enrichment of platinum by copper. Contrary to such hypothesis it can be noticed a decrease of this selectivity at very low copper coverage. This result points out that the evolution of the selectivity in a competitive hydrogenation reaction on partially poisoned catalysts cannot be defined only by a change of the electronic properties of the metal. Such reactions including a lot of elementary steps are too complex to be used to evaluate in an unequivocal way the "ligand effect" of an adsorbed poison..

In conclusion the variation of the free energy of adsorption of different compounds is the more suitable parameter to study the electronic effects of poisons on the catalytic properties of platinum.

REFERENCES

1 J.K. Sass,
Vacuum, 33, (n°10-12) (1983) 741-751.
2 Ph. N. Ross, Jr,
Surface Science, 102 (1981), 463-485.

3 J. Clavilier and J.P. Chauvineau
J. Electroanal. Chem., 100 (1979), 461-462.
4 Ernest Yeager,
J. of the Electrochem. Society, 128 (n°4) (1981) 160C-171C
5 J.L. Stickney, S.R. Rosasco, B.C. Schardt and A.T. Hubbard
The Journal of Phys. Chem., 88 (1984) 251-258.
6 P. Stonehart and P.N. Ross,
Catal. Rev.-Sci.Eng, 12(1) (1975), 1-35.
7 Yu.B. Vassiliev, V.S. Bagotzxy, O.A. Khazova,
V.V. Cherny and A.M. Meretsky
J. Electroanal Chem., 98 (1979), 273-282.
8 K. Shimazu and H. Kita,
Electrochimica Acta, 24, (1979), 1085-1093.
9 E. Lamy, J. Barbier et C. Lamy,
J. de Chimie Physique 77 (10), (1980), 967-972.
10 E. Lamy-Pitara, L. Bencharif et J. Barbier,
Electrochimica Acta., 30(7), (1985), 971-979.
11 E. Lamy-Pitara, L. Bencharif and J. Barbier,
Applied Catalysis, 18 (1985), 117-131.
12 R. Woods in A.J. Bard (Ed), "Electroanal. Chemistry"
Marcel Dekker Inc., New York, 1976, Vol 9, Ch 1, 1-162.
13 D.M. Kolb in H. Gerischer and C.W. Tobias (edition)
"Advances in Electrochemistry and Electrochemical Engineering"
John Wiley, New York, 1978, Vol 11, p 125-271.
14 E. Lamy et J. Barbier,
Electrochimica Acta 27 (6) (1982), 713-719.
15 N. Furuya and S. Motoo,
J. Electroanal. Chem., 98 (1979), 189-194.
16 A.Q. Contractor and Hira Lal,
J. of Electroanal Chem., 96 (1979) 175-81.
17 G. Horanyi and E.M. Rizmayer,
J. of Electroan Chem, 206 (1986), 297-305.
18 E. Lamy-Pitara et J. Barbier
Electrochimica Acta, 31 (6) (1986), 717-721.
19 A.N. Buckley, I.C. Hamilton and R. Woods,
J. Electroan-Chem. 216 (1987), 213-227.
20 T. Wang, A Vazquiez, A. Kato and L.P. Schmidt,
J. Catal. 78 (1982), 306.
21 E. Gileadi, in E. Gileadi (ed),
Electrosorption, Plenum Press 1967, ch I, p 1
22 G. Horanyi, J. Solt and Nagy,
Acta Chim. Acad. Scient. Hung 64(2) (1979) 113-124.
23 J.W. Schultze and F.D. Koppitz,
Electrochimica Acta 21 (1976), 327-336.
24 a) R. Maurel et J. Tellier,
Bull. Soc. Chim. France, n°10 (1968), 4191-4194.
b) R. Maurel et J. Tellier
Bull. Soc. Chim. France n° 11 (1968), 4650-4653.
25 a) J. Cosyns, J.P. Franck et J.M. Gil
C.R. Acad. Sci., Paris 287 (serie C) (1978) 85-88.
b) J. Cosyns, J.P. Franck et J.M. Gil
C.R. Acad. Sci., Paris 288 (serie C) (1979), 25-28.
26 R. Szymanski, H. Charcosset, P. Gallezot, J. Massardier
and L. Tournayan
J. of Catalysis 97 (1986), 366-373.
27 P. Marecot, C. Tifouti and J. Barbier,
React. Kin. and Catal. Letters in press.
28 C.R. Apesteguia, C.E. Brema, T.F. Garetto, A. Bergna
and J.M. Parera, J. of Catalysis 89 (1984), 52-59.
29 L. Cerveny, M. Kuncova, J. Mojzisova and V.P. Ruzicka
J. Chem. Tech. Biotech., 32 (1982), 877-81.

B. Delmon and G.F. Froment (Editors), *Catalyst Deactivation 1987*

COKE DEPOSITION ON HZSM-5 TYPE ZEOLITES

M. BÜLOW[1], J. CARO[1], J. VÖLTER[1] and J. KÄRGER[2]

[1]Zentralinstitut für physikalische Chemie der Akademie der Wissenschaften der DDR, Rudower Chaussee 5, 1199 Berlin (German Democratic Republic)

[2]Sektion Physik der Karl-Marx-Universität Leipzig, Linnéstr. 5, 7010 Leipzig (German Democratic Republic)

ABSTRACT

Coking of HZSM-5 samples of polycrystalline spherical and polyhedral morphology was studied during n-hexane and mesitylene cracking. By measuring the influence of coke deposits on molecular self-diffusion, it is possible to distinguish between intracrystalline and surface coke. Coking with n-hexane exhibits two periods: During an initial period, coke is deposited in the intracrystalline channel network and during the final period, coke is deposited mainly near the external surface of the zeolite crystals. In contrast, coke from mesitylene is predominantly deposited near the external surface from the very beginning of the cracking reaction. Combining this finding with the measurement of the chemisorption of pyridine on coked samples, via the loss of acidity it is demonstrated that coking of HZSM-5 causes a combination of pore blocking and acid site poisoning. From comparing HZSM-5 samples of polycrystalline structure and polyhedral morphology, it is concluded, that in addition to the first order pores of the regular zeolite channel network, polycrystalline grains contain second order pores. The second order pores exhibit two remarkable properties: self-diffusion is enhanced, and coke is deposited preferentially within them.

INTRODUCTION

Coking is a main obstacle in the application of zeolite catalysts. Hence, the elucidation of the mechanism of coke formation on pentasil type zeolites represents a challenging task to both basic and industrial research workers. Recently, selected problems of coke deposition on HZSM-5 have been resolved, e.g. the interdependence of coking and deactivation rates (refs. 1-3), the role of zeolite pore structure in determining the chemical composition of the coke (refs. 1-3) and the poisoning of acid sites by coke (ref. 4). Contradictory are the results from experiments examining the influence of crystal size and morphology (ref. 5) on the coking behaviour of HZSM-5 and those tackling where the coke is deposited.

Whereas in some previous papers HZSM-5 was assumed to produce coke preferentially on the external surface of the crystals (refs. 6,7) recent studies give clear evidence of the existence of coke inside the crystals. Such intracrystalline coke deposits in the channel network have been detected by different techniques, e.g. by a dissolution technique of the coked zeolites in hydrofluoric acid (refs. 1,2), by changes in the ^{29}Si and ^{27}Al MAS NMR spectra of the zeolites during the generation of coke (ref. 8), by a decrease of acidity due to acid site blockage by coke (ref. 4), by a loss of sorption capacity for guest molecules on coked samples (ref. 9) and by the changes of the X-ray diffraction patterns of HZSM-5 containing coke deposits (ref. 9). Furthermore, in a recent paper (ref. 10) we have demonstrated the influence of intracrystalline and surface coke on the diffusion behaviour of guest molecules, sorbed on coked zeolites.

Going on to contribute to this topic, in this paper we present information regarding the influence of crystal morphology on coking of HZSM-5, the coke distribution throughout the crystal and the interdependence of pore blocking and acid site poisoning by coke. For coke production, n-hexane and mesitylene cracking have been used.

EXPERIMENTAL

Zeolite preparation

All specimens of ZSM-5 type zeolites were prepared in the presence of TPA according to established procedures (ref. 11). In recent literature (refs. 12-15), the cracking activity of HZSM-5 was found to be strictly proportional to the concentation of lattice Al and, hence, to the Bronsted acid site density. Therefore, in our experiments we have used only HZSM-5 originating from a synthesis batch with a Si/Al ratio of appr. 35. By means of the ^{1}HMAS NMR technique (ref. 16) the Si/Al ratio in the resulting HZSM-5 samples were determined. They were found to be between 21 and 34. After calcination in air (550°C, 24 h), the zeolites were converted into the H-forms via repeated NH_4-ion exchange (at 90°C) followed by further calcination (550°C, 2 h).

Coking by cracking

Coke was deposited by n-hexane cracking at 500^{0}C in a fixed bed-type glass reactor at atmospheric pressure with a continuous stream of hydrogen (2 l/h.g_{cat}) saturated at 16^{0}C with n-hexane. In the case of mesitylene coking, more severe conditions had to be used for the deposition of a sufficient amount of coke: a temperature of 530^{0}C and nitrogen stream (9 l/h.g_{cat}) saturated at 40^{0}C with mesitylene. The HZSM-5 zeolite (0.5 g) was supported on a glass frit The amount of hydrocarbon reacted into coke and volatile cracking products has been determined by gas chromatography. The coke content of the zeolites was measured by combustion of the coke and microanalysis of the products.

^{1}H NMR diffusion measurements

The coked zeolites were heated in vacuo up to a temperature of 350^{0}C. Methane and propane, respectively, were admitted into the tubes, and these were then sealed. The sorbed amounts of hydrocarbons were determined both volumetrically and gravimetrically. For the determination of the intracrystalline self-diffusion coefficients D_i, the r.m.s. molecular displacement $\langle \vec{r}^{\,2}(\Delta) \rangle^{1/2}$ of the sorbed molecules during an observation time have been measured by means of the NMR pulsed field gradient technique (ref. 17): $D_i = \langle \vec{r}^{\,2}(\Delta) \rangle^{1/2} / 6 \cdot \Delta$.

Whereas diffusion obstacles such as coke deposited on the external surface of the zeolite crystal do not influence D_i, transport resistances like carbonaceous residues within the intracrystalline channel network, cause a severe reduction of the intracrystalline self-diffusivity D_i of sorbed guest molecules. On the other hand, NMR tracer desorption experiments give information on the fraction γ of those molecules which leave the crystals during the observation time Δ . By fitting the corresponding solution of Fick's diffusion law for diffusion limited desorption to the tracer desorption curves, an effective diffusion coefficient D_d was determined (refs. 17,18), $\lim (\partial\gamma/\partial\sqrt{\Delta}) = 2A/V\,(D_d/\pi)^{1/2}$, where V/A denotes the volume to surface ratio of the crystals. Obviously, D_d is influenced by coke deposits on the external surface as well as inside the crystals.

Pyridine chemisorption

The amount of pyridine chemisorbed on coked samples was determined by the following procedure. The activated samples were saturated at 150°C with pyridine. Then they were heated up to 350°C and evacuated up to a final pressure of p $\lesssim 10^{-1}$ Pa. The remaining amount of chemisorbed pyridine was determined gravimetrically.

RESULTS AND DISCUSSION

Determination of the coke positions resulting from n-hexane and mesitylene cracking

The reduction of molecular diffusion due to coke can be used to determine the position of the coke deposits: Within the intracrystalline channel network or near the external surface of the zeolite crystals. If molecular exchange between the crystals as detected by the NMR tracer desorption technique is limited by the intracrystalline self-diffusion, the value of the thus determined tracer desorption diffusivity D_d must be equal to that of the directly measured NMR intracrystalline self-diffusion coefficient D_i. A lower value of D_d compared with D_i indicates mass transport barriers due to coke deposits near the external surface of the crystals.

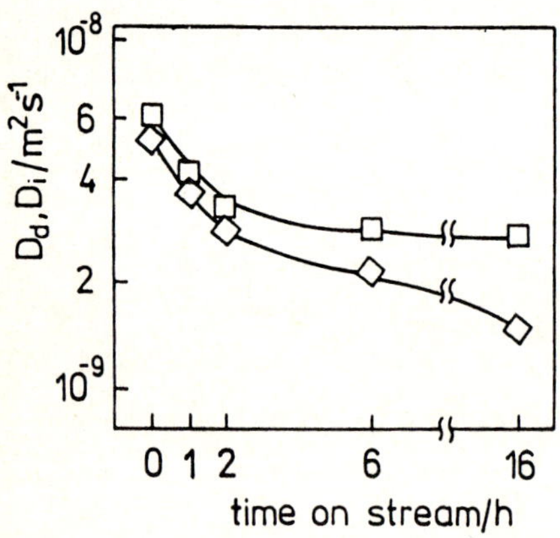

Fig. 1. Intracrystalline self-diffusion coefficient D_i (□) and tracer desorption diffusivity D_d (◇) of methane in HZSM-5 coked by n-hexane.

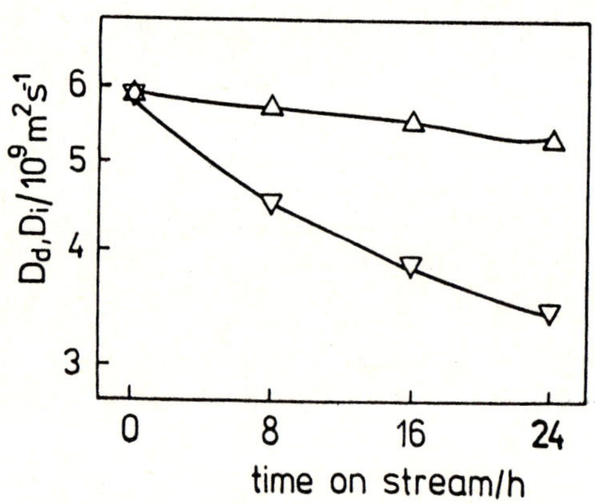

Fig. 2. Intracrystalline diffusivity D_i (△) and desorption diffusion coefficient D_d (▽) of methane in HZSM-5 coked by mesitylene.

Fig. 1 shows the decrease of D_d and D_i for HZSM-5 of polyhedral morphology (twinned shape) as a function of time on n-hexane stream. After appr. 2 h time on stream, the intracrystalline mobility of the guest molecule methane remains practically constant. In contrast, the desorption rate continues to slow down, indicating an increasing transport resistance near or on the external surface. Obviously, with increasing blockage of the intracrystalline channel system by coke, further coke is preferably deposited in the outer regions of the zeolite crystals blocking the mouths of pores.

In contrast to n-hexane coked HZSM-5, Fig. 2 shows that the intracrystalline mobility D_i in mesitylene coked samples is nearly unaffected by the coking procedure. On the other hand, the tracer diffusivity D_d decreases regularly with increasing time on stream. This latter behaviour could also be observed for n-hexane coked HZSM-5. But in the case of mesitylene coking, D_d becomes much less than D_i, even in the initial period of deactivation. As Fig. 3 shows, the ratio D_d/D_i decreases from the very beginning of the reaction. The conclusion is obvious: Mesitylene coking leads to a pronounced formation of a surface barrier, i.e. to a preferential deposition of coke near the external surface of the zeolite crystals. Since the mesitylene molecules are too large to penetrate into the intracrystalline channel system, this result is in accordance with the expected behaviour. Thus a controlled coke deposition can be performed using more or less bulky hydrocarbons for the reaction.

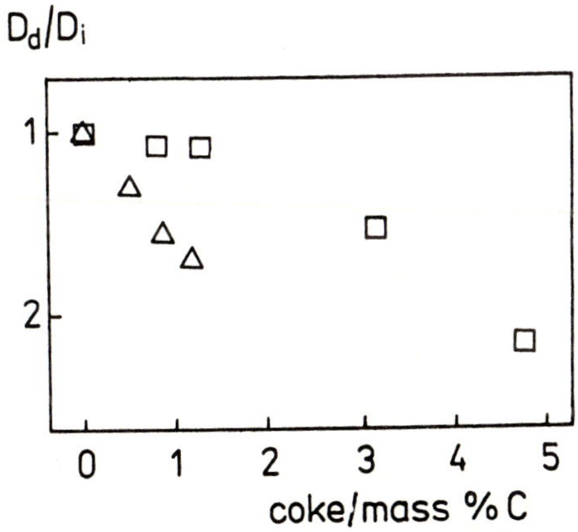

Fig. 3. Ratio D_d/D_i (experimental values of Figs. 1 and 2) as a function of the amount of coke deposited: □ n-hexane coke, △ mesitylene coke.

Chemisorption of pyridine on coked HZSM-5 and methane diffusion in HZSM-5 containing coke and chemisorbed pyridine

The chemisorption of pyridine was determined both on n-hexane and mesitylene coked samples. The results are shown in Fig. 4.

A distinct difference in the amount of chemisorbed pyridine is to be seen between the two types of samples. Whereas coke from mesitylene only slightly inhibits the chemisorption, coke from n-hexane leads to a much stronger inhibiting effect. This result supports the above given model of coke deposition. Mesitylene coke is concentrated near the external surface of the zeolite crystals and the main intracrystalline space remains unaffected. In contrast, coke from n-hexane is distributed homogeneously throughout the crystal. This homogeneous distribution of coke blocks more acidic sites and, hence, inhibits pyridine chemisorption more strongly than the concentration of coke in the outer region of the crystal.

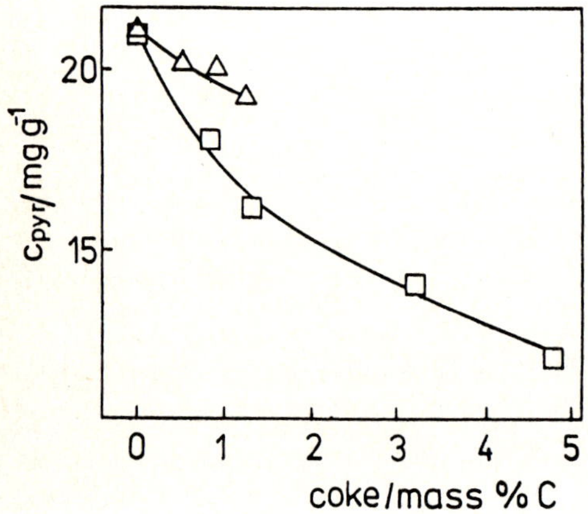

Fig. 4. Amount chemisorbed pyridine as a function of the coke content: □ n-hexane coke, △ mesitylene coke.

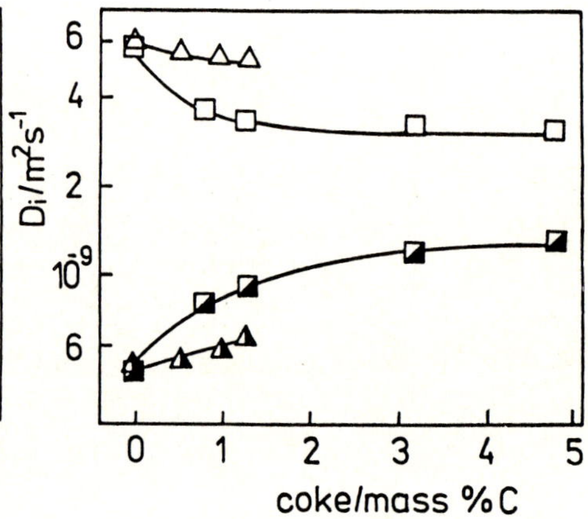

Fig. 5. Intracrystalline diffusivity D_i of methane in coked HZSM-5 after chemisorption of pyridine: ◪ n-hexane coke, ▲ mesitylene coke. For comparison, D_i of methane in the coked samples without pyridine: □ n-hexane coke, △ mesitylene coke.

Fig. 5 displays the result of diffusion studies on the combined effect of chemisorbed pyridine and coke deposits on the molecular transport properties of HZSM-5. The data for the uncoked material reflect the significant influence of the chemisorbed pyridine molecules. In agreement with the preceding considerations, after mesitylene coking this influence remains unchanged. With n-hexane coking, however, the blocking effect of the chemisorbed pyridine is progressively reduced, corresponding to the decrease of its total amount. One has to conclude, therefore, that the coking process is initiated at these very positions, which act as sorption sites for pyridine. Once again, two periods of coke formation can be distinguished. In the first period, the ratio D_d/D_i remains approximately equal to unity.

Coke deposition on HSM-5 of different morphology

Fig. 6 shows the ratio D_d/D_i for HZSM-5 crystals of different morphology as a function of the amount of coke deposited: polycrystalline spherical particles with the habit of "intergrown discs" (ref. 19) and several twinned polyhedral crystals of different size with an elongated hexagonal form (ref. 19). Once again, two periods of coke formation can be distinguished. In the first period, the ratio D_d/D_i remains approximately equal to unity. In the second period, D_d/D_i decreases indicating an enrichment of coke in the surface region. The beginning of the second period is virtually the same for all polyhedral crystals, however, a distinct delay of this onset is to be seen with the polycrystalline grain. From this experimental finding, we are led to the supposition that there is an additional pore system inside the grain which can be filled up by coke. This additional amount of coke is deposited on "neutral" spots outside the zeolite channel network, hence causing a delay to the onset of the second period of coke formation. This assumption will be proved in the following by further experiments.

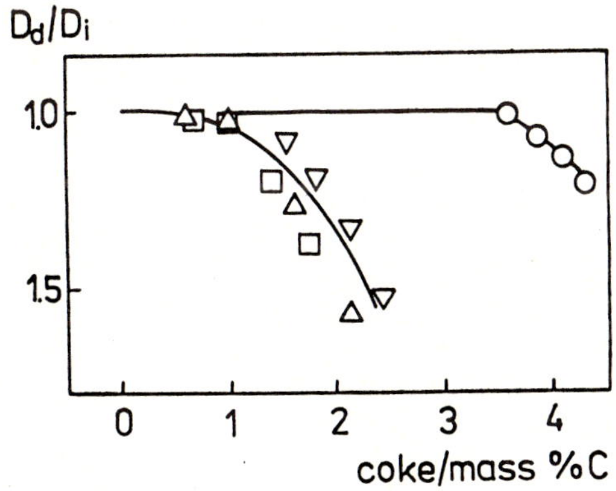

Fig. 6. Ratio D_d/D_i for HZSM-5 samples of different morphology as function of coke amount deposited: polycrystalline grains (○, 6.5 um), twinned polyhedral crystals (△, 8.5 um; ▽, 14 um; □, 28 um)

Firstly, the self-diffusion of methane and propane in the polycrystalline grains an in the polyhedral crystals are compared in the uncoked state. The corresponding data are given in Tab. 1.

It follows from inspection of these data that the intracrystalline self-diffusion coefficient in the polycrystalline grain is by a factor 2...3 higher than in the polyhedral crystals. This experimental finding is explained by a promotion of molecular transport due to additional fast diffusion paths originating from the polycrystalline structure of the grain. Hence, the increase in diffusivity can simply be considered as a higher molecular mobility in the void volume between the intergrown discs forming the substructure of the grain. Obviously, the interfacial voids between adjacent discs have the nature of transport pores. It is concluded therefore, that the polycrystalline grains indeed contain second order pores in addition to the first order pores represented by the channel network of the zeolite.

TABLE 1

Intracrystalline self-diffusion coefficients D_i of methane and propane in uncoked HZSM-5 of different morphology (loading 2.3... 2.5 molecules per 1/4 u.c., 23°C)

morphology	D_i (CH_4) / m^2 s^{-1}	D_i (C_3H_8) / m^2 s^{-1}
polyhedral crystals	$6 \cdot 10^{-8}$	$1.5 \cdot 10^{-10}$
polycrystalline grains	$18 \cdot 10^{-8}$	$3 \cdot 10^{-10}$

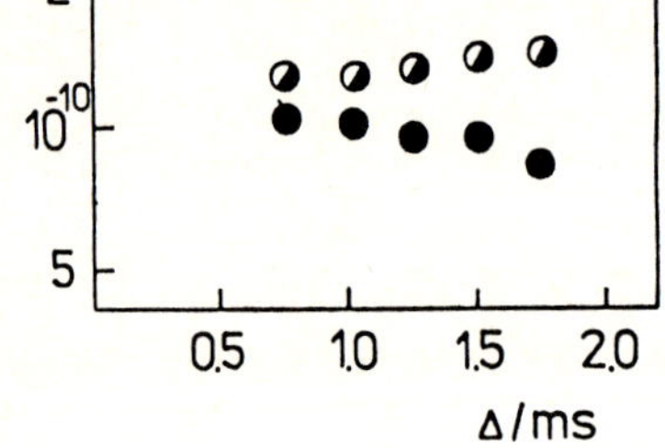

Fig. 7. Self-diffusivity D_i of propane (loading appr. 2.5 molecules per 1/4 u.c., 23°C) as dependence on the observation time Δ of self-diffusion in polycrystalline grains: ○ fresh HZSM-5, ◐ after 1 h on n-hexane stream corresponding to 3.6 mass% coke, and ● after 12 h on n-hexane stream, 4.3 mass% coke.

From this diffusion model for polycrystalline grains, an enhancement of molecular mobility with increasing observation time is to be expected. Results of corresponding experiments are displayed in Fig. 7, revealing the self-diffusion coefficient of propane in polycrystalline grain. For the uncoked sample, an increase of D_i is indeed observed with increasing observation time. This finding can be understood by the following mechanism. During short observation times, the propane molecules move preferentially within the substructure of the polycrystalline grain. With increasing time intervals allowed for diffusion, an increasing number of molecules will enter the interface between the discs, a region of transport enhancement, and will travel over longer distances there.

Consideration of the self-diffusivity of propane in coked grains affords details of the pecularities of coke formation on polycrystalline particles. Fig. 7 shows that after a coking time of 1 h only a slinght increase of D_i with the observation time occurs, however, after 12 h a decrease was observed. This behaviour can easily be explained if one assumes that coke is preferentially incorporated in the second order pores. This means that the interfaces between the discs progressively loose their transport promoting character. Finally, the second order pores, when filled up with coke, become a transport hindrance.

n-Hexane cracking on coked HZSM-5

The realtionship between the total amount of n-hexane converted and the amount of coke deposited is shown in Fig. 8.

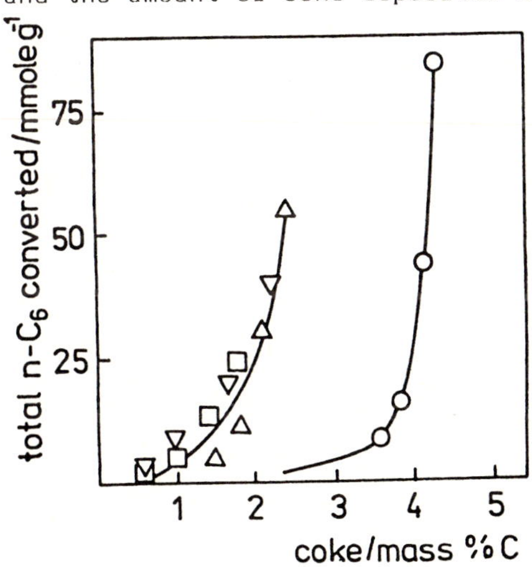

Fig. 8. Total amount of n-hexane converted as a function of the amount of coke deposited (symbols see Fig. 6)

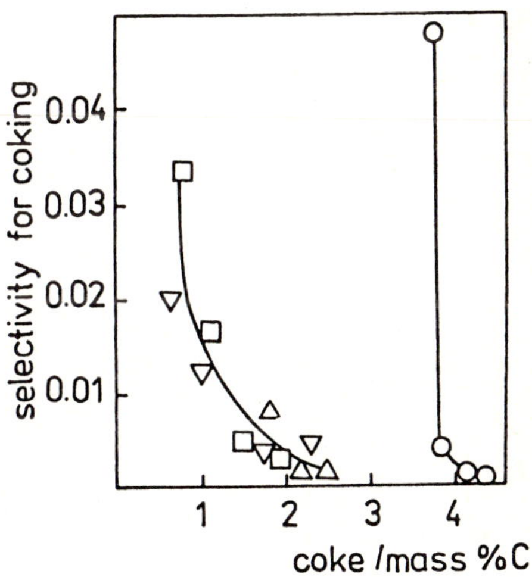

Fig. 9. Selectivity of coke formation during n-hexane cracking as dependence on the amount of coke deposited (symbols see Fig. 6)

The shape of the curves is remarkable. A straight line is to be expected in the case of a sonstant selectivity of coke formation. However, these curves reveal two different sections corresponding to the two periods of coke formation. During the first period, a relatively small increase in n-hexane cracking is accompanied by a relatively large increase in coke production. This is characteristic of the beginning of the reaction. The second period displays the opposite case, a large increase in cracking products is accompanied with only a small increase in coke deposition. Once again, the curves for the polyhedral samples are very similar, only the curve for the polycrystalline grain is exceptional. For this sample the period of enhanced coking is prolonged. This exceptional behaviour corresponds very well with the diffusion pecularities of this sample, hence, the reason for these features should be the same. In contrast to the polyhedral crystals, the polycrystalline grain can accomodate more coke, until the cracking and diffusion properties are dramaticly changed. Obviously, the location of this coke is on "neutral" spots outside the channel network, i.e. in the second order pore system as detected in this sample.

The influence of coke deposition on the selectivity of coking is to be seen in Fig. 9. The selectivity is defined as the mole ratio of n-hexane transformed into coke, divided by the amount of n-hexane converted. The selectivity curves in Fig. 9 are very similar for the polyhedral crystals but again the polycrystalline grain behaves exceptionally. The amount of coke necessary for the same poisoning effect, i.e. for the same selectivity level, is much higher for this sample than for the other ones. This is a further demonstration that the polycrystalline grains can accomodate coke on "neutral" spots in the second order pore system inside the grain. Furthermore, the selectivity curves for all four samples investigated distinctly decrease with increasing coke content. This proves a self-poisoning of the coking in the course of the reaction. Hence, two effects of the deposited coke are to be seen: the total conversion is inhibited and, in addition, the selectivity of coking is inhibited, too. Selective blocking of the coking route could be a transport phenomenon. Coke precursors are formed inside the channel network on catalytically active sites. These move to regions where they form fixed coke deposits. This movement could become increasingly difficult as increasing amounts of coke are deposited.

CONCLUSIONS

- Diffusion and cracking experiments reveal two periods of n-hexane cracking on HZSM-5: In the first period coke is homogeneously distributed throughout the crystal. In the final period an enrichment of the coke near the external surface of the HZSM-5 crystals takes place.

- In contrast, coke from mesitylene cracking is mainly deposited near the external surface even during the initial period of coking. This finding is explained by the larger size of the mesitylene molecule preventing a penetration into the intracrystalline channel network.

- In accordane with this controlled coke deposition, the amount of chemisorbed pyridine is higher on mesitylene coked samples than on n-hexane coked ones. The combination of pore blocking and acid site poisoning is evident.

- Coking of polycrystalline grains reveals that coke is preferentially deposited in the second order pores of the grain as demonstrated by diffusion and catalytic experiments. Due to the coke deposition outside the intracrystalline channel network, the initial coking rate on the polycrystalline grains is higher than on the polyhedral crystals.

- The selectivity of coke formation in n-hexane cracking decreases with increasing amounts of coke deposited. This self-poisoning starts on polycrystalline grains only at higher amounts of deposited coke. This result is explained by deposition of coke in "neutral" positions in the second order pores of the grain.

ACKNOWLEDGMENT

The authors wish to thank Profs. H. Pfeifer (Leipzig), G. Öhlmann (Berlin), W. Schirmer (Berlin) and L.V.C. Rees (London) for stimulating discussions. Mrs. W. Ziesche (Berlin) is thanked for experimental assistance, DP J. Richter-Mendau (Berlin) for SEM and Dr. W. Heink (Leipzig) for the development of the sophisticated NMR pulse spectrometer used in the self-diffusion measurements.

LITERATURE

1 M. Guisnet, P. Magnoux and C. Canaff, Proc. 7th Int. Conf. Zeolites, Tokyo 1986, pp. 701-707.
2 M. Guisnet, P. Magnoux and C. Canaff, Chem. Reactions in Organic and Inorganic Constraint Systems, D. Reidel Publ. Comp., 1986, pp. 131-140.

3 H. Schulz, W. Boehringer, W. Baumgarter and Zhao Siwei, Proc. 7th Int. Conf. Zeolites, Tokyo 1986, pp. 915-922.
4 G.D. McLellan, R.F. Parker, R.F. Howe and D.M. Bibby, J. Catal., 99 (1986) 486-491.
5 V. Ducarme and J.C. Vedrine, Appl. Catal., 17 (1985) 175-184.
6 P. Dejaifve, A. Auroux, P.C. Gravelle, J.C. Vedrine, Z. Gabelica and E.G. Derouane, J. Catal., 70 (1981) 123-136.
7 D.H. Olson and W.O. Haag, ACS Symp. Ser., No. 248 (1984) 275-307.
8 R.H. Meinhold and D.M. Bibby, J. Catal., submitted for publication
9 D.M. Bibby, N.B. Milestone, J.E. Patterson and L.P. Aldrige, J. Catal., 97 (1986) 493-502.
10 J. Kärger, H. Pfeifer, J. Caro, M. Bülow, H. Schlodder, R. Mostowicz and J. Völter, Appl. Catal., 29 (1987) 21-30.
11 R.M. Lago, W.O. Haag, R.J. Mikovsky, D.H. Olson, S.D. Hellring, K.D. Schmitt and G.T. Kerr, Proc. 7th Int. Conf. Zeolites, Tokyo 1986, pp. 677-684.
12 W.O. Haag, Proc. 6th Int. Conf. Zeolites, Reno 1984, pp. 466-478.
13 D.H. Olson, W.O. Haag and R.M. Lago, J. Catal. 61 (1980) 390-396.
14 S. Namba, K. Sato, K. Fujita, J.H. Kim and T. Jashima, Proc. 7th Int. Conf. Zeolites, Tokyo 1986, pp. 661-668.
15 R.J. Argauer and G.R. Landolt, US Patent 3.702.886, 1972.
16 H. Pfeifer, D. Freude and U. Hunger, Zeolites, 5 (1985) 274-286.
17 J. Kärger, H. Pfeifer and W. Heink, Proc. 6th Int. Conf. Zeolites, Reno 1984, pp. 184-200.
18 J. Kärger, AIChE J., 28 (1982) 417-423.
19 J. Kärger, H. Pfeifer, J. Caro, M. Bülow, J. Richter-Mendau, B. Fahlke and L.V.C. Rees, Appl. Catal., 24 (1986) 187-198.

B. Delmon and G.F. Froment (Editors), *Catalyst Deactivation 1987*

PREDICTION OF REACTOR PERFORMANCE UNDER CONDITIONS OF PORE-DIFFUSION-LIMITED CATALYST DEACTIVATION - NICKEL-CATALYZED METHANATION OF RESIDUAL CARBON MONOXIDE IN EXCESS HYDROGEN

R. CHRISTOPH and M. BAERNS

Chair of Technical Chemistry, Ruhr-University Bochum
P.O.B. 10 21 48, D-4630 Bochum 1, FRG

ABSTRACT

The performance of an adiabatic catalytic plug-flow reactor with deactivating catalyst pellets under conditions of external and internal mass-transport limitation is predicted by applying a heterogeneous reactor model for simulation. The simulation is based on the intrinsic kinetics of the chemical reaction i.e. the methanation of CO in excess hydrogen and of the deactivation as well as of the kinetics of the various transport processes. The simulations at close-to-real conditions agree quite well with experimental data obtained in an adiabatic bench-scale reactor during up to ca 60 hrs of operating time.

INTRODUCTION

For the methanation of residual carbon monoxide in excess of hydrogen alumina-supported nickel catalysts are used which may deactivate depending on operating conditions. The deactivation is due to a decrease of the catalytic surface area which can be attributed to a chemically induced nickel particle growth via nickel-carbonyl formation at low temperatures ($T < 553$ K) and to thermally induced nickel recrystallization (sintering) at high temperatures ($T > 573$ K) (ref. 1). With catalyst particle sizes where the methanation reaction is not limited by pore diffusion deactivation occurs rather rapidly to a steady-state activity (ref. 2) while for real-size catalyst pellets the process may be much slower.

In the present paper the performance of an adiabatic catalytic plug-flow reactor with deactivating catalyst pellets under conditions of external and internal mass-transport limitation is predicted on the basis of the intrinsic methanation kinetics, of the kinetics of deactivation as determined when no transport limitation occurs, and of the kinetics of the external and internal transport processes using a heterogeneous reactor model. The results obtained hereby for various conditions are compared with experimental data on the relationship between time of reactor operation and the axial profiles of temperature and CO partial pressure as well as of CO conversion which were obtained in a bench-scale reactor. It should be mentioned that simulation of deactivation behaviour of individual catalyst pellets has been already experimentally verified as reported elsewhere (ref. 3).

BASES OF REACTOR SIMULATION

In the following the reactor model applied for simulation, the numerical solution of the corresponding differential equations and the required data are presented.

Reactor model

Under close-to-real conditions the methanation reaction carried out adiabatically is affected by inter- and intraparticle transport processes; only intraparticle heat-transport limitations could be excluded by Anderson's criterion (ref. 4). Therefore a heterogeneous reactor model had to be applied; the resulting differential heat and mass balances were coupled via their boundary conditions. Carbon monoxide was chosen as the key component for the mass balances. The cylindrical shape of the catalyst pellets is approximated by a sphere with equal characteristic length.

Mass and heat balances:

(1) Pellet

$$\frac{-D^{e}_{CO}\,p_{CO,o}}{\rho_{cat}\,r_p^2\,r^{*2}}\,\frac{d}{dr^*}\left[r^{*2}\,\frac{dp^*_{CO}}{dr^*}\right] = R\,T_o\,T^*_s\,a(t)\,R_{CO}(t=0) \qquad (1)$$

$$\frac{3\,(-\Delta H_R)\,\rho_B\,D^{e}_{CO}\,p_{CO,o}}{\rho_{cat}\,r_p^2\,R\,T^*_s\,T_o}\,\left.\frac{dp^*_{CO}}{dr^*}\right|_{r^*=1} = h_f\,a_V\,T_o\,(T^*_s - T^*) \qquad (2)$$

(2) Fluid

$$-\frac{u_s}{L_R}\,\frac{dp^*_{CO}}{dz^*} = k_g\,a_V\,(p^*_{CO} - p^*_{CO,s}) \qquad (3)$$

$$\frac{u_s\,\rho_g\,c_p}{L_R}\,\frac{dT^*}{dz^*} = h_f\,a_V\,(T^*_s - T^*) \qquad (4)$$

Boundary conditions:

(1) Pellet

$$r^* = 0: \quad \left.\frac{dp^*_{CO}}{dr^*}\right|_{r^*=0} = 0 \tag{5}$$

$$r^* = 1: \quad -\frac{D^e_{CO}}{r_p} \left.\frac{dp^*_{CO}}{dr^*}\right|_{r^*=1} = k_g \, (p^*_{CO,s} - p^*_{CO}) \tag{6}$$

(2) Fluid

$$z^* = 0: \quad p^*_{CO} = 1; \quad T^* = 1 \tag{7}$$

Numerical solution

The system of coupled differential equations was solved numerically using the orthogonal collocation method (ref. 5). For the calculation of the axial profiles of carbon monoxide and of temperature eleven collocation points were used. For the determination of the carbon monoxide profiles inside the catalyst pellet the spline collocation method was applied; the pellet was divided into four finite elements each containing five collocation points. The strategy of calculation has been described in detail elsewhere (ref. 6). (A simulation of 10,000 hours of reactor operation takes approximately 16 min of computation time on a CDC Cyber 855.)

Required data for reactor simulation

The kinetics of the methanation reaction and of catalyst deactivation as well as data for the effective heat and mass transport parameters are presented.

(i) Intrinsic methanation kinetics. The rate law as suggested by Klose and Baerns (ref. 7) was applied:

$$-R_{CO}\ (t=0) = \frac{k_{CH_2} K_C K_H^2 \,(p_{CO,o}\, p^*_{CO})^{0,5}\, p_{H_2}}{(1 + K_C\, (p_{CO,o}\, p^*_{CO})^{0,5} + K_H\, p_{H_2}^{0,5})^3} \tag{8}$$

The kinetic parameters are given in Table 1.

TABLE 1
Kinetic parameters for the methanation of CO according to eq. (8) at operating time t = 0 (ref. 7)

k_{CH_2}	E_{CH_2}	K_C	ΔH_C	K_H	ΔH_H
mol h^{-1} g^{-1}	kJ mol^{-1}	$bar^{-0.5}$	kJ mol^{-1}	$bar^{-0.5}$	kJ mol^{-1}
6.2 10^{10}	103	5.77 10^{-4}	-42	1.60 10^{-2}	-16

(ii) Deactivation kinetics. The activity coefficient a(t) is related to the activity of the fresh catalyst (a(t=0) = 1). Its time dependence is given by an overall kinetic equation valid for conditions of no transport limitations taking also into account that initial catalyst activity decreases to a steady state value a_{ss} which subsequently remains constant.

$$-\frac{da}{dt} = k_d^o \exp(-E_d/RT)\,(p^{*}_{CO}\,p_{CO,o})^{m_1}\,p_{H_2}^{m_2}\,(a - a_{ss})^{m_3} \qquad (9)$$

The parameters of this equation (cp. Table 2) differ somewhat from those formerly reported (ref. 2) due to accounting for additional kinetic data obtained subsequently at higher temperatures (473 to 543 K).

TABLE 2
Kinetic parameters for catalyst deactivation according to eq. (9)
(experimental basis: p_{CO}: 5 to 40 kPa, p_{H_2} : 1 to 1.5 MPa, T = 473 to 543 K)

m_1/-	m_2/-	m_3/-	E_d/kJ mol^{-1}	k_d^o/h^{-1}
-1.40	0.56	4.24	63.33	1.95 10^5

(iii) Transport parameters. Many correlations for determining external heat and mass transfer coefficients have become known. Some selected results for the respective Sherwood and Nusselt numbers corresponding to the reaction conditions of the present study are given in Table 3; they differ by about 30 %.

TABLE 3
Sherwood and Nusselt numbers according to various correlations
(experimental conditions: p_{CO} = 40 kPa, p_{H2} = 1 MPa, ε = 0.44, Re = 386, Sc = 0.81, Pr = 0.37)

Reference	(8)	(9)	(10)	(11)	(12)
Sh = $k_g\,d_p/D_{CO}$	38.58		26.05		30.72
Nu = $h_f\,d_p/\lambda_g$		33.16	24.23	44.87	

In modelling the adiabatic tubular reactor Wakai's and Funazkri's relationship (ref. 8) was chosen for estimating the mass transfer coefficient k_g and Gnielinski's relationship (ref. 9) to calculate the heat transfer coefficient h_f. These more recent correlations take into account the effect of void fraction in the packing on the interparticle transport coefficients.

To determine the effective pore-diffusion coefficient

$$D_{eff} = (\varepsilon/\tau)\,D_{CO,m} \qquad (10)$$

an ε/τ value of 0.086 was used (ref. 13).

EXPERIMENTAL

Catalyst

The size of the cylindrical methanation catalyst pellets (RCH 18/10 of Ruhrchemie AG, Oberhausen, 18 wt.-% Ni on Al_2O_3) was 6 mm in diameter and 5 mm in height. The nickel oxide containing precursor was activated by reduction with hydrogen at 623 K for 17 hrs. (for details comp. ref. 2).

Equipment

Deactivation measurements were carried out in an adiabatic fixed bed reactor equipped with tappings for gas analysis online by ir absorption and for thermocouples to measure the adiabatic temperature increase along the reactor length. Before entering the reactor the gas mixture was preheated. The dimensions of the reactor are summarized in Table 4. To achieve adiabatic operation of the reactor and to minimize for unavoidable heat losses the following procedure was applied (ref. 14): The reactor wall was covered with a 4 cm-thick insulation on which various electrical heating circuits were fixed in several sections along the reactor length. The temperatures of the various heating sections were controlled in such a way that they were equal to the averaged temperature along those sections inside the reactor. Hereby the loss of heat through the reactor well amounted to less than 2 % of the heat of reaction.

TABLE 4
Dimensions of the fixed bed reactor

reactor length	1.0 m
length of catalytic bed L_R	0.3 m
length of each inert bed	0.35 m
reactor diameter d_R	2.5 cm
tapping distance	0.1 m
number of tappings	8

Experimental conditions

Total pressure was 2 MPa, total flux was kept constant at 4 m^3_{STP} h^{-1}. Nitro-

TABLE 5
Operating conditions of the adiabatic fixed-bed reactor

T_o/K	$p_{CO,o}$/kPa	$p_{H_2,o}$/MPa	time of operation
473	41	1	60 h
476	20	1	60 h
523	20	1	60 h

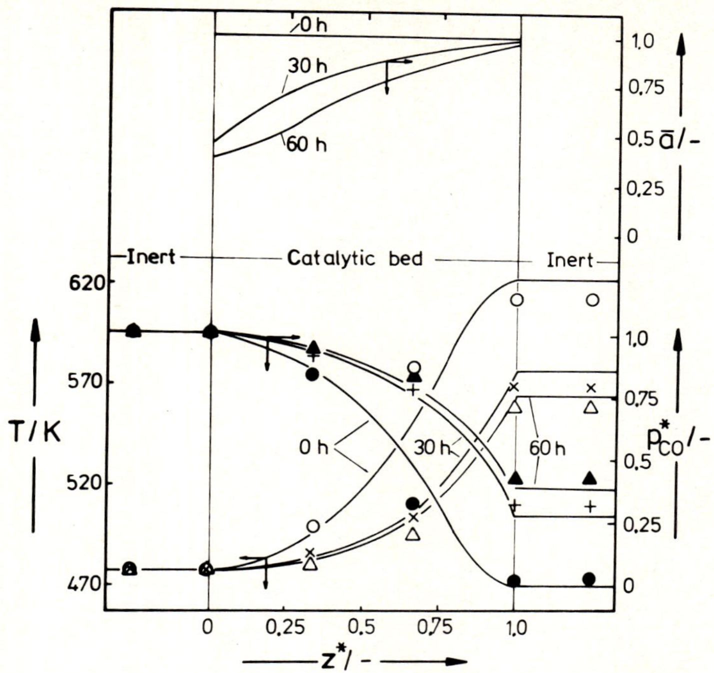

Fig. 1. Profiles of CO partial pressure $p^*_{CO}(z^*)$ (●: 0h, + : 30 h, ▲ : 60 h) and of temperature $T(z^*)$ (○: 0h, × : 30 h, △ : 60 h) in the gas phase and overall activity $\bar{a}(z^*)$ along the reactor length during 60 hrs of operation; inlet conditions: $p_{CO,o}$ = 41 kPa, $p_{H2,o}$ = 1 MPa, T_o = 473 K; simulation: ——— ; experimental data: symbols

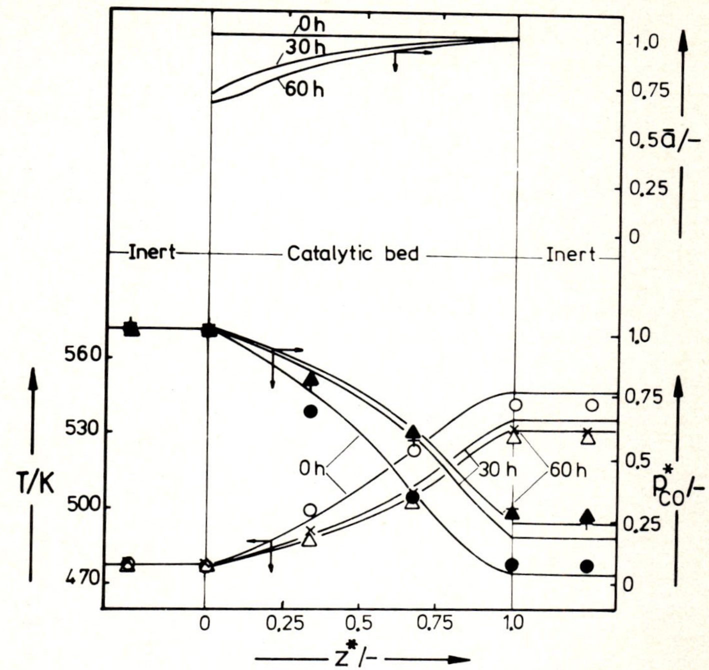

Fig. 2. Profiles of CO partial pressure $p^*_{CO}(z^*)$ (●: 0h, + : 30 h, ▲ : 60 h) and of temperature $T(z^*)$ (○: 0h, × : 30 h, △ : 60 h) in the gas phase and overall activity $\bar{a}(z^*)$ along the reactor length during 60 hrs of operation; inlet conditions: $p_{CO,o}$ = 20 kPa, $p_{H2,o}$ = 1 MPa, T_o = 476 K, simulation ——— ; experimental data: symbols

gen was added to the reactants to provide a constant overall pressure with various partial pressures of carbon monoxide and hydrogen. Inlet conditions are summarized in Table 5.

RESULTS AND DISCUSSION

Axial profiles of temperature and CO partial pressure as experimentally measured and calculated by reactor simulation for different conditions (cp. Table 5) and times of reactor operation are plotted in Figures 1 to 3. Corresponding CO conversions at the reactor outlet are presented in Figure 4. There exists quite a good agreement between experiments and simulations with respect to the qualitative pattern for the various dependencies; the quantitative deviations will be discussed further below.

Depending on inlet conditions the general pattern of the profiles for the axial temperature and CO pressure varied considerably in the catalytic bed with time of operation: When a low inlet temperature (473 K) and a high CO partial pressure (41 kPa) was applied the maximum axial temperature and the minimum CO concentration moved through the catalytic bed towards the outlet of the reactor (cp. Fig. 1) during operation. At a lower CO partial pressure of 20 kPa only moderate changes of the temperature and CO profiles occurred (cp. Fig. 2). When introducing the reactants at a high temperature (T = 523 K) the temperature and concentration profiles remained unchanged (cp. Fig. 3).

Carbon monoxide conversion achieved at the outlet of the catalytic fixed bed was affected correspondingly: At the onset of reactor operation at t = 0, i.e. when all the catalyst pellets exhibited an activity a(t=0) of 1 the carbon monoxide was completely converted to methane (cp. Fig. 4). During operation the degree of conversion remained constant when the gas mixture was entering the reactor at a high temperature (T = 523 K). At low temperature (476 K) and low CO partial pressure (20 kPa) CO conversion changed from 97 % for the fresh catalyst (a = 1) to 80 % after 60 hrs of operation (experiment) or to 70 % respectively after 10.000 hrs of operation (simulation); an even greater drop in CO conversion from initially 95 % to 65 % after 60 hrs (experiment) or to 26 % respectively after 10.000 hrs of operation (simulation) occurred at the same temperature but at a higher CO inlet partial pressure of 41 kPa.

The decrease in CO conversion with time of operation as illustrated in Figure 4 is to be attributed to the loss of activity along the reactor length as shown in Figures 1 to 3; the activity presented in the three figures is value of an individual catalyst pellet at location z^* obtained by averaging over the whole pellet (for details cp. ref. 5).

Quantitative deviations between experimental and simulated profiles of temperature and CO partial pressure along the reactor length (cp. Figures 1 to 3

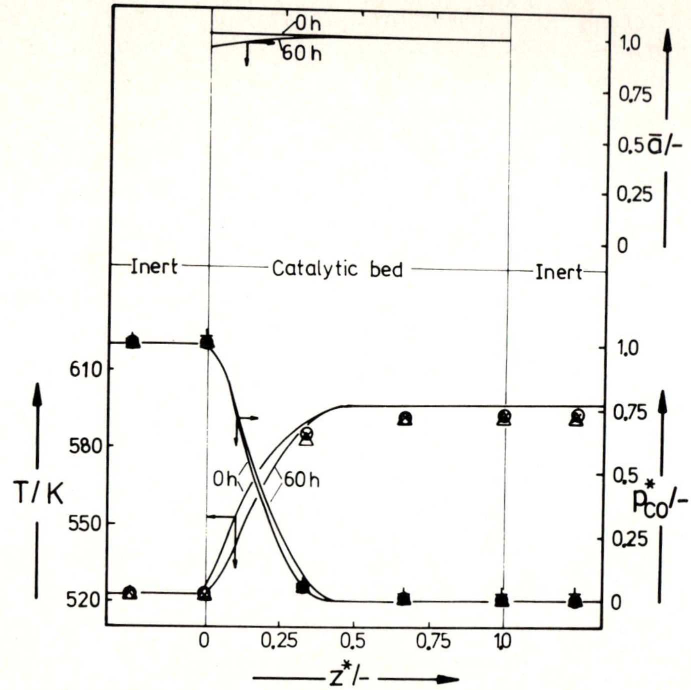

Fig. 3. Profiles of CO partial pressure $p^*_{CO}(z^*)$ (●: 0h, +: 30 h, ▲: 60 h) and of temperature $T(z^*)$ (○: 0h, ×: 30 h, △: 60 h) in the gas phase and overall activity $\bar{a}(z^*)$ along the reactor length during 60 hrs of operation; inlet conditions: $p_{CO,o}$ = 20 kPa, $p_{H2,o}$ = 1 MPa, T_o = 523 K; simulation: ———; experimental data: symbols

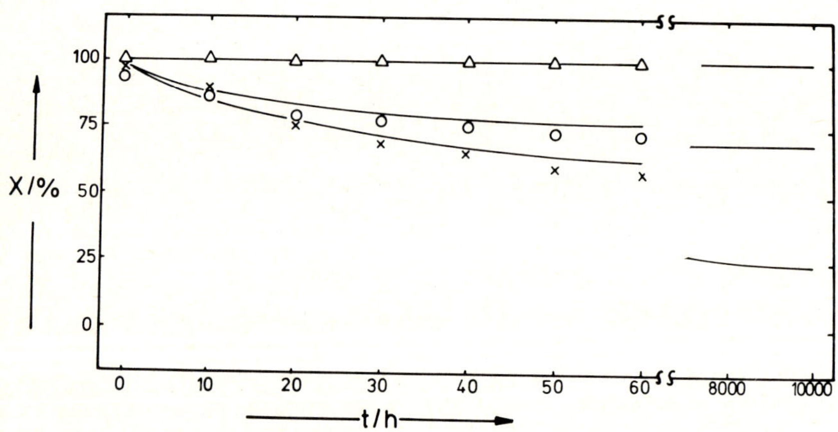

Fig. 4. Relationship between degree of CO conversion X at the reactor outlet and time of operation (simulation: ——— ; experimental data: △ : $p_{CO,o}$ = 20 kPa, $p_{H2,o}$ = 1 MPa, T_o = 523 K; ○ : $p_{CO,o}$ = 20 kPa, $p_{H2,o}$ = 1 MPa, T_o = 476 K; × : $p_{CO,o}$ = 41 kPa, $p_{H2,o}$ = 1 MPa, T_o = 473 K)

but also Figure 4) may be explained as follows: Deactivation kinetics applied in simulation of the reactor performance have been experimentally derived for a temperature range from 473 to 543 K. In this range deactivation decreases with increasing temperature; that is to say the steady-state activity a_{ss} increases. Although the inlet temperatures are within this temperature range the temperatures in the reactor exceed this range significantly due to the adiabatic operation applied (cp. Figures 1 to 3). Since thermal sintering may become important at the elevated temperatures (ref. 1) deactivation is most probably somewhat stronger than predicted by eq. (9); in more recent experiments which are, however, not yet incorporated in the quantitative treatment of deactivation of the applied alumina-supported nickel catalyst this preposition was confirmed.

CONCLUSIONS

The results described above suggest that an industrial reactor should be operated at an elevated inlet temperature ($\geqslant$500 to 530 K) to avoid excessive deactivating due to chemically induced sintering considering, however, that at significantly higher temperatures deactivation may be caused by thermal sintering (cp. above).

From a general point of view the method of simulation of reactor performance under conditions of catalyst deactivation appears to be a suitable tool for accelerated evaluation of catalyst deactivation particularly when transport processes affect the chemical reaction. The application of this method requires, however, quantitative information on the intrinsic kinetics of the chemical reaction and the deactivation process as well as on the inter- and intraparticle transport coefficients. The procurement of such data should commonly need less time than deactivation tests under real conditions which have often to be extended over the whole anticipated life time of an industrially used catalyst.

ACKNOWLEDGEMENT

We thank Fonds der Chemischen Industrie for financial support.

FREQUENTLY USED NOMENCLATURE

a	activity coefficient	-
a_v	specific external particle surface area	m^2/m^3
c_p	specific heat	J/(kg K)
D_i^e	effective pore-diffusion coefficient	m^2/s
ΔH_R	heat of reaction	J/mol
h_f	heat transfer coefficient gas/pellet	$J/(m^2 s\ K)$

K_i	equilibrium constant of gas adsorption	$bar^{-0,5}$
k	reaction rate constant	$mol/(g_{cat}\ s)$
k_g	mass transfer coefficient gas/pellet	m^2/s
L_R	reactor length	m
p_i	partial pressure of species i	bar
R_i	rate of reaction of species i	$mol/(g_{cat}\ s)$
r	radial position in a spherical pellet	m
T	temperature	K
t	operating time	s
u_s	superficial gas velocity	m/s
z	axial coordinate in the reactor	m
ρ	density	g/m^3

REFERENCES

1 R.D. Kelley, G.A. Candela, T.E. Madey, D.E. Newbury and R.R. Schehl, J. Catal., 80 (1983) 235-248
2 R. Christoph and M. Baerns, Chem. Ing. Tech., 57 (1985) 775-778
3 R. Christoph and M. Baerns, Chem. Ing. Tech., 58 (1986) 494-496
4 J.B. Anderson, Chem. Eng. Sci., 18 (1963) 147-156
5 J. Villadsen and M.L. Michelsen, Solution of Differential Equation Models by Polynomial Approximation, Prentice Hall, Englewood Cliffs N.J., 1978, pp. 143-296
6 R. Christoph and M. Baerns, Ber. Bunsenges. Phys. Chem., 90 (1986) 981-985
7 J. Klose and M. Baerns, J. Catal., 85 (1984) 105-116
8 N. Wakao and T. Funazkri, Chem. Eng. Sci., 33 (1978) 1375-1384
9 V. Gnielinski, Chem. Ing. Tech., 52 (1980) 228-236
10 J. de Acetis and G. Thodos, Ind. Eng. Chem., 52 (1960) 1003-1006
11 E.B. Baumeister and C.O. Bennett, AIChE J., 4 (1958) 69-74
12 A. Sen Gupta and G. Thodos, Chem. Eng. Progr., 58 (1962) 58-62
13 E.G. Christoffel, L. Tran-Vinh and M. Baerns, Chem. Ztg., 107 (1983) 349-355
14 J.R. Rostrup-Nielsen, A. Skov and L.J. Christiansen, Appl. Catal., 22 (1986) 71-83

B. Delmon and G.F. Froment (Editors), *Catalyst Deactivation 1987*

STOCHASTIC MODELING OF CATALYST DEACTIVATION BY SITE COVERAGE.

J.W. BEECKMAN[1], IN-SIK NAM and G.F. FROMENT

Laboratorium voor Petrochemische Techniek, Rijksuniversiteit, B9000 Gent (Belgium)

[1]presently with W.R. Grace & Co, Washington Research Center, 7379 Route 32, Columbia, Maryland 21044 (U.S.A.)

ABSTRACT

The state of a catalyst surface on which the main reaction and the coking reaction occur simultaneously is described rigorously, based upon a stochastic approach. This approach, combined with a Boolean reaction matrix, has the advantage that it lends itself to solving complex reaction mechanisms because the RHS of the governing stiff differential equations can easily be generated by computer. Several reaction schemes have been explored and confirm results obtained by a less general model proposed by Nam and Froment (1987). When all reaction steps require only one site to proceed, the system belongs to the class of structure-insensitive reactions. When all or some reaction steps require more than one site, the system can become structure sensitive. The influence of the site coverage on the selectivity for the main reaction in a more complex reaction and the optimization of the cluster size are also illustrated.

INTRODUCTION

The Hougen and Watson (ref. 1) approach has been widely used to express the rate of reaction as a function of reaction conditions and the concentration of sites on a catalyst surface. Froment (ref. 2) extended their approach to accommodate catalyst deactivation through irreversible coverage of sites by coke precursors. The effect of this phenomenon on the rates of both the main and deactivating reactions is generally accounted for by deactivation functions, ϕ_A and ϕ_C respectively, which multiplied with the initial rates, yield the rates at a given coke content. These functions mathematically express the reduction in number of sites, but nevertheless implicitly assume unlimited availability for dual- or multi-site formation. This availability obviously decreases as more sites are irreversibly covered. Nam and Froment (ref. 3) refined what they called the phenomenological approach of Hougen and Watson by accounting for the variation in availability. They used a probabilistic approach and revealed the influence of the number of sites in a given cluster upon the deactivation of the main and coking reaction. The mathematical approach used by Nam and Froment only permits a single main reaction to be dealt with and does not explicitly relate the surface coverage configuration to the gas phase composition. Their approach further assumes that the state of a site is independent of the state of neighboring sites which is, strictly speaking, not necessarily true for multi-site reactions.

The present paper casts the problem in a rigorous general mathematical form and extends Nam and Froment's results to complex reactions, so that selectivity aspects can be included.

THEORETICAL DEVELOPMENT

Let the cluster of reaction sites be defined as a set of sites on the catalyst which are sufficiently close to one another to form the multi-site arrangement required for the given reactions.

Let the number of sites comprised in each cluster on the catalyst surface be the same, so that the behavior of the catalyst under reaction conditions is identical to the behavior of a single cluster. Based on a general single site and dual site reaction mechanism, a certain number of surface species can be generated. Table 1 considers seven possible surface species for the simple reversible reaction $A \rightleftharpoons B$. Note that a reversible reaction is considered as two separate reactions. Surface species occupying two sites, like Al_2, are said to be Type 2 species, in contrast to species of Type 1, like Al, which occupy only one site. In the following the components A, B and C will each generate only one type of surface species. More specifically, the coking reactions will yield either Type 1 or Type 2 species but never the two simultaneously.

Suppose that at time t the cluster contains : i_1 free sites, i_2 sites reversibly covered by A, i_3 sites reversibly covered by B, i_4 sites irreversibly covered by coke, i_5 site-pairs reversibly covered by A, i_6 site-pairs reversibly covered by B and i_7 site-pairs irreversibly covered by coke. The probability of this surface configuration is represented by P_i $(l_{i_1}, Al_{i_2}, Bl_{i_3}, Cl_{i_4}, (Al_2)_{i_5}, (Bl_2)_{i_6}, (Cl_2)_{i_7})$.

For further theoretical development, some important functional quantities are introduced. E(i,j) represents the full cluster combination matrix. Each row of this matrix is dedicated to a particular cluster configuration. The column index specifies the surface compound and E(i,j) holds the information on the number of these surface compounds found in the cluster configuration i :

$$E(i,j) = i_j \qquad j = 1, \ldots, 7$$

TABLE 1

General mechanism for single site and dual site reactions of a reactant A and a product B

(Surface Compounds : 1, A1, B1, C1, $A1_2$, $B1_2$, $C1_2$)

		Type
1. Single site chemisorption	$A + 1 \longrightarrow A1$	1
	$B + 1 \longrightarrow B1$	1
2. Dual site chemisorption	$A + 21 \longrightarrow A1_2$	2
	$B + 21 \longrightarrow B1_2$	2
3. Single site main reaction	$A1 \longrightarrow B1$	1
4. Dual site main reaction	$A1 + 1 \longrightarrow B1 + 1$	1
	$A1_2 \longrightarrow B1_2$	2
	$A1 + 1 \longrightarrow B1_2$	2
	$A1_2 \longrightarrow B1 + 1$	2
5. Single site desorption	$A1 \longrightarrow A + 1$	1
	$B1 \longrightarrow B + 1$	1
6. Dual site desorption	$A1_2 \longrightarrow A + 21$	2
	$B1_2 \longrightarrow B + 21$	2
7. Single site parallel coking	$A1 \longrightarrow C1$	1
8. Dual site parallel coking	$A1 + 1 \longrightarrow C1 + 1$	1
	$A1 + 1 \longrightarrow C1_2$	2
	$A1_2 \longrightarrow C1 + 1$	1
	$A1_2 \longrightarrow C1_2$	2
9. Single site consecutive coking	$B1 \longrightarrow C1$	1
10. Dual site consecutive coking	$B1 + 1 \longrightarrow C1 + 1$	1
	$B1 + 1 \longrightarrow C1_2$	2
	$B1_2 \longrightarrow C1 + 1$	1
	$B1_2 \longrightarrow C1_2$	2

The total number of configurations N_C for a cluster containing a total of N sites can easily be calculated from :

$$N_C = \sum_{i_7=0}^{N/2} \sum_{i_6=0}^{N/2-i_7} \sum_{i_5=0}^{N/2-i_7-i_6} \sum_{i_4=0}^{N'} \sum_{i_3=0}^{N'-i_4} \sum_{i_2=0}^{N''} 1 \qquad (1)$$

with $N' = N-2i_7-2i_6-2i_5$ and $N'' = N'-i_4-i_3$

An analytical expression for N_C is easily derived, but the summation technique yields an important advantage, since it provides all the necessary information on the values of the coefficients i_1 through i_7 at each step of the summation. The computer generation of all cluster configurations is conveniently performed through the use of a DO-loop.

R(m,j) represents the matrix of stoichiometric coefficients. Each row stands for a particular step out of a scheme with a total of M steps. The column index specifies the surface compound and R(m,j) is the number of species involved in that step. Stoichiometric coefficients for reactants are taken to be positive, those for products negative. Columns 8 and 9 specify the amount of gas phase A, respectively B involved in each step.

$k(m)$ is the reaction probability vector, $k(m)dt$ is the probability that reaction m proceeds once on the surface in a time interval dt, provided that the initial cluster configuration allows reaction m to proceed.

$D(i,m)$ is a matrix with elements zero or unity. It states whether or not a configuration i can be converted into any other through reaction m. This matrix can easily be generated through :

$$D(i,m) = 1 \text{ if } E(i,j) - R(m,j) \geqslant 0 \text{ for all } R(m,j) > 0 \tag{2}$$
$$D(i,m) = 0 \text{ if not}$$

$W(i,m)$ is a matrix in which each element contains the number of possibilities that configuration i can lead to any other configuration through step m. The matrix $W(i,m)$ can be calculated from :

$$W(i,m) = \prod_{j=1}^{7} \frac{E(i,j)}{R(m,j)} \tag{3}$$

for $R(m,j) > 0$

$D(i,m) > 0$

$W(i,m) = 0$ for $D(i,m) = 0$

$Q(i,i',m)$ is a three-dimensional field with elements zero or unity. It states whether or not configuration i can be formed from configuration i' through reaction m. It can be calculated from :

$$Q(i,i',m) = 1, \text{ if } E(i,j) = E(i',j) - R(m,j) \text{ for all } j \tag{4}$$
$$Q(i,i',m) = 0 \text{ if not}$$

Applied to the present problem the multiplication law of probabilities can be written : $(P_i)_{t+dt} = (P_i)_t$ x (probability that no reactions occur during the time interval dt in configuration i) + (probability of formation of configuration i out of other configurations in the time interval dt).

The probability that no reaction step occurs during the time interval dt equals unity minus the probability that the step does occur, so that :

$$(P_i)_{t+dt} = (P_i)_t(1 - \sum_{m=1}^{M} D(i,m)W(i,m)k(m)dt)$$
$$+ \sum_{\substack{i'=1 \\ i' \neq i}}^{N_C} P_{i'} \sum_{m=1}^{M} Q(i,i',m)W(i',m)k(m)dt \tag{5}$$

Rearrangement of the above equation finally leads to :

$$\frac{dP_i}{dt} = - P_i \sum_{m=1}^{M} D(i,m)W(i,m)k(m) + \sum_{\substack{i'=1 \\ i'\neq i}}^{N_C} P_{i'} \sum_{m=1}^{M} Q(i,i',m)W(i',m)k(m) \qquad (6)$$

Since the sum of probabilities of all combinations has to be one at any time, the number of differential equations can be reduced by one.

The above approach is quite general for the solution of complex reaction mechanisms, including those leading to deactivation by site coverage, as encountered e.g. in deactivation by coke formation.

The reaction mechanism doesn't need to be limited to the reactions listed in Table 1. Any reaction, when properly introduced into the reaction matrix can be handled. Also, surface compounds other than Type 1 and Type 2 can be easily dealt with after incorporation into the full cluster configuration matrix. Although the number of DE's is quite large and cumbersome to handle analytically, the straightforward automatic generation of the RHS of the DE's allows the investigation of complex mechanisms.

The rate of the various steps involved in the main reaction, the rate of coking and the degree of coverage can then be calculated from :

1) Net rate of adsorption of A :

$$r_1 = \sum_{i=1}^{N_C} P_i \sum_{m=1}^{M} D(i,m)W(i,m)k(m)R(m,8) \qquad (7)$$

2) Rate of surface reaction :

$$r_2 = \sum_{i=1}^{N_C} P_i \sum_{m=1}^{M} D(i,m)W(i,m)k(m)[R(m,2) + R(m,3) + R(m,5) + R(m,6)] \qquad (8)$$

3) Net rate of desorption of B :

$$r_3 = \sum_{i=1}^{N_C} P_i \sum_{m=1}^{M} D(i,m)W(i,m)k(m)R(m,9) \qquad (9)$$

4) Rate of coking :

$$r_C = \sum_{i=1}^{N_C} P_i \sum_{m=1}^{M} D(i,m)W(i,m)k(m)[R(m,4) + R(m,7)] \qquad (10)$$

5) Degree of coverage :

$$\omega = 1/N \sum_{i=1}^{N_C} P_i[E(i,4) + E(i,7)] \qquad (11)$$

The set of equations (6) to (11) permits the calculation of reaction rates and the degree of coverage for the given reaction mechanism.

When the rate of coke formation is slow with respect to the main reaction pseudo steady-state can be assumed, so that the rate of adsorption of A, surface reaction A→B and desorption of B become identical :

$$r_1 = r_2 = r_3 = r_A \tag{12}$$

The deactivation functions for the main reaction and the coking reaction are defined by :

$$\phi_A = (r_A)_t/(r_A)_{t=0} \tag{13}$$

$$\phi_C = (r_C)_t/(r_C)_{t=0} \tag{14}$$

By way of example, consider a cluster consisting of two sites and let the main reaction take place on dual sites and the Type 1 coking on a single site.

$$A + 1 \xrightarrow{k_1} A1$$

$$A1 \xrightarrow{k_2} A + 1$$

$$A1 + 1 \xrightarrow{k_3} B1 + 1$$

$$B1 + 1 \xrightarrow{k_4} A1 + 1$$

$$B1 + 1 \xrightarrow{k_5} B1_2$$

$$B1 \xrightarrow{k_6} B + 1$$

$$A1 \xrightarrow{k_7} C1$$

A total of ten cluster configurations $P(1_i, A1_j, B1_k, C1_m)$ can be identified :

P(2,0,0,0), P(1,1,0,0), P(1,0,1,0), P(1,0,0,1), P(0,2,0,0), P(0,1,1,0), P(0,1,0,1), P(0,0,2,0), P(0,0,1,1), P(0,0,0,2)

The differential equation for the rate of change of configuration $P(1_0, A1_1, B1_1, C1_0)$ is as follows :

$$\frac{dP}{dt}(1_0, A1_1, B1_1, C1_0)$$
$$= - P(1_0, A1_1, B1_1, C1_0)(k_1 + k_5 + k_3 + k_4 + k_7)$$
$$+ P(1_1, A1_1, B1_0, C1_0)(k_5)$$
$$+ P(1_1, A1_0, B1_1, C1_0)(k_1)$$

The equation expresses that configuration $P(1_0, A1_1, B1_1, C1_0)$ can disappear through adsorption of A or B (k_1, k_5), surface reaction (k_3, k_4) or coking (k_7). Only two configurations $P(1_1, A1_1, B1_0, C1_0)$ and $P(1_1, A1_0, B1_1, C1_0)$ can lead to the desired configuration $P(1_0, A1_1, B1_1, C1_0)$ through adsorption of A and B with rate coefficients resp. k_1 and k_5.

FRESH CATALYST; NO DEACTIVATION

The steady state prcbabilities of the different configurations for fresh catalyst can be calculated from the set of equations (6) in which $dP_i/dt = 0$ and $k(m) = 0$ for deactivation reactions. To illustrate the influence of the cluster size on the main reaction rate, Figure 1 shows the reaction rates for a single and a dual site mechanism as a function of the number of sites in the cluster.

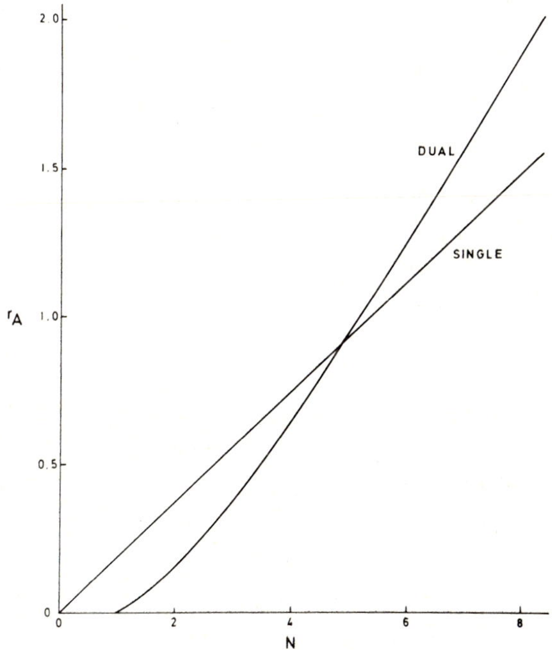

Fig. 1. Global reaction rate for a single and a dual site mechanism as a function of the number of sites in the cluster.

For the single site mechanism, the reaction rate varies linearly with the number of sites in the cluster, in agreement with the phenomenological approach (ref. 1). For the dual site mechanism with the surface reaction as rate determining step, it can be shown that the reaction rate is proportional to N(N - 1)/2. According to the phenomenological approach, the dual site reaction rate is proportional to the square of the total concentration of reaction sites. This is arrived at under the assumption that every site can form a dual pair with every other site on the catalyst surface, disregarding any distance restrictions. In the present approach, distance restrictions apply between clusters on the catalyst surface, but not in the cluster itself. Consider now a catalyst consisting of a support impregnated with metal. With such a catalyst the cluster size may reflect the degree of metal dispersion. In other words, the higher the metal dispersion for a given metal loading, the smaller the cluster size. Figure 2 shows that the single site reaction rate per site is independent of the cluster size, indicating the structure insensitive nature of the reaction (ref. 5).

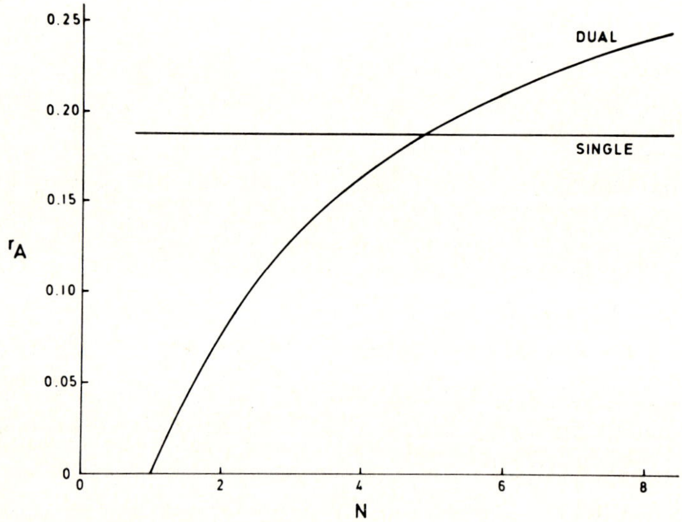

Fig. 2. Reaction rate per site for a single and a dual site mechanism as a function of the number of sites in the cluster.

The dual site reaction rate per site depends upon the cluster size, leading to structure sensitivity. It should be stressed that the reaction sites do not necessarily coincide with the metal atoms of the cluster.

DEACTIVATING CATALYST; STRUCTURE SENSITIVITY

When deactivation is accounted for the system of DE's is stiff. It was solved by means of a GEAR-routine (ref. 6). The simulations were carried out using rate coefficients for the deactivation reactions two orders of magnitude smaller than the rate coefficient of the rate determining step in the main reaction. The observed close agreement of the rates of the various steps involved in the main reaction shown in equations (7), (8) and (9) justifies the pseudo-steady state assumption. It is worthwhile comparing the values of the deactivation functions obtained from this rigorous approach with these obtained from the model of Nam and Froment (ref. 3).

Only the relations ϕ_A and ϕ_C versus the degree of coverage, ω are shown here in Figs. 3, 4, 5 and 6. They confirm the results obtained by Nam and Froment (ref. 3) through a less general approach which does not generate the rates of the main and deactivating reactions.

When both the main and the coking reaction occur on single sites $\phi_A = \phi_C$ linearly depends upon ω. When the main reaction occurs on dual sites and the coking on single sites (Fig. 3) $\phi_A = (1 - \omega)^2$ and $\phi_C = 1 - \omega$, as in the phenomenological approach.

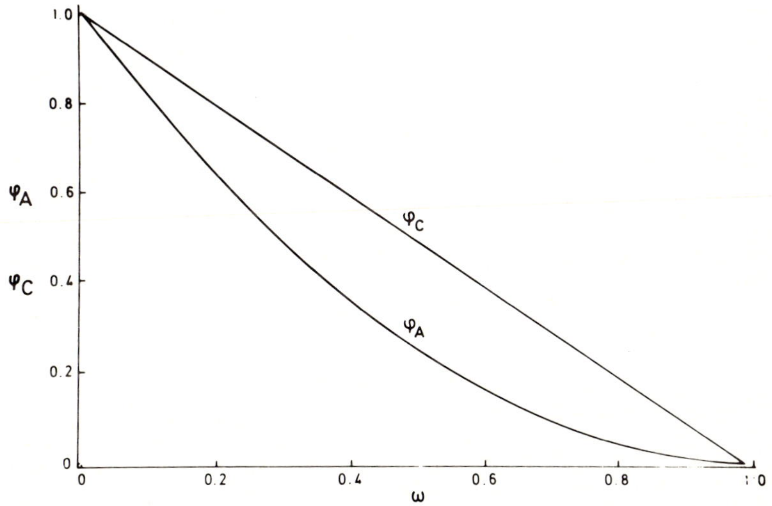

Fig. 3. Deactivation functions versus surface coverage. Main reaction on dual, coking on single sites.

When the main reaction occurs on single sites and the Type 1 coking on dual sites $\Phi_A = 1 - \omega$ and Φ_C versus ω develops a dependence on the number of sites in the cluster (Fig. 4).

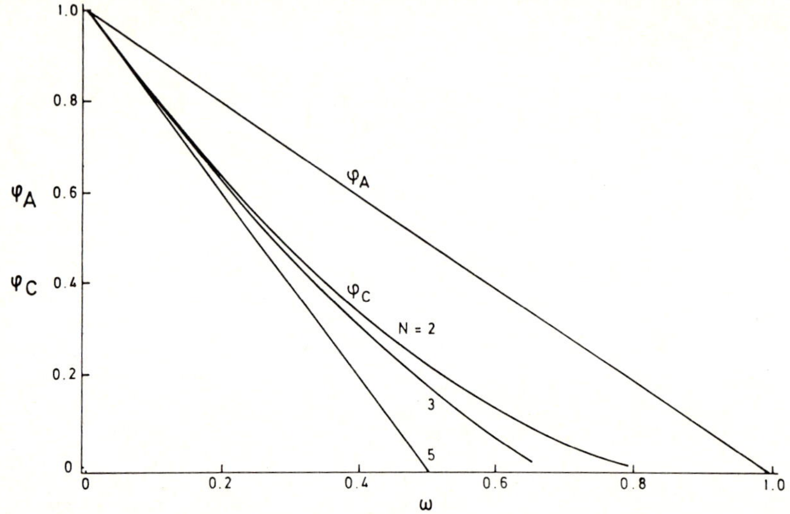

Fig. 4. Deactivation functions versus surface coverage. Main reaction on single, coking on dual sites.

When both the main and the Type 1 coking require dual sites $\Phi_A = \Phi_C$ and again a dependence with respect to the number of sites in the cluster develops (Fig. 5). Figures 4 and 6 illustrate that a catalyst with higher metal dispersion (smaller cluster size in the present study) is more resistant to deactivation than a catalyst with large cluster size (low dispersion) when the coking reaction occurs on dual sites and the main reaction on single sites (ref. 3). Such a trend is well known and was recently experimentally observed by Barbier et al (ref. 4). The opposite is true when both reactions require dual sites, though.

DEACTIVATING CATALYST; SELECTIVITY BEHAVIOR

Changes in selectivity caused by deactivation can also easily be evaluated with the approach presented here. When a reactant A is converted into two products, say B and E, through a single site, respectively a dual site mechanism, the selectivity of A towards B and E changes when deactivation occurs. On the other hand, when both B and E are formed through the same type of mechanism the selectivity remains constant throughout the life of the catalyst. Figure 7 shows the ratio of the deactivation functions, which is a measure of selectivity for the formation of B and E, for a single site coking mechanism.

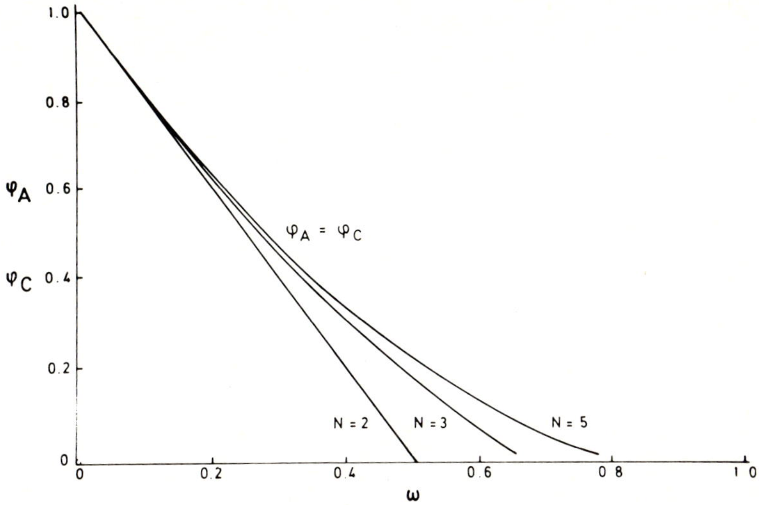

Fig. 5. Deactivation functions versus surface coverage. Main and coking reactions on dual sites.

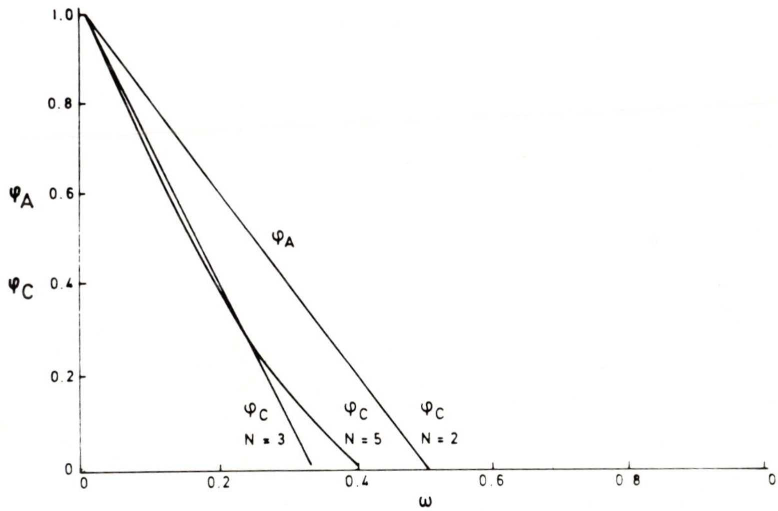

Fig. 6. Deactivation functions versus surface coverage. Main reaction on single, Type 2 coking on dual sites.

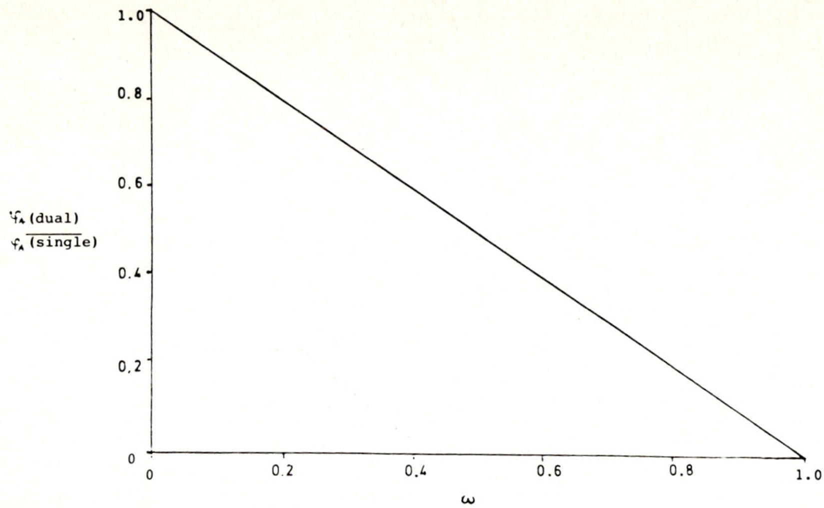

Fig. 7. Ratio of deactivation functions for main reactions versus surface coverage. Coking on single sites.

A linear decline of the ratio of the deactivation functions with the degree of coverage is observed. At the end of the catalyst's life, the single site main reaction is fully favored over the dual site main reaction. Fig. 8 illustrates the trend in the case of dual site coking. Again the single site main reaction is favored over the dual site reaction. The drop in the ratio of deactivation functions becomes steeper at the end of the catalyst life : a dual site coking mechanism Type 1 always leaves one site active at the end of life, so that the single site main reaction continues at a finite rate.

An interesting situation develops with a Type 2 coking mechanism and is presented in Figure 9. When the total number of sites in the cluster is uneven, one active site is left at the end of the catalyst's life, making the ratio of deactivation functions drop to zero. When the total number of sites in the cluster equals 2, however, the ratio of deactivation functions remains constant at 1.0 throughout the catalyst life. This is not surprising since both the single site and the dual site mechanism are in fully active state in the case of fresh catalyst or both in a fully deactivated state when a Cl_2 compound has been formed on the cluster. In the case of 4 sites, the ratio of deactivation functions drops linearly, but levels out to a value of 1/3 at the end of the catalyst's life. This can easily be explained : for fresh catalyst, the number of dual site pairs over the number of single sites is 6/4. At the end of the catalyst's life, when the probability of finding 4 active sites is negligible, the ratio of the number of dual sites and single sites is 1/2. Dividing the end of life ratio by the fresh catalyst ratio yields 1/3.

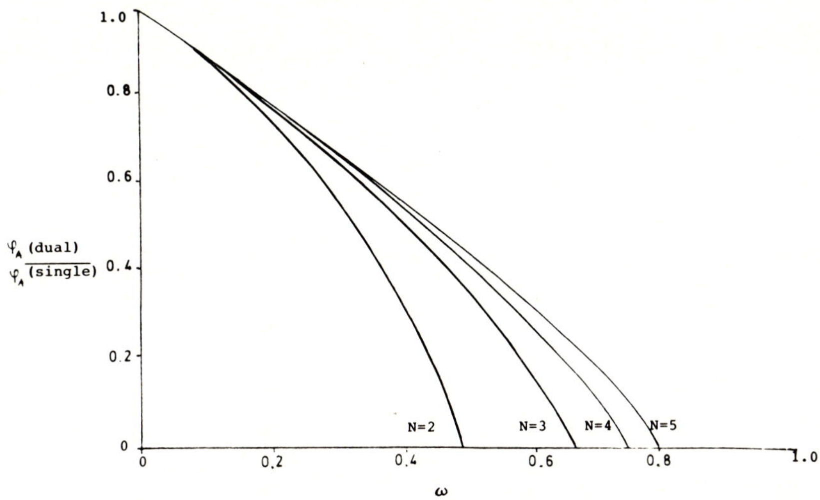

Fig. 8. Ratio of deactivation functions for main reactions versus surface coverage. Coking on dual sites.

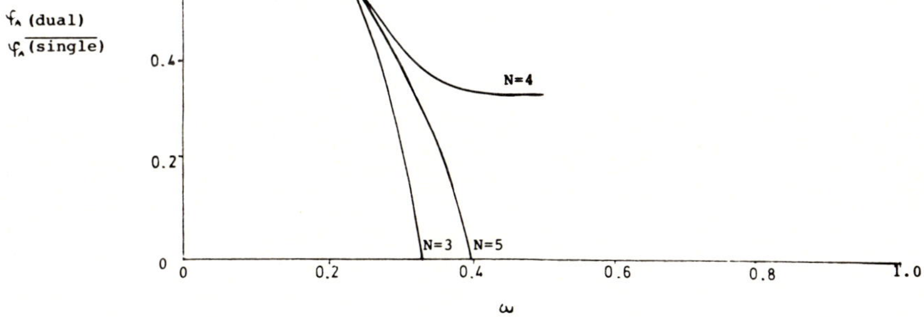

Fig. 9. Ratio of deactivation functions for main reactions versus surface coverage. Type 2 coking on dual sites.

DEACTIVATING CATALYST; CLUSTER SIZE OPTIMIZATION

An important question to be raised is what the optimal cluster size should be to obtain a maximum global conversion throughout the catalyst life for a given loading of active material on the catalyst surface. In the case of a single site main reaction and a single site coking reaction, the system is structure insensitive, so that the cluster size has no effect on the rate.

For a dual site main reaction and a single site coking mechanism, increasing the number of sites per cluster increases the reaction rate per cluster, but reduces the total number of clusters for a given metal loading on the catalyst. The increase in rate per cluster is more important, however, and more than compensates for the reduction in the number of clusters. In this case it is obvious that the number of sites per cluster should be maximized, keeping in mind the site distance restrictions for the given reaction mechanism.

For a single site main reaction and a dual site coking reaction, the choice is obviously towards minimizing the number of sites per cluster, where unity would be optimal, since it would eliminate coking.

A dual site main reaction and a dual site coking reaction represents an interesting case, since maximizing the number of sites per cluster obviously maximizes the main reaction rate, yielding a very active fresh catalyst. At the same time, the coking rate is also maximized, however, so that the catalyst deactivates faster. For a small number of sites per cluster the initial rate of the main reaction is low, but on the other hand, deactivation is also slow. The calculations show that at a sufficient deactivation level the global rates cross-over, favoring the clusters with a small number of sites. Due to the very large initial benefit of large clusters, the maximization of the area below the global rate versus time curve optimizes the cluster size still towards maximum number of sites.

For a single site main reaction and a dual site Type 2 coking reaction, the optimum is obtained for a minimum number of sites per cluster and preferably uneven. For a dual site main reaction and a dual site Type 1 coking reaction, the number of sites per cluster should be maximized and preferably even.

LIST OF SYMBOLS

Al	: site covered with reversibly adsorbed A
Al_2	: site pair covered with reversibly adsorbed A
Bl	: site covered with reversibly adsorbed B
Bl_2	: site pair covered with reversibly adsorbed B
Cl	: site covered with irreversibly adsorbed coke precursor

Cl_2	:	site pair covered with irreversibly adsorbed coke precursor
D(i,m)	:	matrix stating whether reaction m can proceed on cluster configuration i
E(i,j)	:	cluster configuration matrix
k(m)	:	reaction rate vector
1	:	free site
M	:	total number of reactions
N	:	total number of sites in a cluster
N_C	:	total number of cluster configurations
P_i	:	probability of occurrence of cluster configuration i
Q(i,i',m)	:	3-dimensional field stating whether configuration i can be formed from configuration i' through reaction m
R(m,j)	:	reaction matrix of stoichiometric coefficients
r_1	:	net rate of adsorption of A
r_2	:	net surface reaction rate
r_3	:	net rate of desorption of B
r_C	:	rate of coking
W(i,m)	:	matrix containing the number of times that reaction m can proceed on configuration i
ϕ_A	:	deactivation function for the main reaction
ϕ_C	:	deactivation function for the coking reaction
ω	:	degree of coverage

REFERENCES

1 O.A. Hougen and K.M. Watson, Chemical Process Principles, Part III, John Wiley & Sons, 1947.
2 G.F. Froment, Proc. Int. Cong. Catal. 6th, London, 1976, 10.
3 In-Sik Nam and G.F. Froment, Catalyst Deactivation by Site Coverage through Multi-site Reaction Mechanisms (in preparation).
4 J. Barbier, G. Corro, Y. Zhang, J.P. Bournonville and J.P. Frank, Applied Catalysis, 13 (1985) 245.
5 M. Boudart, I. & E.C. Fundamentals, 25 (1986) 656.
6 A.C. Hindmarsh, Gear-Stiff DE system solver, UCID-30001, Rev. 3, Lawrence Livermore Laboratory, Livermore, CA 94550, Dec. 1974.

B. Delmon and G.F. Froment (Editors), *Catalyst Deactivation 1987*

JOINT EFFECTS OF INTRAPARTICLE DIFFUSION RESISTANCE AND CATALYST DEACTIVATION

K.KUMBILIEVA[1] , M.M.KOSTYUKOVSKY[2], L.PETROV[1], and S.L.KIPERMAN[2]

[1]Institute of Kinetics and Catalysis, Bulgarian Academy of Sciences, Sofia 1040 (Bulgaria)
[2]Zelinsky Institute of Organic Chemistry, USSR Academy of Sciences, Leninski Prospect 47, Moscow (USSR)

ABSTRACT

The joint effects of intraparticle diffusion and catalyst deactivation on the rate of catalytic processes are examined.The analysis performed considers different deactivation laws for a class of processes accompanied by consecutive deactivation. The results obtained show that under certain conditions,the catalytic reaction accompanied by catalyst deactivation proceeds with a higher rate in the intraparticle diffusion region than in the kinetic region.

INTRODUCTION

The problem of improving the design of catalytic processes accompanied by catalyst deactivation is of great importance for industry. When considering the optimum conditions of these processes, diffusion effects should also be taken into account. Up to now little attention has been paid to the probability for the diffusion-controlled regime on a deactivating catalyst to be more favourable than the kinetic one.

FORMULATION OF THE PROBLEM

The case of external diffusion control on the process is trivial, and for this reason we shall not discuss it here.

The influence of intraparticle diffusion can lead to a change in rate of both the catalytic and the deactivation reactions.The decrease in rate of the catalytic reaction can be more or less compensated by the drop of the deactivation rate. Under certain conditions the effective rate of the catalytic reaction in the diffusion region may exceed the rate in the kinetic region. The possibility to use this fact for optimization of the process design has not been, up to now, a subject of detailed qualitative or quantitative analysis. Wojciechowski et. al. have suggested in ref.1 that the aging process might be slower under diffusion limitations since the increased intraparticle diffusion resistance would decrease the concentration of poisons in the interior of the catalyst particles. Such a distribution of the poisoning agent in catalyst pellets as well as the aging function discussed in ref.1 (where the fraction of unblocked active sites is considered independent of the degree of conversion) correspond to the case when the aging agent is present in the initial reaction mixture.

The aim of the present paper is to analyse another case: the proceeding of a catalytic reaction accompanied by consecutive catalyst deactivation in (i) the kinetic and (ii) the intraparticle diffusion region. A typical example of consecutive catalyst deactivation is the blocking of the catalyst surface by coke formation. It is well known that the concentration of coke precursors depends on the degree of conversion.

In order to elucidate the effect of diffusion resistance, we have analysed, on the basis of a classical model reaction, the changes in rate of the catalytic reaction and the deactivation of the catalyst in presence and absence of diffusion resistance. Different laws of deactivation have been simulated taking into account that the deactivation rate is a function of the degree of conversion.

MODEL REACTION

Consider a simple model reaction

$$A \rightleftharpoons B \tag{1}$$

proceeding according to the scheme

$$A + Z \underset{k_{-1}}{\overset{k_1}{\rightleftharpoons}} AZ \underset{k_{-2}}{\overset{k_2}{\rightleftharpoons}} B + Z \tag{2}$$

where Z and AZ stand for catalyst surface sites free of and occupied by surface intermediate species, respectively, and k_1, k_2, k_{-1}, and k_{-2} denote the rate constants of the elementary steps in forward and back directions.

We shall consider the quasistationary proceeding of the reaction (including the process of the catalyst deactivation) in an open system (see ref.2). In the case of the so-called "separable deactivation" (ref.3), the reaction rate at a given moment θ can be presented as the product of the initial rate r_0 and the deactivation function F:

$$(r_K)_\theta = (r_K)_0 \cdot (F_K)_\theta \qquad (3)$$

$$(r_d)_\theta = (r_d)_0 \cdot (F_d)_\theta \qquad (4)$$

The subscripts "K" and "d" relate to the proceeding of the catalytic reaction in the kinetic and in the diffusion regions, respectively.

If at a given moment $\theta 1$ the decrease in catalyst deactivation rate due to diffusion limitations becomes larger than the initial decrease in the catalytic reaction rate, i.e.

$$\frac{(F_d)_{\theta 1}}{(F_d)_{\theta 1}} > \frac{(r_K)_0}{(r_d)_0} \qquad (5)$$

then, from (3) and (4) it follows that at the moment under consideration

$$(r_d)_{\theta 1} > (r_K)_{\theta 1} \qquad (6)$$

i.e., the rate of the catalytic reaction under diffusion limitations will be higher than the rate in the kinetic region. Obviously, this possibility may be realized under certain conditions depending on the nature of the deactivation and the catalytic reaction.

In the case of the so-called "non-separable deactivation" (ref.4), the changes of both the kinetic law and and the deactivation rate caused by diffusion limitations cannot be described in an explicit form, but their superposition can also lead to their mutual compensation and in some cases to the state satisfying the inequality (6).

In terms of the degree of conversion x, the rate of the catalytic reaction (1) proceeding in the kinetic region on an ideal adsorbed layer (ref.2) can be presented as follows:

$$r_K = \frac{(H1 - H2.x)}{(H3 + H4.x)} \; F(x) \qquad (7)$$

where:

$$H1 = k_1 . k_2$$

$$H2 = k_1 . k_2 - k_{-1} . k_{-2}$$

$$H3 = k_1 + (k_2 + k_{-1})/(C_A)_0 \qquad (8)$$

$$H4 = k_{-2} - k_1$$

The expression for the function F(x) represents the catalyst deactivation law in the kinetic region in terms of the degree of conversion.

To derive the expressions for the catalytic reaction rate under internal diffusion limitations, we shall use the Pshezhetsky-Rubinstein formula (ref.5) correlating the reaction rate under diffusion limitations, r_d, with the intrinsic reaction rate r_k:

$$r_d = \frac{1}{R}\sqrt{2\int_{(c_j)_{eq}}^{(c_j)_s} D\, r_k dc_j} \qquad (9)$$

where D is the effective diffusion coefficient, R is the ratio of the catalyst pellet volume to its external surface, and c_j is the concentration of the j-th reagent.The subscripts "s" and "eq" correspond to the surface and the center of the catalyst pellet , respectively. The relation (9), derived on accepting the quasi-homogeneous model of the processes in the pellet pores, proves to be correct in cases when the pore radius is much smaller than the pellet radius.

On substituting the expression (7) for r_k, we can write for the process under diffusion limitations:

$$r_d = \frac{\sqrt{2D}}{R}\sqrt{\int_{x_s}^{x_{eq}} \frac{(H1 - H2.x)}{(H3 + H4.x)} F(x)dx} \qquad (10)$$

Evidently, under diffusion limitations, the separable deactivation function is converted to a non-separable deactivation function. This is an indication that there is no physical background defining separable and non-separable deactivation kinetics as already stated in ref. 6 by Froment for some simple cases.

We shall consider the following types of the deactivation law:

$$F(x) = 1 - \beta_K\sqrt{x} \quad , \tag{11}$$

modelling deactivation through dissociative adsorption;

$$F(x) = 1 - \beta_K x \quad , \tag{12}$$

modelling deactivation through one-center adsorption;

$$F(x) = 1 - \beta_K x^2 \quad , \tag{13}$$

modelling deactivation through two-center adsorption;

$$F(x) = \exp(-\beta_K x) \quad , \tag{14}$$

modelling deactivation through product adsorption on an exponentially non-homogeneous surface.

Here, β_K is a parameter whose value is, as a first approximation, independent of x.

The effect of diffusion limitations on the deactivation kinetics depends on the expression for the function F(x) in equation (10). The values of the parameter β_d characteristic of the diffusion region can remain the same as β_K or have other values determined by the condition $\beta_d < \beta_K$.

RESULTS AND DISCUSSION

To compare the rates of the reaction in the absence and in the presence of diffusion resistance, i.e. in the kinetic and in the diffusion resistance regions, we calculated r_K and r_d from the relations (7) and (10) using different types of equations for the deactivation law ((11) - (14)). The "conversion curves" (ref.6) plotted in Fig.1 show how the reaction rate depends on the conversion degree in the kinetic and in the diffusion resistance regions for various cases of reversibility of the steps in scheme (2). The curves refer to the deactivation function $F(x) = 1 - \beta\sqrt{x}$ and to the parameter values R = 0.2 cm, D = 0.01 cm²/s, and $(C_A)_O$ = 1 mol/g. Evidently, on attaining a definite "threshold" degree of conversion, the effective rate under diffusion resistance conditions exceeds the rate in the kinetic region.An analogous intersection of the conversion curves for the kinetic and the diffusion region is also observed with the other expressions for the function F(x) . The results obtained for two different β_d/β_K ratios and different cases of reversibility of the steps are presented in Table 1. Obviously, for all deactivation laws under consideration, there is a domain of conversion values where the rate of the catalytic reaction under diffusion limitations exceeds the rate in the kinetic region. The lower limit of conversion values where diffusion limitations prove to be favourable, varies with the different deactivation laws. The strongest effect is observed with the expression $F(x) = 1 - \beta\sqrt{x}$, which corresponds to deactivation due to surface blocking by dissociative adsorption of the blocking agent. This result is not unexpected and has a reasonable explanation. However, it should be pointed out that with all discussed functions of consecutive deactivation the conversion curves in the kinetic and in the diffusion controlled regions have a similar behaviour: above a certain conversion degree, the intraparticle diffusion resistance regime is more favourable for the process. The existance of such domains

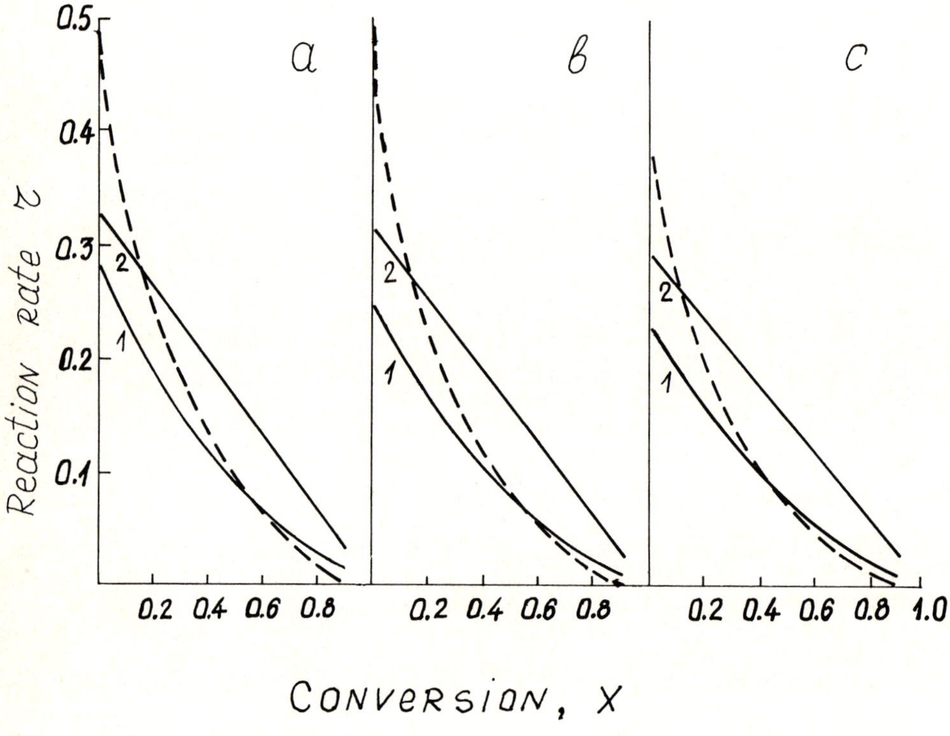

Fig. 1. Reaction rate vs conversion for the deactivation function $F(x) = 1 - \beta\sqrt{x}$ in the kinetic (-----) and the diffusion (______) regions when $\beta_d = \beta_K$ (curves 1) and $\beta_d = 0.5\ \beta_K$ (curves 2). (a) Both steps irreversible. (b) Step 1 irreversible, step 2 reversible. (c) Step 1 reversible, step 2 irreversible.

TABLE 1

Variation of the ratio (r_d/r_K) with degree of conversion x for different deactivation laws.

Deactivation Law	x	Both steps irreversible: Ratio r_d/r_K		Step 1 irreversible Step 2 reversible: Ratio r_d/r_K		Step 1 reversible step 2 irreversible: Ratio r_d/r_K	
		$B_d=B_K$	$B_d=B_K/2$	$B_d = B_K$	$B_d = B_K/2$	$B_d = B_K$	$B_d=B_K/2$
	0.1	0.64	0.75	0.62	0.72	0.70	0.82
	0.2	0.65	0.80	0.65	0.78	0.73	0.88
	0.3	0.67	0.86	0.68	0.86	0.76	0.96
	0.4	0.70	0.94	0.72	0.96	0.79	1.06
$1-Bx$	0.5	0.74	1.06	0.78	1.10	0.84	1.20
	0.6	0.79	1.24	0.85	1.32	0.92	1.42
	0.7	0.88	1.53	0.97	1.68	1.02	1.78
	0.8	1.02	2.12	1.16	2.40	1.21	2.50
	0.9	1.37	3.89	1.61	4.57	1.65	4.67
	0.1	0.67	0.72	0.65	0.69	0.74	0.79
	0.2	0.65	0.71	0.64	0.69	0.72	0.78
	0.3	0.63	0.71	0.63	0.71	0.71	0.79
	0.4	0.62	0.72	0.64	0.74	0.71	0.81
$1-Bx^2$	0.5	0.63	0.76	0.66	0.79	0.72	0.86
	0.6	0.65	0.83	0.70	0.88	0.75	0.95
	0.7	0.69	0.96	0.76	1.05	0.80	1.11
	0.8	0.77	1.23	0.88	1.40	0.91	1.46
	0.9	1.00	2.10	1.18	2.47	1.20	2.53
	0.1	0.68	0.75	0.66	0.73	0.75	0.83
	0.2	0.71	0.79	0.69	0.78	0.78	0.88
	0.3	0.73	0.83	0.73	0.83	0.81	0.93
	0.4	0.75	0.87	0.76	0.89	0.84	0.98
$\exp(-Bx)$	0.5	0.77	0.91	0.80	0.95	0.87	1.03
	0.6	0.79	0.94	0.84	1.00	0.90	1.08
	0.7	0.80	0.98	0.88	1.08	0.93	1.14
	0.8	0.81	1.01	0.92	1.15	0.96	1.19
	0.9	0.82	1.04	0.97	1.22	0.99	1.25

means that for part of the operating time of the catalyst the yield of the desired product on the deactivating catalyst in the internal diffusion region will be higher than the yield obtained in the kinetic region. Since high conversion degrees are usually desirable in industrial processes (unless selectivity is affected), a domain of conversion values within which the intraparticle diffusion resistance will be advantegous, seems to be quite plausible. Such reaction conditions are easily realized in practice.

The domain of conversion values where diffusion limitations have a positive effect will be more pronounced when $\beta_d < \beta_k$. This domain can be clearly perceptible with some deactivation functions even at $\beta_d = \beta_k$. This is, for example, the case of the $F(x) = 1 - \beta\sqrt{x}$ type of the deactivation equation, although the "profitable" conversion domain begins at higher conversion values. As to the remaining approximations of the deactivation law, for the case when $\beta_d = \beta_k$, it may be stated that above a definite conversion value, $r_d \approx r_k$, i.e. the intraparticle diffusion resistance produces no drop of the reaction rate. Therefore, even in these cases the realization of the process on large catalyst pellets (favourable with respect to reducing the hydraulic resistance) would cause no losses due to a decrease in the reaction rate.

The data in ref. 1 on the average conversion of gas oil during cracking over aging zeolite catalysts with different particle sizes refer to another type of selectivity, and yet, they may be considered an experimental confirmation of our general conclusion about the probability for the intraparticle resistance to contribute to the optimum proceeding of some reactions.

Our results show that the retardation of catalyst deactivation in the diffusion region could prolong the operation time of the catalyst, and hence, increase the total yield of the product.

We have used this approach in investigating the influence of intraparticle resistance on the process of isoprene production over a commercial catalyst deactivated by consecutive coke formation (refs. 8, 9). As a result, improved operation conditions have been found.

CONCLUSIONS

For a class of catalytic processes accompanied by consecutive deactivation, the intraparticle diffusion resistance regime could lead to a decrease in catalyst deactivation rate and, as a consequence, an increase in catalytic reaction rate and yield.For this reason, in some cases intraparticle diffusion control may be intentionally provoked in order to improve the effectiveness of the catalyst.

REFERENCES

1 D.Best and B.Wojciechowski,Can.J.Chem.Eng., 54 (1976) 197-202.
2 S.L.Kiperman, Introduction to Kinetics of Heterogeneous Catalytic Reactions, Nauka, Moscow, 1964.
3 O.Levenspiel, J.Catalysis, 25 (1972) 265-272.
4 J.B.Butt, C.K.Watcher and R.H.Billimora, Chem. Eng. Sci.,33 (1978) 1321-1326.
5 S.Ya.Pshezhetsky and R.N.Rubinstein, Zh. Fiz. Khim., 20 (1946) 1127-1131.
6 G.F.Froment, in B.Delmon and G.F.Froment (Editors), Catalyst Deactivation, Elsevier, Amsterdam, 1980, 1-19
7 S.Bashkhirova and S.L.Kiperman,Kinet.Catal.,11 (1970) 631-637.
8 K.Kumbilieva, M.M.Kostyukovsky and S.L.Kiperman, Proc. Second Czech.Conf. on Preparation and Properties of Heterogeneous Catalysts, Bechyne near Tabor, Czechoslovakia, June 3-7, 1985, pp. 93-95.
9 K.Kumbilieva, M.M.Kostyukovsky, L.Petrov and S.L.Kiperman, Chem. Eng.Sci., in press.

B. Delmon and G.F. Froment (Editors), *Catalyst Deactivation 1987*

TEMPERATURE PROGRAMMED OXIDATION AS AN ANALYSIS TECHNIQUE FOR DEACTIVATED HYDROTREATING CATALYSTS

J. VAN DOORN, J.L. BOSCH, R.J. BAKKUM and J.A. MOULIJN

Institute of Chemical Technology, University of Amsterdam,
Nieuwe Achtergracht 166, 1018 WV Amsterdam

ABSTRACT

Temperature Programmed Oxidation (TPO) is used for determination of the amount and the chemical state of carbon and sulfur on deactivated hydrotreating catalysts. The determination of sulfur on sulfided catalysts appeared to be quite accurate. Sulfided $CoMo/Al_2O_3$ and $NiMo/Al_2O_3$ are oxidized in three steps. In the first step Mo-sulfide and part of the Co- or Ni-sulfide is oxidized, whereas in the two other steps the remaining part of the Co- or Ni-sulfide is oxidized. The second oxidation step may also contain a Mo-sulfide phase. Carbon is oxidized to a mixture of CO and CO_2 and therefore it is advisible to measure the carbon content separately by elemental analysis. The carbon deposits on spent catalysts have a low reactivity, despite of the high hydrogen content.

INTRODUCTION

Deactivation of catalysts by carbon deposition is a severe problem in many processes. In order to get a better understanding of the mechanism(s) of carbon deposition, quantitative and qualitative techniques are needed for determination of the amount and chemical structure of carbon on deactivated catalysts.

Besides carbon, deactivated hydrotreating catalysts contain sulfur, nitrogen, hydrogen and metal deposits. These elements are incorporated in the carbon deposit, whereas sulfur is also present in the form of metalsulfides.

A relatively simple method for simultaneous detection of carbon and sulfur is Temperature Programmed Oxidation (TPO). With this technique both the amount and the reactivity of the different forms of sulfur towards oxygen can be determined. As will be shown only qualitative information on carbon is obtained.

In this study the applicability of TPO on "spent" commercial catalysts is tested by comparing TPO of sulfided catalysts and coked catalysts.

EXPERIMENTAL

Catalysts

Two sets of catalysts were used in this study. The first set consisted of home-made γ-Al_2O_3 (Ketjen 000-1.5E (CK 300)) supported Mo, Ni-Mo and Co-Mo. The specific area of the support was 195 m^2/g; the pore volume was 0.50 cm^3/g and the particle size was 100-200 μm. These catalysts were prepared by pore volume impregnation of the alumina with solutions of $(NH_4)_6Mo_7O_{24}.4H_2O$, $Co(NO_3)_2.6H_2O$ or $Ni(NO_3)_2.6H_2O$ in demineralized water. After drying at 383 K for 18 h all catalysts were calcined in a flow of air at 773 K for 2 h. Bimetallic catalysts were calcined after impregnation with Mo and subsequently the second component was added by a repeated impregnation and calcination procedure.

The second set of catalysts consisted of 2.1 wt% NiO/15.5 wt% MoO_3 and 3.8 wt% CoO/15.2 wt% MoO_3 on Al_2O_3 (specific area was 220 m^2/g). These catalysts were donated by AKZO chemie, Amsterdam, both in the oxidic form and after being used for hydrodesulfurization of VGO. The latter catalysts will be referred to as spent catalysts.

Before these spent catalysts were submitted to TPO experiments the remains of the feed were removed by Soxhlet extraction with dichloromethane at 313 K for 18 h (ref. 1).

The home-made catalysts and the oxidic $NiMo/Al_2O_3$ were sulfided in-situ with a mixture of 15 % H_2S in H_2 in a lineair temperature program (10 K/min) up to 673 K. After 30 min at 673 K the sulfiding mixture was replaced by Ar and the sample was cooled down to room temperature. Directly after the sulfiding procedure the sample was submitted to TPO.

TABLE 1
Catalysts studied

code	MoO_3		CoO		NiO	
	wt%	at/nm^2	wt%	at/nm^2	wt%	at/nm^2
Mo(10.4)	10.4	2.2	-	-	-	-
Co(2.0)Mo(10.4)	10.4	2.2	2.0	0.8	-	-
Co(4.0)Mo(10.4)	10.4	2.2	4.0	1.6	-	-
Co(10.0)Mo(10.4)	10.4	2.2	10.0	4.1	-	-
Co(3.8)Mo(15.2)	15.2	2.9	3.8	1.4	-	-
Ni(2.1)Mo(15.5)	15.5	2.9	-	-	2.1	0.8

Coked catalysts were prepared by passing a flow of pure propene (22 μmol/s) over the oxidic catalysts at 673 K or 773 K for 30 min. Subsequently the propene flow was replaced by N_2 and the sample was cooled to room temperature.

Coked and spent catalysts were analyzed for C and H content by means of a Carlo Erba elemental analyzer (model 1106).

The metal contents and the code used are listed in table 1.

Temperature Programmed Oxidation

A schematic diagram of the apparatus is shown in figure 1. The sample was held between two quartz wool plugs in a quartz tube (internal diameter 4-5 mm). The temperature of the sample was increased lineairly from room temperature to 1175 K (heating rate 5 K/min). The feed consisted of 20 % O_2 in He (2.5 μmol O_2/s). The reaction products (CO_2, SO_2 and H_2O) were trapped in a 5A molecular sieve column.

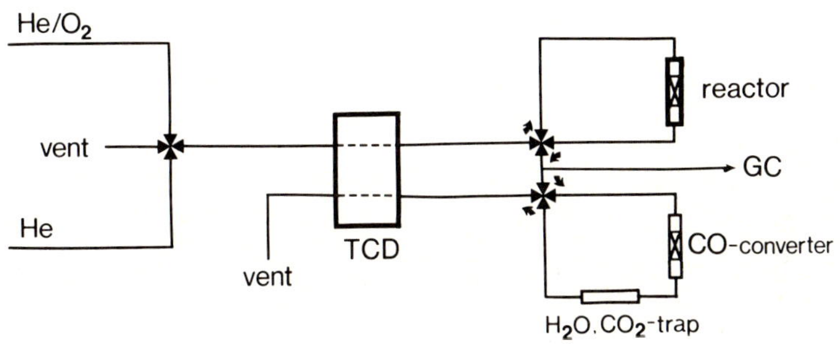

Figure 1: Diagram of the experimental set-up used for Temperature Programmed Oxidation.

All CO formed was converted to CO_2 by an on-line converter. The O_2 content of the remaining mixture was monitored continuously by means of a thermal conductivity detector (TCD). Directly after the reactor, before the product traps, small aliquots of the reaction mixture were injected on a gaschromatograph (carrier gas: He, column: Porapak QS). In this way CO_2 and SO_2 production were measured.

Calibration of the TCD was performed by oxidizing V_2O_3, Mo, MoS_2 and Mo_2C. The latter two compounds were also used for calibration of the GC.

RESULTS

Bulk compounds

In figure 2 the three TPO patterns of the bulk molybdenum compounds are shown. Oxidation of Mo shows a maximum in O_2 consumption at 755 K, while oxidation of MoS_2 gives a maximum at 850 K. The shoulder in the TPO pattern of MoS_2, coinciding with a small CO_2 production peak, is due to a carbon impurity in the MoS_2 used. The maximum for oxidation of Mo_2C is situated at somewhat higher temperature (895 K).

In figure 3 the area under the TCD curve (representing the amount of consumed O_2) is plotted vs. the calculated amount of O_2 needed for the reactions listed in table 2.

TABLE 2
Reactions used to calculate the amount of consumed O_2

V_2O_3	+	O_2	=	V_2O_5		
MoS_2	+	7/2 O_2	=	MoO_3	+	2 SO_2
Mo_2C	+	4 O_2	=	2 MoO_3	+	CO_2
Mo	+	3/2 O_2	=	MoO_3		

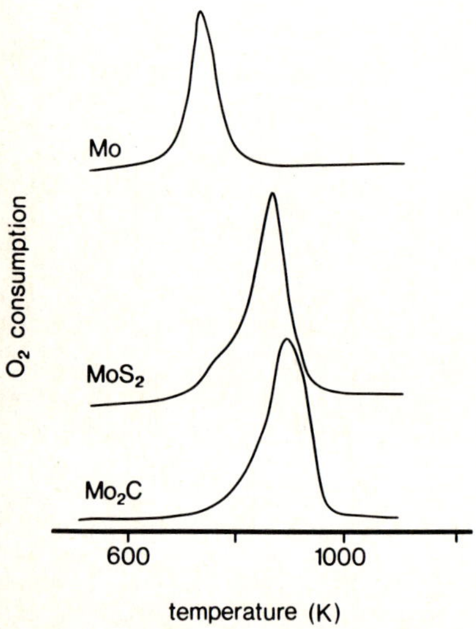

Figure 2: Temperature Programmed Oxidation patterns of bulk Mo, MoS_2 and Mo_2C.

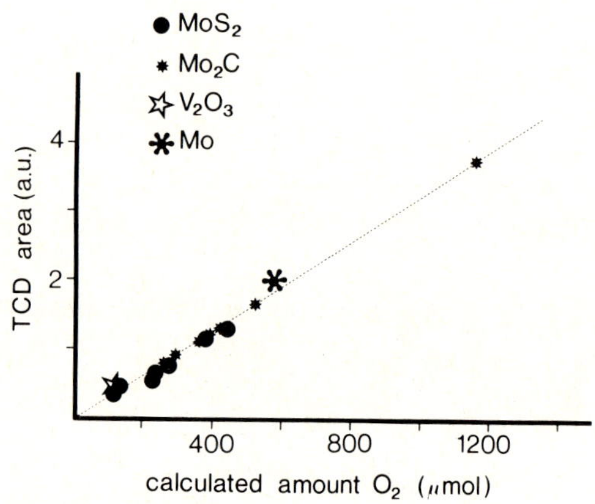

Figure 3: Calibration graph obtained by TPO of V_2O_3, Mo, MoS_2 and Mo_2C. The area under the TPO curve is plotted vs. the amount of O_2 calculated.

From the slope of the line in figure 3 a conversion factor was determined with which the TCD area was translated to the number of μmol O_2 consumed during one experiment.

The signal of the gaschromatograph was calibrated in an analogous way.

Sulfided catalysts

TPO patterns of sulfided Mo/Al_2O_3 and $CoMo/Al_2O_3$ catalysts are shown in figure 4 (O_2 consumption) and figure 5 (SO_2 production). Oxidation of sulfided $Mo(10.4)/Al_2O_3$ started at low temperature (ca. 330 K) and gradually increased with increasing temperature. In the low-temperature region, it was not possible to determine, whether the O_2 consumption was due to formation of SO_2 or to O_2 uptake for the formation of some oxy-sulfide, because of limited SO_2 detection sensitivity. At ca. 500 K the SO_2 production became detectable and was maximal at 600 K. The TPO patterns of sulfided $Co(2.0)/Mo(10.4)/Al_2O_3$ showed two maxima, both in O_2 consumption and SO_2 production. The first maximum was situated at 520 K and was of similar shape as the peak in the pattern of sulfided $Mo(10.4)/Al_2O_3$.

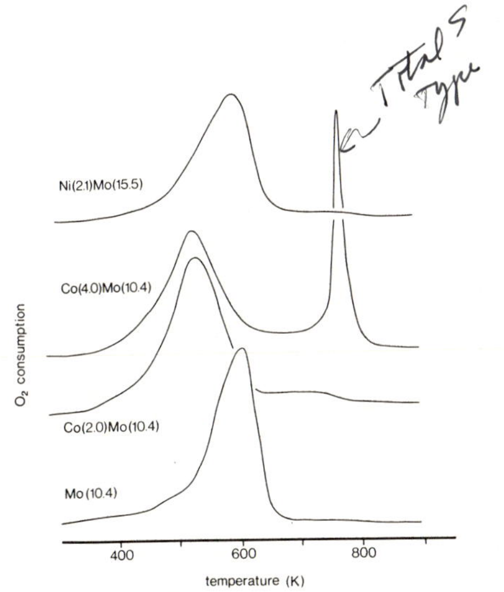

Figure 4: TPO patterns (O_2 consumption) of sulfided Mo/Al_2O_3, $CoMo/Al_2O_3$ and $NiMo/Al_2O_3$.

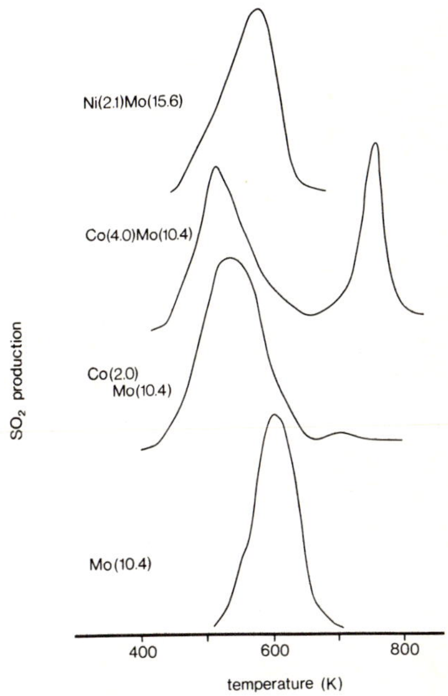

Figure 5: TPO patterns (SO_2 production) of sulfided Mo/Al_2O_3, $CoMo/Al_2O_3$ and $NiMo/Al_2O_3$.

The second maximum occured as a broad plateau in the O_2 consumption and a small maximum in SO_2 production at 700 K. The TPO patterns of sulfided $Co(4.0)/Mo(10.4)/Al_2O_3$ exhibited, besides the two maxima as found in the

TPO pattens of Co(2.0)Mo(10.4)/Al_2O_3, an additional relatively sharp maximum at 765 K.

The temperature of the first maximum shifted from 600 K (Mo(10.4)/Al_2O_3) to 520 K (Co(2.0)/Mo(10.4)/Al_2O_3) and 510 K (Co(4.0)/Mo(10.4)/Al_2O_3). As can be seen from table 3 the total O_2 consumption agrees very well (within 2 %) with the calculated O_2 values, based on the existence of MoS_2 and CoS after sulfiding.

TABLE 3
TPO data of sulfided catalysts

catalyst	O_2 measured	O_2 calculated
Mo(10.4)	384 μmol	387 μmol
Co(2.0)/Mo(10.4)	453 μmol	451 μmol
Co(4.0)/Mo(10.4)	522 μmol	514 μmol
Ni(2.1)/Mo(15.5)	349 μmol	432 μmol

In table 4 the amount of O_2 consumed and SO_2 produced are subdivided for the separate maxima. To quantify the data for the separate maxima the patterns were deconvoluted by hand, which introduced an additional inaccuracy.

TABLE 4
TPO data of sulfided catalysts [a]

			peak I		peak II/III	
catalyst	Mo calc[b]	Co calc[b]	O_2 meas	SO_2 meas	O_2 meas	SO_2 meas
Mo(10.4)	111	-	384	220	-	-
Co(2.0)/Mo(10.4)	111	41	419	250	55	b.d.l.[c]
Co(4.0)/Mo(10.4)	112	83	332	168	191	93

a = values are given in μmol.
b = calculated from the composition of the catalyst.
c = below detection limit.

From this table it can be seen that the total O_2 uptake and SO_2 production are in agreement with the stoichiometry.

The uppermost curves in figure 4 and figure 5 are the TPO patterns of sulfided Ni(2.1)/Mo(15.5)/Al_2O_3. This catalyst is the oxidic precursor of the spent catalyst. Oxidation started at low temperature (ca. 330 K) leading to a maximum in O_2 consumption at 600 K. The main peak was followed by a plateau up to 750 K. Table 3 shows that the O_2 uptake was less than the theoretical value.

Coked catalysts

Propene treatment at 773 K of Mo(10.4)/Al_2O_3 resulted in the deposition of 10.4 wt% carbon, propene treatment at 673 K of Co(10.0)Mo(10.4)/Al_2O_3 resulted in the deposition of 2.0 wt% carbon, as determined with elemental analysis. In figure 6 the TPO patterns (CO_2 production) of coked Mo(10.4)/Al_2O_3 and Co(10.0)/Mo(10.4)/Al_2O_3 are shown. CO_2 production started at 600 K for the coked Mo/Al_2O_3 catalyst, with a maximum at 760 K and a small peak around 840 K. The CO_2 production pattern of coked CoMo/Al_2O_3 showed a broad maximum around 680 K. The O_2 consumption patterns of these coked catalysts were similar to the CO_2 production patterns (not shown). The TPO results are summarized in table 5. The C/H ratio's were calculated by substracting the number of μmol O_2 consumed for CO_2 production and metal oxidation from the total O_2 consumption measured. For this calculation it was assumed that propene treatment reduced the metaloxides. The remaining amount of O_2 is than the amount of O_2 consumed by reaction with hydrogen to H_2O. The carbon content determined by TPO appeared to be much lower compared with the carbon content from elemental analysis. Therefore carbon values obtained by TPO were replaced by the carbon values determined from the weigth percentage carbon measured by elemental analysis. These values were used for further calculations.

TABLE 5
TPO results of the coked catalysts [a]

catalyst	prop. T[b]	O_2 meas	CO_2 meas	C/H[c]	C/H[d]
Co(10.0)Mo(10.4)	673 K	123.6	59.1	0.3	0.6
Mo(10.4)	773 K	387.5	239.9	1.5	1.7

a = all values are given in μmol.
b = propene treatment temperature.
c = C/H ratio calculated from TPO ($C + O_2 = CO_2$ assumed)
d = C/H ratio determined by elemental analysis

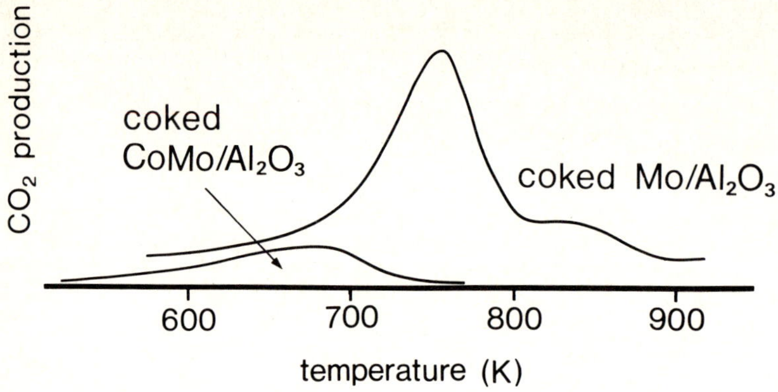

Figure 6: TPO patterns (CO_2 production) of coked Mo/Al_2O_3 and $CoMo/Al_2O_3$. Mo/Al_2O_3 had been treated with propene at 773 K, $CoMo/Al_2O_3$ had been treated with propene at 673 K.

Spent catalysts

In figure 7 the SO_2 and CO_2 production patterns of spent $Ni(2.1)/Mo(15.5)/Al_2O_3$ and $Co(3.8)/Mo(15.2)/Al_2O_3$ are vizualized. The SO_2 production patterns exhibited large maxima at 540 K (CoMo) and 580 K (NiMo) and broad, less pronounced maxima at ca. 750 K (CoMo) and 730 K (NiMo). CO_2 production started below 600 K with maxima around 700 K for both catalysts. The data, subdivided for the individual maxima are listed in table 6.

TABLE 6

TPO results of the spent catalysts [a]

catalyst	Mo[b]	Co/Ni[b]	O_2	SO_2(I)	SO_2(II)	CO_2	C/H[c]	C/H[d]
Co(3.8)Mo(15.2)	103	49	1000	103	53	172	0.5	0.3
Ni(2.1)Mo(15.5)	104	27	1314	103	35	321	0.3	0.4

a = values are given in μmol.
b = calculated from the composition of the catalyst.
c = C/H ratio calculated from TPO ($C + O_2 = CO_2$ assumed)
d = C/H ratio determined by elemental analysis

The amount of carbon determined with elemental analysis is higher compared with the TPO results. The actual carbon contents were 5.5 wt% for spent $CoMo/Al_2O_3$ and 6.6 wt% for spent $NiMo/Al_2O_3$. For calculation of the C/H ratio's the carbon contents as determined by elemental analysis were used.

The number of µmol SO_2 produced appeared to be more or less the same as the number of µmol Mo, Co and Ni.

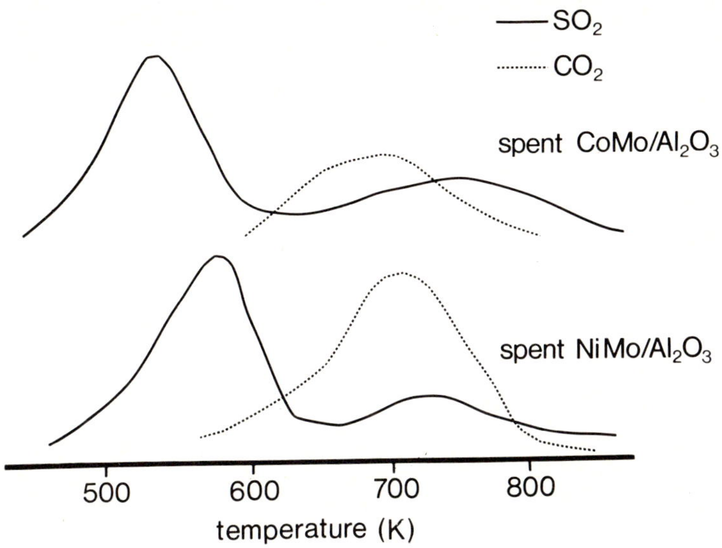

Figure 7: TPO patterns (CO_2 and SO_2 production) of spent Co(3.8)Mo(15.2)/Al_2O_3 and Ni(2.1)Mo(15.5)/Al_2O_3.

DISCUSSION

Since a plot of the TCD area vs. the calculated amount of consumed O_2 is a straight line one can conclude that the oxidation of MoS_2 and Mo_2C has taken place following the reactions listed in table 2. This means that no or little SO_3 is formed, although thermodynamic calculations show that SO_3 formation under the experimental conditions is possible. One should be careful when using V, Fe or Pt catalysts, which are known to be good SO_2 oxidation catalysts, in TPO. The formation of COS from CO_2 and SO_2 is not to be expected on the basis of thermodynamic calculations.

From the figures 2 and 4 it can be seen that supported MoS_2 oxidizes at considerable lower temperatures (T_{max} = 600 K) than bulk MoS_2 (T_{max} = 850 K). This is probably caused by diffusional limitations. In the case of bulk MoS_2 a surface metaloxide layer might be formed in the early stages of oxidation. Bartholomew et al. (ref 2) reported that at O_2 pressure of 1-100 kPa the formation of an oxide layer on top of the bulk sulfide can prevent bulk oxidation. From the good agreement of the measured and calculated O_2 values for the molybdenum compounds it is concluded that in the experiments bulk oxidation of the sulfides takes place.

From the TPO patterns of sulfided Mo/Al_2O_3 and $CoMo/Al_2O_3$ it can be seen that at increasing Co loadings an additional maximum emerged, so peak III is attributed to a Co-sulfide phase. Similar results were obtained for a series of sulfided $NiMo/Al_2O_3$ (results not shown). Peak I is due to the oxidation of a phase consisting of Mo-and Co-sulfide, because O_2 uptake exceeds the amount expected for MoS_2. The maximum around 700 K (peak II) is attributed to a Co-sulfide phase or a Co-Mo-sulfide phase. Further investigations to elucidate this important point are in progress.

The maximum in the oxidation pattern of Mo-sulfide shifts to lower temperature with increasing Co or Ni loadings. This agrees with the conclusion that a mixed phase is present, although a catalytic effect of CoS on oxygen dissociation is not excluded.

From the data, listed in table 4 S/Mo and S/Co ratio's could be determined. The S/Mo ratio's vary from 1.5 to 2.3, depending on Co loading. From literature it is known that the S/Mo ratio is normally slightly below 2 (ref. 3-4).

The TPO profiles after sulfiding of $NiMo/Al_2O_3$ show that sulfiding for 30 min at 673 K is not sufficient for complete sulfidation of this catalyst. From the measured and calculated values it appeared that this catalyst was sulfided up to 80% completion.

The patterns of the spent catalysts clearly show a low and a high temperature SO_2 production maximum. In table 7 the temperatures of the SO_2 maxima of the spent catalysts and sulfided catalysts are listed.

TABLE 7
Peak temperatures (SO_2 production) of sulfided and spent catalysts

catalyst		peak I	peak II	peak III
Mo(10.4)	sulfided	600 K	-	-
Co(2.0)Mo(10.4)	sulfided	520 K	700 K	-
Co(4.0)Mo(10.4)	sulfided	510 K	600-700 K	765 K
Ni(2.1)Mo(15.5)	sulfided	600 K	650-750 K	-
Co(3.8)Mo(15.2)	spent	540 K	-	750 K
Ni(2.1)Mo(15.5)	spent	580 K	-	730 K

The temperatures of the maxima in SO_2 production of the sulfided and related spent catalysts are comparable, suggesting a similar chemical state of sulfur. Yoshimura et al. (ref 5), explained identical patterns for spent catalysts by assuming that the high temperature SO_2 production originates mainly from sulfur incorporated in the carbon deposit. Our results indicate that the high temperature SO_2 production peak is caused, at least partially, by metal sulfide oxidation.

Quantifying the data of TPO of spent catalysts showed that much more O_2 was consumed than could be accounted for by summation of O_2 used for SO_2 production, CO_2 production and oxidation of the metal to metal oxide. From the weight percentage of carbon determined by elemental analysis it appeared that the actual carbon content was higher than found with TPO. The low carbon recovery can be attributed to CO formation, which could not be detected. The C/H ratio's calculated from the corrected TPO data are in agreement with the C/H ratio's measured by elemental analysis. No correction was made for the water content of the catalysts, so the observed C/H ratio's are upper limits.

The carbon deposits on the spent catalysts react at ca. 700 K. At this temperature we believe that the Mo is in oxidic form. MoO_3 is known to be a good oxidation catalyst (ref. 6) and one would expect that all carbon in the vicinity of the molybdenum would be oxidized. CO_2 production however starts at the same temperature where Ni- and Co sulfides are oxidized. A similar CO_2 production profile was found for coked $CoMo/Al_2O_3$. Whether this is an indication for preferred location of the carbon deposit near Co- or Ni is not clear at present. The reactivity of the carbon deposit is low, even compared with the reactivity of graphitic filaments on Co/Al_2O_3 and Ni/Al_2O_3 (ref. 7).

The CO_2 production of the coked Mo/Al_2O_3 is maximal at 760 K, with a second maximum at 840 K. Both maxima are located at higher temperature compared with the maxima in CO_2 production of the coked $CoMo/Al_2O_3$. Two explanations are possible for this fact. The catalytic influence on the $C-O_2$ reaction can be different for both catalysts or the carbon deposit on $CoMo/Al_2O_3$ is more reactive towards O_2. From the data of the coked catalysts we calculated the C/H ratio's. The found values indicates that the carbon deposit on $Co(10.0)Mo(10.4)/Al_2O_3$ must contain short aliphatic chains or alicyclic units.

CONCLUSIONS

Temperature Programmed Oxidation is a useful technique for analysis of sulfided, coked and spent catalysts. Information on the sulfur source, vizualized as separate maxima in the SO_2 production profiles makes an estimation of S/Mo and S/Co or S/Ni ratio's possible, although part of the Ni- or Co sulfide is oxidized at lower temperature. Quantification of the data is good in the case of sulfided catalysts. In quantifying the TPO data of spent catalysts the formation of CO has to be taken into account. Quantitative TPO should be supported by elemental analysis.

Oxidation of the major part of Ni- or Co-sulfide coincides with the oxidation of the carbon deposit. The reactivity of the carbon deposit is low, despite the fact that the deposit contains a high amount of hydrogen.
The catalytic effect of the metal can play an important role on the temperature at which the carbon reacts with O_2 and as a consequence a comparison between carbon deposits only based on oxidation temperatures can lead to erroneous conclusions.

ACKNOWLEDGEMENTS

These investigations were supported (in part) by the Netherlands Technology Foundations (STW). AKZO Chemie, Amsterdam, is gratefully acknowledged for the supply of the catalysts; ECN Petten for the use of the Elemental Analyzer.

REFERENCES

1 J. van Doorn, J.L. Bosch and J.A. Moulijn, in preparation.
2 C.H. Bartholomew, P.K. Agrawal and J.R. Katzer, Adv. in Catal., 31 (1982) 135.
3 F.E. Massoth, K.S. Chung and R. Ramanchandran, Fuel Proc. Techn., 2 (1979) 57.
4 P. Arnoldy, J.A.M. van den Heykant, G.D. de Bok and J.A. Moulijn, J. Catal., 92 (1985) 35.
5 D.W. McKee, Carbon, 8 (1970) 623.
6 Y. Yoshimura and E. Furimsky, Fuel, 65 (1986) 1388.
7 J. van Doorn, R.C.S. Verheul, L. Singoredjo and J.A. Moulijn, Fuel, 65 (1986) 1383.

B. Delmon and G.F. Froment (Editors), *Catalyst Deactivation 1987*

HIGH-PRESSURE GRAVIMETRIC STUDY OF CARBON FORMATION DURING CO HYDROGENATION OVER Fe/Al_2O_3

D. Schanke* and A. Holmen

Department of Industrial Chemistry, University of Trondheim, N-7034 Trondheim-NTH (Norway)

ABSTRACT

Carbon formation on an alumina-supported iron catalyst has been studied under CO hydrogenation conditions in a combined high-pressure microbalance/microreactor. The carbon formation process is characterized by an initial, very rapid period of carbon formation, followed by a period of significantly slower carbon deposition. Typically, the amount of carbon deposited exceeded the amount corresponding to bulk carbide formation after only a few minutes of reaction. The initial rate of carbon deposition increased with increasing reaction temperature and CO partial pressure, and decreased with increasing partial pressure of hydrogen. Transient experiments revealed the presence of several types of surface carbon with different reactivity towards hydrogen.

INTRODUCTION

The conversion of iron catalysts into bulk carbides under Fischer-Tropsch conditions has been reported by several authors (refs. 1-5). It has also been suggested that the iron carbide is the active iron phase in the Fischer-Tropsch synthesis (ref. 6). In addition, many investigations have indicated that surface carbon or partially hydrogenated carbon may play an important role in the reaction mechanism of the Fischer-Tropsch synthesis on Ru, Co, Ni and Fe catalysts (refs. 7-10).

Recently, Bennett et al. (refs. 1, 11-14) characterized the bulk and surface of supported iron catalysts during CO hydrogenation. Various forms of surface carbon were formed after only a few seconds on stream. The surface carbon was found to consist of a reactive CH_x-species ($x \simeq 1$) and a less reactive surface carbide. After longer exposures to synthesis gas, bulk carbides and inactive (graphitic) carbon were also formed. Oxygen-

*Present adress: SINTEF, Div. of Applied Chemistry, N-7034 Trondheim-NTH (Norway) containing intermediates were not detected. The existence of surface carbon with different reactivity has also been shown by surface spectroscopic methods (refs. 15-16).

Carbon formation can conveniently be studied by gravimetric methods, and the kinetics of carbon formation on iron catalysts at atmospheric pressure have been reported by several investigators (refs. 17-20). A high-pressure gravimetric study of carbon formation on iron catalysts have also recently been published (ref. 21).

In the present communication, the kinetics of carbon formation on an alumina-supported iron catalyst are reported. The experiments have been carried out in a combined high-pressure microbalance/microreactor. Thus, the kinetics of carbon formation could be studied while simultaneously monitoring catalytic activity.

EXPERIMENTAL

Catalyst preparation

The alumina-supported iron catalyst used in the present study was prepared by aqueous impregnation on γ-Al_2O_3 (Johnson Matthey Chem., BET-area 334 m^2/g), using excess water (i.e. not the incipient wetness method). The solvent was removed by rotary evaporation under reduced pressure, and the catalyst was dried in air at 383 K for 25 hours. After drying, the catalyst was calcined in flowing air at 673 K for 2 hours. For the microbalance experiments, the 35-50 mesh fraction was used. The iron content of the catalyst was determined to 9.5 weight% by chemical analysis. CO chemisorption indicated a CO(ads)/Fe ratio of 0.008, as measured by the dual-isotherm technique and assuming 1:1 adsorption stoichiometry (ref. 22).

Apparatus

The central part of the apparatus is an integrated microbalance/microreactor. The catalyst was placed in a perforated stainless steel basket and hung from one arm of the microbalance by a quartz fibre. The basket was positioned inside an electrically heated 1.0 inch O.D. stainless steel tubular reactor, connected to the 3/8 inch O.D. tubing of the microbalance. The microbalance is a Sartorius model 4436 with 0.1 μg sensitivity. The experimental equipment has been described elsewhere (ref.22).

Procedure

Before experiments, the microreactor/microbalance was purged with He and heated to 723 K with He flowing. The catalyst was normally reduced in flowing H_2 (P_{H_2}= 11 bar, T = 723 K) for 16-18 hours. After reduction, the catalyst was cooled in hydrogen to the desired reaction temperature and the feed was switched to synthesis gas. The space velocity of the synthesis gas was normally regulated to keep total CO conversion below 15%. CO hydrogenation was usually continued for 2-3 hours. The feed was then switched to pure H_2, in order to investigate the reactivity of the deposited material. The reactivity of the deposited material in H_2 could also be studied by programming to higher temperatures with flowing H_2. In addition to the procedure described above, short periods (10 sec.- 5 min.) of exposure to synthesis gas with H_2-treatment between the H_2/CO exposures, were also used. For studying the influence of reaction conditions on C-deposition rate and catalytic activity, a fresh catalyst was used for each set of experimental conditions.

RESULTS AND DISCUSSION

Kinetics of carbon formation

Typical examples of carbon formation on 9.5%Fe/Al_2O_3 are shown in Fig. 1. The carbon content of the catalyst after 2-3 hours of CO hydrogenation is very high, exceeding the C/Fe-ratios corresponding to bulk carbide formation. The most carbon-rich iron carbide has a C/Fe-ratio of 0.5 (Fe_2C), while measured C/Fe-ratios are typically larger than unity. Furthermore, the carbon formation process can be divided into at least two regimes. An initial, very rapid weight increase typically results in a C/Fe-ratio of 0.7-0.9 within less than 5 minutes of reaction. The C/Fe-ratio corresponding to bulk carbide formation has therefore already been exceeded at this stage.

The initial, rapid weight increase, is followed by a period of slower carbon deposition, after which the carbon deposition rate again increases. After this second increase in carbon deposition rate, the rate slowly decreases, and at certain reaction conditions the C/Fe-ratio reaches a constant level. The existence of two regimes of carbon formation is clearly visible for H_2/CO=2 in Fig. 1. The initial period of rapid carbon formation normally resulted in a C/Fe-ratio of 0.7-0.9. The location (with respect to time) of the second (slower) regime of carbon deposition, appeared to be strongly affected by the reaction conditions. Increasing temperatures caused the second regime of carbon deposition to begin earlier, while increasing H_2/CO-ratios displace the start of the second regime to a later point of time. For H_2/CO=4, the second regime of carbon deposition is almost absent (Fig. 1).

The initial rates of carbon deposition for different reaction conditions are shown in Table 1. The initial rate of carbon deposition increases with increasing temperature and CO partial pressure, and decreases with increasing partial pressure of hydrogen.

TABLE 1
Kinetic data for carbon deposition on 9.5%Fe/Al_2O_3.

CO hydrogenation conditions			Initial C - deposition rate
T (K)	P_{tot} (bar)	H_2/CO	(mol C/mol Fe·sec)·10^4
548	11.0	2	45.2
573	11.0	2	69.0
598	11.0	2	141.0
573	14.7	3	55.1
573	11.0	1*)	84.0
573	9.2	4	45.4

*) Nitrogen added as inert ($P_{CO}= P_{H_2}= P_{N_2}=$ 3.7 bar).

Nature of the carbonaceous deposits

In general, a substantial part of the material accumulated during CO hydrogenation could be removed by H_2-treatment at 573 K (Fig. 2). H_2-treatment of the catalyst after exposure to synthesis gas for 2-3 hours produced mainly methane, but significant amounts of C_2-C_4 hydrocarbons were also detected. Increasing the temperature to 723 K after ≈1 hour of H_2-treatment at 573 K, indicated that virtually all of the carbon could be removed by hydrogen at this temperature (Fig. 2).

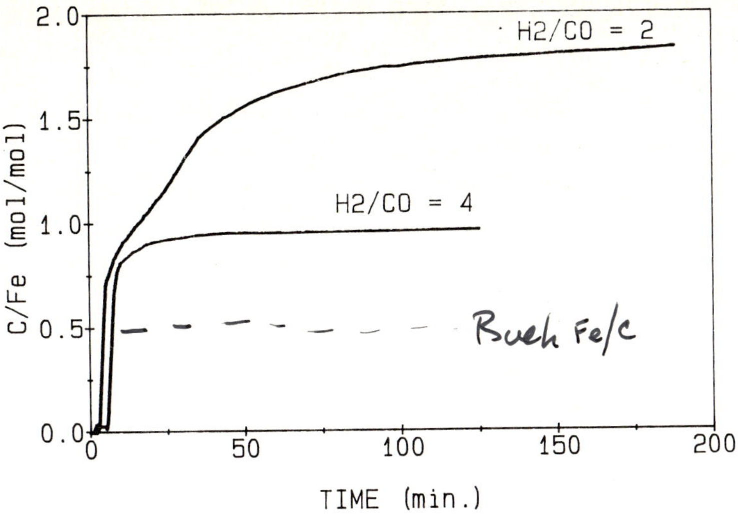

Fig. 1. Carbon formation during CO hydrogenation over 9.5%Fe/Al_2O_3 at different partial pressures of CO. T = 573 K , Partial pressure of H_2= 7.3 bar.

A blank run with pure Al_2O_3 revealed a small but significant weight increase when H_2/CO was passed over the sample at 573 K, although CO conversion was negligible (Fig. 2). A control experiment with glass-spheres produced negligible weight changes (Fig. 2). From Fig. 2 it can be seen that the weight curve for Al_2O_3 lacks the initial, very rapid increase observed on Fe/Al_2O_3. Apparently CO (or CO + H_2) interacts with the alumina to form carbon or another surface compound. It is possible that this phenomenon is connected to the formate/carbonate structures observed by IR-spectroscopy over Al_2O_3 or Al_2O_3-supported metals during CO hydrogenation (Refs. 22-23).

As noted in the previous section, the observed C/Fe-ratios exceeded the value expected for bulk iron carbides (Fe_xC, x = 2-3). Very high C/Fe-ratios during CO hydrogenation over supported Fe-catalysts have also been reported by Unmuth et al. (ref. 17) and Sommen et al. (ref. 20). Sommen et al. showed by transmission electron microscopy that this was caused by filamentous carbon growing out from the iron particles. We have found that the catalytic activity of the 9.5%Fe/Al_2O_3 catalyst generally decreased by less than 50% from 0.5 hour to 2 hours of reaction time (ref. 22). It is therefore likely that the relatively slow

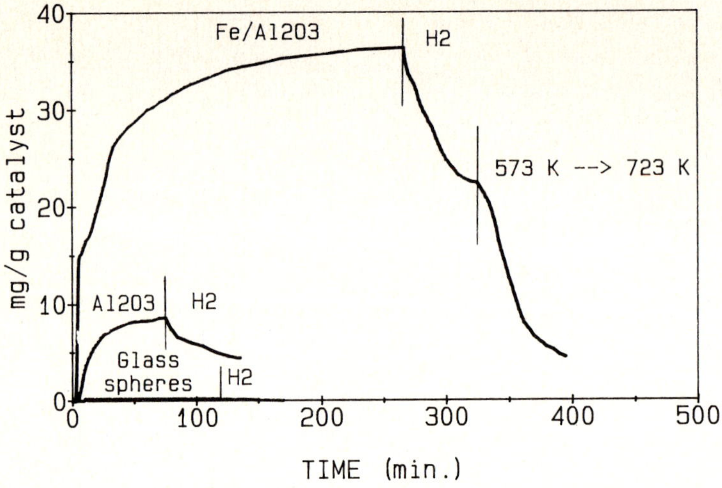

Fig. 2. Weight changes during CO hydrogenation and subsequent H_2-treatment of 9.5%Fe/Al_2O_3, pure Al_2O_3 and glass spheres.
T = 573 K , H_2/CO = 2.7 , P = 11 bar.
Hydrogenation conditions: T = 573 K , P_{H_2} = 11 bar.
Hydrogenation conditions for 9.5%Fe/Al_2O_3: 573 K for 1 hour, then 5 K/min. to 723 K.

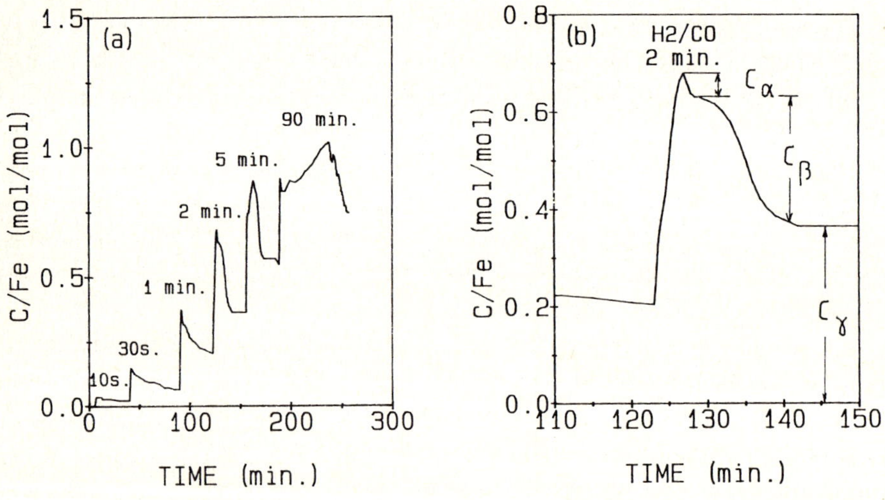

Fig. 3. Carbon deposition and removal on 9.5%Fe/Al_2O_3.
(a) Successive transient exposures to synthesis gas. (b) Part of Fig. 3a expanded.
T = 573 K , H_2/CO = 3.3 , P = 11 bar.

region of carbon deposition observed for longer reaction times in the present study corresponds to carbon deposits growing away from the iron particles, since the catalytic activity is not drastically reduced during this period. With respect to the CO hydrogenation mechanism over iron catalysts, the initial period of rapid carbon formation may therefore be of greater interest. To investigate this, a freshly reduced catalyst was exposed to synthesis gas ($H_2/CO = 3.3$, GHSV $\simeq$ 35000 h^{-1}) for short periods of time (10 sec. - 5 min.) at 573 K and 11 bar and kept in a H_2-stream between H_2/CO - exposures. The results are shown in Fig. 3.

Fig. 3a shows that each H_2/CO-exposure results in rapid carbon deposition, and the amount of carbon deposited increases with the size of the H_2/CO-dose. Furthermore, each dose of H_2/CO apparently produces an additional amount of carbon that can not be easily removed by H_2. For the 5 min. H_2/CO - dose, the second regime of slower carbon deposition (described in the previous section) is clearly entered at C/Fe $\simeq$ 0.75. The subsequent H_2-treatment and 1.5 hour exposure to H_2/CO produces only a small additional amount of carbon by the initial, rapid deposition period. Closer inspection of the initial rates for carbon deposition and carbon removal reveals that the initial carbon deposition rate increases with the size of the H_2/CO - dose (Fig. 4), until reaching an approximately constant value. The initial rate of carbon removal goes through a maximum and then decreases for increasing duration of the H_2/CO - exposures (Fig. 4). In addition, a second rate maximum for carbon removal is observed (Fig. 3b). From Fig. 4 it can be seen that the second maximum in carbon removal rate increases with the size of the H_2/CO doses, and for exposures >2 min. the 2nd. rate maximum becomes larger than the initial carbon removal rate.

Fig. 3b indicates that at least three types of carbon is formed during the initial period of CO hydrogenation over iron catalysts. After 2 min. of H_2/CO - exposure, a reactive form of carbon (C_α) is quickly removed in H_2. A second rate maximum occurs after C_α has been removed, indicating the removal of a second carbon species, designated C_β. After C_β has been removed by H_2, a third species still remains on the catalyst and is quite resistant to hydrogenation at 573 K. This is indicated by the flat portions in the weight curves in Fig. 3. This species can

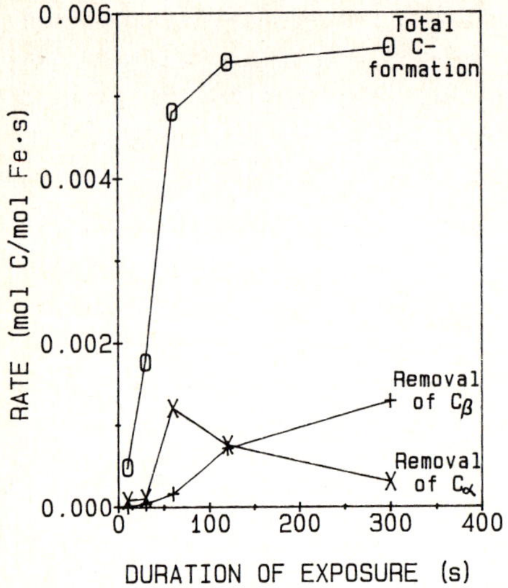

Fig. 4. Rates of carbon formation and removal on 9.5%Fe/Al_2O_3 during transient exposures to synthesis gas.

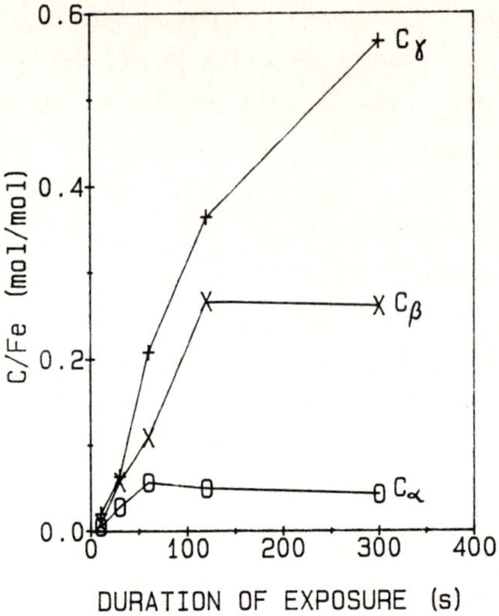

Fig. 5. Amount of different C-species on 9.5%Fe/Al_2O_3 after transient exposures to synthesis gas.

be referred to as C_γ . The amounts of C_α, C_β and C_γ is shown in Fig. 5 for increasing H_2/CO - doses.

The variation in the amounts of C_α, C_β and C_γ, and their rate of hydrogenation in a pure H_2-atmosphere can be interpreted in terms of a general rate expression for hydrogenation of carbon:

$$r_i = k_i \theta_H \theta_i \qquad , i = \alpha, \beta \text{ or } \gamma \tag{1}$$

, where θ_H and θ_i are the surface coverage of H_2 and carbon type i, respectively. k_i is the rate constant for hydrogenation of carbon type i, or the "reactivity" of that type of carbon. Since C_α is hydrogenated first (Fig. 3b) and $\theta_\alpha < \theta_\beta$ (Fig. 5), k_α is obviously larger than k_β (and k_γ). As the amount of C_α increases with increasing H_2/CO - doses, its rate of removal also increases, as predicted by Eq. 1 and confirmed by Fig. 4 & 5. The amount of C_α passes through a maximum and then decreases for H_2/CO - exposures >1 min. As predicted by Eq. 1, the rate of hydrogenation of C_α also decreases, but at a higher rate than the amount of C_α. A likely explanation for this is that the coverage of hydrogen decreases for larger doses of H_2/CO. The decrease in θ_H and θ_α is probably caused by the increasing amounts of C_β and/or C_γ, as shown in Fig 5. For a 2 min. H_2/CO - dose, the initial rate of carbon removal and the second rate maximum are of approximately equal magnitude (Fig. 4). Since it has been established that $k_\alpha > k_\beta$, this must imply that the hydrogen coverage is increased after C_α has been removed, thereby increasing r_β. Thus, the reactions occuring during a short exposure of iron to H_2/CO and subsequent H2-treatment can be described as follows:

i) Introduction of H_2/CO results in rapid deposition of C_α, C_β and C_γ. The amounts of the different types of carbon depend on the duration of the exposure (and the reaction conditions).

ii) The most reactive carbon type (C_α) is quickly removed by H_2, thereby cleaning the Fe-surface and increasing θ_H. This results in the removal of a larger amount of less reactive C_β. Finally, the least reactive species, C_γ, is hydrogenated at a much lower rate.

As shown in Fig. 5, the ratio C_α/total Fe is approximately 0.05, and its high reactivity in H_2 suggests that C_α is a surface species. The dispersion of the 9.5%Fe/Al_2O_3 catalyst has been estimated to 0.8% by chemisorption of CO. The amount of C_α therefore corresponds to approximately 5 monolayers of carbon on iron, if the dispersion has been correctly measured and the surface species contains only carbon. Bennett et al. (refs. 1,12) have shown that the carbon species present on Fe/Al_2O_3 after short H_2/CO-exposures does not contain oxygen. If C_α is a partially hydrogenated species CH_x ($x = 1$-3), this will not contribute significantly to the calculated C/Fe-ratios.

The possibility that C_α represents growing hydrocarbon chains has been considered. GC-samples taken 5 - 10 min. after a H_2/CO exposure gave nearly 100% CH_4 for H_2/CO - exposures <1 min., with only traces of C_2 and C_3 hydrocarbons. For exposures >2 min., significant amounts of C_2-C_4 hydrocarbons were also detected, accounting for ≃ 15% (carbon atom%) of the total hydrocarbon product detected after a 5 min. H_2/CO exposure. If C_α consisted of hydrocarbon chains with several C-atoms, a larger fraction of C_2+ hydrocarbons would be expected to appear in the products during H_2-treatment.

Bennett et al. (ref. 1) claim that CO chemisorption using the dual isotherm method (and assuming 1:1 adsorption stoichiometry) underestimates the specific iron surface area by a factor of ≃ 6 for 10%Fe/Al_2O_3. If this correction factor is used, the observed amount of C_α will correspond approximately to monolayer coverage. (In fact, recent X-ray diffraction and H_2-desorption measurements indicate that the iron dispersion is significantly higher than the 0.8% value from CO chemisorption (ref. 24).)

Bennett et al. (refs. 1,12) found the following bulk and surface species after 3 min. of exposure of 10%Fe/Al_2O_3 to H_2/CO = 2 (T = 558 K):

"CH"	:	C/Fe = 0.03
"Surface carbide"	:	C/Fe = 0.21
Bulk carbide	:	C/Fe = 0.12

By comparison with Fig. 5, it can be seen that amounts of "CH" and "surface carbide" agree closely with the amounts of C_α and C_β reported in the present study. Bennett et al. also reported similar behavior for the amounts of "CH" and "surface carbide" for increasing doses of H_2/CO, in agreement with the observations in the present study. It is therefore reasonable to assume that these are the same species.

The nature of C_β is an intrigueing question, since the amount by far exceeds monolayer capacity on iron. Although less reactive than C_α, the high rate of hydrogenation of C_β after C_α has been removed suggests that it is a surface species. It is also reasonable to assume that it is associated with the iron surface, in order to facilitate hydrogen-transport from the iron surface to C_β. The work of Bennett et al. showed that this species contained very little hydrogen, proving that it is not growing hydrocarbon chains. It is possible that C_α can "communicate" with C_β, i.e. that C_α can be converted to C_β (or vice versa). The possibility that C_β could represent a bulk carbide was rejected due to its high rate of removal in H_2. Fig. 5 also shows that C_β reaches a maximum C/Fe-ratio lower than expected for bulk iron carbides. In addition, the amount of C_β decreases for larger doses of H_2/CO, while the bulk carbide should be expected to continue to grow.

The variation in the amounts of C_α, C_β and C_γ with the size of the H_2/CO-dose shows that the initial, very rapid carbon deposition observed during CO hydrogenation is caused by rapid formation of a very reactive surface carbon (C_α), a less reactive surface carbon (C_β) and bulk carbide(s). At the conditions used in the transient experiments (T = 573 K , H_2/CO = 3.3 , P = 11 bar), this process is completed within approximately 5 minutes. This implies that C_γ, in addition to bulk carbide, also contains a fourth carbon species, formed during the second regime of slower carbon deposition. At the conditions used for H_2-treatment after H_2/CO - exposures, this species is hydrogenated at an even lower rate than the bulk carbide. Fig. 2 indicated that higher temperatures are needed to remove this species. If the amounts of C_α, C_β and bulk carbides do not change drastically for longer exposures to H_2/CO, the amount of inactive carbon reached C/Fe-ratios of $\simeq$ 1 during some of the experiments with 2-3 hour exposures to H_2/CO (Fig. 1). It is reasonable to attribute this inactive species to graphitic carbon extending away from the iron particles, since formation of such quantities of inactive carbon otherwise would be expected to block the iron surface completely and thereby drastically reduce the catalytic activity.

The maximum initial rate of hydrogenation of C_α was measured to $12\cdot10^{-4}$ mol C/mol Fe·sec. (Fig. 4). Based on the measured iron dispersion (0.8%), the rate of hydrogenation of C_α then becomes 0.15 s^{-1}. This can be compared with the steady-state rate of CO hydrogenation $N_{HC} \simeq 0.7\ s^{-1}$ at similar conditions (ref. 22). Although the measured rate of hydrogenation of C_α still is lower than N_{HC}, it can not be excluded that C_α represents an important reaction intermediate in CO hydrogenation over iron catalysts.

CONCLUSIONS

The following types of carbon have been detected during CO hydrogenation over 9.5%Fe/Al_2O_3:

- Reactive carbon present on the iron surface (C_α).
- Less reactive surface carbon, also associated with the iron

surface (C_β).
- Bulk iron carbide.
- Inactive carbon (graphite).
- Carbon-containing species formed independently on Al_2O_3.

It is suggested that C_α, and possibly also C_β, are important in the mechanism for hydrocarbon formation from H_2/CO on Fe/Al_2O_3.

ACKNOWLEDGEMENT

The authors are grateful to NTNF (The Royal Norwegian Council for Scientific and Industrial Research) for financial support.

REFERENCES

1 Bianchi, D., Borcar, S., Teule-Gay, F. and Bennett, C.O., J. Catal., 82 (1983) 442.
2 Niemantsverdriet, J.W., Flipse, C.F.J., van der Kraan, A.M. and van Loef, J.J., Appl. Surf. Sci., 10 (1982) 302.
3 Le Caer, G., Dubois, J.M., Pijolat, M., Perrichon, V. and Bussiere, P., J. Phys. Chem., 86 (1982) 4799.
4 Amelse, J.A., Schwartz, L.H. and Butt, J.B., J. Catal., 72 (1981) 95.
5 Raupp, G.B. and Delgass, W.N., J. Catal., 58 (1979) 348.
6 Raupp, G.B. and Delgass, W.N., J. Catal., 58 (1979) 361.
7 Biloen, P. and Sachtler, W.M.H., Adv. Catal., 30 (1981) 165.
8 Sachtler, W.M.H., Proc. 8th Int. Congress Catal., I (1984) 15
9 Ponec, V., Coal Sci., 3 (1984) 1.
10 Leith, I.R. and McCormack, C.G., CHEMSA, 8(3) (1982) 2.
11 Tau, L.M. and Bennett, C.O., J. Catal., 89 (1984) 285.
12 Bianchi, D., Tau, L.M., Borcar, S. and Bennett, C.O., J. Catal., 84 (1983) 358.
13 Tau, L.M., Borcar, S., Bianchi, D. and Bennett, C.O., J. Catal., 87 (1984) 36.
14 Tau, L.M. and Bennett, C.O., J. Catal., 89 (1984) 327.
15 Bonzel, H.P., Izv. Khim., 17(1) (1984) 20.
16 Dwyer, D.J. and Hardenbergh, J.H., J. Catal., 87 (1984) 66.
17 Unmuth, E.E., Schwartz, L.H. and Butt, J.B., J. Catal., 63 (1980) 404.
18 Sancier, K.M., Isakson, W.E. and Wise, H., Adv. Chem. Ser., 178 (1979) 129.
19 Jensen, K.B. and Massoth, F.E., J. Catal., 92 (1985) 109.
20 Sommen, A.P.B., Stoop, F. and van der Wiele, K., Appl. Catal., 14 (1985) 277.
21 Papp, H. and Wieczorek, Thermochim. Acta, 103 (1986) 187.
22 Schanke, D., Ph. D. Thesis, Univ. of Trondheim (1986)
23 Kellner, C.S. and Bell, A.T., J. Catal., 71 (1981) 296.
24 Schanke, D. and Holmen A., in preparation.

B. Delmon and G.F. Froment (Editors), *Catalyst Deactivation 1987*

ACCELERATION OF DEACTIVATION OF Ag CATALYST BY PERIODIC PULSE TECHNIQUE FOR RAPID ESTIMATION OF CATALYST LIFE

T. HATTORI,* S. KOMAI, T. HANAICHI,+ A. MIYAMOTO and Y. MURAKAMI

Department of Synthetic Chemistry, Faculty of Engineering, Nagoya University, Chikusa-ku, Nagoya 464, Japan. +Central Laboratory for Electron Microscopy, School of Medicine, Nagoya University, Showa-ku, Nagoya 466, Japan.

ABSTRACT

In order to examine the possibility of the rapid estimation of catalyst life by a periodic pulse technique, the deactivation of Ag catalyst in the oxidation of C_2H_4 was examined. In the periodic pulse technique, O_2+N_2 mixture and C_2H_4+N_2 mixture were fed alternately to subject a catalyst to forced redox cycle, which is expected to accelerate the sintering of catalyst under the reaction condition. As expected, the deactivation was faster in the periodic pulse technique than in the continuous flow technique. TEM also indicated that the particle size of Ag increased faster in the periodic pulse run. Although the deactivation was the fastest in O_2+N_2 environment, the deactivation behavior was different from that under the reaction condition. It was shown that the deactivation should be accelerated under the reaction condition for the rapid estimation of catalyst life, and that the periodic pulse technique is useful for such purpose.

INTRODUCTION

The problem in investigating the deactivation of catalysts is that prolonged experiment is required, especially for good catalysts. It is frequently attempted to accelerate the deactivation by treating catalysts under severe condition, such as high temperature, high concentration of poison and so on. However, special care should be taken not to apply too severe treatment for the catalysts. Although extensive acceleration will effectively reduce the time required to complete experiments, it may also result in a different type of deactivation from the "real" one under the actual reaction condition; for example, it is sometimes observed that the sintering in a different atmosphere results in a different morphology of crystallites.

We have proposed a novel method to accelerate the sintering for the rapid estimation of catalyst life (ref. 1). The method is based on the following hypothesis. Many oxidation reactions proceed via a reduction-oxidation, or redox, cycle. Thus, surface atoms or ions are repeatedly reduced by hydrocarbon and oxidized by O_2, while the oxidation state of catalyst bulk remains constant. The repeated reduction and oxidation leads to repeated rearrangement of surface atoms or ions, which would promote the diffusion of surface atoms, resulting in the sintering. If this is the case, a forced redox cycle will result in more rearrangement of lattice atoms and faster sintering (ref. 2). The periodic pulse reaction technique (ref. 3) was utilized to subject a catalyst to the forced redox cycle. In the technique, hydrocarbon flowed over the catalyst for a certain period of time, and then O_2 flowed for another period of time. This alternate feed of hydrocarbon and O_2 was repeated cyclically. When O_2 is fed, the catalyst undergoes forced oxidation. And the catalyst is forcedly reduced, when hydrocarbon is fed. This forced redox cycle may promote the sintering of catalyst under the reaction condition, leading to the rapid estimation of catalyst life. The method has been applied for the oxidation of C_2H_4 on a Cu/SiO_2 catalyst, and it has been shown that the deactivation in the periodic pulse technique was, at the maximum, ten times as fast as the continuous flow run (ref. 1).

In the present paper, the method has been applied to the oxidation of C_2H_4 on an Ag catalyst supported on silica gel. It has been said that the catalytic properties of Ag is quite sensitive to the pretreatment condition (ref. 4), which might be resulted in by the difference in morphology obtained by sintering (ref. 5). It is also reported that the sintering behavior is very sensitive to gas environment (ref. 6). These features of Ag catalysts will enable us to examine if the accelerated sintering occurs in the same way as the "real" sintering under the reaction condition.

EXPERIMENTAL

In the periodic pulse reaction, catalyst was exposed to O_2+N_2 mixture and to C_2H_4+N_2 mixture alternately, as shown by a diagram in Fig. 1. O_2+N_2 mixture was fed over the catalyst bed for a certain period of time (t_O, pulse width of O_2 pulse), and then C_2H_4+N_2 mixture was fed for another period of time (t_R, pulse width of C_2H_4 pulse). This alternate feed of O_2 and C_2H_4 was repeated cyclically. The period (t_p) is equal to the sum of the pulse

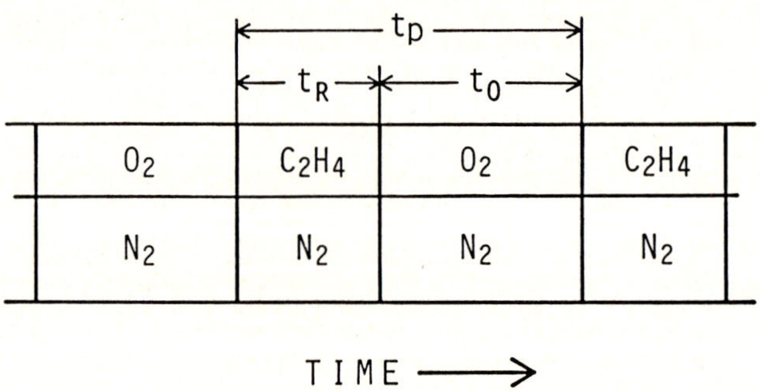

Fig. 1. Time diagram of periodic pulse technique.

widths, i.e., $t_p = t_0 + t_R$. Period 150+30s means the periodic pulse experiment of t_0 = 150s, t_R = 30s and t_p = 180s.

The reactor was a Pyrex glass tubing with an inside diameter of 10mm, at the center of which a Pyrex tubing with an outside diameter of 4mm was installed as a sheath for the thermocouple. Two reactors were installed in an electrically heated fluidized sand bath: one for the periodic pulse technique and another for the continuous flow reaction to monitor the change in experimental condition such as the bath temperature. Standard reaction condition was as follows; the catalyst weight was 2.00g, the reaction temperature was 473K, the flow rates of C_2H_4, O_2 and N_2 in the periodic pulse technique were 21.0, 21.0 and 79.0 cm^3/min, respectively, and the flow rates of C_2H_4 and O_2 in the flow reaction were halves of them. The continuous flow reaction under such a condition corresponds to the periodic pulse reaction of t_p = 0 (refs. 1,3).

The catalyst used in the present study was a supported Ag on silica gel, prepared by the impregnation of silica gel (ID-gel, Fuji-Davison) with an aqueous solution of silver nitrate and by the evaporation to dryness. The resulting materials was reduced in a flow of H_2 at 423K. Ag content was 13.4wt%.

Transmission electron micrograms of catalysts were taken with Hitachi H-800 electron microscope. Samples were prepared by embedding a catalyst particle in capsule containing Epon followed by polymerization and by ultrathin sectioning using a diamond knife on a LKB microtome. The electron microscope was operated at magnification of 100,000 and further magnification to about 150,000 was obtained by photographic enlargement.

RESULTS

Deactivation in Periodic Pulse Technique

Figure 2 shows the change of C_2H_4 conversion with time-on-stream. The open circles represent the results in the continuous flow reaction, in which a mixture of C_2H_4, O_2 and N_2 flowed continuously, and the time-on-stream represents the time elapsed since the run has started. On the other hand, in the periodic pulse technique, C_2H_4+N_2 mixture and O_2+N_2 mixture were fed alternately to give the forced redox cycle. The alternate feed of C_2H_4 and O_2 was interrupted several times a day, and a mixture of C_2H_4, O_2 and N_2 was fed continuously. The effluents of continuous feed of mixture were analyzed to measure the conversion of C_2H_4. The time-on-stream in the periodic pulse run does not involve the time for the continuous feed of the mixture, and, therefore, it represents the time for which the catalyst was subjected to the forced redox cycle.

As shown in Fig. 2, the conversion of C_2H_4 decreased faster in the periodic pulse experiment than the continuous flow reaction in accordance with the above-mentioned expectation. The rate of deactivation appeared to depend on the period. In 15+15s run, the conversion in the periodic pulse technique was essentially equal to that in the continuous flow technique, indicating no acceleration of deactivation. The deactivation in the periodic pulse technique became fast with increasing the period, but the deactivation rate seemed to decrease when the period increased further; the deactivation in 90+90s run was slower than that in 60+60s run.

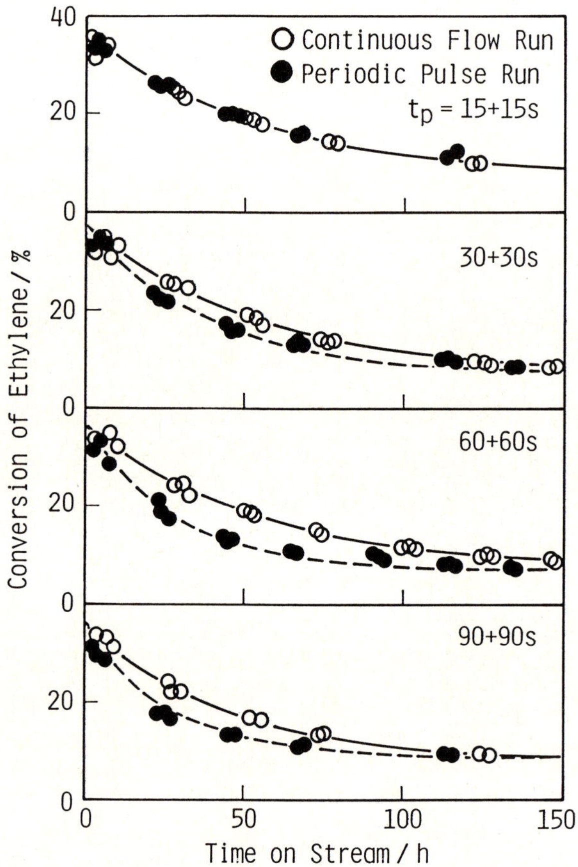

Fig. 2. Deactivation of Ag catalyst in periodic pulse run (closed circles) and in continuous flow run (open circles) at 473 K. Curves represent decay curves calculated from Equation (2).

Effect of Redox Ratio

Figure 3 shows the effect of the redox ratio on the rate of deactivation. As shown by the open circles, the deactivation was the fastest in a flow of a mixture of O_2 and N_2 which was interrupted several times a day and the oxidation of C_2H_4 was conducted to measure the catalytic activity. This run, referred to as O_2+N_2 run, corresponds to one of the periodic pulse runs of infinite pulse width. In another run corresponding to the infinite pulse width, a mixture of C_2H_4 and N_2 was continuously fed with several interruptions a day for the measurement of catalytic activity. This run, referred to as C_2H_4+N_2 run, gave the slowest deactivation, as shown by the open triangles.

The decay curves for the periodic pulse runs lay between the two extremes. The open squares represent the results in 60+60s run which gave the fastest deactivation among the periodic pulse runs of $t_O = t_R$ shown in Fig. 2. The run of t_O = 150s and t_R = 30s, referred to as 150+30s run, resulted in faster deactivation than that of t_p = 60+60s, while 30+150s run resulted in slower deactivation. After all, the deactivation seems to be faster in more oxidizing atmosphere. It should be emphasized that the decay curves in O_2+N_2 and C_2H_4+N_2 runs to approach the abscissa, but the others do not.

Figure 4 shows the change in the selectivity of ethylene oxide with time-on-stream. The results in the continuous flow runs lay in the hatched band; it increased steeply in the initial 20 hours and then it increased only

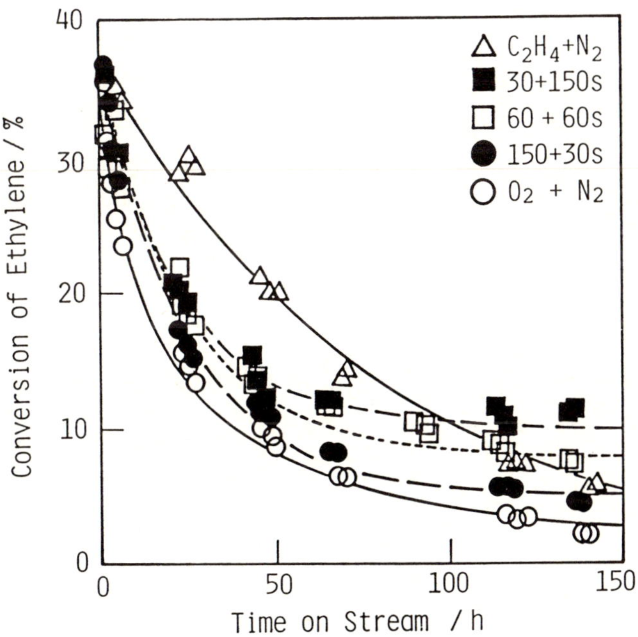

Fig. 3. Effect of redox ratio on the deactivation rate. Curves were calculated from Equations (1) and (2).

slightly. The periodic pulse runs of $t_O = t_R$ gave essentially the same results with somewhat larger scatter.

The redox ratio in the deactivation process also had a remarkable effect on the selectivity; the reducing treatment increased the selectivity and the oxidizing treatment decreased. The selectivity remarkably increased in $C_2H_4+N_2$ run, and the selectivity attained about 60% in 30+150s run. The periodic pulse run of t_p = 150+30s gave essentially the same selectivity as those in the continuous flow run and the periodic pulse run of $t_O = t_R$, and O_2+N_2 run resulted in the lowest selectivity.

The trend agrees well with the results reported by Nault et al (ref. 7). In their results, both of the activity and selectivity were higher after the pretreatment with C_2H_4 than that pretreated with O_2.

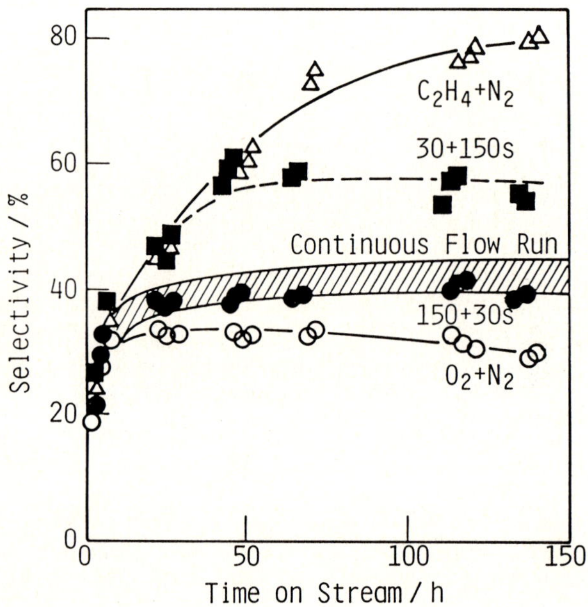

Fig. 4. Effect of redox ratio on the selectivity.

Growth of Ag Particles

Transmission electron micrograms (TEM) indicated that a few Ag particles were clustered together, and some of them were in contact with each other. But the clustered particles appeared to have the same distribution of particle size as that of homogeneously dispersed particles. In a histogram of the fresh catalyst shown in Fig. 5a, the highest peak was observed in the second lowest band of particle size, i.e., 3.3 to 6.7 nm, suggesting the presence of a large number of undetectable particles less than 3.3 nm. After the continuous flow reaction for 150 hours, the distribution was broadened and the highest peak in the histogram shifted to the range of 6.7 to 10 nm, indicating that the sintering occurred during the reaction. The periodic pulse runs, especially, the run with larger t_0 than t_R, resulted in the sintering to larger extent, and the C_2H_4+N_2 run and the O_2+N_2 run resulted in more extensive sintering. Mean particle size increased in the following order: fresh catalyst < continuous flow run < 60+60s run < 150+30s run < C_2H_4+N_2 run < O_2+N_2 run. (25 nm). This order of sequence agrees well with the order of deactivation rate except the deactivation in C_2H_4+N_2 run.

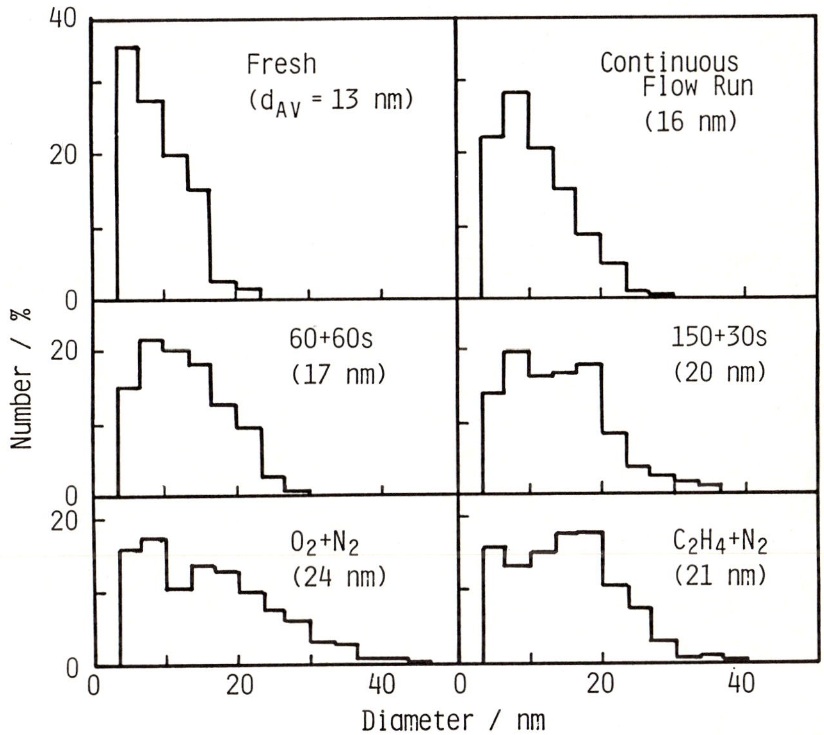

Fig. 5. Particle size distribution of fresh and deactivated Ag catalyst.

DISCUSSION

Rate Equation of Deactivation

A power law rate expression shown below is one of the most frequently used equations to describe the deactivation process:

$$-dA/dt = k_d \cdot A^n \qquad (1)$$

where k_d is a deactivation rate constant and A is a relative activity of catalyst (ref. 8). In the case of the deactivation of CuO/SiO_2 catalyst in the oxidation of C_2H_4, Equation (1) of n=3 could well describe the change of the conversion with time-on-stream in both the continuous flow and the periodic pulse runs (ref. 1).

In the present case, at first, it was attempted to apply Equation (1) to the results shown in Figs. 2 and 3, but only a poor fit was obtained. Then, another equation of the following form was applied:

$$-dA/dt = k_d \cdot (A-a)^n \qquad (2)$$

Equation (2) of n=1 fitted well the deactivations in both the continuous flow and the periodic pulse runs. But $C_2H_4+N_2$ run and O_2+N_2 run showed different deactivation behavior. Equation (1) of n=1 well fitted the former, and that of n=2 fitted the latter. The curves in Figs. 2 and 3 show the decay curves calculated from these equations.

Figure 6 shows the effect of the period on k_d calculated on the basis of Equation (2). k_d at t_p = 0 represent the rate constants in the continuous flow technique. It has been shown in the previous paper (refs. 1,3) that, when the period is extrapolated to zero, the periodic pulse technique

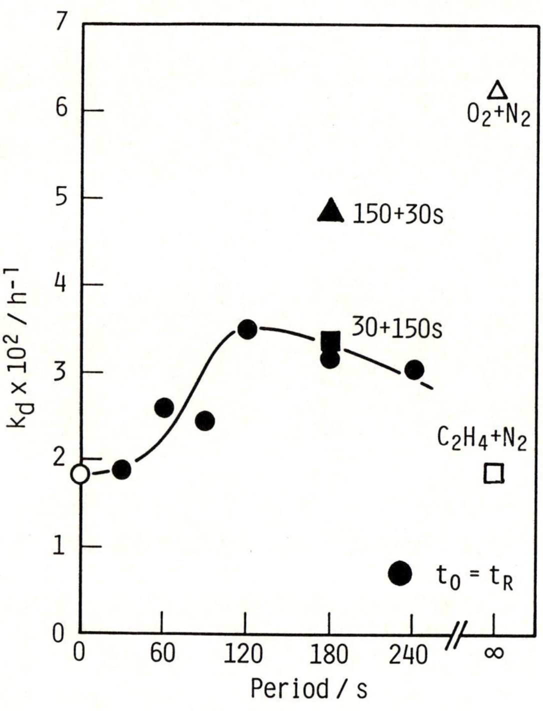

Fig. 6. Deactivation rate constant calculated from Equation (1).

coincides with the continuous flow technique in which the partial pressures of reactants are identical to the averaged pressure in the periodic pulse technique. k_d at infinite period represent the deactivation rate constants obtained in C_2H_4+N_2 run and in O_2+N_2 run. k_d for the latter shown in Fig. 6 was calculated from Equation (2) of n=1 for the comparison, though it gave only a poor fit.

In the periodic pulse runs of t_0 = t_R, the deactivation rate constant increased with the period, but further increase in the period was accompanied with the decrease in k_d. k_d for 30+150s run was almost identical to that for 90+90s run, but that for 150+30s run was significantly larger. C_2H_4+N_2 run resulted in k_d close to that for the continuous flow run, while k_d for O_2+N_2 run was the largest. This tendency agrees with that obtained by Presland et al (ref. 9). They reported that the sintering of a model Ag catalyst occurred in O_2 environment, but not in C_2H_4.

Sintering in Forced Redox Cycle

It has been reported that the sintering certainly affects the performance of Ag catalyst in industrial run (ref. 10). In the present case also, the deactivation can be regarded as a result of the sintering. TEM indicated that the sintering occurred during the continuous flow reaction and the periodic pulse run brought about more sintering, as shown in Fig. 5.

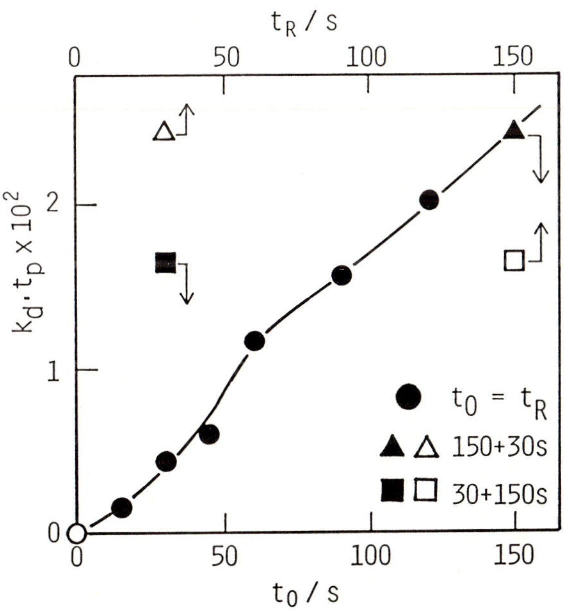

Fig. 7. Deactivation rate per period as a function of pulse width.

Many oxidation reactions proceed via a redox cycle, which brought about the microscopic rearrangement of the lattice of catalyst, at least, the lattice of surface. Although the rearrangement of the lattice occurs repeatedly, atoms or ions do not necessarily return to their initial position. They will move to occupy the thermodynamically stable position, which results in the sintering of catalyst. In the periodic pulse technique, the catalyst is subjected to the forced redox cycle. The longer period will cause the oxidation and reduction of catalyst with larger amplitude, and thus atoms will transfer longer distance in one redox cycle. This may result in the increase of k_d at small period. However, longer period is accompanied with smaller number of cycles in unit time, and it may result in the decrease in k_d at large period. Thus, the effect of the period may consist of two factors; the amplitude of redox cycle and the number of redox cycles. The latter effect can be ignored, when one consider the deactivation rate per period. Since the period is inversely proportional to the number of cycles, the deactivation rate per period is proportional to the product of k_d and t_p.

In Fig. 7, the deactivation rate per period, $k_d \cdot t_p$, was plotted against the width of O_2 pulse (lower abscissa) and that of C_2H_4 pulse (upper abscissa). When $t_0 = t_R$, the plot gave a gentle S-shaped curve, indicating that the rate of deactivation per period increased with increasing pulse widths. However, because $t_0 = t_R$, it is not clear which O_2 pulse or C_2H_4 pulse mainly affects the deactivation. The runs of 30+150s and 150+30s has been conducted to examine it. The results of 30+150s run did not fit the curve, even when it was plotted against either the width of O_2 pulse or that of C_2H_4 pulse. The selectivity of 30+150s run was significantly higher than that in the continuous flow run, as shown in Fig. 4. Since it has been said that the selectivity depends on the crystallographic plane and/or the morphology of Ag particles (ref. 5), higher selectivity suggests that the 30+150s run resulted in different morphology from that in the continuous flow run, or, in other words, the 30+150s run results in the different type of sintering. Thus, 30+150s run did not give any information about the problem.

In the case of 150+30s run, the plot of $k_d \cdot t_p$ against the width of O_2 pulse agreed well with the curve, while the plot against the width of C_2H_4 pulse did not agree. This suggests that the sintering occurs mainly when the catalyst is exposed to O_2. This is in agreement with the result that the fastest deactivation was obtained in O_2+N_2 run, as shown in Figs. 3 and 6.

Rapid Estimation of Catalyst Life

As mentioned above, the deactivation rate per period increases with the width of O_2 pulse, but long pulse width is accompanied by the long period, resulting in the decrease of the number of redox cycles. Thus, long period of O_2 pulse and short width of C_2H_4 pulse will result in fast deactivation. Actually, 150+30s run resulted in the fastest deactivation among the periodic pulse run, and O_2+N_2 run which corresponds to the extremely long width of O_2 pulse and short width of C_2H_4 pulse gave the fastest deactivation.

However, the deactivation in O_2+N_2 run appears to be too much accelerated. The deactivation rate could not be described well by Equation (2) of n=1 which fitted very well the deactivation under the reaction condition. This may indicate that O_2+N_2 run results in a different type of deactivation from the others. Furthermore, the selectivity in O_2+N_2 run was lower than the others. The difference in the selectivity may be indicative of the difference in the morphology of the catalyst, as mentioned above. One might suspect that low selectivity is due to highly oxidized state of Ag catalyst which has been treated in O_2+N_2 flow. But this is not the case, because the selectivity was not recovered even after by the prolonged reduction of catalyst with ethylene. After all, the accelerated sintering in O_2+N_2 environment can not be useful for the rapid estimation of catalyst life, even if the fastest sintering could be obtained. For such purpose, it is necessary to accelerate the sintering under the reaction condition.

In the periodic pulse run of t_p=150+30s which gave the fastest deactivation among the periodic pulse runs, the selectivity agreed well with that in the continuous flow run, and the equation which is identical to that for the continuous flow reaction fitted the deactivation rate. Thus, the sintering process in the run can be regarded as the "real" one under the reaction condition. Long O_2 pulse may accelerate the sintering and short C_2H_4 pulse may prevent the change in morphology of Ag crystallites, resulting in the acceleration of " real" deactivation. Thus, the periodic pulse technique with balanced redox ratio can be a useful tool for the rapid estimation of catalyst life.

CONCLUSION

For the rapid estimation of catalyst life, it is necessary to accelerate the deactivation under the reaction condition. Excess acceleration may bring about a different type of deactivation; the sintering of Ag catalyst was the fastest in O_2+N_2 environment, but the deactivation behavior was entirely different from that in the continuous flow reaction. The periodic pulse run with long O_2 pulse and short C_2H_4 pulse led to the "real" sintering under the reaction condition, which may enable the rapid estimation of catalyst life.

ACKNOWLEDGMENT

This work was partially supported by a Grant-in-Aid for Scientific Research (No. 58550644) and for Encouragement of Classroom Teachers (No. 60918036) from the Ministry of Education, Science and Culture, Japan.

REFERENCES

1 S.Komai,T. Hattori, A. Miyamoto and Y. Murakami, J. Catal., submitted, T. Hattori, S. Komai, A. Miyamoto and Y. Murakami, Proc. World Congr. III Chem. Eng., IV (1986) 350.
2 S.Komai, T.Hattori, A. Miyamoto and Y. Murakami, Chem. Lett., (1983) 1749.
3 M. Niwa and Y. Murakami, J. Catal., 26 (1972) 359, 27 (1972) 26, T. Hattori, T. Hori, M. Maeda, M. Ii and Y. Murakami, J. Japan Petrol. Inst., 23 (1980) 158.
4 J.C. Wu and P. Harriott, J. Catal., 39 (1975) 395.
5 X.E. Verykios, F.P. Stein and R.W. Coughlin, J. Catal., 66 (1980) 368.
6 S.R. Seyedmonir, D.E. Strohmayer, G.J. Guskey, G.L. Geoffroy and M.A. Vannice, J. Catal., 93 (1985) 288.
7 L.G.Nault, D.W. Bolme and L.N. Johanson, Ind. Eng. Chem., Process Des. Dev., 1 (1962) 285.
8 S. Szepe, and O. Levenspiel, Chem. React. Eng., Proc. Eur. Symp., 4th, Pergamon, London, p265, 1971.
9 A.E.B.Presland, G.L.Price and D.L. Trimm, J. Catal., 26 (1972) 313, Surface Sci., 29 (1972) 424, 435.
10 G.L.Montrasi, G.R. Tauszik, M. Solari and G. Leofanti, Appl. Catal., 5 (1983) 359.

B. Delmon and G.F. Froment (Editors), *Catalyst Deactivation 1987*

"STOPPED-FLOW DESORPTION" ANALYSIS OF THE NATURE OF STRONGLY ADSORBED SPECIES DURING n-BUTANE OXIDATION IN A FLOW REACTOR

G. BUSCA[1], G. CENTI[2] and F. TRIFIRO'[2]

[1]Istituto Chimico, Facoltã Ingegneria, Fiera del Mare Pad. D, Genova (Italy).

[2]Dipartimento di Chimica Industriale e dei Materiali, Viale Risorgimento 4, 40136 Bologna (Italy).

ABSTRACT

The presence and the evolution as a function of time of strongly adsorbed species during n-butane oxidation in a flow reactor was studied by "stopped-flow desorption" experiments and by thermogravimetric and Fourier-transform infrared analyses on a $(VO)_2P_2O_7$ catalyst highly active/selective in the conversion of n-butane to maleic anhydride. In particular, the presence of an adsorbed species was found which desorbs as crotonaldehyde only at temperatures around 100 K higher than the reaction temperature (573 K). The parallel increase in the amount of this species formed with the change in catalytic behavior (a decrease in the rate of n-butane depletion with a parallel increase in the rate of maleic anhydride formation) suggests that due to the reduced turnover number, the formation of strongly adsorbed species causes catalyst deactivation by site blocking, but at the same time allows controlled reactivity of the surface which prevents the consecutive oxidation of maleic anhydride to carbon oxides.

INTRODUCTION

Obtaining an understanding of the real working state of catalyst surfaces has become a frontier of heterogeneous catalysis. In particular, it has been shown that in several cases strongly adsorbed species, i.e. organic molecules-surface complexes with turnover numbers lower than that of intermediates of reaction, are present during steady-state conditions (1). However their role in surface modifications associated with deactivation phenomena is not a well investigated area of research. Coking phenomena and deactivation related aspects are well documented (2), but in this case the hydrogen-deficient carbonaceous residues that form may not be correctly interpreted as strongly adsorbed species and basically they overlie the active sites, physically blocking access of the reactants to the active sites.

In previous studies on the selective conversion of C_4 hydrocarbons to maleic anhydride on VPO catalysts (3-6) we noted (i) a substantial worsening of the catalytic performances when a pulse reactor method was adopted and (ii) a significant loss of carbon balance in the tests with pulse reactor. Similar features also have been found by other authors (7-9). Furthermore, in a recent infrared study of n-butane interaction with PVO catalysts (10), the presence of adsorbed species whose amounts increase with the time of exposure under reaction conditions was observed, suggesting that they are not intermediates, but rather probably strongly adsorbed species. All these effects suggest the idea that strongly adsorbed species also may be present on the surface of $(VO)_2P_2O_7$ (the active phase in n-butane oxidation to maleic anhydride (11,12)) during steady-state oxidation in a flow reactor and that a substantial change in the working state of the catalyst surface may derive from this effect.

In order to better characterize the nature and evolution of strongly adsorbed species as well as their implication in the change of catalytic performances we have adopted the "stopped-flow desorption" method of analysis .This technique (called hereinafter SFD) consists in the gas chromatographic analysis of the products of thermal desorption from a catalyst subjected to a rapid switching from flow steady-state catalytic conditions to those for the desorption. This technique allows (i) a quali-quantitative analysis of the products formed by desorption from a catalyst surface operating in steady-state flow conditions, (ii) characterization of the variation in the adsorbed species vs. the time on stream of the catalyst and (iii) information to be obtained on the energetics of the adsorbate-surface interaction based on the range of desorption temperatures.

EXPERIMENTAL

Catalyst preparation. Thirty grams of V_2O_5 were suspended in a 1:2 benzyl/isobutyl alcohol mixture (0.6 L); after 5 h under boiling, the slurry was cooled to 298 K and 99% o-H_3PO_4 added in order to obtain a P:V=1.1 atomic ratio. The mixture then was heated to boiling for 2 h and the resulting solid, filtered, washed, dried, and activated at 670 K in a flow of 1% n-butane in air for 12 h. After the activation both XRD and IR analyses indicated the presence of only the $(VO)_2P_2O_7$ active phase in the catalyst (11-13).

SFD apparatus. Figure 1 shows a schematic scheme of the apparatus and the gas flow distribution used for SFD and steady-state (SS) experiments. In the (A) configuration the system operates in the usual SS reaction conditions with gas chromatographic analyses of the reaction products through the six-way valve (n.7). The valve is placed in an oven maintained at 500 K in order to avoid condensation of the reaction products. In order to simplify the reading of the scheme, analogo-

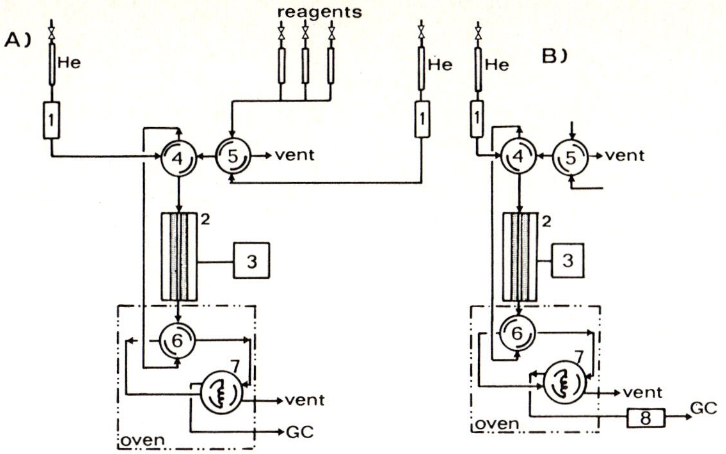

FIG. 1 Scheme of the apparatus used for SS and SFD experiments : detail of gas flow distribution during steady-state (SS) studies (A) and during "stopped-flow desorption" (SFD) studies (B).

us valves for the analysis of reagent composition and of permanent gases (O_2,N_2, CO and CO_2) are omitted.

The first gas chromatograph (GC) utilized a flame ionization detector and a Porapak QS column. The second GC operate instead with a thermoconducibility detector and a Carbosieve-II column. For both GC the carrier gas was deoxygenated helium. The reactor consisted of a stainless steel tube (ϕ=4 mm) placed in a Cu bar in which the heating elements were inserted. The latter were controlled by a linear temperature programmer which read the reactor temperature through an axial thermocouple placed in the catalytic bed. 0.5-0.7 grams of sample were used. The reagent composition was 1.3% n-butane, 16.7% O_2 with the remaining part He.

After attainment of SS catalytic behavior at the chosen reaction temperature (usually 573 K), an equal flow of deoxygenated He instead of the reagent mixture was sent to the reactor through four-way valve number 5, in order to purge the line and also to remove weakly adsorbed species from the catalyst surface. After this time, through contemporaneous switching of the four-way valves numbers 4 and 6, the reactor was placed directly on line to the gas chromatograph. The substances that desorb from the catalyst surface were cut off from the He stream in the cold trap (n. 8). The trap usually consisted of a small portion of the same GC column utilized for the separation, maintained at low temperature; the temperature was rapidly raised immediately before analysis of the trapped products. If only the valve n. 4 is switched , the same apparatus may be used for TPD experiments; the products formed are analyzed through valve n. 7 as a function of the desorption temperature. On the contrary, using configuration (B), the system may be used also as a pulse reactor, if the cold trap is not maintained at low temperature. In general, we adopted the following sequence for SFD experiments : I) the catalyst was maintained for 4 h in the reagent mixture stream with periodic testing of the catalytic behavior, II) the He flow was sent to the reactor by switching valve n. 5, and after 5 min, valve n. 4 and n. 6 were switched, thus connecting the reactor on line to the GC column, III) under isothermal conditions (the same of reaction, usually 573 K) the products of desorption were concentrated in the cold trap for 2 h and after this time analyzed after rapid heating of the cold trap, IV) upon completation of the GC analysis, the trap was again cooled and the reactor temperature increased to 720 K. Finally, the products collected in the cold trap in this second part of the experiment were analyzed.

Fourier-transform infrared (FT-IR) and thermogravimetric (TG) experiments. Self-supporting disks were used for infrared examination with a Nicolet MX-1 Fourier-transform spectrometer . The infrared cell was connected with conventional gas manipulation and evacuations ramps (13).

Thermogravimetric tests were carried out in a flow system using a Perkin-Elmer TG-2 computer controlled apparatus; 4 mg of activated $(VO)_2P_2O_7$ were usually used for the tests.

RESULTS

SFD experiments. Reported in Table I are the amounts of the principal products of thermal desorption obtained from the catalyst surface after attainment of steady-state (SS) catalytic behavior in n-butane oxidation at 573 K. The data refer to products collected (a) after isothermal conditions (573 K) and (b) after a consecutive heating of the reactor up to 723 K still under He flow.

TABLE I Main products (except carbon oxides) found during desorption in a deoxygenated He stream after SS catalytic tests in n-butane oxidation (T=573 K).

Desorption conditions	Products of partial oxid., moles$\times10^7$/$g_{cat.}$				
	CA*	AC*	MA*	CR*	PH*
(a) isothermal, 2 h§ at 573 K	1.6	0.5	5.1	-	-
(b) heating up to 723 K after step (a)	-	0.4	0.5	4.3	1.7

Notes on Table I :
(*) C4: C4 hydrocarbons (mainly butadiene); AC: acetic acid and acetaldehyde; MA: maleic anhydride; CR: crotonaldehyde: PH: phthalic anhydride and acid.
(§) After the initial 5 min treatment, in order to purge the line and to remove weakly adsorbed species; see experimental part.

TABLE II Main products(except CO_x) found during desorption in a deoxygenated He stream after SS catalytic tests in butadiene oxidation (T=573 K).

Desorption conditions	Products of partial oxidation, moles$\times10^7$/g_{cat} CA*	FU*	CR*	MA*	PH*
(a) isothermal, 2 h§ at 573 K	25.2	2.1	0.1	9.8	0.1
(b) heating up to 723 K after step (a)	0.6	0.1	27.7	1.5	8.1

(*) C4: butadiene; FU: furan; CR: crotonaldehyde; MA: maleic anhydride; PH: phthalic anhydride and acid.
(§) see note on table I.

Two main considerations derive from this Table : 1) A significant amount of adsorbed species is present on the surface of the catalyst working in SS conditions, which is not removed with the preliminary treatment (5 min in helium flow - see experimental part). Assuming a mean surface coverage of 20×10^{-20} m^2 for one adsorbed molecule, the total amount of adsorbed species would cover 1-2% of the surface area of the catalyst . 2) In respect to the products formed in the SS oxidation, in addition to carbon oxides, maleic anhydride and low yields of acetic acid, significant amounts of butadiene in the case (a) and of crotonaldehyde and phthalic anhydride in the case (b) also were observed. A more close examination of the temperature at which the different substances desorb indicates that the C4 hydrocarbons (mainly present as butadiene), furan and maleic anhydride desorb at the lower temperatures, in the 573-623 K range. At higher temperatures, in the 643-683 K range, crotonaldehyde and phthalic anhydride desorb.

The same substances were observed when the products of desorption were analyzed after reaching SS catalytic behavior in butadiene oxidation to maleic anhydride (Table II). The main differences lie in the general higher amount of all the products of desorption and, in particular, of the C4 hydrocarbons at the lower temperatures and again of crotonaldehyde at the higher temperatures of desorption. Furthermore, as compared to n-butane, significant amounts of furan also were detected. These data show the higher degree of interaction of butadiene with the catalyst surface as compared with n-butane, and the substantial ana-

TABLE III Main products (except CO_x) found during desorption in He stream after 8 pulses of 2.1% hydrocarbon in He at 573 K (6.95×10^{-6} total moles of hydrocarbon sent) (tests in the absence of O_2). Desorption by heating up to 723 K.

Hydrocarbon	Products of oxidation, moles$\times10^8$/g_{cat}				
	CA*	FU*	MA*	CR*	PH*
n-butane	1.2	0.1	0.6	6.3	0.3
butadiene	13.1	1.1	1.0	12.8	1.7

(*) See note on table II.

logy of the reaction mechanism.

Crotonaldehyde also is the principal product of desorption as seen when the catalyst surface was analyzed after some pulses at 573 K of only n-butane in He (Table III). Although the amounts of the desorption products were higher, similar results were found also using butadiene instead of n-butane in the tests in the pulse reactor in the absence of gaseous oxygen. These data indicate that the formation of crotonaldehyde as a product of desorption occurs both in the presence and the absence of gaseous oxygen in the inlet reagent mixture and furthermore confirm the strict analogy in the results with the two hydrocarbons.

Reported in Figure 2 are the activity and the selectivity in n-butane oxidation to maleic anhydride as a function of time on stream in a flow reactor in the presence of gaseous O_2. Before the catalytic tests, the catalyst was conditioned with the following procedure : (a) holding for 6 h at 573 K in a flow of n-butane/air, (b) removal of strongly adsorbed species from the catalyst surface by heating up to 723 K in a deoxygenated He stream inside the reactor, (c)

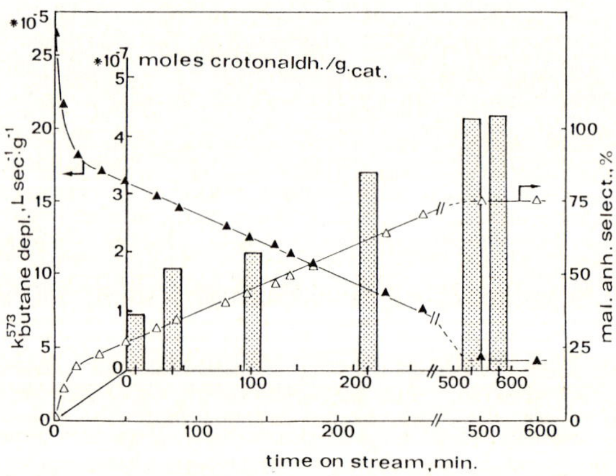

FIG. 2 Effect of time on stream at 573 K on the first order rate constant of n-butane depletion and on the selectivity to maleic anhydride in a flow reactor and on the amount of crotonaldehyde found in parallel SFD experiments.

bringing the temperature to 573 K still under the He stream. After this pretreatment, the n-butane/air reagent mixture was sent to the catalyst and the changes in catalytic behavior against time on stream were followed. Parallel experiments were done in order to determine the amount of strongly adsorbed species on the catalyst surface as a function of time on stream. Also reported in figure 2 is the amount of crotonaldehyde found in these SFD experiments. Comparable behavior in the change of catalytic activity/selectivity and in the amount of strongly adsorbed species was found in the SFD tests, in particular for the crotonaldehyde. Thus the adsorbed complex that desorbs at high temperature as crotonaldehyde seems to have a central role in the modification of the reactivity of the catalyst.

Thermogravimetric tests. The increase in weight of the catalyst at 573 K in a flow of 1% n-butane, 11% O_2 and 87% He in shown in Figure 3. The pretreatment of the catalyst in case (A) was the same used for the tests of Figure 2 [(a) reaching SS conditions at 573 K, (b) desorption at 723 K in He flow, (c) bringing the temperature of catalyst once again to 573 K in a He flow]. In the

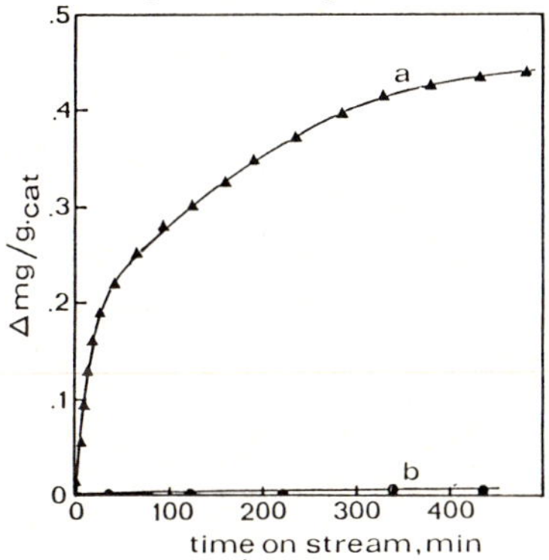

FIG. 3 Effect of time in TG tests (1% n-butane, 11% O_2 , 87% He flow) on weight increase for the $(VO)_2P_2O_7$ catalyst after the high temperature (723 K) (A) or low temperature (573 K) (B) pretreatments (see text).

case (B) (Fig. 3) only the (a) step of the pretreatment was done. It is shown that in the case of higher temperature pretreatment (A), the weight of the catalyst increases reaching constant weight after about 6 h, in good agreement with the data reported in Figure 2. This effect is not present in the case (B) where the high temperature treatment was not done. The overall weight increase is around three times higher than that deduced from the SFD experiments (Table I) showing that there is a significant contribution to the weight increase by weakly adsorbed species.

Fourier-transform infrared spectra. The presence of adsorbed species may be confirmed by infrared spectroscopy. The spectrum (a) obtained in the 1300-2200 cm^{-1} region after interaction at 573 K with butadiene (150 torr for 10 min) and subsequent evacuation at the same temperature is shown in Figure 4. The spectrum of $(VO)_2P_2O_7$ evacuated ($P<10^{-5}$ torr) at 573 K (spectrum b) has been subtracted from spectrum (a). The interaction of butadiene with the catalyst leads to the formation of one or more species characterized by an intense band centred near 1620 cm^{-1}, two shoulders at higher frequencies (1715 and 1770 cm^{-1}) and by a broad absorption centred at 1420 cm^{-1}.

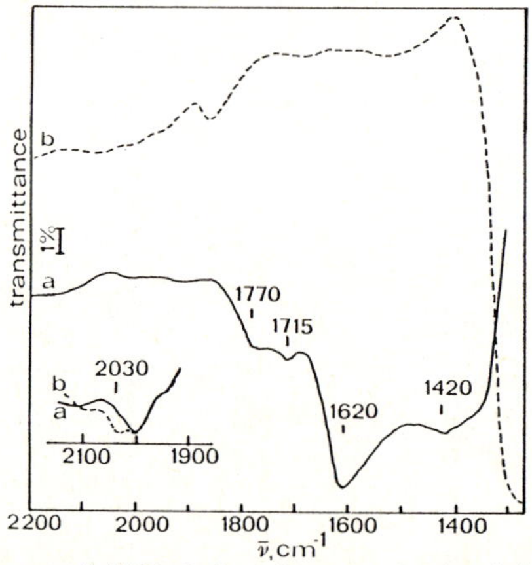

FIG. 4 (a): spectrum of $(VO)_2P_2O_7$ after contact with butadiene (10 min at 573 K) and subsequent evacuation at the same temperature . Spectrum (b) has been subtracted from spectrum (a).
(b): spectrum of $(VO)_2P_2O_7$ evacuated at 573 K.

An unambiguous attribution is difficult. It is worth noting, however, that the interaction with butadiene leads to the disappearence of a weak band near 2030 cm^{-1} attributed (14) to the first overtone of $\nu V{=}O$. The same spectrum of adsorbed species may be obtained by interaction of n-butane with the catalyst in the same conditions as for butadiene (Fig. 5); however, in this case the intensity of the adsorbed species is much lower. Both for n-butane and butadiene, the adsorbed species disappear by evacuation only at temperatures higher than 673 K. The spectrum does not correspond to adsorbed maleic anhydride or other anhydrides, whose characteristic bands at 1785 and 1860 cm^{-1} ($\nu_{C=O}$ in anhydrides) appear only in the presence of O_2. Taking into account (i) the disappearence of the $2\times\nu V{=}O$, (ii) the analogy of the spectra from n-butane and butadiene, (iii) the results of the SFD experiments and (iv) the analogy with the spectrum of adsorbed furan [main band in this region at 1740(w), 1710(w), 1600(vs), 1550(w)

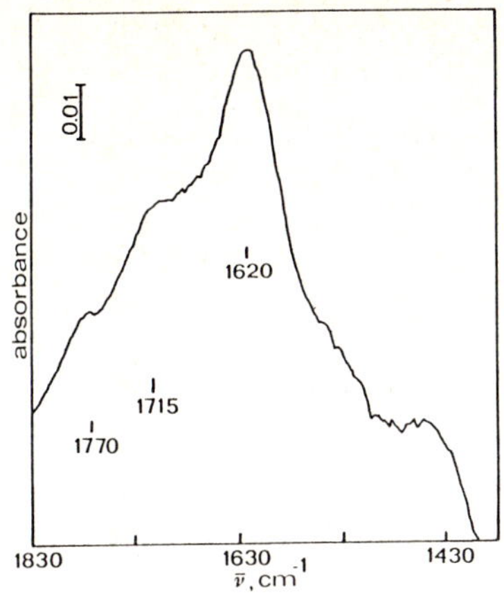

FIG. 5 Spectrum of $(VO)_2P_2O_7$ after contact with n-butane (10 min at 573 K) and subsequent evacuation at the same temperature. The spectrum of $(VO)_2P_2O_7$ evacuated at the same temperature has been subtracted from this spectrum.

1486(w), 1380(vs) cm^{-1}, the bands can be attributed to combinations of ring vibrations (15) - with respect to furan, the strong band at the lower frequencies is not present in the spectra reported in fig.s 4 and 5], a possible interpretation of the adsorbed species is based on the following reaction scheme:

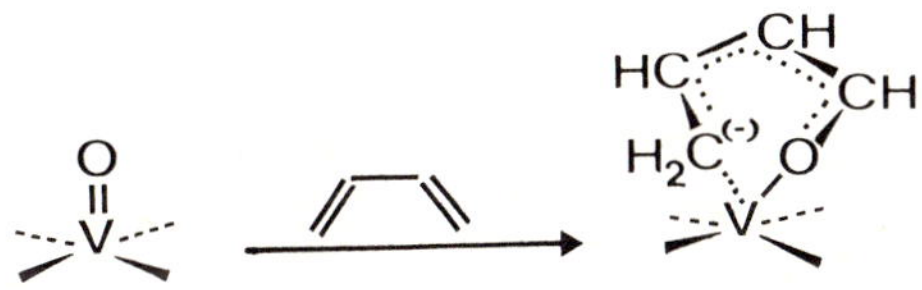

At high temperature in the absence of O_2 this species may desorb as crotonaldehyde through hydrogen transfer from terminal carbon atoms.

Reported in Figure 6 is the variation of the intensity of the band at 1620 cm^{-1} and of the two shoulders at 1725 and 1770 cm^{-1} as a function of the time of exposure during FT-IR tests with butadiene at 573 K. The intensities of the three bands increase as time in contact with butadiene increases, suggesting that they are not due to an intermediate but rather to a strongly adsorbed species (in agreement also with the high temperature of thermal desorption). The variation of the band intensities agree well with the variation of strongly adsorbed species previously observed with the other techniques in the presence of gaseous O_2 (Fig.s 2 and 3), although the kinetic rate of formation is slighly lower in the presence of O_2. Furthermore the parallel change of the three bands suggests that they are all due to the same intermediate.

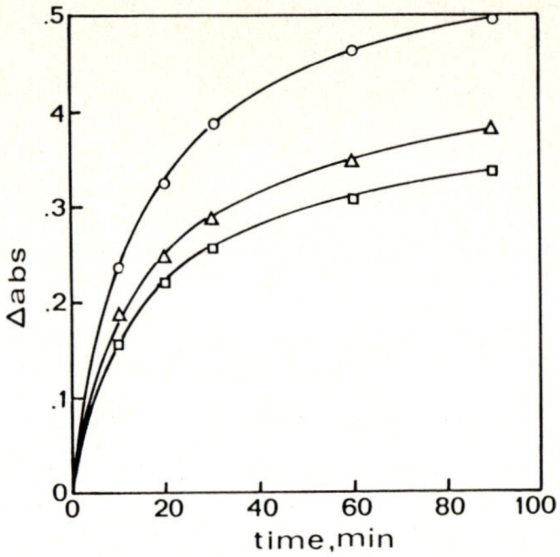

FIG. 6 Variation of the intensity of the infrared bands at 1620 cm^{-1} (○), at 1715 cm^{-1} (△) and at 1770 cm^{-1} (□) as a function of time in contact with butadiene at 573 K.

DISCUSSION

As shown in Figure 2, during steady-state oxidation of n-butane the $(VO)_2P_2O_7$ catalyst works in a partially deactivated state, even though the selectivity to maleic anhydride increases as deactivation increases. If, after steady-state conditions have been reached, the strongly adsorbed species are removed by thermal desorption, the same variation of activity/selectivity vs. time on stream is found, showing that this effect is not due only to surface oxidation. In correspondence to the change of the surface reactivity, the SFD, TG and FT-IR experiments showed the formation of strongly adsorbed species, whose amounts increased at the same time as the change in catalytic behavior, indicating the strong relationship between the two phenomena. These strongly adsorbed species that desorb only at temperatures higher than the reaction temperature form both in the presence and the absence of gaseous oxygen. The most significant product of desorption in the SFD tests is the crotonaldehyde, which is not a reaction product in the case of n-butane and forms only with low yields from butadiene. Phthalic anhydride, on the contrary, is probably a product of secondary reactions, such as the Diels-Alder reaction of butadiene with adsorbed maleic anhydride followed by dehydrogenation. In fact, phthalic anhydride, even if in low amounts, is found also in butadiene oxidation to maleic anhydride and in traces from n-butane. FT-IR experiments, furthermore, evidence that in the absence of gaseous oxygen, anhydrides do not form; probably only one strongly adsorbed species is formed (as shown by the increase as a function of time) that thermally desorbs at the same temperatures found for crotonaldehyde in SFD experiments (around 673 K). This adsorbed species can be considered as an adsorbed precursor of crotonaldehyde which forms through a specific reaction of V=O double bonds with butadiene, an intermediate also in the mechanism from n-butane. In agreement, the same adsorbed species is found also from n-butane. This species is very stable, as shown from the high temperature of desorption, suggesting that its turnover number is probably very low. Thus the formation of this strongly adsorbed species prevents or limits the reactivity of the vanadium site, inducing a deactivation by site blocking. On the other hand, this phenomenum allows the control of the surface reactivity itself preventing overoxidation of reaction products and increasing the productivity to maleic anhydride.

In conclusion, all the present data suggest that the real working state of the $(VO)_2P_2O_7$ surface in steady-state conditions differs from that of the discharged catalyst. Strongly adsorbed species, and in particular an adsorbed precursor of crotonaldehyde, are present in these conditions. Their reduced turnover number induces catalyst deactivation by site blocking, but at the same time allows a controlled surface oxidation power deriving from this deactivation mechanism, finally leading to an increase in the formation of maleic anhydride.

ACKNOWLEDGEMENTS

This work was realized with the financial support from the Ministero Pubblica Istruzione (Rome, Italy).

REFERENCES

1 B.E. Koel, G.A. Somorjai, In "Catalysis - Science and Techn." Vol. 7; J.R Anderson, M. Boudart Eds.; Springer-Verlag Berlin 1985; p. 159.
2 E.E. Wolf, F. Alfani, Catal. Rev. -Sci. Eng., 24 (1982) 613.
3 F. Cavani, G. Centi, F. Trifirò, A. Vaccari, In "Adsorption and Catalysis on Oxide Surfaces"; M. Che and G.C. Bond Eds.; Elsevier Pub. Amsterdam 1985; p. 287.
4 F. Cavani, G. Centi, F. Trifirò, Appl. Catal., 15 (1985) 151.
5 F. Cavani, G. Centi, I. Manenti, F. Trifirò, Ind. Eng. Chem. Prod. Res. Dev., 24 (1985) 221.
6 L. Morselli, F. Trifirò, L. Urban, J. Catal., 75 (1982) 112.
7 M.A. Pepera, J.L. Callahan, M.J. Desmond, E.C. Milberger, P.R. Blum, N.J. Bremer, J. Am. Chem. Soc., 107 (1985) 4883.
8 V.A. Zazhigalov, Yu.P. Zaitsev, V.M. Belousov, N. Wüstnek, H. Wolf, React. Kinet. Catal. Lett., 24 (1984) 375.
9 S. Szukacs, W. Wolf, G. Mink, I. Bertoti, N. Wüstnek, B. Lücke, H. Seeboth, Proceedings 1st Symposium "New Developments in Selective Oxidation", Louvain

la Neuve, March 1986.
10 R.W. Wenig, G.L. Schrader, J. Phys. Chem., 90 (1986) 6480.
11 G. Busca, F. Cavani, G. Centi, F. Trifirò, J. Catal., 99 (1986) 400.
12 G. Centi, F. Trifirò, Chim. Ind.(Milan), 68 (1986) 74.
13 G. Busca, G. Centi, F. Trifirò, V. Lorenzelli, J. Phys. Chem., 90 (1986) 1337.
14 G. Busca, J.C. Lavalley, Spectrochim. Acta, 42A (1986) 443.
15 C. Pouchan, J. Raymond, H. Sauvaitre, M. Chaillet, J. Molec. Struct., 21 (1974) 253.

B. Delmon and G.F. Froment (Editors), *Catalyst Deactivation 1987*

CATALYST DEACTIVATION STUDIES BY MEANS OF A CONCENTRATION-CONTROLLED RECYCLE REACTOR

A. LÖWE and U. TANGER

Institut für Technische Chemie der TU Braunschweig, Hans-Sommer-Str. 10, D-3300 Braunschweig, FRG

ABSTRACT

A concentration-controlled recycle reactor is described. It was used to investigate methanation over a Ni-based catalyst at 30 bar and 320 °C. Methanation was confirmed to proceed via a triangular reaction network consisting of hydrogenation steps for carbon monoxide and carbon dioxide, and the water gas shift reaction. By adjusting partial equilibrium for the latter step in some experiments, the rates of the individual reactions could be derived. These rate data were utilized to study in particular (i) separability of the kinetics of the individual reaction steps, (ii) activity and selectivity changes with time on stream, and (iii) some more qualitative features felt to be of general interest.

INTRODUCTION

Adjusting the feed rate to a gradientless recycle reactor so as to maintain conversion over a decaying catalyst constant enables the experimentalist to uncouple concentration and activity effects upon the reaction rate (ref. 1). This basic concept has been extended to multiple reactions, and appropriate control strategies have been developed (ref. 2). Particularly important is the possibility to investigate whether the kinetics of a reaction is separable or not (refs. 3-4).

When it has proved that the kinetics of a reaction is separable or can at least be treated as separable in the concentration and temperature region of interest, reaction as well as deactivation kinetics are much easier to model. Therefore any kinetic investigation of a reaction system should start with tests for separability. In the following it will be described how such tests may be performed, not only for single reactions but also for reaction steps in a reaction network.

TEST FOR SEPARABILITY

By its very definition, separability of a catalytic rate equation means that the activity

$$a = \frac{r(\underline{c}=\underline{c}_k,\ T=T_k,\ t=t_u)}{r^0(\underline{c}=\underline{c}_k,\ T=T_k,\ t=0)} \tag{1}$$

must be independent of the concentration vector $\underline{c}_k$ and the temperature T_k applied to measure the initial rate r^0 and the rate r after a definite time on stream, t_u, or more generally spoken at any activity state of the catalyst. Only in this case the complete rate equation $r(\underline{c},T,h)$, which takes into account the history (h) of the catalyst sample, can be written in the separated form

$$r = r^0(\underline{c},T)\cdot a(h) \tag{2}$$

(see ref.1). It should perhaps be pointed out that $(\underline{c},T)$ in eqn. 2 should be read as "function of $\underline{c}$ and T", whereas ($\underline{c} = \underline{c}_k$ etc.) in eqn. 1 means "measured at $\underline{c}_k$ etc.".

With a single reaction, a test for separability appears most simple: At any activity state of the catalyst, e.g. after some time on stream (in principle under arbitrary conditions), the rate should be measured at several conditions of concentrations and temperature and related to corresponding rate values measured at t=0 under the very same conditions of $\underline{c}_k$ and T_k. This may be repeated at several different activity states.

Finding the activity **a** independent of the applied conditions $\underline{c}_k$ and T_k indicates separable kinetics. Choosing the reference time t=0 may be a subtle problem (see ref. 5); usually the first contact between the catalyst sample and the reaction gas mixture will be chosen.

Adjustment of the same gas compositions at t=0 and at any other activity state is best done by means of a concentration-controlled recycle reactor. Performing a sufficient number of experiments at a given activity state so as to decide safely about separability in view of some inevitable experimental scatter will not always be possible, particularly at the beginning of a run where deactivation may often occur too rapidly. (Even with "rapid" deactivation, the mean residence time in the recycle reactor must be slow compared with the time constant of the deactivation process so that quasi-steady state conditions always prevail.) In such cases, some modifications of the basic method just outlined should be developed. For example, when the deactivation rate is concentration-independent, activity data obtained in an isothermal run at different activity states may be grouped to give an activity-time curve for each composition $\underline{c}_k$. If these smoothing curves agree closely, the kinetics is separable, otherwise it is not. This procedure would give reliable results also with concentration-dependent deactivation rates provided that the concentration effect is not too strong and, what is more important, the different compositions are adjusted in turn as frequently as possible.

With multiple reactions where the number of reactions (nr) exceeds the number of independent stoichiometric relationships (ns), tests for separability are more difficult to perform. In principle, unless nr ≥ 2·ns, the activities $\mathbf{a}_j$ of the individual reaction steps of a network can be evaluated from a sufficient number of concentration-controlled experiments; some simulation studies have shown, however, that unusual accuracy of the experimental data is required to give reliable results (ref. 6). If the network contains reversible steps, then the method of partial equilibrium offers the chance to uncouple the network and measure rates and activities of individual steps independently of each other. This method has been applied in the present work.

EXPERIMENTAL

Reaction system

Subject of the present studies was the catalytic methanation of synthesis gas. According to Fig. 1, three reaction steps should be considered in a mixture of CO, H_2, CO_2, H_2O, and CH_4 reacting over a typical supported Ni catalyst. It will become clear from the following how concentration-controlled experiments have contributed to establish the triangular network of Fig. 1.

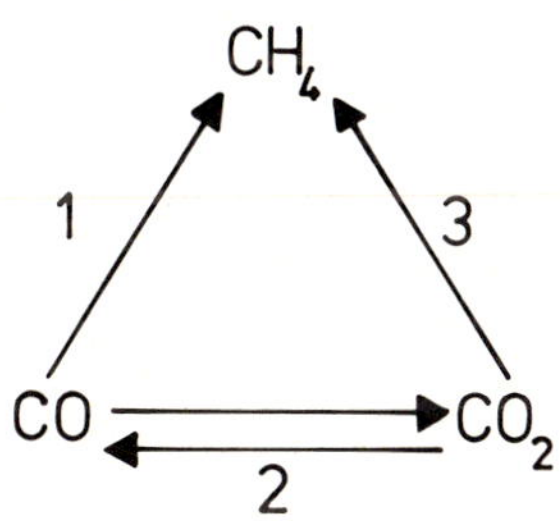

Fig. 1. Reaction network.

Apparatus

A scheme of the concentration-controlled recycle reactor used for the present deactivation studies performed at 30 bar and 320 °C is shown in Fig. 2. Its main parts are the gas feeding system, the reactor itself, the gas analysis system, and the computer-aided control system. The individual gaseous reaction

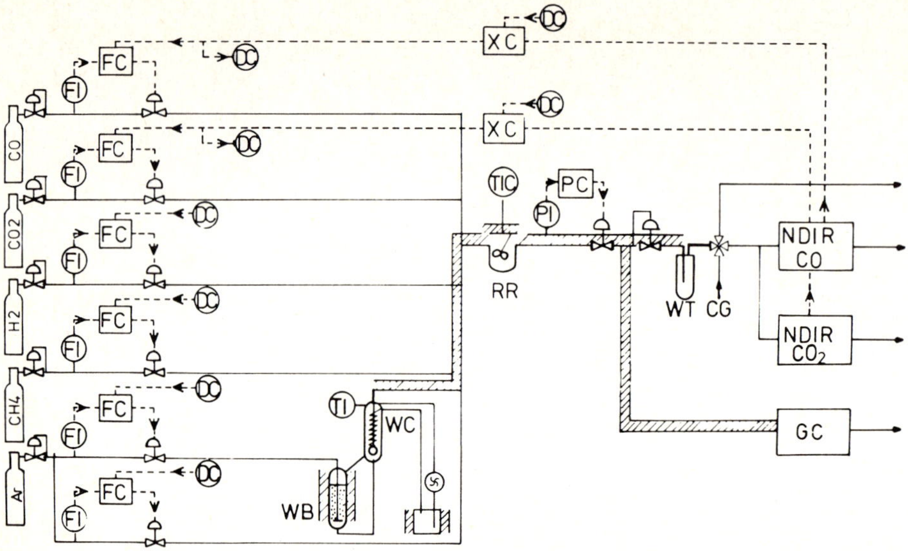

Fig. 2. Experimental set-up
DC desk computer, WB water bubbler, WC water condenser, RR recycle reactor, WT water trap, CG calibration gas.

components were fed by means of thermal mass flow meters (VI) and mass flow controllers (VC). The flow controllers for CO and CO_2 were cascaded by analogue PI-controllers (XC) in feedback circuits, the set points of which were calculated from the preselected composition within the reactor by the process computer (DC) for each experiment and transferred via D/A converters. The set points for the flow controllers (FC) of the other components were computed on-line both from the measured x_{CO}- and x_{CO_2}-values and the stoichiometry of the reaction system as detailed in ref. 2. Water vapour was fed by bubbling a controlled part of the inert gas stream Ar through a saturator system maintained at an appropriate temperature, as may be seen from the figure.

For operation up to at least 30 bar and 500 ^{o}C, a self-designed reactor with internal recycle was used (ref. 7). Its main difference to similar reactors of this type is that the magnetic clutch for driving the turbine is located in a water-cooled housing away from the hot reactor. For this reason it was possible to use common material for bearings and magnets.

CO and CO_2 were continuously measured with non-dispersive infra-red analyzers (NDIR), their values being used for the feedback control loops as mentioned above. The values were also used as external standards for GC analyses of the whole gas mixture including H_2O, which were performed from time to time in order to check the prescribed composition; it should be noted that no other products, particularly no higher hydrocarbons were detected by these analyses.

A desk computer stored the calibration curves for the flow meters and gas analyzers as well as the whole experimental program to be run. It registered all measured concentrations, flows, temperatures etc., computed set points and transferred them to the analogue controllers as mentioned above. The digital processing considerably improved the accuracy of the data.

Catalyst

If not otherwise noted, experiments were performed with a Girdler's G65-type catalyst, a Ni/Al_2O_3 catalyst with some 25% Ni content; its main commercial application is in the purification of NH_3 synthesis gas. Some experiments were performed with a commercially available catalyst for SNG production from CO-rich synthesis gas. In the experiments, crushed material with particle diameters between 0.18 and 0.20 mm were used to avoid any pore diffusional effects. The oxidic form of the catalysts was reduced in situ with 20% H_2 in Ar. The temperature was increased from room temperature to 450 ^oC with a rate of 80 $^oC/hr$, remained there for about 2 hrs, and was then decreased to 250 ^oC, the whole procedure being performed under full computer control.

Procedure

During an actual experimental run at a desired temperature, an experimental program consisting of 30 to 50 experiments at different gas compositions was repeated several times. At least 30 experiments were part of such a program, 17 of which were in accordance with a 2^4-factorial plan including a center point. A further 13 experiments were planned where two concentrations were varied at a time, while the remaining ones were held at a center point. The constraint for this second "factorial plan" was that the equilibrium conditions for the shift reaction (step 2 in Fig. 1)

$$x_{H_2} \cdot x_{CO_2}/(x_{CO} \cdot x_{H_2O}) = K_2 \tag{3}$$

had to be fulfilled in each experiment. Additional compositions were established mainly by varying the mole fractions of CO and H_2. In preliminary runs, the influence of CH_4 had been found to be negligible in the concentration range of the experiments shown in Table 1; its concentration was therefore fixed at 15% in all runs.

The two center points served as reference conditions, which were adjusted many times in order to follow the decaying activity of the catalyst. In the sequel they are referred to as center point 1 and center point 2.

It lasted about 5 minutes until the feedback and feedforward control loops

TABLE 1

Concentration range of the individual components

CO:	0.5 - 4.0 mol-%
CO_2:	0.8 - 4.0 mol-%
H_2:	2.0 - 20 mol-%
H_2O:	1.5 - 3.5 mol-%
CH_4:	5.0 - 25 mol-%
Ar:	balance

had adjusted a new gas composition in the reactor. A steady state however was reached only after some 20 minutes in most cases, most probably because of slow responses in the adsorption layer of the catalyst. Separate experiments with a microbalance have shown that indeed the catalyst needs considerable time to adapt its surface coverage to changes in the surrounding gas atmosphere. A steady state in the strict sense was of course never reached, because deactivation continued to occur all the time. The computer accepted quasi-steady state conditions, when the drift of the Ar carrier gas stream for H_2O, being the most sensitive variable, had fallen beneath a prescribed small value for a prescribed time. Then the computer stored all relevant data, read a new composition from a program file, and started the next experiment.

RESULTS AND DISCUSSION

Rates and activities

In accordance with the network in Fig. 1, evaluation of all experiments was based upon the following two independent mass balances:

$$f \cdot x_{CO} - f^{o}_{CO_2} = - r_1 - r_2 = R_{CO} \tag{4}$$

$$f \cdot x_{CO_2} - f^{o}_{CO_2} = - r_3 + r_2 = R_{CO_2} \tag{5}$$

where f is the total exit molar flow rate per mass of catalyst, f^o is the molar feed rate per mass of catalyst of the indicated component, x is mole fraction, and $r_2 = r_2$(forward) - r_2(back) denotes the net rate of the shift reaction. It may easily be seen from these equations that if partial equilibrium for step 2 has been established in the recycle reactor, i.e. when r_2 vanishes, the rates r_1 and r_3 can be calculated, since all quantities on the left hand sides are measurable.

Results for step 3 at the center point 2 are presented in Fig. 3 as an ac-

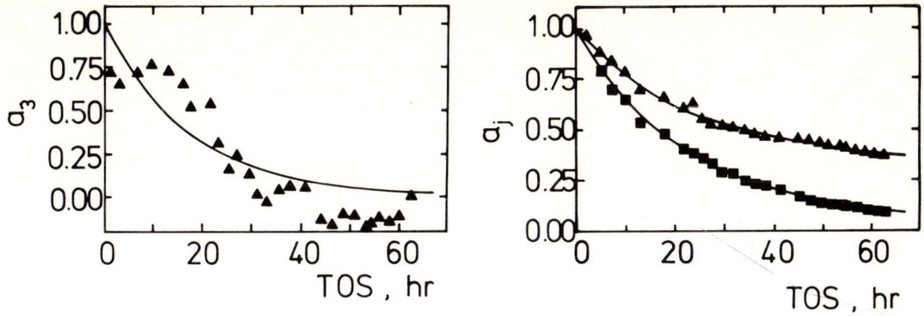

Fig. 3. Activity vs time on stream (TOS)
left: center point 2; rigth: center point 1, ■ a_1, ▲ a_2.

tivity-time plot. As the rate of step 3 is slow, the relative error in r_3 is large causing considerable scatter. Nevertheless, a complete rate equation of the form

$$r_3 = k_r \cdot x_{CO_2} \cdot \exp(-k_d t) \tag{6}$$

could be satisfactorily fitted to the r_3-data. Eqn. 6 was used to purge component rate data, R_{CO} and R_{CO_2}, measured outside equilibrium conditions of step 2, from contributions of step 3 so as to obtain rate data r_1 and r_2. Since r_3 contributed only about 10% to the methanation rate R_{CH_4}, r_1 was not markedly affected by inaccuracies of eqn. 6. Rate data for step 2, however, are stronger influenced, espesially for conditions near equilibrium, where r_2 is small itself and therefore prone to larger relative errors. Nevertheless, in sufficient distance from equilibrium, r_2-data look quite reliable. This may be seen from the right graph in Fig. 3, where the rates of steps 1 and 2 at the center point 1 are plotted in an a-t diagram.

The qualitative behaviour of the reaction system represented by Fig. 3 has been found in numerous runs, at 320 ^{o}C as well as at somewhat lower and higher temperatures. In all cases, the rate of step 3 decayed more rapidly than the rates of the other two steps; also, the slight selectivity change between steps 1 and 2 was observed in all runs.

When the different distances from equilibrium of the steps are properly taken into account, the catalyst is as active for step 2 as for step 1.

Over catalyst 2 no direct hydrogenation of CO_2 was observed; its activity for the shift reaction was roughly 20% of its methanation activity.

Separability

Separability of the rate equation for r_3 (eqn. 6) was assumed but could not be proved, whereas tests for separability for steps 1 and 2 were performed as outlined above: All rate data obtained with the same composition during a run were smoothed by fitting the integral deactivation equation

$$r_{jk} = r^{o}_{jk}\cdot(1 - k_{1jk}\cdot(1 - \exp(- k_{2jk}t))) \tag{7}$$

by means of the parameter r^{o}_{jk}, k_{1jk}, and k_{2jk}; here again the subscript k denotes all experiments with the same composition. In its differential form, eqn. 7 resembles a special case of a deactivation rate law as proposed in ref. 8, that makes allowance for a residual activity, $\mathbf{a}_{ss}$:

$$- \dot{\mathbf{a}} = k_d\cdot(\mathbf{a} - \mathbf{a}_{ss}) \tag{8}$$

While for step 1 all activity data $\mathbf{a}_{1k} = r_{1k}/r^{o}_{1k}$ fall close to a common regression line as may be seen from Fig. 4, the $\mathbf{a}_{2k}$-data lie within a rather broad band. For the sake of clarity, the results for only three different compositions including the center point 1 are shown in Fig. 4; the two outer curves span the range of all activity data of the run. The solid lines in Fig. 4 represent the regression equation 7. At present we have no explanation to offer why step 1 obeys separable kinetics while step 2 does not.

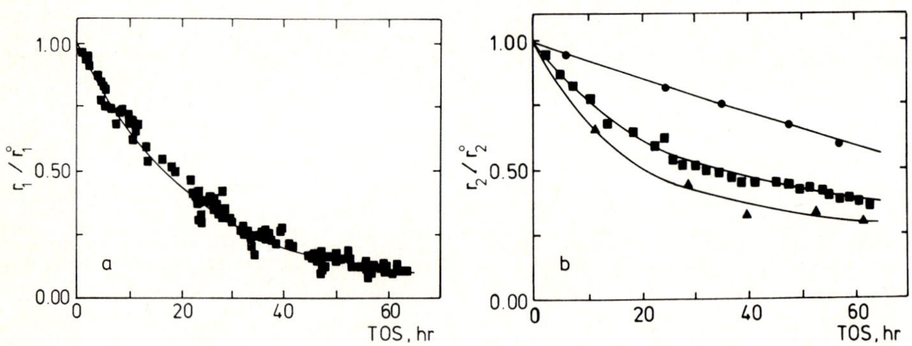

Fig. 4. Activity vs time on stream (ref. 9)
left: ■ all gas compositions; right: ■ center point 1,
● ▲ two different gas compositions.

So far the question of separability has been restricted to concentration effects. Deactivation was too rapid and the response of the reactor to temperature steps too slow to include different temperature levels in the experimental program. There is strong evidence, however, that at least in the small temperature interval between 300 and 330 ^{o}C a_1 is also independent of temperature while a_2 is not. This was concluded from the observation that the temperature dependence of step 1 remains constant with decaying activity, while the overall activation energy of step 2 drops to about half its initial value (ref. 9).

Influence of gas concentrations upon the deactivation rate

By its very definition, separable kinetics means that the activity **a** does not depend on the present measuring conditions. The next question to discuss is whether **a** depends on past conditions of concentrations (and temperature in the general case), i.e. whether the deactivating process is concentration-dependent or not. The **a**-t curves presented so far should be related to some mean composition of the experimental program; the time intervals between two experiments (some 20 minutes on the average) were long enough to sometimes cause slight but noticeable decay, but too short to reveal any concentration effect.

Some time ago deactivation runs of the kind presented here had been performed at very similar conditions except for the total pressure, which was only 1 bar (ref. 10). At this low pressure, no deactivation could be detected at all. Hence the partial pressures have a strong effect when varied about more than one order of magnitude. However, even within the much smaller range of the present conditions, a concentration effect could be detected. The lower curve in Fig. 5 shows the results of a run with catalyst 2, where for the first three hours no hydrogen was fed to the recycle reactor, and hydrogen production in the reactor was counteracted by a high CO_2 level. Then, at the point marked by a full square, the usual experimental program was started. The single square

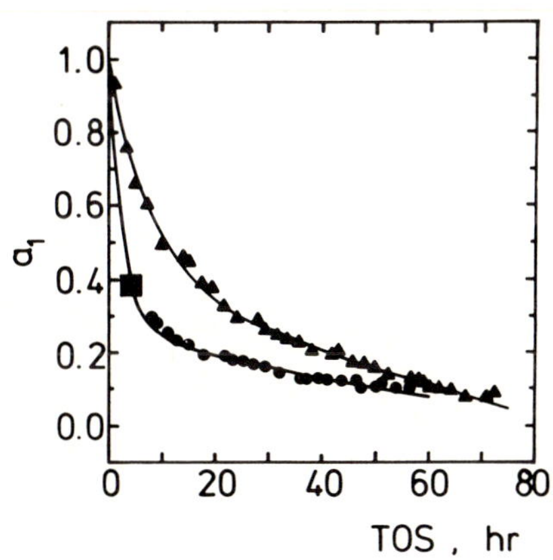

Fig. 5. Activity vs time on stream for catalyst 2
● ▲ center point 1; lower curve: no H_2 feed up to ■ .

and the following full circles represent the activity a_1 at the center point 1, as do the full triangles for a usual run.

The results presented here for step 1 are in qualitative agreement with those reported in the literature: The deactivation rate of step 1 increases with the partial pressure of CO and with decreasing H_2/CO ratio. Despite this agreement regarding the concentration effect, the underlying mechanism may be quite different for different Ni catalysts. For example, in refs. 11-12 growth of Ni cristallites via carbonyls is proposed. For catalyst 2 of the present study, we found only slightly increased cristallites. Instead fouling occurred by less than 1 weight-% of carbonaceous deposits. These deposits could be removed by hydrogen treatment at elevated temperatures, whereby the initial activity could be restored to some 60%. Similar results are reported in ref. 13.

Particle size effect

As mentioned above, catalyst 2 was a commercially available catalyst for SNG production from synthesis gas. Its short life of only about two days under typical methanation conditions is therefore somewhat surprising at a first glance. There is experimental evidence, however, that at very similar reaction conditions larger pellets remain at least one order of magnitude longer active. A qualitative reasoning is as follows: With particles as small as 0.1 to 0.2 mm in diameter, methanation occurs in the kinetic regime. (Avoiding any diffusional effects was in fact an absolute prerequisite for the present measurements, above all to ensure that equilibrium of step 2, when adjusted in the gas phase, existed throughout the whole catalyst particle.) With larger particles, the CO concentration may drop to such small values towards the particle's interior that deactivation ceases to occur any longer. In addition, the CO de-

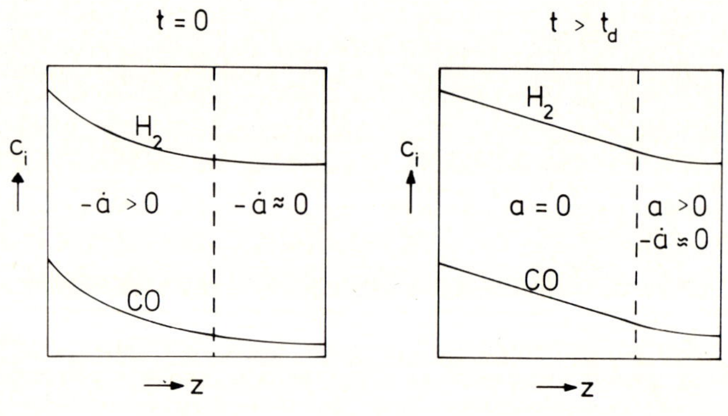

Fig. 6. Concentration profiles in a catalyst particle (schematic)

crease will be supported by an increase of the H_2/CO ratio. Then, after some time on stream, (t_d in Fig. 6), a large particle would consist of an inactive outer shell and a core that would remain active for a rather long time. This is shown in Fig. 6 in a qualitative manner. Very recently, Christoph and Baerns (ref. 11) have presented detailed calculations regarding this point.

SUMMARY AND CONCLUSIONS

The main intention of the present study was to develop the method of concentration-controlled experiments in recycle reactors and to apply it to a multiple reaction system. It could be shown that concentration control will be of considerable value to treat some crucial questions of any kinetic investigation, for example, which reaction steps do actually occur and whether their kinetics is separable or not. The right answer to these questions is thought to be an extremely important prerequisite for all subsequent modelling work on reaction and deactivation kinetics for a particular system.

Though catalytic methanation served mainly as a test system for the methodical approach, some specific results are thought to be quite interesting. (i) The method of partial equilibrium applied to this system revealed the occurrence of three reaction steps (Fig. 1) over a particular catalyst. The contributions of the shift reaction and of the direct hydrogenation of CO_2 may vary from catalyst to catalyst. (ii) The rates of the three steps decayed differently with time on stream, or, in other words, a selectivity change of the catalyst was observed. (iii) Moreover, and most important, step 1 could be shown to obey separable kinetics, while the kinetics of the shift reaction proved non-separable. (A statement about step 3 was not possible.) Selectivity as well as the different behaviour regarding separability should be a challenge for more mechanistically oriented research work.

Under usual reaction conditions, the dominating step of the network is of course the CO-methanation step. Some features of its deactivation kinetics were highlighted and found to be in qualitative agreement with the main body of the vast literature.

A more detailed kinetic modelling of reaction and deactivation could doubtless be supported and facilitated by concentration-controlled experimental strategies. Even then considerable experimental effort would be required, which seems best devoted to specific applications.

REFERENCES

1 O. Levenspiel, J. Catal. 25 (1972) 265-272.
2 A. Löwe, Ind. Eng. Chem. Fund. 19 (1980) 160-166.
3 A. Löwe, Ger. Chem. Eng. 4 (1981) 106-112.
4 A. Löwe, Chem. Eng. Sci. 37 (1982) 944-945.

5 S. Szepe and O. Levenspiel, Proc. 4th European Symposium on Chemical Reaction Engineering, Brussels, Belgium, September 9-11, 1968, Pergamon Press, Oxford, 1971, pp. 265-274.
6 A. Löwe and R.J. Cantaro, Chem.-Ing.-Tech. 58 (1986) 439.
7 U. Tanger, Doctoral Thesis, TU Braunschweig, 1984.
8 G.A. Fuentes, Appl. Catal. 15 (1985) 33-41.
9 A. Löwe and U. Tanger, Chemical Engineering and Technology, in press.
10 A. Löwe and R. Krokoszinski, Chem.-Ing.-Tech. 52 (1980) 809-811.
11 R. Christoph and M. Baerns, Chem.-Ing.-Tech. 58 (1986) 494-496.
12 W. Lommerzheim and K. Hedden, Proc. 1st International Gas Research Conference, Chicago, Illinois, June 9-12, 1980, pp. 704-721.
13 H.H. Gierlich, M. Fremery, A. Skov and J.R. Rostrup-Nielsen, in B. Delmon and G.F. Froment (Editors), Catalyst Deactivation, Elsevier, Amsterdam, 1980, pp. 459-469.

B. Delmon and G.F. Froment (Editors), *Catalyst Deactivation 1987*

PROMOTER DEACTIVATION OF PLATINUM GROUP METALS PROMOTED CRACKING CATALYSTS

P. STEINGASZNER, A. SZÜCS and L. MÉRI

Department of Chemical Technology, Technical University of Budapest
H-1521 Budapest, Budafoki u. 8. (Hungary)

ABSTRACT

The physical and chemical factors influencing the regeneration improving promoter function of platinum group metals containing cracking catalysts have been investigated. Promoter function was characterized by the carbon monoxide conversion activity of the catalyst preparations. Commercial catalysts showed characteristic differences upon thermal and hydrothermal treatments. Transition metals - nickel, iron and vanadium - reduced the carbon monoxide conversion activity in different ways. Sulphidation by hydrogen sulphide treatment did not affect the regeneration activity , while sulphur dioxide, derived from sulphur containing coke, caused reversible poisoning

INTRODUCTION

Catalytic cracking units are very important in the refining industry, since they convert heavier feedstocks (heavy gas oils, residua) into more valuable fractions, such as high octane gasoline, LPG and distillate fuel.

The feed is introduced into the reactor of the cracking unit mixed with hot, regenerated catalyst, during that cracking cycle coke is deposited on the catalyst. The coke formed has to be removed in the regenerator by burning. Highly efficient regeneration is very important with regular channel structure zeolite cracking catalysts, where a coke level of 0.1 by weight, or less on the regenerated catalyst is imperative.

Proper coke removal can be effected by high temperature regeneration (ref. 1), by two-step regeneration (ref. 2) and/or by the use of coke oxidation improvers incorporated into the catalyst or by adding coke oxidation improvers in a concentrated form to the catalyst (refs. 1, 3-6).

Oxidation promoters belong to the class of platinum group metals, their presence in ppm amounts, related to the catalyst, makes a practically complete oxidation of coke possible leading to higher gasoline yields, lower carbon monoxide emission, etc.

Cracking catalysts are exposed during their lifetime within the cracking unit to repeatedly changing thermal and hydrothermal effects, and, additionally metals from the feed - nickel, vanadium and iron are deposited on them. Further, sulphur compounds, mainly as thiols and hydrogen sulphide in the cracking reactor and sulphur oxides in the regenarator influence their catalytic activity (refs. 1, 7, 8).

The aim of the investigations reported in the present paper was the determination of the effects of these factors on the carbon monoxide conversion activity of platinum metal promoted cracking catalysts.

EXPERIMENTAL

Regeneration behaviour of cracking catalysts and effectiveness of oxidation improvers is tested either by determining the carbon monoxide/carbon dioxide ratio in the flue gas of a batch regeneration experiment with the coked catalyst (ref. 1), or by measuring the carbon monoxide conversion of a carbon monoxide and oxygen containing gas led over the catalyst under specified conditons (refs. 5, 9). In the present work this latter method has been used by introducing a gas stream, containing 2 % by volume of carbon monoxide in air into an electrically heated upflow isothermal quartz reactor, at a flow rate of 30 liters/hour, using 6,2 ml catalyst samples in the reactor. The CO-content of the feed gas as well as that of the effluent from the reactor has been measured by means of infrared gas analyzers.

Catalyst samples have been stabilized by heating the catalyst for 2 hours at 500 ^{o}C in air and then pretreating at 500 ^{o}C for 30 min. with air containing 2 % of CO by volume. Measurements with the same batch of the catalyst have been carried out at different temperatures, and the curves of CO-conversion plotted against the temperature have been used for the characterization of the CO-burning activity. The measured CO-conversion was corrected by substracting the CO-oxidation activity of the empty reactor at the same temperature.

TABLE 1

Data of the catalysts used

Catalysts	A	B	C
Chemical composition, % by wt.			
Al_2O_3	28.0	46.8	32.0
Na_2O	0.20	0.25	0.70
Fe	0.08	0.76	0.35
Physical properties			
Apparent bulk density (g/ml)	0.53	0.84	0.85
Pore volume (ml/g)	0.50	0.27	0.19
Surface area (m^2/g)	390	122	200

Industrial fluid cracking catalysts from three different manufacturers have been used, containing oxidation improvers of unspecified concentration. Data of the catalysts are summarized in Table 1.

Thermal treatment has been carried out at 700 ^{o}C for 3 hours in air. Hydrothermal effects, occuring during the catalytic cracking have been simulated by treating the catalyst at 750 ^{o}C for 6 hours with 100 % steam. In order to test the effect of transition metals on the regenerability, catalyst B has been impregnated with aqueous solutions of $Ni(NO_3)_2$, $Fe(NO_3)_3$ and NH_4VO_3 to different metal concentration levels, dried at 120 ^{o}C for 3 hours and calcined at 700 ^{o}C for 3 hours.

RESULTS AND DISCUSSION

Effect of thermal and hydrothermal treatment

Figure 1. shows the carbon monoxide conversion vs. temperature curves for the catalysts investigated. The samples tested were the following:

- fresh catalysts A_F, B_F and C_F
- equilibrum catalysts A_E and B_E, obtained from industrial fluid catalytic cracking units
- thermally treated catalysts A_T, B_T and C_T
- hydrothermally treated catalysts A_H, B_H and C_H

where subscripts F, E, T and H refer to fresh, equilibrum, thermally and hydrothermally treated catalysts, respectively.

Figure 1 shows that different promoted catalysts behave differently on hydrothermal and thermal treatment. With catalyst A the equilibrium form A_E is much more active than the fresh catalyst A_F whereas the equilibrated catalyst B_E is less active than fresh catalyst B_F. The CO-conversion activity of fresh catalyst B_F is improved by thermal treatment and even more by hydrothermal treatment. Similarily, the CO-conversion activity of fresh catalyst A_F is increased by thermal treatment, even more by hydrothermal treatment whereas equilibrium catalyst A_E shows the highest activity. Catalyst C shows opposite trends as both thermal and hydrothermal treatment decreases its CO-converting activity considerably.

Effect of transition metals

Equilibrum cracking catalysts contain a certain amount of transition metals (nikkel, iron and vanadium) deposited on the catalyst surface from the feed, containing metals in the form of organic complexes. Usual levels of this metals on the equilibrum catalysts vary from a few hundred up to several thousand ppm, depending on the feedstock processed (refs. 7, 10, 11). Transition metals, being dehydrogenation catalysts have a disadvantageous impact on the product composition, enhancing coke make and hydrogen

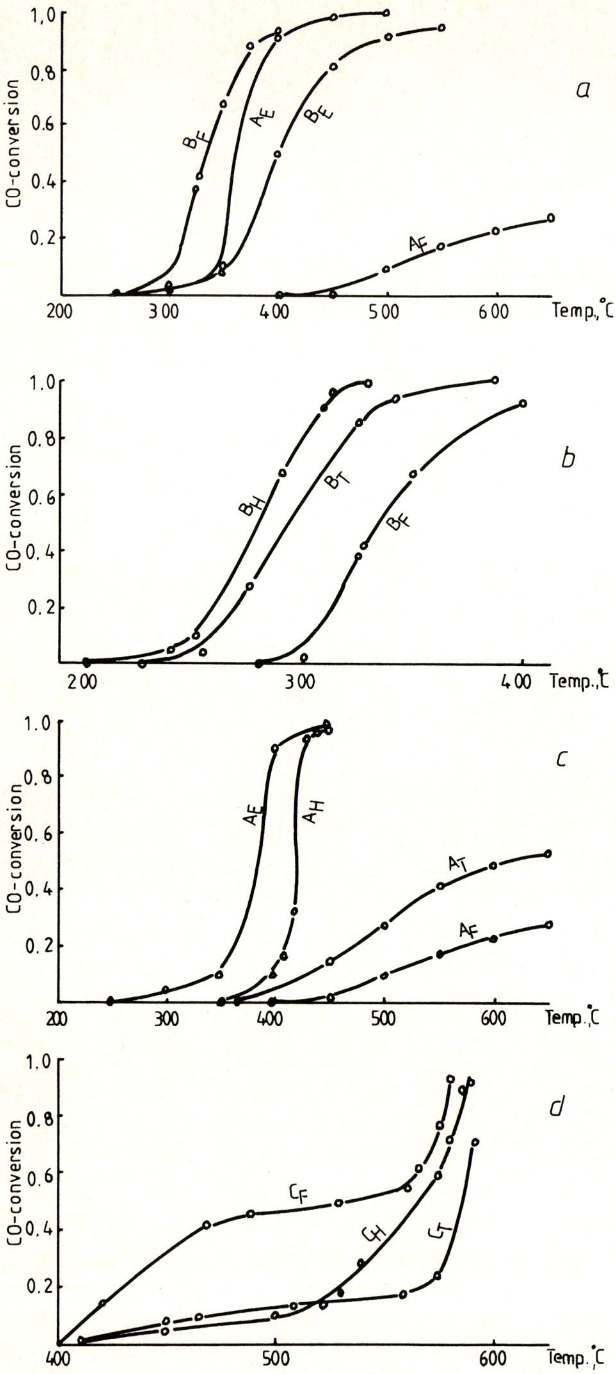

Fig.1. Carbon monoxide conversion vs. temperature with fresh, equilibrum, thermally and hydrothermally treated cracking catalysts

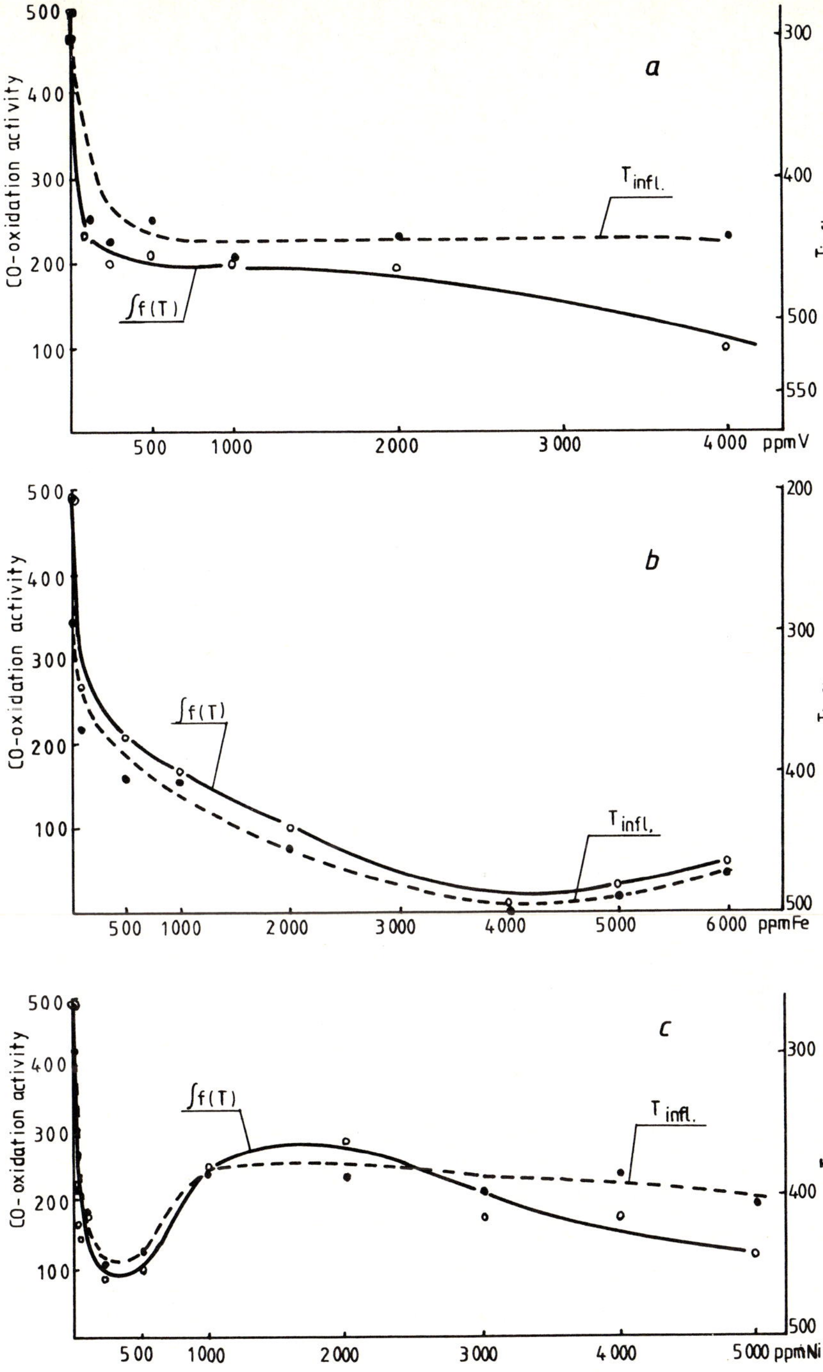

Fig.2. Influence of different transient metals on the regeneration behaviour of the promoted cracking catalyst B

production, decreasing conversion and gasoline yield (ref. 7). In some cases, transition metals may enhance the regenerability of cracking catalysts (ref. 12), but there is hardly any information on the effect of these metals on the regeneration behaviour of promoted cracking catalyst and on the interaction of the promoter and the transition metals content.

Experimental data prove that the carbon monoxide conversion activity of promoted catalysts decreases with increasing transition metal content in a way specific to the transition metal in consideration and especially at high transition metal contents these samples show modest carbon monoxide conversion even at high temperatures. In order to compare the effect of transition metal poisoning, two empirical evaluation methods have been used. CO-oxidation activities were expressed by integrating the CO-conversion curves over a selected temperature interval and the areas divided by the length of the interval. These values are plotted in function of the transition metal content of the catalysts on Figure 2, points are connected with a solid line. Inflexion points of the CO-oxidation vs. temperature curves were also determined and plotted on Figure 2 and points were connected with a broken line.

Lines of Figure 2 show that both evaluation methods yield similarly shaped curves with characteristic maxima or minima at the same metal content.

Figure 2/a shows that in the case of vanadium, CO-oxidation activity sharply drops with the first few hundreds ppm of metal loading and from there on activity further declines slightly with increasing metal content, up to cca 4000 ppm.

Figure 2/b shows a much more gradual decrease for iron, however promoted catalyst samples containing cca 4000 ppm of iron loose their activity completely. Increasing the iron content up to 6000 ppm, activity slightly increases.

As shown on Figure 2/c, nickel behaves completely differently from the other transition metals: CO-oxidation activity sharply declines up to cca 350 ppm of nickel content, then rises again up to 1500-2000 ppm of nickel content, where it reaches a maximum then it declines slightly.

Effect of sulphur compounds

Feedstocks of catalytic cracking usually contain several thousand ppm (0.3-1.0 % by weight) of sulphur, in form of organic compounds. In the cracking reactor, these compounds are partially converted to coke, and in the oxidizing atmosphere of the regenerator are converted to sulphur oxides.

In order to test the effect of sulphur compounds on the activity of the promoter, promoted cracking catalyst B_F had been exposed to 5000 ppm H_2S in hydrogen gas stream at 490 ^{o}C for 1 hour and then its CO-oxidation activity has been checked. The catalyst did not show any change in the CO-conversion

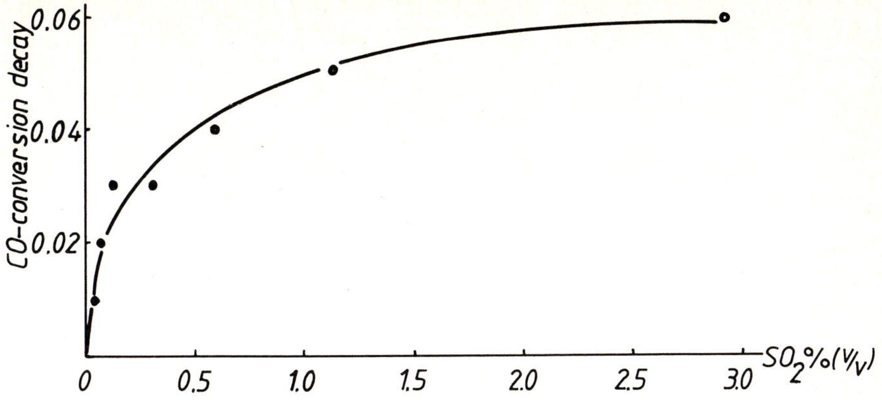

Fig.3. Effect of SO_2-content on the regenerability of catalyst B

activity compared to the unsulphided catalyst, i.e. sulphidation does not effect the activity of the promoter.

The effect of sulphur dioxide on CO-oxidation activity of promoted catalyst B_F has been measured, by determining the CO-conversion at different SO_2-concentrations in the CO/air stream. Results are shown in Figure 3. Sulphur dioxide causes a slight but sharp decrease in the CO-conversion. The shape of the curve in the SO_2-concentration interval 0.03-3 % by volume is logarithmic. Over 3 % by vol. SO_2-content, the CO-conversion does not decrease any more.

The decrease in the CO-oxidation activity, caused by SO_2 was reversible: after having stopped the SO_2-feed, CO-conversion was re-established, i.e. promoter/sulphur compounds formed on the surface are not stable and exist only in the presence of SO_2.

REFERENCES

1 A.W. Chester, A.B. Schwartz, W.A. Stover, CHEMTECH, 1 (1981) 50-58
2 J.R. Murphy, M. Soudek, Oil Gas J. 75 (3) (1977) 70-76
3 USP 4.064.039
4 F.D. Hartzell, A.W. Chester, Hydrocarbon Processing 58 (7) (1979) 137-140
5 L. Rheaume, R.E. Ritter, J.J. Blazek, J.A. Montgomery, Oil Gas J. 74 (20) (1976) 103-110
6 L. Rheaume, R.E. Ritter, J.J. Blazek, J.A. Montgomery, Oil Gas J. 74 (21) (1976) 66-70
7 E.T. Habib, Jr., H. Owen, P.W. Snyder, C.W. Streed, P.B. Venuto, Ind. Eng. Chem., Prod. Res. Dev., 16 (1977) 291-296
8 A.W. Chester, W.A. Stover, Ind. Eng. Chem., Prod. Res. Dev., 16 (1977) 285-289
9 AKZO Ketjen Technical Information FCC 79/53
10 R.R. Edison, J.O. Siemssen, G.P. Masologites, Hydrocarbon Processing 55 (5) (1976) 133-138
11 G.H. Dale, D.L. McKay, Hydrocarbon Processing 56 (9) (1977) 97-102
12 W.F. Pansing, A.I.Ch.E. Journal 2 (1956) 71-76

B. Delmon and G.F. Froment (Editors), *Catalyst Deactivation 1987*

OPTIMAL CATALYST DISTRIBUTION IN PELLETS WITH SHELL PROGRESSIVE POISONING: THE CASE OF LINEAR KINETICS

T. BACAROS, S. BEBELIS, S. PAVLOU and C.G. VAYENAS*

Institute of Chemical Engineering and High Temperature Chemical Processes, Department of Chemical Engineering, University of Patras, GR-26110, Patras, Greece

ABSTRACT

The problem of finding the optimal activity distribution in isothermal catalyst pellets is investigated for linear kinetics and shell progressive poisoning. It is found that when the rate limiting step is the chemical reaction then the optimal distribution is an appropriately chosen Dirac delta function, i.e. the optimal strategy is to concentrate the active component in a thin shell located inside the pellet. However, in the case of large Thiele numbers the uniform distribution is not substantially inferior to any other catalyst distribution.

INTRODUCTION

It has been shown both theoretically and experimentally that catalyst pellets with nonuniform distribution of the active catalyst within the porous support exhibit enhanced yield, selectivity and durability characteristics. A comprehensive review of work in this area prior to 1986 has been given by Dougherty and Verykios (ref. 1).

The problem of finding the optimal catalyst activity distribution in pellets which are not poisoned has been solved for single reactions with Langmuir-Hinshelwood (refs. 2-4) and arbitrary (ref. 5) kinetics and for some cases of consecutive and parallel reaction networks (ref. 6). In all these cases it was found that the optimal catalyst distribution is an appropriately chosen Dirac delta function, i.e. all the active component must be concentrated in a specific location within the pellet. Analytical expressions for the optimal catalyst location have been obtained in terms of the pertinent physicochemical parameters. For a single reaction occuring in an isothermal pellet, which is the case considered in the present communication,but without catalyst poisoning, the generalized optimal catalyst location equations of ref. 5 reduce to

$$\int_{s_{opt}}^{1} s^{-n} ds = \frac{1-u_{opt}}{\Phi^2 \varphi(u_{opt})} - \frac{1}{Bi} \qquad (1)$$

*Author to whom correspondence should be addressed

where s_{opt} is the dimensionless optimal catalyst location, n=0,1,2 for the infinite slab, cylinder and sphere respectively, Φ and Bi are the Thiele and Biot numbers respectively and u_{opt} is the value of the dimensionless reactant concentration u which maximizes the kinetic expression $\varphi(u)$ in a specific subinterval of [0,1] (ref. 5). Equations which are formally similar to eqn. 1 have been shown to give the optimal catalyst location for selectivity maximization in isothermal pellets with simple consecutive and parallel reaction networks (ref. 6).

The poison resistance characteristics of catalyst pellets with nonuniform catalytic activity profiles have been the focus of many studies, because of the industrial importance of the phenomenon of poisoning. In selecting the most advantageous activity profile one may have to tolerate a certain degree of diffusion resistance in order to avoid rapid deactivation by poisoning and this makes the selection more complicated compared to the case of catalyst pellets not being poisoned.

DeLancey (ref. 7) used Pontryagin's continuous maximum principle to optimize the distribution of catalytic material within a particle for an isothermal first order reaction accompanied by homogeneous poisoning. The optimal activity distribution, that maximized the average reaction rate over the operating time for a given catalyst quantity, was found to consist of an outer region of uniform activity to a certain depth from the external surface followed by a totally inert core.

Becker and Wei (ref. 8) studied the case of a first order reaction in spherical catalyst pellets and compared the durability against poisoning of pellets with the same quantity of active material, for different modes of deposition of the active phase on the porous support. They concluded that catalyst spheres with an exterior distribution are optimum for uniform poisoning, while in the case of shell-progressive poisoning and little diffusion limitation for the main reaction an interior catalyst distribution is preferable. They also gave a criterion for catalyst selection based on durability and efficiency.

Varghese and Wolf (ref. 9) studied the case of a first order reaction in a catalyst pellet containing microspheres of active material imbedded in an inert porous structure under conditions of shell-progressive poisoning. They showed that the fall in the reaction rate due to poisoning is smaller in the case of a diluted catalyst. They also concluded that, for shell-progressive poisoning in diffusion limited cases, diluting the catalyst and producing more uniform profiles is beneficial in terms of durability.

The effect of poisoning on the consecutive reaction scheme $A \rightarrow B \rightarrow C$, where B is the desired product, has been investigated by Shadman-Yazdi and Petersen (ref. 10) for the case of self-deactivation and by Corbett and Luss (ref. 11) for the case of independent poisoning.

In the present communication we study the problem of finding the optimal activity distribution in a catalyst pellet for the case of a first order reaction under pore-mouth poisoning conditions. The optimization criterion used is maximization of total reactant conversion up to the point of full catalyst deactivation.

PROBLEM FORMULATION

Consider a first order reaction A → B occuring isothermally in a symmetric porous catalyst pellet (slab, cylinder or sphere) with negligible external mass transfer resistance. The local density of the active component in the pellet is a function g(x) of the distance from the symmetry element of the pellet. The reaction is accompanied by a shell-progressive type of poisoning of the catalyst, i.e., the catalyst at any moment can be visualized as divided into two regions. From the external surface up to a distance x_p from the center, the catalyst is completely poisoned and thus inactive, while the reaction occurs only in the remaining fraction of the pellet. Under the quasi-steady-state assumption, the mass balance for the reacting component A in the nondeactivated region can be written in terms of dimensionless variables as follows:

$$\frac{1}{s^n}\frac{d}{ds}\left(s^n\frac{du}{ds}\right) = (n+1)\Phi^2 u\ a(s) \tag{2}$$

where s=x/L is the dimensionless distance from the center of the pellet with L the distance of the external surface from the center of the pellet; $u=C/C_0$ is the dimensionless concentration of the reactant with C_0 the concentration at the external surface; $a(s) = g(x)/g_0$ is the dimensionless distribution of the active component with g_0 the volume averaged active component density; $\Phi=L[g_0k/(n+1)D_e]^{\frac{1}{2}}$ is the Thiele modulus with D_e the effective diffusivity of the reactant in the nondeactivated region, k the kinetic constant of the reaction and n=0,1,2 for the infinite slab, infinite cylinder and sphere, respectively. The quasi-steady-state assumption is valid provided that the rate of catalyst poisoning is much slower than the rate of diffusion within the pellet. From its definition, the activity distribution function a(s) satisfies the following equation:

$$\int_0^1 a(s)s^n ds = \frac{1}{n+1} \tag{3}$$

The boundary conditions corresponding to eqn. 2 are

$$\text{BC1}: \quad \left(\frac{du}{ds}\right)_{s=0} = 0 \tag{4}$$

$$\text{BC2 : } \left(\frac{du}{ds}\right)_{s_p} = \begin{cases} \dfrac{1-u_p}{1-s_p} & \text{for } n=0 \quad (5a) \\ \dfrac{u_p-1}{s_p \ln s_p} & \text{for } n=1 \quad (5b) \\ \dfrac{1-u_p}{s_p(1-s_p)} & \text{for } n=2 \quad (5c) \end{cases}$$

where s_p is the location of the deactivation front and u_p is the reactant concentration at this location. The second boundary condition results from a mass balance of the reactant in the deactivated region with the assumption of continuity of the concentration gradient du/ds at $s=s_p$. Namely, it is assumed that the poison concentration is low enough so as not to affect the diffusivities of the chemical species present. Thus, the effective diffusivity of the reactant is the same in both the active and the deactivated region.

The position of the deactivation front s_p changes with time and thus solution of eqn. 2 with the boundary conditions given by eqns. 4 and 5 yields the concentration profile of the reactant in the pellet at a given time instant. Hence, the reactant concentration u in the pellet is dependent on the position of the deactivation front s_p as well as on the location s in the pellet. The effectiveness factor of the pellet, defined as the global reaction rate at a given time instant divided by the global rate obtainable with a fresh catalyst in the absence of diffusion resistance, is given by the following equation:

$$\eta(s_p) = (n+1)\int_0^{s_p} u(s,s_p)a(s)s^n ds \qquad (6)$$

The effectiveness factor η depends on time through its dependence on s_p.

The total dimensionless reactant conversion until complete deactivation of the catalyst is given by the following equation:

$$H = \int_0^1 \eta(\tau)d\tau \qquad (7)$$

where $\tau=t/t_0$ is the dimensionless time from the setup of the reaction and t_0 the total elapsed time until complete deactivation. In order to be able to substitute eqn. 6 into eqn. 7 one needs to define the dependence of s_p on time τ.

In the present work a linear relation is assumed, i.e.

$$1 - s_p = \tau \qquad (8)$$

Using eqn. 8 in eqn. 7, the total dimensionless reactant conversion can be written as follows

$$H = \int_0^1 \eta(s_p)ds_p \tag{9}$$

or substituting $\eta(s_p)$ from eqn. 6:

$$H = (n+1)\int_0^1 \int_0^{s_p} u(s,s_p)a(s)s^n ds\, ds_p \tag{10}$$

The optimal catalyst activity distribution a(s) is the one which maximizes the objective function H, in which $u(s,s_p)$ is the solution of eqn. 2 with its boundary conditions (eqns. 4 and 5). The function a(s) must also satisfy the constraint given by eqn. 3.

COMPARISON OF ACTIVITY DISTRIBUTIONS

The problem of finding the optimal activity distribution a(s) appears not to have a general analytical solution. To facilitate the analysis, the following two characteristic monoparametric distributions were chosen:

$$a_1(s) = A_{1n}s^{\alpha_1} \tag{11}$$

$$a_2(s) = A_{2n}/(\alpha_2+s)^2 \tag{12}$$

where A_{1n} and A_{2n} are normalization constants such that eqn. 3 is satisfied. The expressions for A_{1n} and A_{2n} for the various pellet geometries are shown in Table 1. Eqns. 11 and 12 cover at least qualitatively a wide range of possible activity distributions. Eqn. 11 corresponds to a decreasing activity profile towards the pellet center, a case generally resulting from partial impregnation of a porous support followed by drying. On the other hand, eqn. 12 corresponds to an increasing activity profile towards the pellet center, a case that can be found in catalysts partially poisoned by impurities in chemical feedstocks.

Using the above activity distributions, eqn. 2 was integrated numerically and the objective function H was computed from eqn. 9 for various values of the parameters α_1 and α_2. The results were also compared with the following two cases:

1. Uniform distribution, a(s)=1. This can be viewed as a limiting case of eqns. 11 and 12 when $\alpha_1=0$ and $\alpha_2 \to \infty$ respectively. The uniform distribution allows analytical solution of eqn. 2 and eqn. 6 resulting in the following expressions for $\eta(s_p)$:

$$\eta(s_p) = \frac{\tanh(\Phi s_p)}{\Phi[1+\Phi(1-s_p)\tanh(\Phi s_p)]} \quad \text{for } n=0 \tag{13a}$$

TABLE 1

Expressions for the normalizing factors A_{1n} and A_{2n}

n	A_{1n}	A_{2n}
0	α_1+1	$\alpha_2(\alpha_2+1)$
1	$\alpha_1/2+1$	$\frac{1}{2}\left[\frac{1}{\ln(\frac{\alpha_2+1}{\alpha_2}) - \frac{1}{\alpha_2+1}}\right]$
2	$\alpha_1/3+1$	$\frac{1}{3}\left[\frac{1}{\frac{2\alpha_2+1}{\alpha_2+1} - 2\alpha_2\ln(\frac{\alpha_2+1}{\alpha_2})}\right]$

$$\eta(s_p) = \frac{\sqrt{2}\, s_p I_1(\sqrt{2}\,\Phi s_p)}{\Phi[I_0(\sqrt{2}\,\Phi s_p) - \sqrt{2}\,\Phi s_p \ln s_p I_1(\sqrt{2}\,\Phi s_p)]} \qquad \text{for } n=1 \tag{13b}$$

$$\eta(s_p) = \frac{\sqrt{3}\,\Phi s_p - \tanh(\sqrt{3}\,\Phi s_p)}{\Phi^2[\sqrt{3}\,\Phi(1-s_p) + \tanh(\sqrt{3}\,\Phi s_p)]} \qquad \text{for } n=2 \tag{13c}$$

In eqn. 13b, I_0 and I_1 are the modified Bessel functions of zero and first order, respectively. The above expressions for $\eta(s_p)$ were used in eqn. 9 to compute numerically the value of H.

2. Dirac-delta-function type distribution,

$$a(s) = \delta(s-s_c)/(n+1)s^n \tag{14}$$

In this case the active component is concentrated in a specific location s_c in the pellet. Such a distribution function is, of course,a mathematical idealization of a narrow shell distribution, but, it has been shown (ref. 2-6) to provide a rather good approximation, if the shell width is less than 4% of the pellet radius. Since we are interested in maximizing H, we choose from all the Dirac type distributions the one that yields the largest H. The location of the active component s_c and the value of H can be computed analytically. The effectiveness factor for a first order reaction in an isothermal pellet with no external mass transfer resistance where the active component has been deposited in a specific location s_c, in the pellet can be computed analytically (ref. 5) to be

$$\eta = 1/(1+\Phi_B^2) \tag{15}$$

where

$$\Phi_B = \Phi \left(\int_{s_c}^{1} s^{-n} ds \right)^{\frac{1}{2}} \tag{16}$$

If the pellet is being poisoned, the effectiveness factor will have the value given by eqn. 15 when $s_p > s_c$, but it will be zero as soon as s_p becomes less than s_c. Thus, introducing eqn. 15 into eqn. 9 and integrating from s_c to 1, one can easily find the value of s_c that maximizes H and the corresponding value of H. The values of s_c and H corresponding to the optimal Dirac type distribution are shown in Table 2 for the three geometries. It is worth noting that only for the slab geometry the catalyst location of the optimal Dirac type distribution is independent of the Thiele modulus Φ.

The results obtained with the various activity distributions are shown in Figure 1 for the three different geometries. Also, in Table 3 the asymptotic behavior of H as $\Phi \rightarrow 0$ or $\Phi \rightarrow \infty$ is summarized. Comparing the results obtained with the various distributions one can make the following general observations:

(i). For low values of Φ (<1, <0.9 and <0.7 for n=0,1,2 respectively) the Dirac type distribution appears to be the optimal one, and yields a total conversion at least twice as much as the uniform distribution does. This is in accord with the observation of Becker and Wei (ref. 8) who found that in pellets

TABLE 2

Catalyst location and reactant conversion corresponding to the optimal Dirac delta function type distribution

n	s_c	H
0	0	$1/(1+\Phi^2)$
1	root of $\Phi^2 s_c \ln s_c - (\Phi^2+1)s_c + \Phi^2 = 0$	$\dfrac{1 - s_c}{1+\Phi^2 \ln s_c}$
2	$\dfrac{\Phi}{1+\Phi}$	$\dfrac{1}{(1+\Phi)^2}$

under pore-mouth poisoning the "egg yolk" distribution is preferable for small Φ values. Actually, it can be easily shown that, when $\Phi \rightarrow 0$, the optimal activity distribution approaches a Dirac type distribution located at the center of the pellet ($s_c \rightarrow 0$). Indeed, it can be seen from Table 3 that, when $\Phi \rightarrow 0$, the Dirac type distribution yields H=1. From eqns. 3 and 10 and since $u(s,s_p) \leq 1$ it is deduced that H is bounded by unity. Therefore, since for $\Phi \rightarrow 0$ the Dirac type distribution yields H=1, it is the optimal distribution. Finally, using

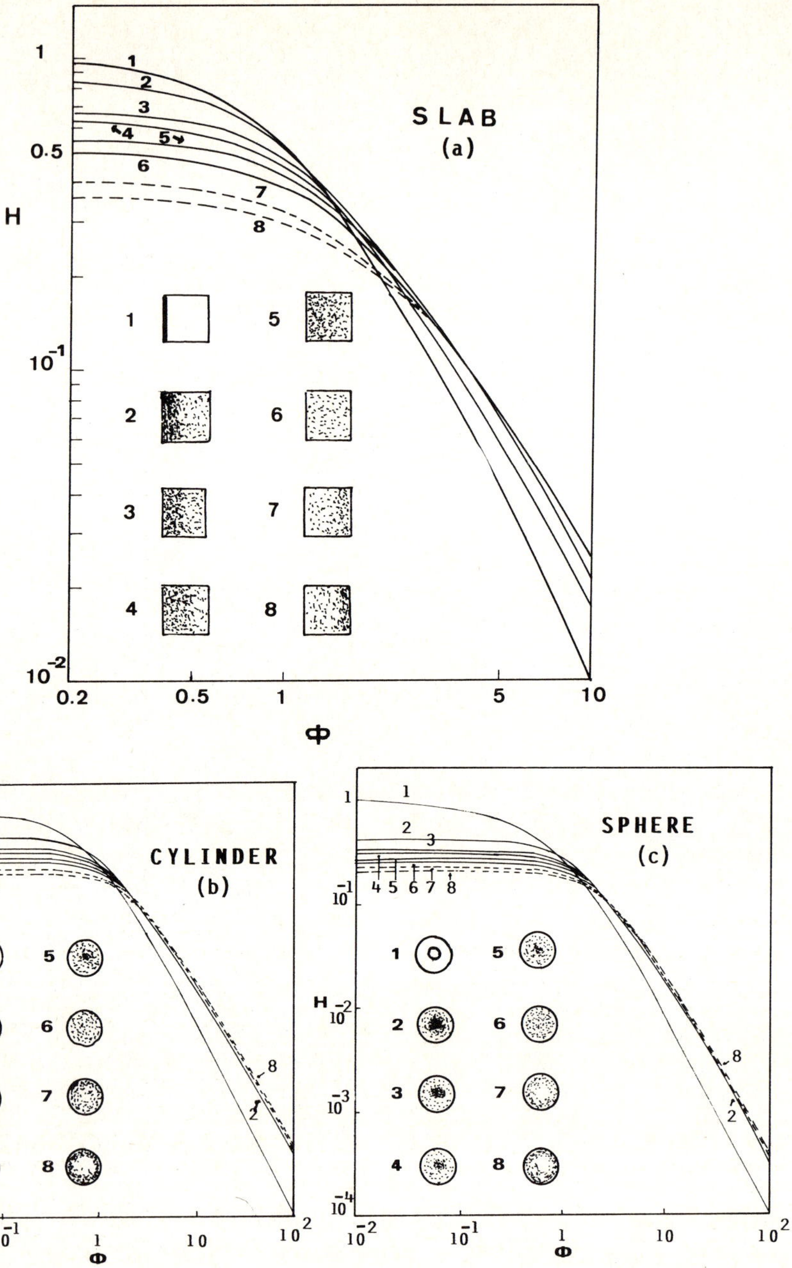

Fig. 1. Dependence of total dimensionless conversion H on Thiele modulus Φ for various activity distributions. Numbers denote: 1. Dirac type distribution; 2,3,4,5. $a_2(s)=A_{2n}/(s+\alpha_2)^2$ with α_2=0.1(2), 0.5(3), 0.9(4), 3(5); 6. Uniform distribution; 7,8. $a_1(s)=A_{1n}s^{\alpha_1}$ with α_1=0.5(7), 0.9(8). (a) Flat pellets (n=0). (b) Cylindrical pellets (n=1). (c) Spherical pellets (n=2).

TABLE 3
Asymptotic behavior of H

		$a(s)=1$	$a(s)=A_{1n}s^{\alpha_1}$	$a(s)=A_{2n}/(\alpha_2+s)^2$	$a(s)=\delta(s-s_c)/(n+1)s^n$
n=0	$\Phi \to 0$	1/2	$1/(\alpha_1+2)$	$(\alpha_2+1)[1-\alpha_2 \ln(\frac{\alpha_2+1}{\alpha_2})]$	1
	$\Phi \to \infty$	$\ln(1+\Phi)/\Phi^2$			$1/\Phi^2$
n=1	$\Phi \to 0$	1/3	$1/(\alpha_1+3)$	$\dfrac{(2\alpha_2+1)\ln(\frac{\alpha_2+1}{\alpha_2}) - 2}{\ln(\frac{\alpha_2+1}{\alpha_2}) - \frac{1}{\alpha_2+1}}$	1
	$\Phi \to \infty$				$1/\Phi^2$
n=2	$\Phi \to 0$	1/4	$1/(\alpha_1+4)$	$\dfrac{3\alpha_2+\frac{1}{2} - (3\alpha_2^2+2\alpha_2)\ln(\frac{\alpha_2+1}{\alpha_2})}{\frac{2\alpha_2+1}{\alpha_2+1} - 2\alpha_2\ln(\frac{\alpha_2+1}{\alpha_2})}$	1
	$\Phi \to \infty$	$\dfrac{\ln(\sqrt{3}\Phi+1)-1}{\Phi^2}$			$1/\Phi^2$

the expressions of Table 2 one can show that in this case $s_c \to 0$.

(ii). For large values of Φ (>3) the uniform distribution gives significantly better results than the Dirac type distribution. Also, there is no significant difference between the values of H calculated with a uniform distribution and the ones calculated with the distributions shown in eqns. 11 and 12, although the distribution with an increasing activity profile towards the pellet surface (eqn.11) gives slightly better results. The observation agrees with the suggestion of Varghese and Wolf (ref. 9) that for a Φ value of 5 or larger it is preferable to disperse the effective activity uniformly over the catalyst volume in order to retard the reaction rate suppression due to poisoning and thus increase the total attained conversion. Becker and Wei (ref. 8) found that for large Φ values an "egg shell" catalyst distribution is preferable in agreement with the observation that a distribution with an increasing activity profile towards the pellet surface gives slightly better results.

When Φ is very large, the suppression of the effectiveness factor owing to the very large diffusion resistance dominates upon its suppression because of poisoning, so that one would not expect large differences in the attained H at least among smooth activity distributions.

(iii). For intermediate Φ values ($1.5<\Phi<3$) there are distributions of decreasing activity profile towards the pellet surface (eqn. 12) that give better results than the uniform or the Dirac type distribution.

(iv). Distributions of increasing activity profile towards the pellet surface (eqn. 11) generally give low values of H for small and intermediate Φ values. It is worth noting that in the limit as $\alpha_2 \to \infty$, the distribution becomes a Dirac type distribution at $s_c=1$, $a(s)=\delta(s-1)/(n+1)$, i.e., all the active component is deposited on the external surface of the pellet. In this case H=0 for all geometries owing to the immediate deactivation of all the active material.

SUMMARY

In a porous catalytic pellet in which a first order reaction occurs isothermally and which is subject to pore-mouth poisoning, the distribution of the active component that yields the maximum overall reactant conversion during the lifetime of the catalyst depends strongly on the value of the Thiele modulus. Thus, for small values of the Thiele modulus, i.e., when the rate determining step is the chemical reaction, a Dirac type distribution is the optimal one. Namely, the active component should be located in a specific position in the pellet. On the other hand, for large values of the Thiele modulus, i.e., when the rate determining step is the internal diffusion, the uniform distribution appears not to be significantly inferior to any other activity distribution. An interesting conclusion of the present analysis is that the optimal activity distribution is not always of the Dirac type, contrary to the case of nondeactivating catalyst pellets for single reactions (refs. 2-5) and also for simple consecutive and parallel reaction networks (ref. 6) where a Dirac type distribution is always the optimal one.

REFERENCES

1 R.C. Dougherty and X.E. Verykios, Catal. Rev.-Sci. Eng. 29(1) (1987) 101-130.
2 M. Morbidelli, A. Servida and A. Varma, Ind. Eng. Chem. Fundam. 21(1982) 278-284.
3 M. Morbidelli and A. Varma, Ind. Eng. Chem. Fundam. 21 (1982) 284-289.
4 M. Morbidelli, A. Servida, S. Carra and A. Varma, Ind. Eng. Chem. Fundam. 24 (1985) 116-119.
5 C.G. Vayenas and S. Pavlou, Chem. Eng. Sci., submitted (1986).
6 C.G. Vayenas and S. Pavlou, Chem. Eng. Sci., in press (1987).
7 G.B. DeLancey, Chem. Eng. Sci. 28 (1973) 105-118.
8 E.R. Becker and J. Wei, J. Catal. 46 (1977) 372-381.
9 P. Varghese and E.E. Wolf, AIChE J. 26 (1980) 55-60.
10 F. Shadman-Yazdi and E.E. Petersen, Chem. Eng. Sci. 27 (1972) 227-237.
11 W.E. Corbett and D. Luss, Chem. Eng. Sci. 29 (1974) 1473-1483.

B. Delmon and G.F. Froment (Editors), *Catalyst Deactivation 1987*
1987 Elsevier Science Publishers B.V., Amsterdam — Printed in The Netherlands

A MODEL FOR ACCUMULATION OF C, FE, AND TI FOULANTS IN COAL LIQUEFACTION CATALYSTS

B.D. Adkins, S.R. Adkins, B.H. Davis, and D.R. Milburn

Kentucky Energy Cabinet Laboratory, University of Louisville, P.O. Box 13015, Lexington, KY 40512 (U.S.A.)

ABSTRACT

A phenomenological model has been developed to describe the accumulation of C, Fe, and Ti in catalysts used in a pilot-plant scale two-stage coal liquefaction operation. Two species for each foulant have been identified on the basis of (a) spatial accumulation profiles and (b) time rate of deposition. The more rapidly diffusing species appears to be associated with plant start-up and is uniformly distributed throughout the catalyst pellet. Accumulation of the more slowly diffusing species has been related to a process stream which is high in non-distillate materials. The effects of coal ash on these foulant species are examined and show that the presence of ash may drastically alter foulant deposition. The effect is consistent with competitive adsorption between ash and catalyst, and in the case of C, the adsorption of the slowly diffusing species appears to be reversible.

INTRODUCTION

Numerous studies of deactivated Ni-Mo coal liquefaction catalysts (refs. 1-9) have identified fouling to be a major cause of activity loss. For Co-Mo catalysts, a decrease of dispersion has also been identified (refs. 10,11). In both cases, fouling by both carbon and trace metals are believed to be prime factors.

Recently, we have developed a phenomenological model to describe the accumulation of C, Fe, and Ti foulants in 1/32" Shell 324 Ni-Mo coal liquefaction catalyst used in the two-stage liquefaction (TSL) pilot plant in Wilsonville, Ala. The model is based on correlations obtained between various plant conditions and the results of the characterization of 85-90 catalyst samples. In all, five separate pilot plant runs were considered (Table 1).

This coal liquefaction pilot plant is equipped with an H-Oil type ebullating bed catalytic hydrotreating unit (HTR) and is normally operated in the ebullating mode. Usually, negligible quantities of the catalyst bed are withdrawn and replaced to provide samples for analysis. These catalyst samples have well-known reactor residence times. However, it must always be kept in mind the operating conditions may be varied widely during a run.

Table 1. *Various Conditions for Wilsonville Pilot Plant Runs and Figure Legend.*

Run No.	Mode	Coal	TR Present	Ash Present	Symbol
242	ITSL	Illinois Bituminous	Yes	No	□
246 (A)	DITSL	Wyoming Sub-bituminous	No	No	□
246 (B)	ITSL	Wyoming Sub-bituminous	Yes	No	○
247	RITSL	Illinois Bituminous	Yes	Yes	△
248 (A)	DITSL	Illinois Bituminous	No	No	□
248 (B)	ITSL	Illinois Bituminous	Yes	No	▲
249	RITSL	Wyoming Sub-bituminous	Yes	Yes	○

EXPERIMENTAL

Catalyst samples were shipped in oil from the Wilsonville pilot plant to our laboratory. These samples were extracted with THF using a Soxhlet apparatus until the THF exiting the extraction thimble was clear. Then, they were dried to a constant weight in a vacuum oven at 60-80°C. The catalysts were ground using a mortar and pestle prior to analysis. The carbon content was determined directly with a LECO CHN-600 analyzer. Dissolution of the ground catalysts prior to analysis for Fe and Ti was achieved using a standard method (ref. 12). A Spectraspan IIIB DCP Atomic Emission Spectrometer was used to determine the Fe and Ti concentrations.

RESULTS

A schematic of the proposed model is shown in Figure 1. The important components of this model are: (a) start-up conditions, (b) thermal resid (TR), and (c) coal ash. Since the presence or absence of coal ash and TR in the HTR (ref. 13) depends on the configuration of the pilot plant, this becomes an important consideration for the model. The configurations examined in developing this model (Figures 2a-c) are Integrated Two-Stage Liquefaction (ITSL), Double Integrated Two-Stage Liquifaction (DITSL), and Reconfigured Integrated Two-Stage Liquifaction (RITSL). Detailed descriptions of these configurations are avaiable (ref. 13). It is important to note that in the DITSL mode TR is recycled from the critical solvent deasher (CSD) to the thermal liquefaction unit (TLU); consequently only the light thermal resid (LTR) and process

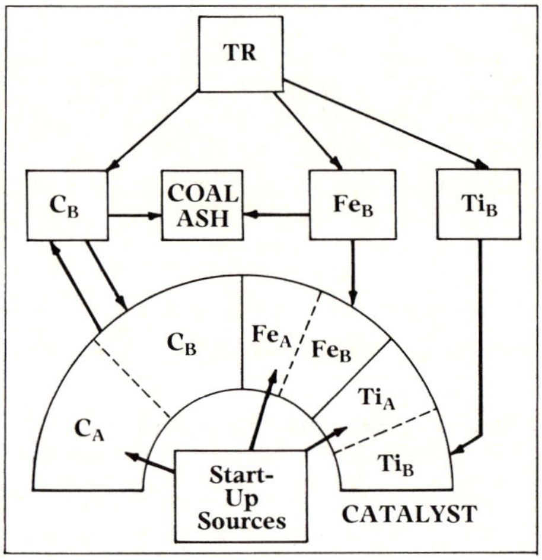

Figure 1. *Schematic of the general phenomenological model.*

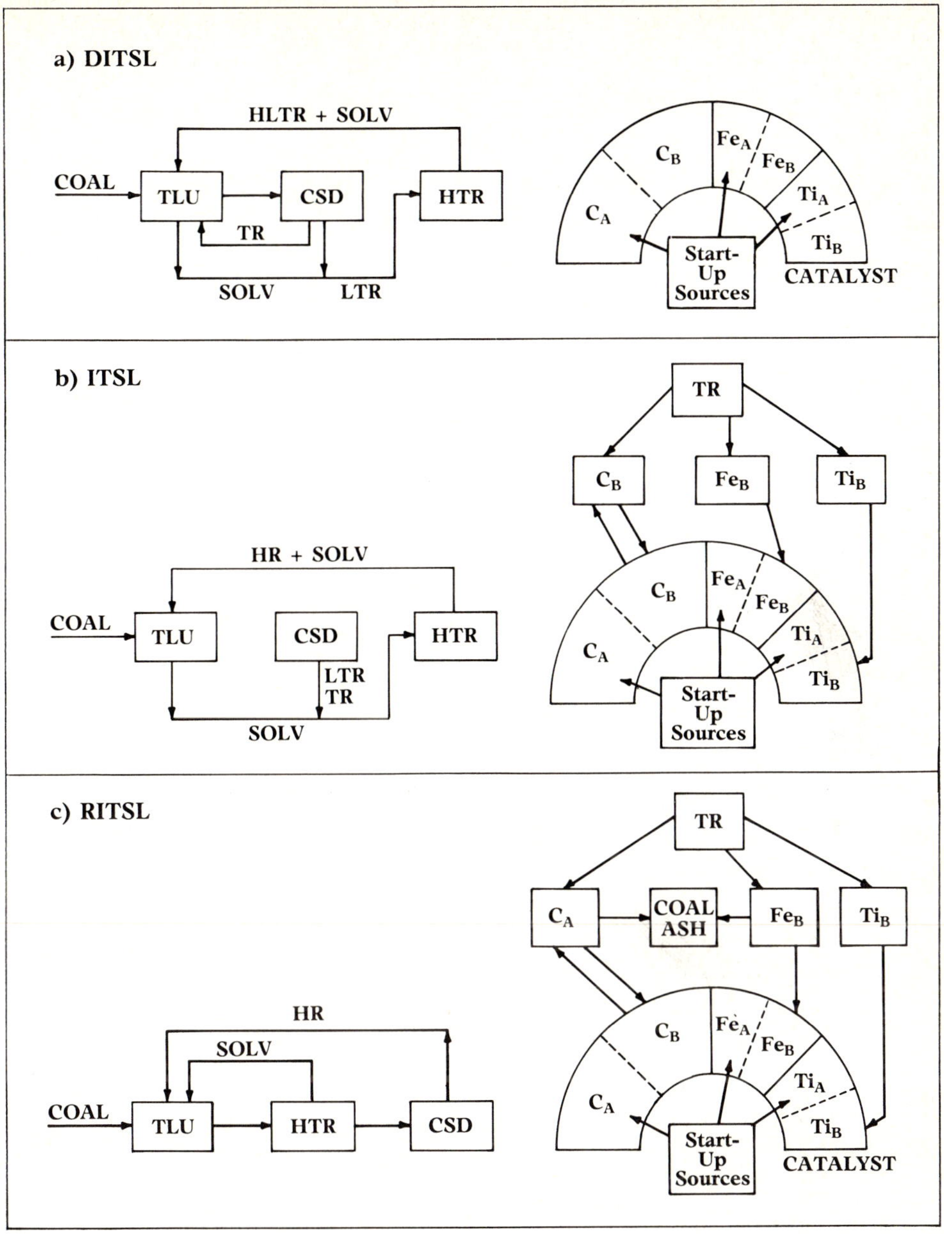

Figure 2. *Pertinent features of the general model for: (a) DITSL, (b) ITSL, and (c) RITSL configurations.*

solvent are sent to the HTR (Figure 2a). In the ITSL configuration, both TR and LTR are sent from the CSD to the HTR (Figure 2b). In RITSL mode, the CSD is placed after the HTR, so that coal ash and unconverted coal as well as the light and heavy portions of the stream from the TLU are present in the HTR (Figure 2c).

Carbon

Total carbon data for catalysts from all five runs are shown in Figure 3. For catalysts in the DITSL mode (Figure 3a) the deposited carbon rapidly increases to approximately 8% w/w and then remains constant. For the catalysts in the ITSL mode (Figure 3b), the C concentration shows a slight but steady increase during the course of the run. In the RITSL mode (Figure 3c) the catalysts initially have high levels of carbon but the carbon content shows a consistent decrease with catalyst age. These observations lead to the proposal, as shown in the model, that there are two types of carbon foulant present on the catalyst. The first species (C_A) is assumed to be a more conventional coke which is rapidly deposited and likely to be associated with start-up conditions and/or LTR (which is low in preasphaltenes). In our model most, if not all, of the carbon from the DITSL configuration is C_A (Figure 3a). When the configuration is changed from DITSL to ITSL, the catalyst is exposed to both LTR and TR streams. The second carbon species, C_B, appears to be a reversibly adsorbed carbon associated with the TR, which is high in preasphaltenes. The carbon associated with the catalyst from the ITSL mode is shown in Figure 3b.

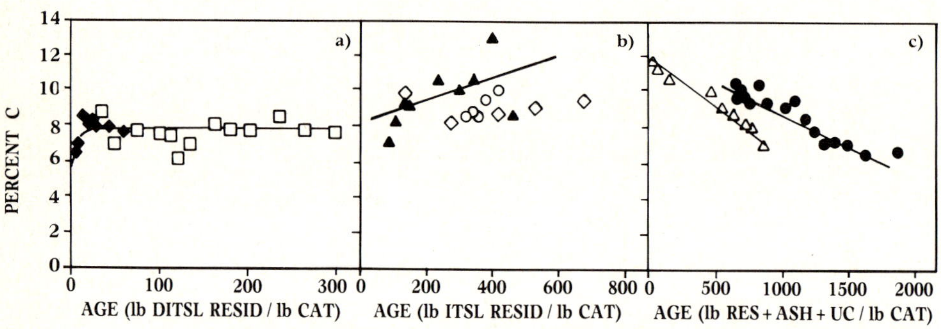

Figure 3. *Weight % carbon versus catalyst age for: (a) DITSL, (b) ITSL, and (c) RITSL configurations.*

The decrease in carbon during catalyst use in the RITSL mode is evidence of desorption of C_B. This desorption is consistent with a model in which there is competitive adsorption of C_B on coal ash and catalyst (the major difference between ITSL and RITSL run conditions is the presence coal ash in the RITSL mode). A clearer picture of adsorption and desorption of C_B is evident from the data shown in Figure 4. Run 246 was first operated in the DITSL mode,and was then changed to the ITSL mode. Catalyst from Run 246 was withdrawn from the reactor, stored in drums and was then reused in Run 249. Thus, Figure 4 shows the carbon accumulation for a single catalyst batch subjected to DITSL, then ITSL and, finally, RITSL operating conditions. During operation in the DITSL mode,C_A rapidly increases to ca. 8% w/w and then stabilizes at this value. Upon switching to the ITSL mode, the carbon continuously accumulates to several percent above the 8% w/w C_A deposited during the DITSL operation. Upon exposure of this catalyst to the RITSL configuration (i.e. ash present in the HTR), carbon, presumably C_B, apparently desorbs from the catalyst and readsorbs on the coal ash during the RITSL mode of operation. There is insufficient data to adequately establish that an equilibrium level is attained during operation at the RITSL conditions and that the same carbon level is ultimately attained for the RITSL and DITSL modes, as the model suggests.

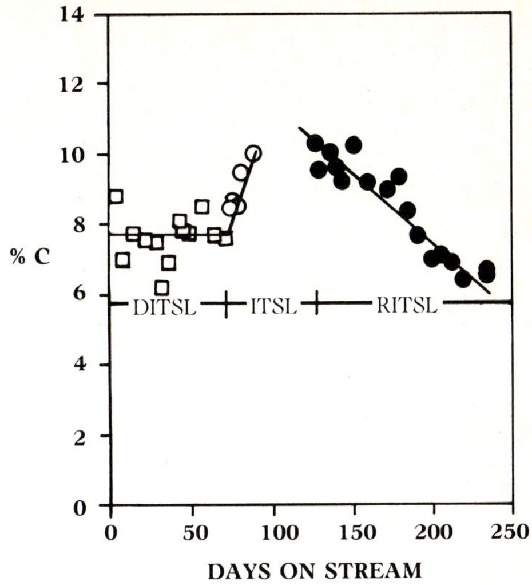

Figure 4. *Weight % carbon versus days on stream for a single catalyst batch subjected to DITSL, ITSL, then RITSL configurations. The coal is a Wyodak sub-bituminous.*

Iron

The model for Fe is similar to that for C (i.e. two species, Fe_A and Fe_B are involved) except that Fe does not desorb under the plant conditions examined. Figure 5 summarizes the data for the bulk analysis for Fe vs. catalyst age for the three plant modes. In the DITSL mode (Figure 5a), the Fe concentration is relatively constant during the run. There is more scatter in this data than for carbon but a distinct increase or decrease in the Fe concentration is not evident. This is observed whether a sub-bituminous Wyodak or a bituminous Illinois #6 coal is used. This iron is associated with the start-up sources and is referred to as the baseline iron, Fe_A. The data (Figure 5b) show clear evidence of Fe_B accumulation when Illinois bituminous coal is used as the feed coal in the ISTL mode. The species responsible for

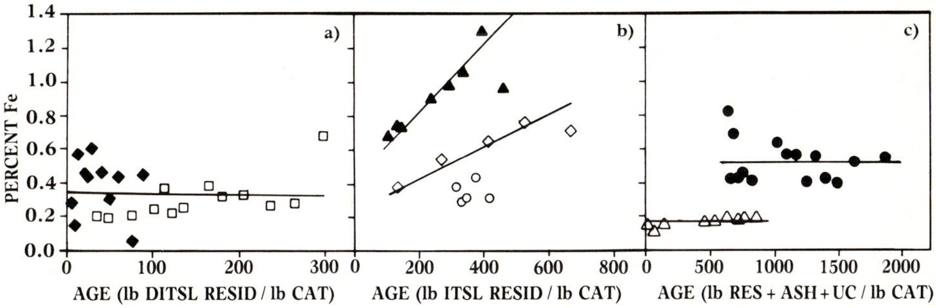

Figure 5. *Weight % iron versus catalyst age for: (a) DITSL, (b) ITSL, and (c) RITSL configurations.*

Fe_B may be coal dependent since there is little evidence of an increase in iron when a Wyodak sub-bituminous coal is used. Under RITSL conditions (Figure 5c), the Fe concentration appears to remain constant with time. Thus, the coal ash present in the RITSL mode appears to be a competing sorbent for Fe in a manner similar to that postulated for carbon except that the Fe_B species apparently does not desorb from the catalyst. Note that the higher level of Fe found in RITSL Run 249 may be either a second dose of Fe_B from start-up sources or from Fe_B accumulation during Run 246.

Examples of SEM line profile analysis (LPA) are shown for catalyst pellets from ITSL (Figure 6a and b) and RITSL (Figure 6c) modes when an Illinois bituminous coal was used as feed. The higher concentration of Fe near the pellet edge for the ITSL samples is further evidence for an Fe_B species. Earlier SEM LPA work on catalysts from Wilsonville had suggested the existence of two Fe species in the ITSL mode. One species is uniformly distributed (Fe_A) while the other (Fe_B) is a slowly diffusing species, and gives a shell progressive type deposition profile (refs. 14,15). We had originally thought the Fe_B species might be due to corrosion products found in the plant under normal operating conditions. Because of the lack of continued iron accumulation in the DITSL mode operation, corrosion derived iron can be ruled out unless it is only transported in the TR fraction and this seems unlikely.

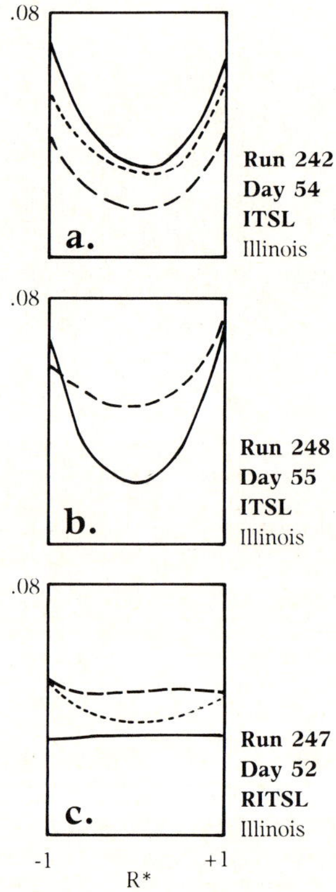

Figure 6. *SEM LPA for iron deposition samples from (a) Run 242, (b) Run 248, and (c) Run 247.*

<u>Titanium</u>

Results of Ti accumulation for each of the three modes are shown in Figure 7. There is a striking similarity between Ti and Fe concentration vs catalyst age when the plant configuration is operated in either the DITSL (Figures 5a and 7a) or ITSL (Figures 5b and 7b) modes. However, the analogy for the metals accumulation does not apply for the RITSL mode (Figures 5c and 7c). Ti continues to accumulate on the catalyst throughout the runs in the RITSL configuration whereas the Fe content remains constant. This is most easily explained by assuming that Ti is not adsorbed by coal ash, although we have no simple explanation for this adsorption selectivity at this time. The increase is pronounced for the Illinois coal but

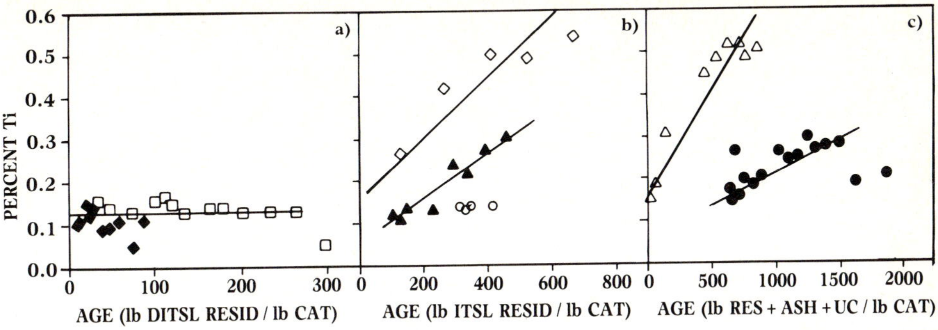

Figure 7. *Weight % titanium versus catalyst age for: (a) DITSL, (b) ITSL, and (c) RITSL configurations.*

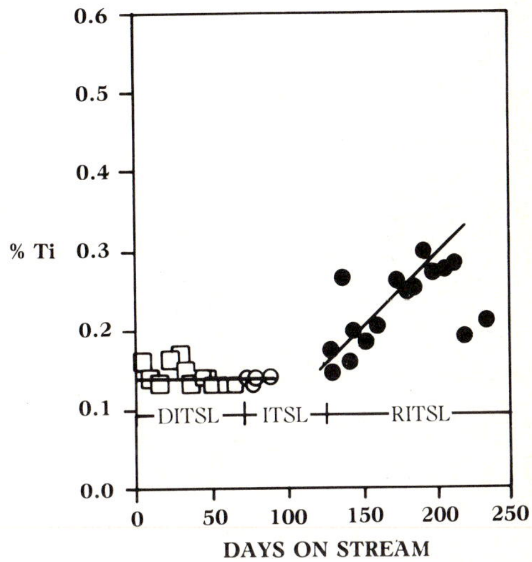

Figure 8. *Weight % titanium versus days on stream for a single catalyst batch subjected to DITSL, ITSL, then RITSL configurations. The coal is a Wyodak sub-bituminous.*

is also present for the Wyoming coal. Figure 8 shows a composite of the Ti data for the same catalyst samples used to obtain the C data shown in Figure 4. There is no apparent increase in Ti concentration with catalyst usage for the DITSL or the ITSL modes with the Wyodak coal. Unfortunately, the duration of the ITSL period is insufficient for the determination of an established trend for Ti content. The only increase for this catalyst series results from the RITSL configuration. This further supports the speculation that coal ash does not adsorb Ti. Figure 9 shows SEM LPA for Run 242 and Run 247. Again, this data supports the existence of the two species of Ti, with Ti_A being a rapidly diffusing species and Ti_B being a more slowly diffusing one. Both species are present in catalysts from runs in the ITSL and DITSL modes with Illinois #6 as the feed coal. One possible source of Ti_B could be titanium porphyrins; Lynch (ref. 1) has reported shell progressive deposition of Ti porphyrins on the Shell 324 catalyst aged in a microflow reactor.

Diffusion-Limited Nature of Adsorption of Fe_B and Ti_B

The evidence of diffusion control in the deposition of Fe_B and Ti_B has been examined in more detail and a mathematical model has been developed for

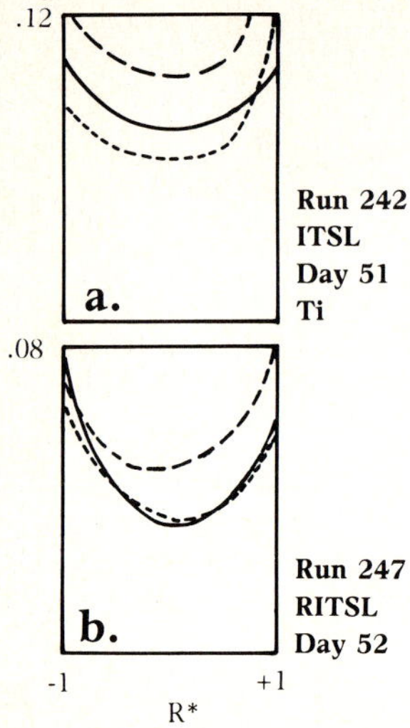

Figure 9. *SEM LPA for titanium deposition on catalyst samples from (a) Run 242 and (b) Run 247.*

this process(ref. 16). The model takes the form of two ordinary differential equations (ODE's) which can be solved using a simple finite difference scheme with time stepping. The model is based on a first order adsorption of contaminant with linear site blocking and their subsequent saturation. The Thiele moduli for both contamination processes have been estimated to be in the range of 3 to 7. Extensive catalyst characterization data was utilized and this allowed us to select this model from a more general partial differential equation (PDE) model which allowed for various orders for the adsorption and site blocking steps.

CONCLUSIONS

1. Irreversibly adsorbed species are present on the spent catalyst (C_A, Fe_A, Ti_A) which are apparently associated with the catalyst sulfidation process and plant start-up.

2. A reversibly adsorbed carbon species (C_B) is associated with the TR present in the ITSL mode. Coal ash competes with catalyst for adsorption of C_B to the extent that the carbon concentration is dramatically decreased when ash is present. Thus, the ash apparently has a higher affinity for C_B than the catalyst. These effects seem to be independent of coal type.

3. Some evidence, suggests that Fe_B and Ti_B may be coal dependent.

4. Coal ash competes with the catalyst for the adsorption of Fe_B. Apparently the Fe_B already adsorbed on the catalyst does not desorb. Coal ash does not appear to adsorb Ti, however.

5. Given the variability of pilot plant conditions, the next step would seem to be studying these depositions with carefully controlled conditions in laboratory scale reactors.

ACKNOWLEDGEMENT

This work was performed at the Kentucky Energy Cabinet Laboratory (KECL) with funding from the Commonwealth of Kentucky, Kentucky Energy Cabinet. The

KECL is administered under contract by the University of Louisville. We would also like to thank Catalytic, Inc. for supplying the samples used in this study.

REFERENCES

1 A.W. Lynch, Appl. Catal., 24 (1986) 227-239.
2 D.S. Thakur and M.G. Thomas, Appl. Catal., 15 (1985) 197-225.
3 D.S. Thakur and M.G. Thomas, Ind. Eng. Chem. Prod. Res. Dev., 23 (1984) 349-360.
4 T.L. Cable, F.E. Massoth and M.G. Thomas, Fuel Proc. Tech., 4 (1981) 265-275.
5 T.L. Cable, F.E. Massoth and M.G. Thomas, Fuel Proc. Tech., 10 (1985) 105-120.
6 D. Garg and E.N. Givens, Fuel Proc. Tech., 9 (1984) 29-42.
7 A. Ocampo, J.T. Schrodt and S.M. Kovach, Ind. Eng. Chem. Prod. Res. Dev., 17 (1978) 56-61.
8 S.M. Kovach, L.J. Castle, J.V. Bennett, and J.T. Schrodt, Ind. Eng. Chem. Prod. Res. Dev., 17 (1978) 62-67.
9 G.J. Steigel, R.E. Tischer, D.L. Cillo and N.K. Narain, Ind. Eng. Chem. Prod. Res. Dev., 24 (1985) 206-213.
10 M.G. Thomas and D.G. Sample, Fuel, 60 (1981) 145-150.
11 G.B. Freeman, J. Heink, N.J. Long, and B.H. Davis, Appl. Catal., 23 (1986) 309-326.
12 R. Bock, Decomposition Methods in Analytical Chemistry, John Wiley and Sons, New York, 1979.
13 Technical Progress Report, Run 249 with Wyodak Coal, Catalytic, Inc., DOE/PC/50041-75, October, 1986.
14 B.D. Adkins, D.R. Milburn, S.R. Adkins, B.H. Davis, Proc. Tenth EPRI Cont. Conf. on Clean Liq. Sol. Fuels, Palo Alto, CA, April 23-25, 1985.
15 B.D. Adkins, K. Cisler, B.H. Davis, Appl. Catal., 23 (1986) 111-127.
16 B.D. Adkins, D.R. Milburn, B.H. Davis, Ind. Eng. Chem. Prod. Res. Dev., submitted for publication.

B. Delmon and G.F. Froment (Editors), *Catalyst Deactivation 1987*

COKE FORMING REACTIONS DURING METHANOL CONVERSION ON ZEOLITE CATALYSTS

H. SCHULZ, ZHAO SIWEI AND W. BAUMGARTNER
Engler-Bunte-Institut, Universität Karlsruhe, Kaiserstr. 12, 7500 Karlsruhe, FRG

ABSTRACT

The changes in detailed product composition with proceeding time on stream have been studied during methanol conversion on H-ZSM-5, RE-Y, H-mordenite and an amorphous silica/alumina catalyst. In parallel experiments the build up of coke has been determined. Results are comparatively evaluated as a function of "Normalized Time on Stream" (NTOS). Catalyst deactivation is kinetically traced with the help of the propane/propene mole ratio and exhibits different deactivation patterns for the examined catalysts. One type of deactivation - slow deactivation in the range NTOS = 0 to 0.5 and fast deactivation in the range NTOS = 0.5 to 1.0 is explained as resulting from mass transport limitations respectively filling of the pore volume with organic deposites (e. g. H-ZSM-5 and RE-Y at 375 ^{o}C). A second type of deactivation - fast deactivation in the range NTOS = 0 to 0.5 and slow deactivation in the range NTOS = 0.5 to 1.0 is related to specific deactivation of the active catalyst sites and observed e. g. at high temperature (475 ^{o}C) with RE-Y.

As one prominent reaction of coke formation from methanol the direct non catalytic alkylation of coke has been observed. As a typical reaction which lowers the hydrogen content of the coke at elevated temperature the formation of methane has been found. The influences of geometric constraints (shape selectivity) and acidity of the catalyst on individual reaction steps in the reactions network are established from the selectivity results.

The deposited coke participates in the overall conversion. The reduced coke selectivity, which is obtained with H-ZSM-5, and its special nature (mainly two ring aromatics have been found) are the reason for inhibition of several important reaction steps, particularly the formation of methane and H_2 plus CO.

INTRODUCTION

The course of deactivation due to coke formation during methanol conversion has comparatively been investigated with 4 types of catalysts. Momentary mass balances are established with the help of a special procedure of instantaneous gas/vapour-total product sampling (refs. 1 - 4) which yields the desired time resolution of product composition. Detailed product composition date are obtained by capillary gas chromatography. The multiplicity of these composition data is grouped so as to correlate with individual reaction steps of the conversion and with the actual state of catalyst activity.

As a kinetic measure of catalyst activity under transient conditions the usage of the molar propane/propene ratio is examined in detail. It is well established in literature that during hydrocarbon reactions like catalytic cracking the paraffin/olefin ratio declines with decreasing catalyst activity (refs. 5 - 6).

Selectivity of coke formation and correspondingly the rate of catalyst deactivation is extremely different with H-ZSM-5 as compared with zeolite catalysts with wider pore dimensions (ref. 7). In order to establish a basis for comparatively evaluating the initial catalyst activity, its function of decline with time on stream and the related time/activity and selectivity changes a "Normalized Time on Stream" (NTOS) has recently been introduced (ref. 4). The underlying concept is, to define a distinct state of catalyst deactivation which is regarded "the same" for different catalysts. In this work normalization of the time axis is related to the point of breakthrough of unconverted methanol from the reactor (NTOS = 1.00) as it is to be observed via continuous monitoring of the methanol in the product stream. However it is also shown that normalization of the time axis to the point of equal catalyst activity e. g. to the molar propane/propene ratio being equal to 1.00) could be a more general approach. From selectivity changes with increasing NTOS individual reaction steps of formation of coke and also of various product compounds are derived as a function of catalyst activity, catalyst coke coverage and spaciousness constraints.

EXPERIMENTAL

The applied catalysts H-ZSM-5, H-mordenite and RE-Y consisted of pure zeolite phases as examined with x-ray diffraction (ref. 4). The Si/Al-ratios were H-ZSM-5: 105, H-mordenite: 13.2, RE-Y: 2.47. The RE-Y sample was obtained by means of exchange with a commercial rare-earth chloride solution containing 19.4 m-% of RE-oxides. The amorphous catalyst was one of the older commercial type cracking catalysts (Durabead I).

The methanol conversion was performed in a fixed-bed reactor without recycle at 375 and 475 °C and two space velocities (WHSV 0.1 and 1.0 h^{-1}). Samples from the hot gaseous product stream were taken in small glass ampoules and analyzed by gas chromatography. Independently the formation of coke and its composition (H/C-ratio) was investigated in separate experiments. After the desired time on stream for methanol conversion, the adsorbed components were eluted and the coke determined via combustion in a diluted oxygen stream and measuring of the concentrations of CO, CO_2, O_2 and H_2 in the effluent stream.

A survey of the experiments is given in Table 1. With the amorphous catalyst at WHSV = 0.99 h^{-1} already in the initial product some methanol is obtained and no NTOS normalization is possible. The NTOS values used for plotting the results in the diagrams (except Fig. 1) have been calculated as the quotients of the actual duration of the experiment at the time of sampling and the duration of the experiment at the time of methanol breakthrough (for which the amount of processed methanol per gram of catalyst is reported in the table).

TABLE 1

Survey of experiments

Methanol conversion of different acidic catalysts (total pressure 5 bar, p_{CH_3OH} = 2.5 bar, p_{N_2} = 2.5 bar

	H-ZSM-5		H-Mordenite				RE-Y				amorphous SiO_2/Al_2O_3			
T, °C	375	475	375	375	475	475	375	375	475	475	375	375	475	475
WHSV, h^{-1}	1.0	1.0	.09	.84	.09	.84	.10	.99	.10	.99	.10	.99	.10	.99
Cat. load at MeOH-breakthrough (g MeOH/g Catalyst)	163	109	1.5	1.5	1.3	.93	1.8	1.6	2.6	1.2	.30	-	1.0	-
Duration of exp. at MeOH-breakthrough, h	163	109	18	1.8	-	1.1	18	1.6	-	1.2	3.0	-	11	-

TIME ON STREAM NORMALIZATION OF DEACTIVATION EXPERIMENTS

Coke selectivity and correspondingly coke formation rates differ up to two orders of magnitude with H-ZSM-5 as compared with RE-Y or H-mordenite (see Figs. 4 and 8). However, though through different durations a similar state of catalyst deactivation is attained, when the catalyst activity is no longer sufficient for the desired conversion.

It has now been tried to define the identical state of catalyst deactivation in order to normalize different runs to this particular time on stream, which is then taken as NTOS = 1.00, so that the deactivation runs are presented on a comparable basis. 3 approaches of time on stream normalization have been regarded.

(1) Catalyst coking up to the same coke load. This appears reasonable at a first glance. However, it was observed, that on H-ZSM-5 combined with an alumina binder much of the coke is deposited on the alumina. Then equal amounts of coke do not correspond to the same extent of deactivation. Furthermore the amount of deposited coke in dependence of time on stream can only be determined in a series of experiments with different lengths of runs, when the

amount of coke is analyzed at the end of each run. This makes the approach also very laborious and impractical.

(2) Breakthrough time of methanol. In the fixed bed version of the MTG process (Methanol to Gasoline), the useful catalyst life time is indicated by the occurence of unconverted methanol in the product stream. The breakthrough time of methanol can then be taken as NTOS = 1.00 as the comparable state of catalyst deactivation. This normalization is applied during this work (except for Fig. 1 and 2).

This approach is, however, restricted to the conversion of methanol and is only applicable to experiments where a breakthrough point occurs and not to such experiments where methanol is already found in the initial reaction product. It is also necessary that the zone of catalyst coking, which slowly moves through the catalyst bed is short in relation to the length of the catalyst bed.

(3) Catalyst coking up to the same low level of activity as indicated by the same value of molar propane/propene ratio in the product stream. This is the simplest and most general approach, applicable to all systems of carbocation reactions in which propane and propene are among the reaction products. It is a well established correlation, that the paraffin/olefin molar ratio in the product stream declines with decreasing activity of the acidic catalyst (refs. 5 - 6).

CATALYST ACTIVITY AND COKE FORMATION AS A FUNCTION OF NORMALIZED TIME ON STREAM

As a kinetic measure of catalyst activity the molar propane/propene ratio is shown in dependence of normalized time on stream for the different catalysts and several reaction conditions in the figures below.

In Figs. 1 and 2 per definition NTOS = 1.00 corresponds to the actual time on stream at which the observed propane/propene ratio is 1.00. (This is roughly equal to the breakthrough point of methanol).

In Fig. 1 the initial activity of the fresh catalyst is represented by the extrapolated propane/propene value at zero time (intersection with the ordinate). The course of deactivation is characterized by the shape of the curves of propane/propene ratio. Apparently the four catalysts differ in initial activity and deactivation functions as well.

The initial activity of RE-Y and H-mordenite is very high as characterized by a propane/propene ratio of about 500. The initial activity of H-ZSM-5 and of the amorphous silica-alumina are comparatively low (propane/propene value of about 30). The deactivation curve for the amorphous catalyst is concavely shaped indicating a fast deactivation in the first part

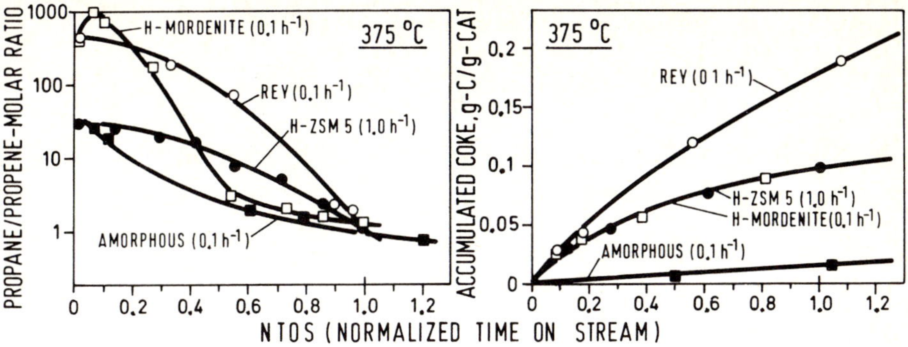

Fig. 1. (left hand) Propane/propene molar ratio as a function of normalized time on stream (NTOS = 1.00 for propane/propene equal to 1.00) for methanol conversion
Fig. 2. (right hand) Accumulated coke on the catalysts as a function of time on stream for the same catalysts as in Fig. 1

of the run. Deactivation of H-ZSM-5 proceeds rather steadily over the run length however faster towards the end of the run. The curve for RE-Y is similarly shaped as that for H-ZSM-5 pointing towards a similar deactivation process which is visualized as a process of mainly pore filling in nature (when taking also into account additional results being discussed later). The curve for H-mordenite (the catalyst with the highest initial activity) shows a miximum at about NTOS = 0.05. The maximum value of propane/propene is about as large as 1000. An explanation of the increase of the propane/propene ratio in the early stage of this experiment is that the formation of propane (from a propyl cation as the precursor) needs a hydride donating species. This can be in common instances an easily accessible coke molecule or a molecule of a coke precursor or a 6-ring naphthene, however, there is no coke on the fresh catalyst surface and therefore in case of particular high initial activity the limited availability of hydrids reduce the propane/propene ratio in the beginning of an experiment.

The kinetic scheme which characterizes the propane/propene molar ratio as a measure of catalyst activity can be understood as follows:

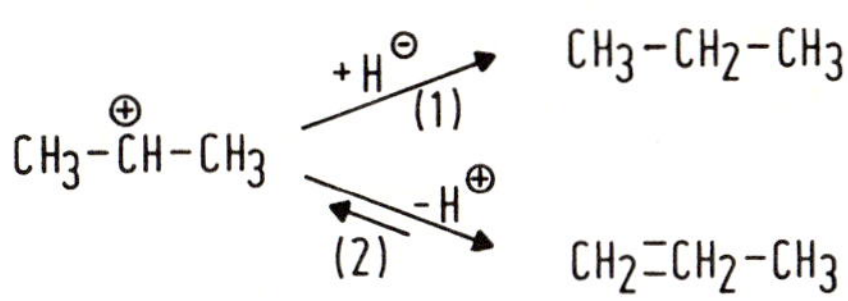

The propyl cation (the precursor of the products propene and propane) can pick up a hydride to form the propane. This reaction is irreversible and demanding in strength of acidity. The propyl cation can on the other hand easily loose one proton to form the propene in a reversible reaction. Thus at high level of activity and long space time finally almost all of the primarily formed propene will be consumed through hydrogenation via proton and hydride addition. At particularly low activity and short space time the olefin will be the favoured product. Of course, as any other kinetic measure of catalyst activity, the molar propane/propene ratio depends also on the various reaction conditions. The kinetic scheme can also be completed by the conversion of the propyl cation to coke and to aromatic compounds. This has been observed by Emmett and coworkers (ref. 8) who introduced ^{14}C-labelled propene in the system of hexadecane cracking and traced the ^{14}C in the products.

Fig. 2 shows the amount of accumulated coke on the catalyst as a function of normalized time on stream. The curves of H-mordenite and H-ZSM-5 are identical. When NTOS is equal to one (and propene/propane thus also equal to one both the catalysts are loaded with 10 grams of coke (only the carbon of the coke is being regarded) per gram of catalyst. The RE-Y obviously has a higher coke capacity of 18 g C per 100 g RE-Y at NTOS = 1.0.

The low level of accumulated coke for the amorphous silica-alumina has to be interpreted in a different way. With this catalyst of small initial activity already a low amount of coke deposition (1.5 g C per 100 g catalyst) diminishes the activity to the reference value of the propane/propene ratio of 1.00.

With the normalization NTOS = 1.00 for the breakthrough point of methanol the diagrams of Figs. 3 and 4 (and all further figures) are obtained.

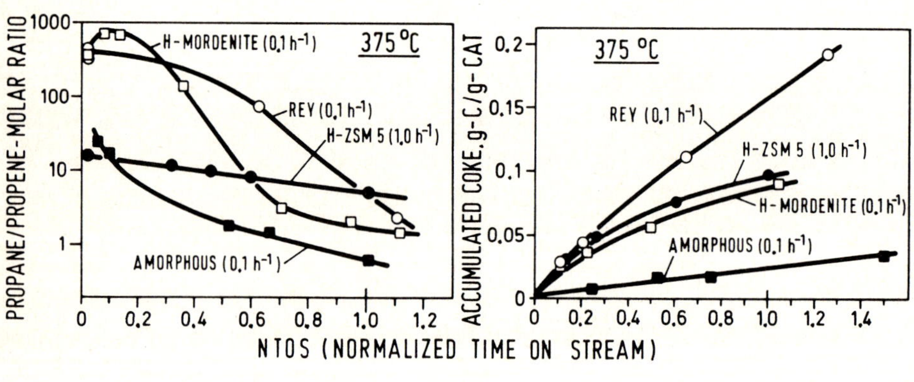

Fig. 3 (left hand). Propane/propene molar ratio as a function of normalized time on stream (NTOS = 1.00 for breakthrough of methanol) for methanol conversion on 4 catalysts at 375 °C

Fig. 4 (right hand). Accumulated coke on the catalysts as a function of NTOS in relation to Fig. 3

They are rather similar to Figures 1 and 2, indicating that normalization of the time coordinate to the same propane/propene ratio or to the breakthrough time of methanol leads in general to the same conclusions.

Deactivation curves for H-ZSM-5 at 325, 350, 375 and 475 °C are shown in Fig. 5. From 350 to 475 °C the propane/propene ratio decreases, however, towards low temperature (form 350 to 325 °) it decreases also. With RE-Y (Fig. 6) the increase of reaction temperature from 375 to 475 °C also lowers the propane/propene value but also the course of deactivation is seriously affected: At the high temperature there is a very fast initial deactivation, which indicates the deactivation of active sites, whereas at the low temperature initial deactivation is not pronounced and the produced coke seems mainly to fill up the pore volume without reducing activity.

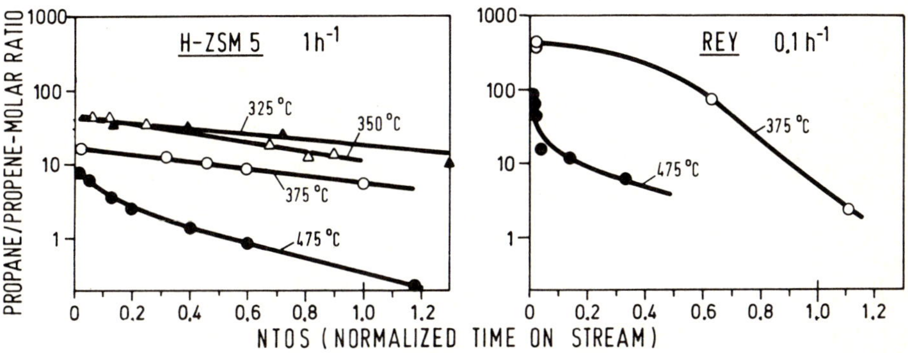

Fig. 5 (left hand). Deactivation of H-ZSM-5 during methanol conversion at 4 different temperatures
Fig. 6 (right hand). Deactivation of RE-Y during methanol conversion at 375 and 475 °C. (Normalization of time on stream to methanol breakthrough)

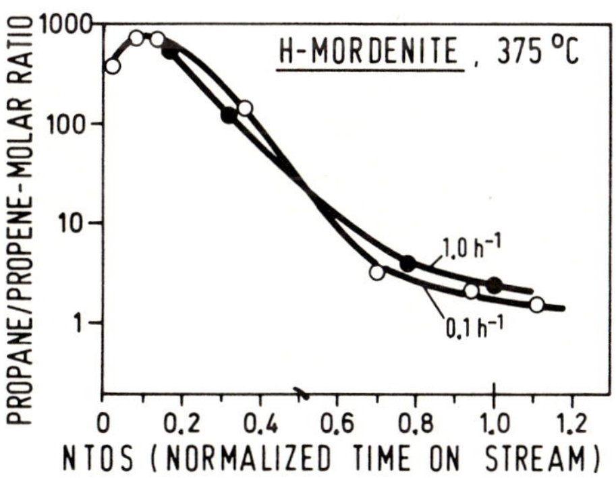

Fig. 7. Deactivation of H-mordenite during methanol conversion at 2 space velocities

The curves of deactivation of H-mordenite at 375 °C at two values of space velocity (WHSV 1.0 and 0.1 h^{-1}) show no noticeable difference (Fig. 7). In this representation (propane/propene ratio over normalized time on stream) deactivation is not substantially influenced by space velocity.

Coke yield as a function of NTOS is shown in Fig. 8 for the 4 catalysts at 375 °C. Coke yield with H-ZSM-5 is about 100 times lower than with the other catalysts. The common behaviour is a relatively high initial coke yield and an almost constant yield during further deactivation. With H-ZSM-5, however, the coke yield declines all over the time of deactivation.

The H/C-ratio of the coke on H-ZSM-5 at 375 °C is substantially higher than that of the coke on H-mordenite and RE-Y (Fig. 9).

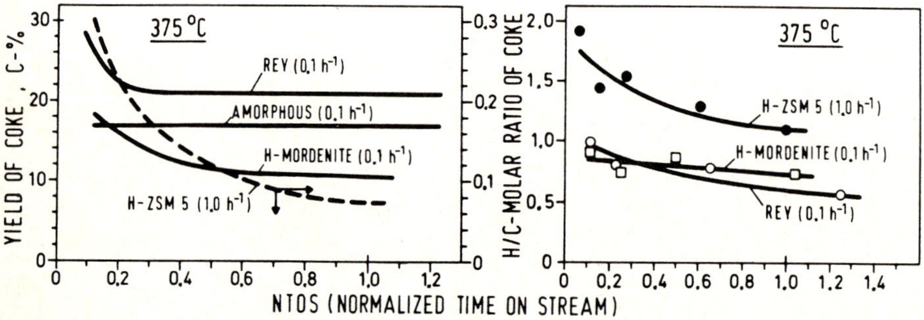

Fig. 8 (left hand). Yield of coke as a function of NTOS for 4 catalysts
Fig. 9 (right hand). H/C-molar ratio of coke as a function of NTOS for 3 catalysts

It declines from ca. 1.7 to 1.0 with increasing time on stream indicating the coke to loose hydrogen during its stay on the catalyst. With H-mordenite and RE-Y the H/C-ratio declines from about 1.0 to about 0.5 with increasing time on stream.

Thus it is concluded that coke on the H-ZSM-5 is of different chemical nature as compared with coke on H-mordenite and RE-Y and it is deduced that coke on H-ZSM-5 mainly is located within the zeolite lattice and not on the crystallites surface.

At high reaction temperature (475 °C) coke formation is favoured with H-ZSM-5, RE-Y and H-mordenite (Fig. 10). At NTOS = 1.00 the coke load is 50 g C / 100 g catalyst with H-ZSM-5 and about 20 g C / 100 g catalyst with RE-Y and H-mordenite. As below, direct thermal reactions of coke formation between already existing coke and methanol are predominant under these conditions and the extremely high coke load of the H-ZSM-5 is then attributed mainly to coke deposition on the outer surface of the catalyst crystallites and due to the very long duration of the experiment as compared with the other catalysts.

With the amorphous catalyst coke formation remains low due to the poor activity and the short duration of the run.

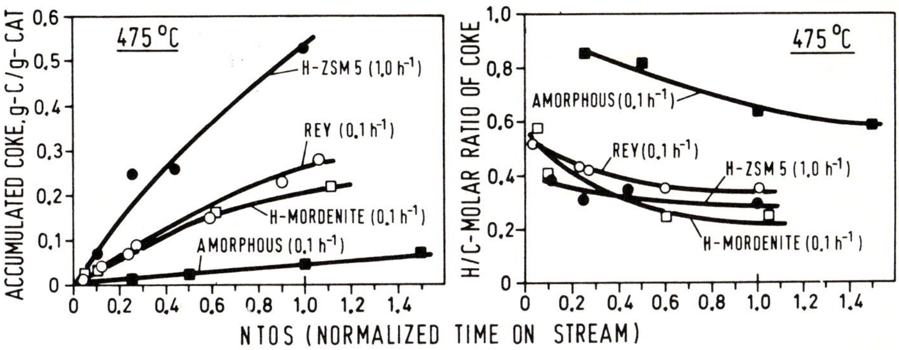

Fig. 10 (left hand). Accumulated coke on 4 catalysts as a function of NTOS during methanol conversion at 475 °C
Fig. 11 (right hand). H/C-molar ratio of coke as a function of NTOS during methanol conversion at 475 °C

The H/C-ratio of the coke at 475 °C (Fig. 11) is generally lower than that of the coke being formed at 375 °C and the coke on H-ZSM-5 shows no higher H/C-ratio than that on RE-Y and H-mordenite which supports the conclusion that now for all the three catalysts the main route of coke formation is equal and as outlined above. (The relatively high H/C-ratio for the amorphous catalyst again reflects its low activity and the short run duration and the already concluded statement, that thermal coke formation mainly appears as a growth reaction of coke which initially was formed on acidic sites and this initiation is poor with the amorphous catalyst of low acidity).

METHANE SELECTIVITY AND COKE FORMATION

Methane is generally not expected to be formed via a cationic intermediate on acidic catalyst sites. Methane selectivity as percent of carbon in methane related to the sum of carbon in all hydrocarbon product compounds is shown as a function of NTOS for the 4 catalysts at 375 and 475 °C in Fig. 12. When comparing the results at 375 °C the unique behaviour of H-ZSM-5 is obvious: Methane selectivity is only about 1 C-%, whereas with H-mordenite it is about 10 - 15 % with RE-Y up to 40 % and with the amorphous catalyst 5 to 10 %.

When increasing the reaction temperature, methane selectivity increases generally seriously. With H-ZSM-5 at 475 °C it is about 10 C-%, however, with the other catalysts methane becomes the major hydrocarbon product. 90 C-% with RE-Y, 70 C-% with H-mordenite, 80 C-% with the amorphous catalyst.

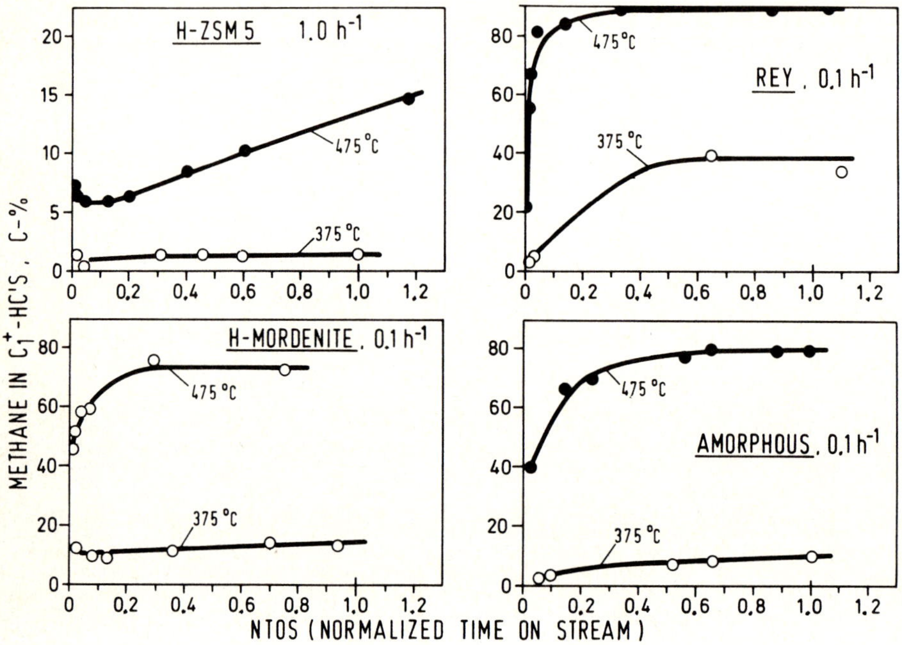

Fig. 12. Methane selectivity as a function of NTOS during methanol conversion on 4 catalysts and at 2 temperatures

When regarding the shape of the curves it can be generally concluded that the fresh catalyst of highest activity and with no coke deposits on it shows low methane selectivity. For instance with the RE-Y at 475 °C the initial methane selectivity is only about 20 C-%, whereas at NTOS = 1.00 the methane selectivity has attained a value of 90 C-%. Then the main route of methanol conversion is now the production of methane and coke together with CO, H_2, CO_2 (and water). Coke formation in this system is coupled with methane formation and because almost no higher hydrocarbons are present, coke formation cannot proceed via olefins or aromatic hydrocarbons (and not at the acidic sites) but proceeds via a direct reaction between the coke and the methanol, e. g.:

$$\text{H-Coke} + CH_3OH \longrightarrow CH_3\text{-Coke} + H_2O$$

On the other hand the H/C-ratio of the coke decreases with increase of temperature and increase of NTOS. The reaction which makes the coke more deficient in hydrogen is visualized as demethanation e. g.

$$CH_3\text{-Coke-H} \longrightarrow CH_4 + \text{Coke}$$

Thus the ultimate stoichiometries of coke and methane formation in this regime would be

$$2\ \text{H-Coke} + 2\ CH_3OH \longrightarrow 2\ CH_3\text{-Coke} + 2\ H_2O \quad (1)$$

$$2\ CH_3\text{-Coke} \longrightarrow CH_4 + \text{H-Coke} + \text{CH-Coke} \quad (2)$$

$$1\ \text{H-Coke} + 2\ CH_3OH \longrightarrow CH_4 + \text{CH-Coke} + 2\ H_2O \quad (3)$$

Due to reaction (1) 1 CH_2 is added to the coke; due to reaction (3) 1 C is added.

Of course, coke formation is a complex process and additional reaction steps of rearrangement and ring closure have to be taken into account. Even in the high temperature range initiation of coke formation on acidic catalyst sites via cationic hydrocarbon species is very probable. This coke then will grow further via direct thermal reaction with methanol. Stabilisation of radicals in the multiring coke system should be a substantial feature of this mechanism.

The explanation of the unique behaviour of H-ZSM-5 as the catalyst for methanol to gasoline conversion does then concern substantially the specific inhibition of distinct reaction steps as:

(1) Methane formation which is inhibited, because coke selectivity is very low and methane is only formed in course of the reaction of methanol with the coke.

(2) Coke formation from hydrocarbons on the acidic sites is inhibited because of the small size of pore dimensions of the H-ZSM-5

(3) As shown below also methanol decomposition to CO and H_2 is accelerated by the coke and thus inhibited on H-ZSM-5.

(4) The last governing inhibition which is well known concerns the restriction of aromatic product compound formation to ones with only one aromatic ring, because of the small pore size dimensions.

(5) Coke within the lattice of H-ZSM-5 is of very different nature as compared with coke which is formed on catalysts with large pores and is only restrictively capable to participate on further reactions. Coke in the H-ZSM-5 lattice as reported below preferentially consists of alkylated two ring aromatics.

METHANOL DECOMPOSITION

Thermodynamically the decomposition of methanol to CO and H_2 is favoured in the range of reaction conditions as applied in this study. In Fig. 13 the yield of $CO + CO_2$ is reported as a function of time on stream for the two temperatures and the different catalysts.

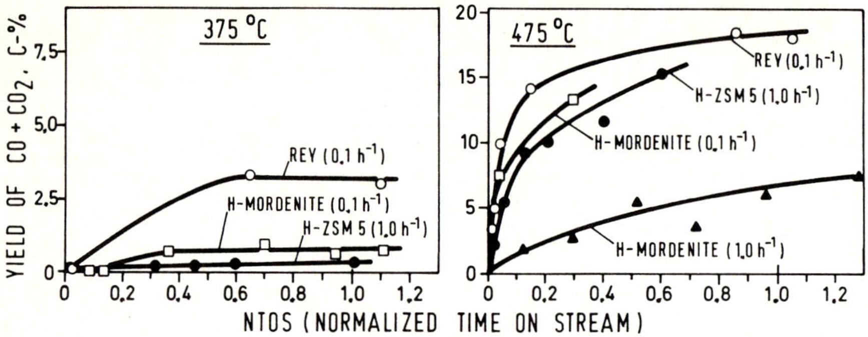

Fig. 13. Yield of $CO + CO_2$ as a function of NTOS during methanol conversion on different catalysts at 375 and 475 °C

The trends are similar as for methane selectivity: Methanol decomposition is favoured by increase of temperature, space time and amount of coke, which is already deposited on the catalyst. The reaction is obviously not catalyzed by acidic sites, however accelerated by the coke, indicating it to proceed as a thermal radical-like reaction. Some of the CO reacts with water according to the water gas shift reaction.

$$CH_3OH \longrightarrow CO + 2\ H_2$$
$$CO + H_2 \longrightarrow CO_2 + H_2$$

Suppression of methanol decomposition and also methane formation in high temperature application of H-ZSM-5 as for olefine production from methanol then means inhibition of coke formation on the outer surface of the H-ZSM-5 crystals.

COMPOSITION OF THE HYDROCARBON PRODUCT EXCEPT METHANE

In Figs. 14 and 15 the composition of the hydrocarbon products is recorded as fraction of aromatics in C_2^+ and fractions of C_2–C_5 HC's in the C_2^+ HC's. Methane is now not taken into account, because it is produced via a different mechanism (see above).

These two fractions constitute almost the total amount of the C_2^+ product, because in the range C_6^+ the hydrocarbons are almost exclusively aromatics and correspondingly the remaining rest are aliphatic hydrocarbons C_2 to C_5.

There are big differences to be notified in selectivity of aromatics fromation for the 4 catalysts as well with respect to the average of the value as with respect to the time on stream changes (Fig. 14). With H-ZSM-5 at 375 °C and also 475 °C the selectivity for aromatics is relatively high (ca. 40 C-% of the C_2^+ products) and does not much alter with time on stream. With

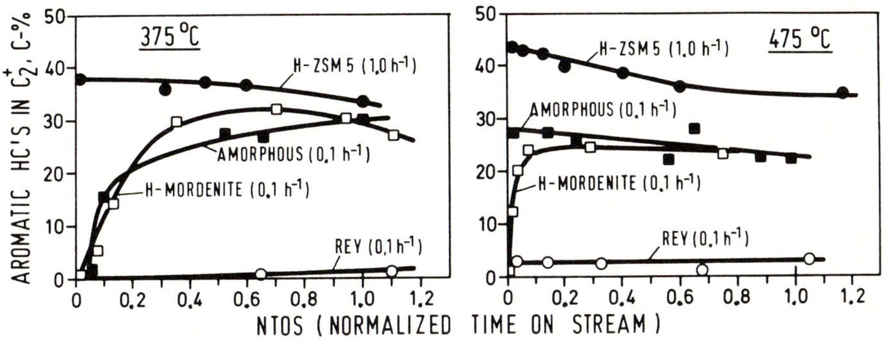

Fig. 14. Selectivity of formation of aromatic hydrocarbons as a function of NTOS during methanol conversion

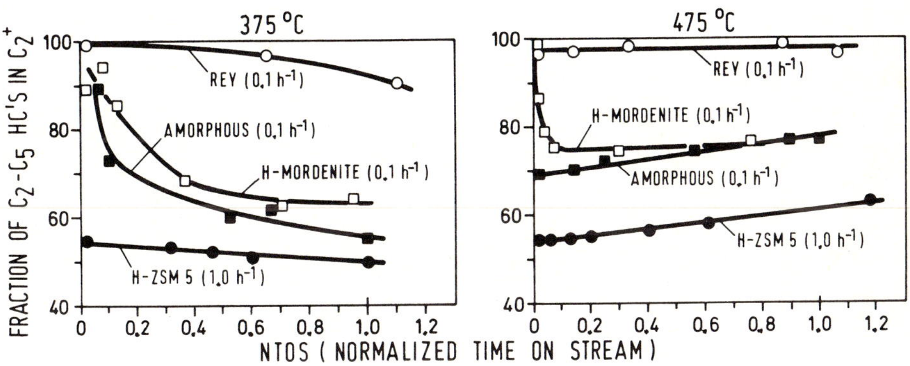

Fig. 15. Selectivity of formation of aromatic hydrocarbons as a function of NTOS during methanol conversion

the H-mordenite initially almost no aromatics are formed and almost exclusively small aliphatic molecules are found (Fig. 15).

With increasing time on stream the selectivity for aromatics increases up to ca. 30 C-% of the C_2^+ hydrocarbons. It is concluded, that the acidity of the fresh catalysts is to high for the formation of aromatics and predominantly the scarcely reactive saturated molecules C_2-C_4 are obtained via hydride transfer. With RE-Y this kinetic situation is valid over the total duration of the experiment, up to NTOS = 1.00. Values of selectivity for the individual compounds C_2-C_4 are reported in (ref. 4).

NATURE OF THE COKE ON H-ZSM-5

After converting methanol on H-ZSM-5 at 375 °C up to NTOS = 1.00 the inorganic matter of the catalyst was dissolved in hydrofluoric acid, the remaining coke extracted with an organic solvent and the solution investigated with GC/MS. Coke extracts, obtained in a similar way, have recently been examined by Guisnet et al. (refs. 9 - 10). Coking of H-ZSM-5 has also been studied by Bibby et al. (ref. 11). As main constituents of the coke we have found dimethyl- and trimethyl naphthalenes like alkylated biphenyl and alkylated biphenyl methane

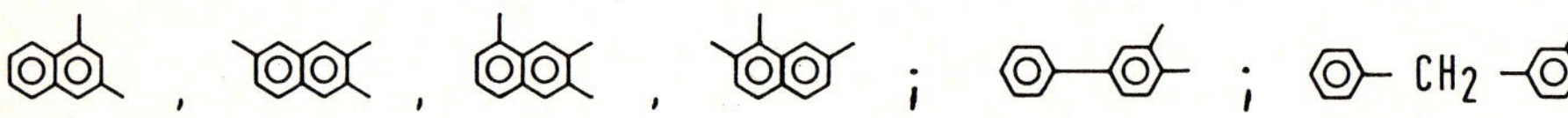

It is concluded that "the coke" in the pores of H-ZSM-5 preferentially consisted of two ring aromatics. (This work will be published in detail in a later paper).

ACKNOWLEDGEMENT

Financial support of part of this work by Ruhrkohle AG (Bottrop) and the Bundesministerium für Forschung und Technologie (Bonn) is gratefully acknowledged.

REFERENCES

1 H. Schulz and S. Nehren, Erdöl und Kohle - Erdgas - Petrochemie vereinigt mit Brennstoff-Chemie, 39, 2 (1986), 93 - 94

2 H. Schulz and A. Geertsema, Erdöl und Kohle, 30 (1977), 313 - 321

3 H. Schulz, E. Bamberger, H. Gorre, Proc. 8th Intern. Congr. on Catalysis, Berlin 1984

4 H. Schulz, W. Böhringer, W. Baumgartner and Zhao Siwei, Proc. 7th Intern. Conf. on Zeolites, Tokyo, 1986, 915 - 922

5 S. C. Eastwood, C. J. Plank and P. B. Weiss, Proc. 8th World Petroleum Congr. 4 (1971), 245

6 H. Schulz and A. Geertsema, Proc. 5th Intern. Conf. on Zeolites, Neapel (1980), 874

7 P. Dejaifve, A. Auroux, P. C. Gravelle and J. C. Védrine, J. Catal. 70 (1981) 123 - 136

8 J. W. Hightower, P. H. Emmett, J. Am. Chem. Soc. 87 (1965) 939

9 M. Guisnet, P. Magnoux and C. Canaff, Proc. 7th Intern. Conf. on Zeolites, Tokyo, 1986, 701 - 707

10 M. Guisnet, P. Magnoux and C. Canaff, in R. Setton (Editor), Chemical Reactions in Organic and Inorganic Constrained Systems, Reidel, Dordrecht, Boston, Lancaster, Tokyo, 1986, 131 - 140

11 D. M. Bibby, Proc. 7th Intern. Conf. on Zeolites, Tokyo, 1986, 1D - 11

B. Delmon and G.F. Froment (Editors), *Catalyst Deactivation 1987*

COKE DEPOSITION ON Y-ZEOLITES IN METHYLNAPHTHALENE ISOMERISATION

V. SOLINAS[1], R. MONACI[1], E. ROMBI[1] and L. FORNI[2]

[1]Dipartimento di Scienze Chimiche, Università di Cagliari, Via Ospedale 72, 09124 Cagliari (Italy)

[2]Dipartimento di Chimica Fisica ed Elettrochimica, Università di Milano, Via Golgi 19, 20133 Milano (Italy)

ABSTRACT

Coke deposition on variously decationated Y-zeolite catalysts, during methylnaphthalene isomerisation, was studied at 573-633 K. Coke deposition rate was found to decrease with increasing temperature and/or ion-exchange degree, tending to zero as time increases. The amount of coke formed and the activity decay were expressed as a function of time-on-stream or of coke content of the catalyst, by means of exponential equations, whose parameters depend on the degree of decationation and on reaction temperature.

INTRODUCTION

Many catalytic reactions of organic compounds are accompanied by the formation of carbonaceous residues referred to as "coke". The rate of this secondary reaction depends both on the operating conditions and on the nature of the catalyst. Generally, it is slower than the main reaction, but sometimes it can be of the same order of magnitude (refs. 1-6). The deactivation of zeolites by coking depends on two factors: the availability of catalytic sites and the spatial constraints acting on the reactions leading to the carbonaceous residues. The effective concentration of acid sites, catalyzing the main reaction and coke deposition at any time during operation, is a function of two independent parameters. The first one is site coverage, occurring when acid sites are poisoned by coke, coke precursors or products, which do not desorb under reaction conditions. The second one is pore blockage, preventing the access of reactants to the active sites. With some zeolites, coke formation may be controlled also by the molecular shape selective properties of the catalyst. In large pore zeolites, e.g. of Y-type, the initial steps, leading to coke precursors, are the alkylation of aromatics and the aromatization of alkyl-aromatics. The rapid and easy regeneration upon air calcination is due to the existence of the channel system, allowing a better access of oxygen to the coke deposits.

In a previous work (ref. 7) it was found that Y-zeolite, totally or partially protonated, is a very active and selective catalyst for the isomerisation of 1-methyl-naphthalene (1MN) to 2-methyl-naphthalene (2MN). However, fouling by carbonaceous deposits brings about a rapid decay of activity. In the present study, coke deposition on Y-zeolites was examined as a function of temperature and surface acidity of the catalyst, looking for correlations with coke content, by means of a deactivation function.

EXPERIMENTAL

Catalyst

Y-zeolite catalysts were prepared from commercial crystalline powder (LZY-52, from Union Carbide), by ion-exchange in the usual way (ref. 8). Surface acidity was measured as reported (ref. 9), by titration with n-butylamine in anhydrous solvent.

Apparatus and procedure

Isomerisation runs were carried out in a continuous, tubular, quartz microreactor. After activation of the catalyst, by heating at 773 K for 12 h in nitrogen, a mixture of carrier gas (H_2) and 1MN at a molar ratio R = 10 was fed at WHSV = 6 (g of 1MN/g cat. x h). Fresh catalyst (0.5 g) was usually charged for each run. Liquid products were analyzed by GC on a capillary glass column, coated with Carbowax 20M. The amount of coke formed was determined at the end of the reaction, after cleaning up and drying the fouled catalyst by a nitrogen stream at the reaction temperature. The coke was then burnt off in oxygen at 353-923 K and the CO_2 evolved was determined by acidimetric titration. In some cases the fouled catalyst was also extracted by refluxing with solvents.

RESULTS AND DISCUSSION

Analysis of coke

The GC analysis of the solution obtained by extraction, with any of the solvents employed (benzene, pyridine or methylene chloride), showed only the presence of the MN isomers, the latter becoming undetectable after 24 h of N_2 purging of the catalyst.

The analysis by XRD and NMR/MAS, carried out on the coke separated from the catalyst, after disgregation of the zeolite with HF, showed only the presence of unresolved systems of fused aromatic rings. This confirms the well known mechanism, usually accepted for the formation of coke (see e.g. ref. 10). Following or simultaneous with adsorption, the naphthalene molecule undergoes protonation to form positive ionic species, starting the coking reaction. The reaction of naphthalene with itself accounts for the formation of perylene and benzofluoranthene. The latter in turn continue to undergo addition and dehydrogenation reactions, ending into the polyaromatic aggregates of the final size.

Coking and isomerisation rates

The isomerisation of 1MN has been studied at 573-633 K and on 30, 55 and 98% protonated zeolite (figures refer to the starting fully Na-form). Standard conditions were chosen so to keep conversion below 20% in any case. Under these conditions, no gaseous byproducts were ever detected. The amount of thermal cracking was determined by replacing the catalyst with quartz particles of the same mesh fraction. It has been found that, even at the highest temperature, thermal cracking can be completely neglected. Figure 1 shows the typical trend of 1MN fractional conversion y and of coke deposited C_c (g/g cat.) vs. time-on--stream.

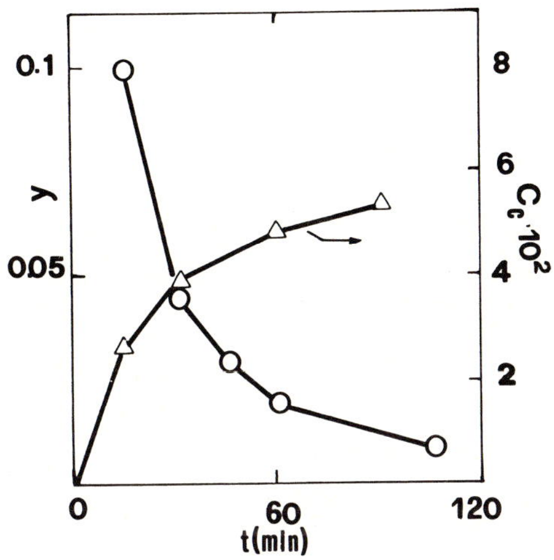

Fig. 1. Fractional conversion of 1MN and coke formation on HNaY-55 catalyst vs. time-on-stream, at 573 K.

Coke formation rate r_c has been expressed as mol of 1MN transformed into coke/h x g cat. Figure 2a shows that, for a given catalyst, r_c is scarcely dependent on temperature, but quickly decreases with time-on-stream, its value after 100 min being less than 20% of the value after 15 min. However, r_c strongly depends on the ion-exchange degree (i.e. on surface acidity). In fact, when comparing the behaviour of differently ion-exchanged zeolites, at the same temperature (Fig. 2b), it may be noticed that the initial (after 15 min on-stream) coking rate of the most acidic catalyst (HNaY-98) is one order of magnitude higher than for the less acidic one (HNaY-30), while the values after 120 min are very low and practically identical for all the catalysts.

It is well-known (ref. 2) that a correlation exists between coking rate and the amount of coke deposited on the catalyst, HNaY-98 catalyst possesses strong acid sites (0.13 mmol/g for $pK_a \leq -1.5$) which are virtually absent in both HNaY-

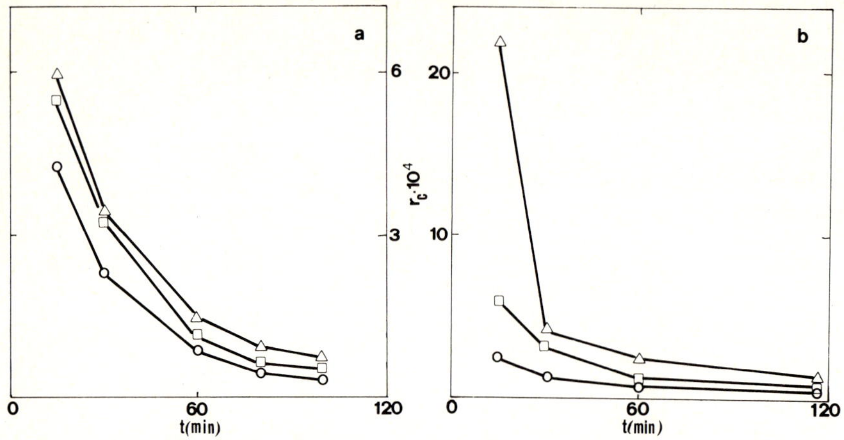

Fig. 2. Coking rate vs. time-on-stream. (a) HNaY-55 catalyst: (△) 633 K, (□) 603 K, (O) 573 K; (b) T = 633 K: (△) HNaY-98, (□) HNaY-55, (O) HNaY-30. Other reaction conditions: standard.

-55 and HNaY-30. These are responsible not only of the high initial rate of coke formation, but also of the rapid decay of activity, because of the high quantity (ca. 7% of the catalyst weight, within the initial 15 min on-stream) of coke, forming on fresh catalyst. The heavy coverage by carbonaceous deposits prevents any further access of the reactant to the active sites, so that r_c decreases more rapidly than on less acidic surfaces. It is interesting to compare the isomerisation rate r_i, defined as mol of 1MN transformed into 2MN/h x g cat., with the coking rate r_c.

Figure 3 shows not only that r_i is always higher than r_c, by one or two orders of magnitude, but also that the higher the temperature (Fig. 3a) and the higher the surface acidity (Fig. 3b), the lower is the (r_c/r_i) ratio. In other words, in spite of a marked increase of coking rate, due to an increase of temperature and/or of surface acidity, isomerisation grows more quickly than coking. Furthermore, Fig. 3b shows that the less acidic catalyst (HNaY-30, surface acidity = 0.16 mmol/g, for $pK_a \leq 6.8$) performs more steadily than the more acidic ones (1.46 and 2.00 mmol/g, for HNaY-55 and HNaY-98, respectively). However, both coking and isomerisation rates being in any case quite low, (ca. 1.1 x 10^{-4} and ca. 0.9 x 10^{-3} mol/h x g, respectively), this catalyst does not perform satisfactorily. On the other hand, with the most acidic catalyst (HNaY-98) both r_i and r_c decrease with time-on-stream. However, within 0.5 h on-stream, the latter drops more quickly (from more than 23 x 10^{-4} to ca. 4 x 10^{-4} mol/h x x g) than the former (from ca. 30 x 10^{-3} to ca. 23 x 10^{-3}). As a consequence,

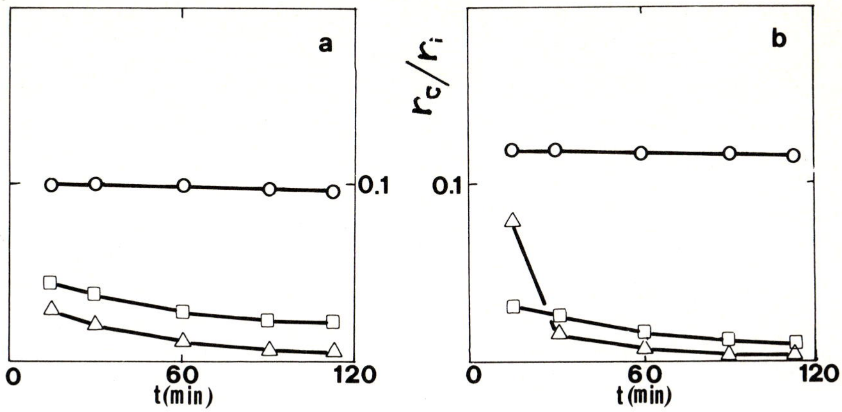

Fig. 3. Coking and isomerisation rates vs. time-on-stream. (a) HNaY-55 catalyst: (△) 633 K, (□) 603 K, (O) 573 K; (b) T = 633 K: (△) HNaY-98, (□) HNaY-55, (O) HNaY-30.

the ratio (r_c/r_i) becomes very low and then remains practically unchanged, due to a further slow decaying of both the rates with similar trends. These facts seem to point to the conclusion that, at least after the initial "flash", coking takes place through a slow and progressive poisoning of the active sites, more than through the pore blocking mechanism.

<u>Coke deposition and deactivation rate</u>

The increase Δp in weight of catalyst, due to coke deposition, may be written as

$$\Delta p = a\theta_d \tag{1}$$

where a is the coke weight deposited at complete deactivation of sites and θ_d the fraction of deactivated sites. The following simple equation

$$\log(a/(a-\Delta p)) = B/2.303\ t \tag{2}$$

was employed to interpret the increase of catalyst weight with time (t) in a similar process (ref. 11). For the present case, by plotting the first member of eqn. 2 vs. t, straight lines were obtained, the slope of which, evaluated by the least-squares method, gave the values of the coefficient B, collected in Table 1. This parameter may be considered only as an index of the amount of coke deposited on catalyst. It may be seen that its value increases with increasing temperature and surface acidity.

A different approach may be followed (ref. 4). If the activity decay is due

TABLE 1

Values of parameter B (eqn. 2).

Catalyst	T,K	$B \times 10^2$, min^{-1}
HNaY-55	573	2.20
HNaY-55	603	2.46
HNaY-55	633	2.82
HNaY-30	633	2.16
HNaY-98	633	3.31

to coke formation, then activity cannot be a simple function of time and the deactivation function should be referred to coke content, rather than to time-on-stream. For the cracking of cumene on Y zeolite, the best deactivation function was found to be (ref. 5):

$$\phi = \exp(-\alpha C_c) \quad (3)$$

where $\phi = r_i/r_i^\circ$, r_i° being the value of r_i for fresh catalyst ($t\to 0$), and α is an empirical constant. By applying such an equation to our data, the plots shown in Fig. 4 were obtained. From the slope of such straight lines (least-squares method) the values of α, shown in Table 2, were calculated.

TABLE 2

Deactivation coefficient α(g cat./g coke).

Catalyst	T,K	α
HNaY-55	573	40
HNaY-55	603	36
HNaY-55	633	31
HNaY-30	633	55
HNaY-98	633	6

One may notice that the value of α decreases with increasing temperature and surface acidity. In other words, the lower the temperature and surface acidity, the less is the amount of coke required for poisoning the active sites. As for the effect of surface acidity, this can be explained by considering that, in zeolitic catalysts both concentration and strength of acid sites decrease with decreasing the ion-exchange degree. The centres present on the less exchanged zeolites being weaker than the ones present on the more exchanged ones, a thinner layer of coke may be reasonably sufficient for poisoning the catalyst. On the other hand, the effect of temperature is easily explainable, by taking into account that the lower the temperature, the more strongly coke precursors are adsorbed on catalyst surface and the less easily they can move out of the zeolite pore system.

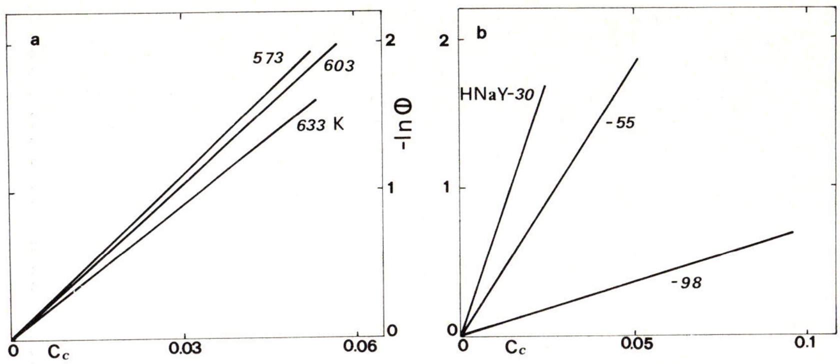

Fig. 4. Effect of coke on catalyst activity. (a) HNaY-55 catalyst, (b) T = 633 K.

CONCLUSIONS

The principal results coming from the present study are: i) in 1MN isomerisation on Y zeolite, the rate of coke formation is relatively fast, but, in any case, it is at least one order of magnitude slower than the main reaction. ii) Coke is very likely formed of polyaromatic, highly condensed systems, which are not significantly volatile, but decompose easily by oxidation. iii) The deactivation process seems to follow a site-poisoning, rather than a pore-blocking mechanism. iv) The lower the reaction temperature and the less acidic the catalyst surface, the lower is the quantity of coke required for poisoning the catalyst.

ACKNOWLEDGEMENT

This work was done within the Italian C.N.R. Project on Fine Chemistry.

REFERENCES

1 E.G. Derouane, in B. Imelik et al. (Editors), Catalysis by Acids and Bases, Elsevier, Amsterdam, 1985, p. 221.
2 C.-C. Lin, S.W. Park and W.Y. Hatchen, Ind. Eng. Chem., Process Des. Dev., 22 (1983) 609.
3 J.E. Wukasch and H.F. Rase, Ind. Eng. Chem., Process Des. Dev., 21 (1982) 558.
4 G.F. Froment and K.B. Bischoff, in Chemical Reactor Analysis and Design, Wiley, New York, 1979.
5 F.J. Dumez and G.F. Froment, Ind. Eng. Chem., Process Des. Dev., 15 (1976) 291.
6 L.D. Rollmann and D.E. Walsh, J. Catal., 56 (1979) 139.

7 V. Solinas, R. Monaci, B. Marongiu and L. Forni, Appl. Catal., 9 (1984) 109.
8 A.P. Bolton, in R.B. Anderson and P.T. Dawson (Editors), Experimental Methods in Catalytic Research, Vol. II, Academic Press, New York, 1976, p. 1.
9 V. Solinas, R. Monaci, B. Marongiu and L. Forni, Appl. Catal., 5 (1983) 171.
10 W.G. Appleby, J.W. Gibson and G.M. Good, Ind. Eng. Chem., Process Des. Dev., 1 (1962) 102.
11 L. Forni, L. Zanderighi, C. Cavenaghi and S. Carrà, J. Catal., 15 (1969) 153.

B. Delmon and G.F. Froment (Editors), *Catalyst Deactivation 1987*

DEACTIVATION AND REACTIVATION BEHAVIOR OF ZEOLITE HYDROCRACKING CATALYST FOR RESIDUAL OIL

KENJI NITA, SATOSHI NAKAI, SETSUO HIDAKA, TAKEHARU MIBUCHI,
HAJIME SHIMAKAWA, KEN-ICHI II, and KAZUHIRO INAMURA

Central Research Laboratories, Idemitsu Kosan Co. Ltd.,
1280 Kamiizumi, Sodegaura, Kimitsu, Chiba 299-02, Japan

ABSTRACT

Deactivation and reactivation behavior of zeolitic catalyst for residual oil hydrocracking has been studied, and especially the change of the catalyst state in the course of the run was investigated. The hydrodesulfurization activity and the hydrocracking activity decreased with time on stream at 400°C for about 500 hours. However after raising the temperature up to 410°C, the cracking activity increased gradually for about 1500 hours, while the hydrodesulfurization activity decreased. The behavior of the hydrocracking activity, deactivation and reactivation, had a good agreement with the change of the acidity of the catalyst installed in a zone from the middle to the bottom of the reactor. The carbon to hydrogen atomic ratio, Laser Raman and FT-IR spectra of the used catalysts suggested that the graphitization of the carbonacious species on the used catalysts taken out from the middle and the bottom of the reactor proceeded during the operation at 410°C, and acidic sites was regenerated.

INTRODUCTION

Hydrocracking catalysts are roughly classified into two groups for its use. One is for distillate oil, naphtha or gas oil, and the other is for residual oil. Hydrocracking catalysts are generally prepared by impregnating group 6B and 8 metals on stable carriers. Amorphous silica-alumina carriers have been widely used in commercial hydrocracking processes. In recent years, crystalline zeolitic carriers have become more important due to high activity and resistance to poisoning by nitrogen compound. However, those zeolitic carriers were not available for hydrocracking residual oils containing a relatively large amount of poisoning species such as asphaltenes and metals.

Idemitus Kosan Co. Ltd. developed the unique zeolitic catalyst, of which surface acidity and porosity were modified for hydrocracking residual oil. The performance of the catalysts and the practical capabilities were confirmed using conventional resid HDS units (ref.1,2). One of the striking characteristic of this catalyst was the behavior of the hydrocracking activity around the specific reaction temperature. Although at 400°C the hydrocracking activity gradually decreased with time on stream, raising the temperature up to 410°C the hydrocracking activity increased with time on stream for 2000 hours and then decreased.

In this paper, we report the results of the studies for the changes of the chemical and physical properties of the catalysts as a function of time on stream to understand the deactivation and reactivation mechanism of the zeolitic catalyst.

EXPERIMENTAL

The hydrocracking catalyst used for this experiment was prepared by impregnating cobalt and molybdenum on carrier consisting of FeHY zeolite and alumina. FeHY zeolite, which has the unique acidic properties under the presence of H_2S, was prepared by the treatment of HY zeolite with ferric nitrate solution (ref.3). The catalyst form was that of cylindrical extrudate particles with L/D = 3.

The residue hydrocracking experiments were carried out using bench scale fixed bed reactors. The reactor had a catalyst volume of 100 ml and a length to diameter ratio of 20. The feedstock mixed with hydrogen was continuously fed to the top of the reactor. The whole product withdrawn from the bottom of the reactor was seperated to liquid and vapor products in separation system. Each experiment was performed at a pressure of 13.5 MPa, a liquid space velocity of 0.3 h^{-1}, and a hydrogen flow rate of 60 l/h. The catalyst was presulfided at a temperature of 250°C and a liquid space velocity of 1.0 h^{-1} for 24 hours using light gas oil. The used catalysts were sampled from three sections, the top,the middle and the bottom of the catalyst bed. Each sample was soxhlet extracted with toluene and dried in vacuum at 120°C before performing elemental analyses and other experiments. The properties of the feedstock, Kuwait atmospheric residue, are shown in Table 1.

TABLE 1

Properties of feedstock, Kw-AR

Gravity, API	13.3
Sulfur, wt%	4.24
Nitrogen, ppm	2,100
Concarbon residue, wt%	12.4
Vanadium, ppm	54
Nickel, ppm	17
n-Heptane insoluble, wt%	3.85
C/H of AR, atomic ratio	0.64

Cumene cracking for evaluating the acidity of the used catalysts was performed using the conventional method of pulse technique under herium stream (ref.4).

The coke deposited on used catalysts has been characterized by means of Raman and Infrared spectroscopies. Laser Raman spectra were obtained using a JASCO NR-1000 spectrophotometer (514.5 nm excitation). IR spectra were recorded using a JEOL JIR-100 FT-IR spectrometer.

RESULTS AND DISCUSSION

Residue hydrocracking

Catalyst performance of FeHY hydrocracking catalyst for residual oil under two operation modes is shown in Figure 1. In MODE 1 the temperature was raised up to 400°C and kept constant for about 400 hours after presulfiding, then the temperature was raised up to 410°C and kept constant during the run. In MODE 2 the temperature was raised up to 410°C after presulfiding and was kept constant during the run. In MODE 1 the

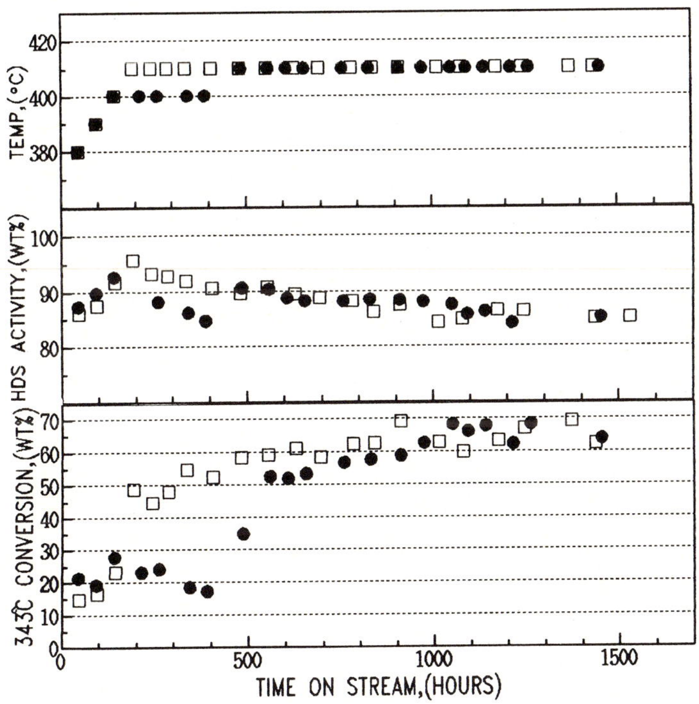

Fig.1. Performance of zeolitic hydrocracking catalyst for Kuwait atmosphric residue under different operation modes. Solid circles and open squars represent MODE 1 and MODE 2.

hydrodesulfurization activity (HDS) and the hydrocracking activity initially decreased with time on stream at 400°C, while after raising the temperature up to 410°C at operation time of 500 hours the cracking activity increased gradually for about 1000 hours nevertheless the temperature was kept constant. Generally, residue hydroprocessing catalysts are known to deactivate in a characteristic manner, as shown in a number of articles (ref.4,5,6). The initial period is characterized by a rapid, but continuously decreasing, deactivation rate. This deactivation phenomenon has been known to be caused by the coke deposition on the catalyst. The HDS activity in this experiment showed the same behavior, while hydrocracking activity showed different behavior. To confirm and reproduce this unusual phenomenon the residue hydrocracking was performed in a different mode, MODE 2, also shown in Figure 1. The hydrocracking activity at 410°C increased in a similar manner as MODE 1 with operation time, and finally the hydrocracking activity reached to the same conversion level as MODE 1 after time on stream of about 1000 hours.

Hydrocracking conversion and product yields as a function of time on stream are shown in Table 2. The conversion gradually increased after raising the temperature up to 410°C in both MODE 1 and 2, and reached the

Table 2

Conversion and product yields as a function of time on stream

Time (hr)	MODE	Temp. (°C)	Conversion[a] (wt%)	Yield (wt%) Naphtha[b]	Kerosene[c]	LGO[d]	H D S (wt%)
150	1	400	28	6	6	14	93
	2	400	23	5	5	13	92
250	1	400	23	4	5	14	88
	2	410	45	13	11	15	93
400	1	400	17	2	3	11	85
	2	410	55	17	13	14	92
500	1	410	35	8	8	16	91
	2	410	58	22	14	15	90
700	1	410	57	16	13	15	88
	2	410	63	24	14	11	86
1000	1	410	63	25	12	12	88
	2	410	63	31	13	11	86
1500	1	410	64	23	12	14	85
	2	410	65	33	10	8	85

[a] $\left(1 - \frac{\text{wt\%, 343°C in product}}{\text{wt\%, 343°C in feedstock}}\right) \times 100$, [b] C5 - 171°C, [c] 171 - 232°C, [d] 232 - 343°C

same level after 1000 hours on stream. The naphtha yield increased as the conversion increased in each MODE. However, the yields of kerosene and LGO(light gas oil), did not increase monotonously with respect to the increase of conversion, even they decreased after the conversion exceed around 60 %. Hydrocracking of atmospheric residue can be explained to proceed successively as follows ;

$$\text{A.R.} \xrightarrow{k_1} \text{middle distillate} \xrightarrow{k_2} \text{naphtha} \xrightarrow{k_3} \text{C4-}$$

The increase of the conversion shall mean the reaction rate constant k_1 becoming larger. The naphtha yields increased and middle distillates yield did not increase in spite of the conversion increase, which suggests that the rate constant k_2 may become larger along with k_1.

Cumene cracking

The change of the catalyst properties with time on stream was studied by repeating the run (MODE 1). Six samples of used catalysts were taken out of the reactor for evaluating the catalyst properties at the indicated points in Figure 2.

Cumene cracking activities of the used catalysts are also shown as a function of time in Figure 2. The change of cumene cracking activities of the catalysts taken out from the middle and the bottom of the reactor had

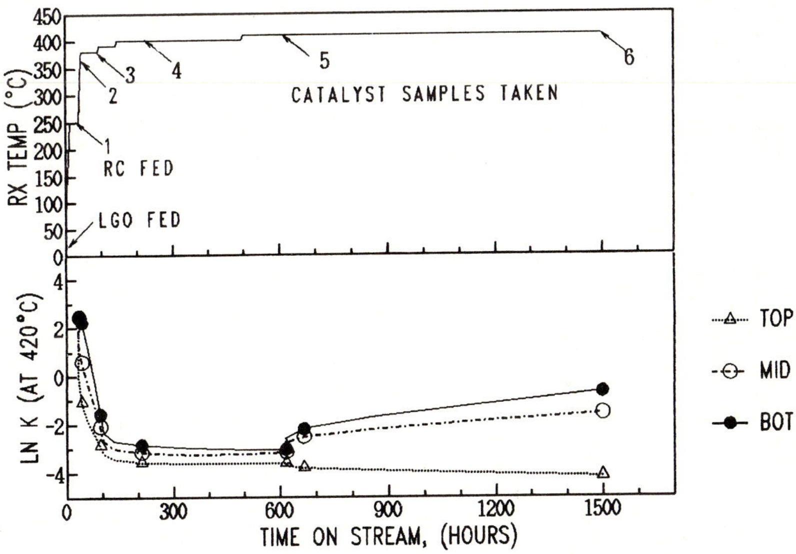

Fig.2. Cumene cracking activities of used catalysts as a function of time on stream(MODE 1).

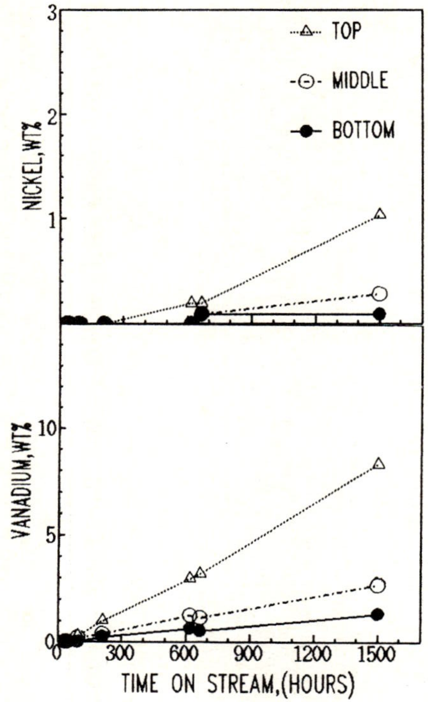

Fig.3. Vanadium and Nikel (wt%,based on fresh catalyst) deposited on the used catalyst as a function of time on stream (MODE 1).

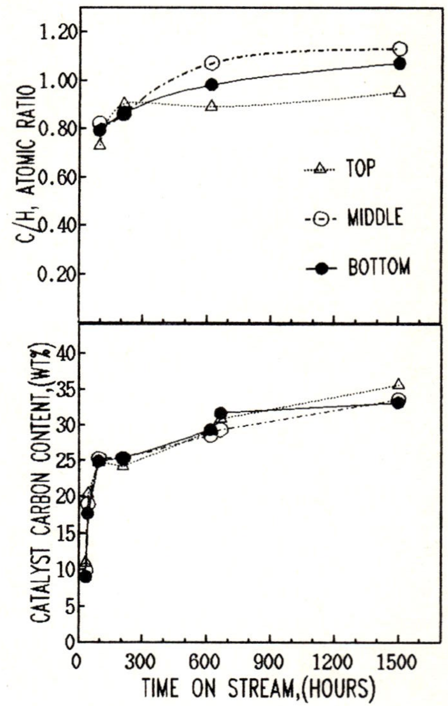

Fig.4. Catalyst carbon content (wt%,based on fresh catalyst) and carbon to hydrogen atomic ratio in the used catalyst as a function of time on stream (MODE 1).

the same behavior as that of residue hydrocracking activity as shown in Figure 1, while the activities of the catalysts taken out from the top of the reactor did not change after time on stream of 100 hours. The behavior of residue hydrocracking activities of zeolite catalyst could be explained by the rejuvenation of the acidity of the zeolite contained in the catalysts from the middle to the bottom of the reactor.

Elemental analysis

The depositional profiles for nickel and vanadium from the top to the bottom of the reactor, as a function of time on stream, are shown in Figure 3. Both the deposition of nickel and vanadium increased with time on stream, and the amount of the deposition was largest at the top of the reactor and smallest at the reactor bottom during the run. Metal sulfide, especially nickel sulfide, is known to have a hydrogenolysis activity (ref.8). The most of nickel sulfide accumulated on the catalysts at the top of the reactor, which had the lowest cumene cracking activity during the run. This result cannot explain the increase in the acidity of the catalysts taken out from the middle and the bottom of the reactor after 500 hours operation.

The change in the amount of coke on the catalysts was also investigated for this set of catalyst samples. As shown in Figure 4 and Table 3, the carbon contents on catalysts increased rapidly during the initial period of the run before time on stream of 45 hours, and after that they increased gradually. There was no remarkable differnce in the carbon content between the catalysts taken out from the reactor top and bottom. However the carbon to hydrogen atomic ratio in the coke on the catalysts showed interesting results, as also shown in Table 3 and Figure 4. The catalysts taken out

TABLE 3

Analyses of used catalysts (MODE 1)

Time on stream (hours)	Carbon (wt%[a])			C/H (Atomic ratio)			Surface Area (m^2/g)		
	Top	Middle	Bottom	Top	Middle	Bottom	Top	Middle	Bottom
① 37 (Presulfiding)	10.8	9.8	8.9	-	-	-	205	247	243
② 45 (AR 370℃)	20.3	18.9	17.6	-	-	-	113	150	220
③ 96 (AR 380℃)	24.7	25.3	24.8	0.73	0.82	0.79	79	81	78
④ 211 (AR 400℃)	24.1	25.3	25.3	0.90	0.86	0.86	78	79	79
⑤ 619 (AR 410℃)	29.1	28.6	29.3	0.89	1.07	0.98	61	63	60
⑥ 1501 (AR 410℃)	35.6	33.5	33.1	0.95	1.13	1.07	54	55	54

[a]Based on fresh catalyst.

from the top of the reactor showed little increase of carbon to hydrogen ratio during the run. However, the catalysts from the middle to the bottom of the reactor had a higher carbon to hydrogen ratio and showed a substantial increase after 500 hours on stream.

Spectroscopic characterization ; Laser Raman and FT-IR spectroscopies

Laser Raman and FT-IR spectroscopies were applied to characterize the properties of the coke on the catalysts. Figure 5 shows a comparison of the Raman spectra for cabonacious species on 200 hours aged catalyst(A) and 1500 hours aged catalyst(B), both taken out from the bottom of the reactor. Both catalysts showed characteristic modes 1600 cm^{-1} and 1350 cm^{-1}. According to previous works (ref.9,10), well crystallized graphite shows a sharp band at 1580 cm^{-1}, while pregraphitic carbon, or crystalline graphite with structural defects, shows another broad composite band with a maximum at about 1355 cm^{-1}. The ratio of the intensity 1355 cm^{-1} and 1580 cm^{-1}, I(1355)/I(1580), has been correlated to the degree of graphitization or the size of graphite crystallites. In the Raman spectrum of the coke on catalyst(B), the ratio I(1355)/I(1600) decreased and the 1600 cm^{-1} became sharper. These results indicate that the coke on the aged catalyst for 1500 hours has a more graphitic structure. In Figure 6, the IR spectrum of the catalyst (A) and (B) showed the absorption bands at 2965 cm^{-1} and 2925 cm^{-1} correlated to assymmetric CH_3- and CH_2- stretching vibrations respectively, and a band at 2860 cm^{-1} being due to the symmetric C-H vibrations. As can be seen from Figure 6, the amount of aliphatic hydrocarbon decreased with time on stream, indicating the progress of aromatization for carbonacious species on the catalyst with time on stream.

Deactivation and reactivation mechanism

The deactivation and reactivation mechanism of the zeolite catalyst around the specific reaction temperature were assumed on the basis of these results. The content of coke on the catalyst increased rapidly during the initial period of the run (Figure 4). As the carbon to hydrogen atomic ratio in the coke on the catalysts used at lower temperature than 400°C was lower than that of asphaltene (Table 3), 0.95 , contained in the atmospheric residue, this coke could be carbonacious species which was asphaltenes or polyaromatic compounds adsorbed on the catalyst acid sites. Aging the catalysts at 400°C, the coke content of the catalysts and the carbon to hydrogen atomic ratio increased gradually (Fig.4). This suggests that the asphaltene adsorption, polymerization and dehydrogenation

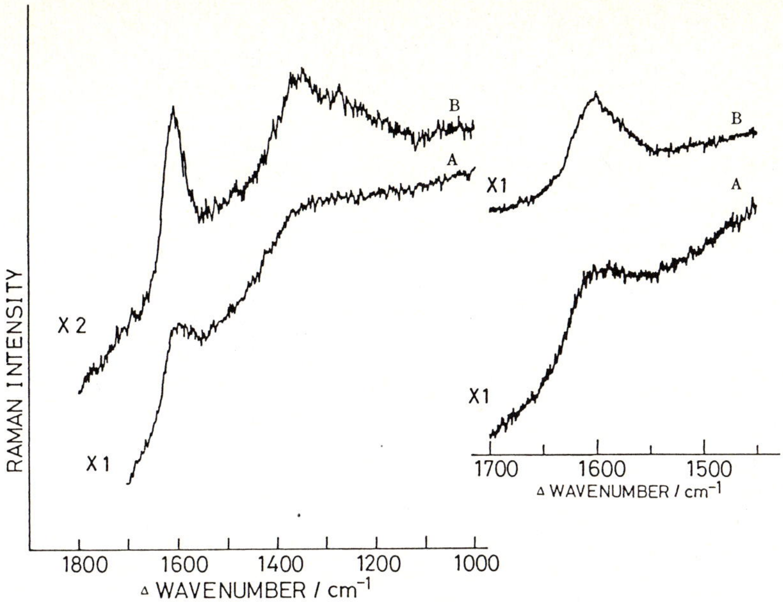

Fig.5. Laser Raman spectra of used catalysts. A ; 200 hours aged catalyst at 400°C. B ; 1500 hours aged catalyst at 410°C.

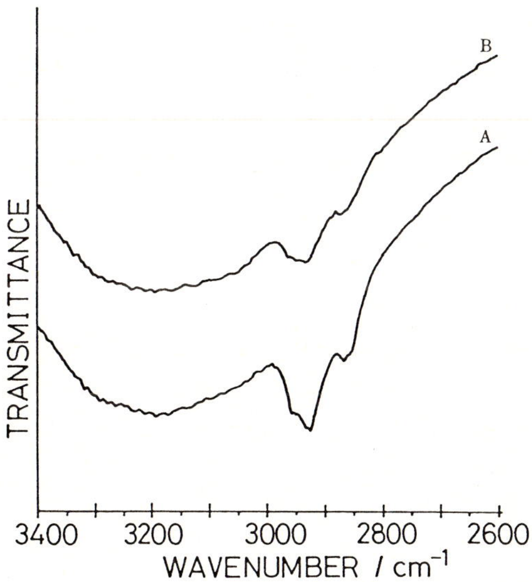

Fig.6. FT-IR spectra of used catalysts. A ; 200 hours aged catalyst at 400°C. B ; 1500 hours aged catalyst at 410°C.

proceeded substantially. The decrease of cracking activity with time on stream at 400°C could be caused by covering the acid sites with carbonacious species(Figure.1,2). Raising the temperature up to 410°C, the rate of the dehydrogenation and the graphitization of carbonacious species adsorbed acid site on the catalyst became larger relatively than that of adsorption. Then the carbonacious species could have changed to graphitic particles, resulting in the exposure of acid sites as shown in Figure 7. The decrease of the surface area of used catalysts during the run(Table 3) suggests that the regeneration of acid sites did not correspond to the internal micropore, but external acid sites of zeolite which is effective for residual oil hydrocracking. Asphaltenes or polyaromatic large molecules, especially containing heteroatoms such as nitrogen and oxygen, tend to be present as basic groups. These groups are readily adsorbed on the surface acid sites of zeolite, and may have caused the unusual phenomenum of zeolitic hydrocracking catalyst activity for residual oil.

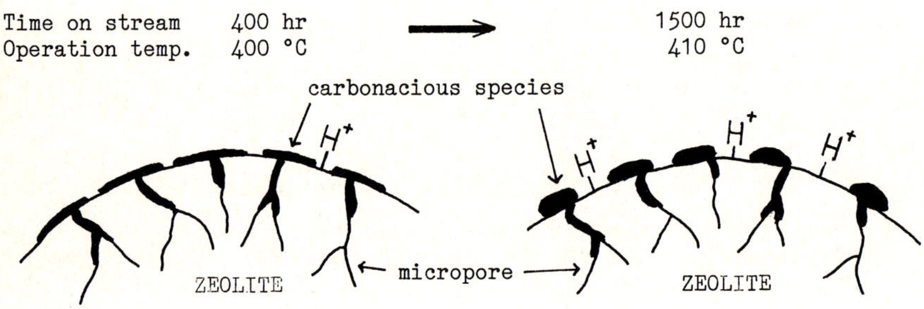

Fig.7. The change of the zeolite surface with time on stream and operation temperature.

Acknowledgment

We wish to thank Professor N. Yamazoe for valuable discussion and the Research Association for Residual Oil Processing (RAROP) for it's sponsorship to this work.

REFERENCES

1. Y. Ito, H. Sugiyama, E. Sarashina and M. Yoshita, the AIChE 1986 Spring National Meeting, April 6-10, 1986.
2. H. Sue and M. Fujita, Oil and Gas J., May 26, 1986.
3. S. Hidaka, A. Iino, K. Nita, Y. Maeda, K. Morinaga and N. Yamazoe, Proc. of the 7th International Zeolite Conference, Tokyo, 1986 pp.329-

336.
4. J. Turkevich and Y. Ono, Molecular Sieve Zeolite-2, ACS 102 (1971), 315-326.
5. A. G. Bridge, E. M. Read, P. W. Tamm, and D.R.Cash, Paper No.14a, 74th National AIChE Meeting, New Orleans, La, March 1979.
6. A. M. Henke, Oil and Gas J., 68(14) (1970) 97 .
7. H. Nitta, T. Takatsuka, S. Kodama and T. Yokoyama, 86th National AIChE Meeting, Houston, Texas, April 1979.
8. R. F. Sullivan, C. J. Egan, G. E. Langlois, and R. P. Sieg, J. Am. Chem. Soc., 83 (1961) 1156.
9. P. Lespade, R. Al-Jishi and M. S. Dresselhaus, Carbon, 20(5) (1982) 427-431.
10. D. Espinat, H. Dexpert, E. Freund and G. Martino, Applied Catalysis, 16 (1985) 343-354.

B. Delmon and G.F. Froment (Editors), *Catalyst Deactivation 1987*
© 1987 Elsevier Science Publishers B.V., Amsterdam — Printed in The Netherlands

"MECHANISMS FOR THIOPHENE POISONING OF NICKEL CATALYSTS: EFFECT OF CRYSTALLITE SIZE"

K. AHMED, D. CHADWICK and L.S. KERSHENBAUM

Department of Chemical Engineering & Chemical Technology, Imperial College of Science and Technology, Prince Consort Road, London, SW7 2BY, U.K.

ABSTRACT

Thiophene adsorption studies were carried out on nickel catalysts of varying crystallite size. The experiments were performed at 298K with a 1000 ppm thiophene/hydrogen mixture, and 10%-20 wt% $Ni/\gamma\text{-}Al_2O_3$ catalysts were used. The crystallite size of nickel in the catalyst was changed by varing its nickel loading and by sintering in hydrogen at elevated temperatures. Nickel areas of the samples were determined from CO chemisorption and their crystallite sizes were determined by X-ray line broadening. Results showed that thiophene adsorption on nickel is structure sensitive: the uptake of thiophene by the different catalyst samples varied with the Ni-crystallite size. The experimental results were consistent with a model which could be represented by two rate processes: one following a 2-site adsorption mechanism and the other following a 5-site mechanism.

INTRODUCTION

The poisoning effect of thiophene on metal catalysts is well documented. However, the mechanism underlying the adsorption of thiophene on the metal surface is still not understood completely. There have been some attempts (refs. 1-3) to characterize the effect of temperature on the poisoning; these and other investigations have led to certain hypotheses regarding the mechanism of thiophene poisoning. Lyubarskii et al. (ref. 1) proposed a scheme according to which a thiophene molecule is strongly bonded with plane orientation to five nickel atoms. At elevated temperatures, they suggested thiophene is hydrogenated to thiophane, which may then be further hydrogenated to butane and other decomposition products. Bourne et al. (ref. 2) suggested that at 100°C, thiophene initially adsorbs flat and then decomposes, taking up hydrogen to liberate butane, leaving a sulphide ion attached to a nickel site. They found that at 30°C to 150°C, the S/Ni ratio ranged from 0.03 to 0.09. At temperatures above 150°C, the S/Ni ratio increased rapidly to reach a value of 0.25 at 200°C, which, if sulphiding were confined to the surface only, corresponds to a fully covered surface. They explained the partial sulphiding by using a geometric model. They also suggested that at high temperatures thiophene may react with nickel to give H_2S. They claimed that the ability of a thiophene-sulphided catalyst to adsorb carbon monoxide confirms the existence of unsulphided sites which results from random poisoning. This, however, is not true as shown by the results of Bartholomew & Pannel (ref. 9) and Viveros-Garcia (ref. 3), who found that the measured uptake of carbon monoxide at 190-298K, by a S-poisoned Ni-catalyst, is increased with the amount of sulphur present on the nickel surface, presumably due to the increased formation of nickel carbonyl; therefore, CO titration is not representative of the free-area of the poisoned samples.

Weng *et al.* (ref. 4) studied the poisoning kinetics of thiophene adsorption on Ni-kieselguhr catalysts at temperatures of 65-175°C and for thiophene concentrations ranging from 50 to 250 ppm. Benzene hydrogenation was used as a model reaction to measure remaining catalytic activity. They found excellent agreement with a power law equation for the rate of deactivation with time. They also considered a model with two types of sites, one active for thiophene chemisorption alone and the other active for hydrogenation as well. Although both models were able to fit the data from an integral fixed-bed reactor, further results on the intrinsic kinetics of thiophene poisoning would be needed in order to represent unambiguously the state of the catalyst surface.

From infrared studies of adsorbed thiophene, Blyholder & Bowen (ref. 5) concluded that although it is generally assumed that adsorption of sulphur compounds is via coordination of the sulphur atom with the surface, adsorption on clean silica-supported nickel is a much more varied and complicated process involving frequent bond rupture in the adsorbing compound even at room temperature. Rochester & Terrell (ref. 6) questioned whether bands reported in previous infrared studies of sulphur compounds on nickel/silica may be correctly attributed entirely to adsorption on the metal surface. They pointed out that some contribution to the spectra probably resulted from chemisorbed species on the oxide support.

Recent studies of thiophene adsorption at room temperature (refs. 3, 7) have given Ni/C_4H_4S stoichiometric ratios of around 3, which indicates that in addition to being adsorbed in the coplanar mode (ref. 1), thiophene can also adsorb on nickel occupying a fewer number of sites. The present work was undertaken to investigate the varying modes of thiophene adsorption and the possible effect of crystallite size on the adsorption.

EXPERIMENTAL

The catalysts studied had compositions of 10, 15 and 20 wt% Ni and were prepared by impregnation of a nickel nitrate solution on gamma alumina. Particle size ranged between 30-50 mesh. Before impregnation the support was treated in air for 2hr at 393K and for 16hr at 673K. The impregnated catalyst was dried in flowing air (150 ml/min) at 393K for 2hr and then calcined in air at 673K; the calcined catalyst was then cooled under air flow. The samples were then reactivated by hydrogen in situ at 600°C prior to either chemisorption of CO for nickel area determination or experiments on poisoning. The properties of the catalysts studied are illustrated in Table 1. Samples of the 20% catalyst were sintered at four different temperatures (650, 700, 750 and 780°C) in order to increase crystallite size. In preparing the sintered catalysts, fresh catalyst samples were charged to a quartz tube and heated for 50hr in flowing hydrogen (100ml/min). The sintered catalyst samples were then cooled under hydrogen flow and then purged with nitrogen prior to exposure to the atmosphere for crystallite size determination by XRD.

Adsorption studies were performed in a microbalance reactor coupled to a flow system. Hydrogen was passed through a saturator containing thiophene at a controlled temperature (-30±0.1°C); this stream was then mixed with a diluent hydrogen stream to obtain the desired feed concentration. The poisoning experiments were all carried out in an atmosphere of hydrogen, with the catalyst initially in its reduced state with chemisorbed hydrogen; the adsorption of thiophene on the catalyst was therefore accompanied by a displacement of chemisorbed hydrogen from the surface. The microbalance was also coupled to a vacuum BET system for in situ measurement of surface area, metal area and pore size distribution.

TABLE 1

Nickel surface area and average crystallite size

Sample	Loading wt% Ni	Sintering Temperature °C	Nickel area m^2/g cat	Crystallite Size Å	Mean Pore Diameter Å
F10	10	(unsintered)	7.31	33	104
F15	15	(unsintered)	9.47	45	102
F20	20	(unsintered)	10.66	59	101
S1	20	650	9.38	64	100
S2	20	700	8.01	71	97
S3	20	750	7.32	80	53
S4	20	780	6.40	92	53

RESULTS

Catalyst Characterisation

Table 1 lists the Ni-area and the crystallite size of the various samples. The Ni-area was determined from CO chemisorption isotherms at 195K. The choice of the adsorption temperature was made from the findings of Viveros-Garcia (ref. 3), who investigated CO adsorption on Ni/γ-Al_2O_3 at three different temperatures and found that at 77K, high physisorption led to poor reproducibility and at 273K, there was substantial nickel carbonyl formation. These difficulties did not arise at 195K. A Ni/CO ratio of 1.4 was used in calculating the area from the CO monolayer uptake. This value is consistent with the finding of a constant saturation coverage of 1.1 x 10^{19} molecules/m^2 for CO chemisorption on nickel (refs. 10-13) and, except for the lowest loading catalyst, was proportional to the area calculated from crystallite size measurements.

The crystallite size of the samples were determined by X-ray line broadening. Some experimental difficulties were experienced in determining the average crystallite size by XRD because of the interference of the support. It was found that the most prominent peak for Ni(111) was almost entirely obscured by a broad peak for alumina. To obviate this problem, the crystallite size was determined from the second most prominent peak for Ni (200), which for the catalyst loading used in this study was of moderate size and most importantly, free from any support interference.

Thiophene Adsorption

Fig. 1 shows typical thiophene adsorption uptake curves for some of the samples and Table 2 lists the overall thiophene uptake and the resultant Ni/C_4H_4S stoichiometry for all the samples.

For catalyst samples with relatively small crystallites (F10, F15, F20, S1 and S2), ninety percent of the adsorption occurs in the first 10 minutes with up to half the uptake in only 30 seconds. Poisoning data at $t < 30$ sec. was not measurable because of the initial fluctuations in microbalance reading when the feed was switched from hydrogen to the thiophene mixture. After an initial period of about 20-30 minutes, the rate of uptake was found to be very slow and continued for up to 2 hours. (The physical adsorption component of the uptake continued for 6-8 hours and has been subtracted away to give the results shown in Fig. 1.) The same behaviour was observed for both catalyst particles (0.4mm) and powders (0.4μm).

In contrast, in the case of catalyst particles with large crystallites (S3 and S4), the rate of uptake was considerably lower - 90% of the total adsorption was completed in 25-30 minutes. However, the rate of adsorption on powdered samples of S3 and S4 was much higher than on the corresponding particles and they approached saturation even more rapidly than did the samples with smaller crystallites.

The saturation uptake of thiophene decreased with increasing crystallite size, to a larger extent than could be accounted for by a corresponding decrease in surface area. Gas chromatographic analysis of the exit-stream from the adsorption experiment did not detect any butane or butene (ref. 7), indicating that at room temperature, thiophene was not undergoing any hydrodesulphurisation. The Ni/C_4H_4S stoichiometric ratios at saturation have been calculated on this basis and are presented in Table 2.

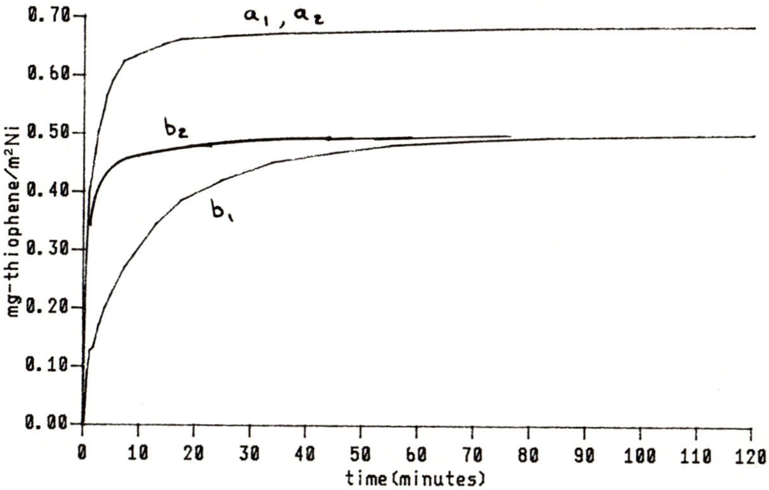

Fig. 1. Thiophene chemisorption uptake: (a_1) sample F20-pellet; (a_2) F20-powder; (b_1) S3-pellet; (b_2) S3-powder.

TABLE 2

Saturation thiophene uptake and Ni/C_4H_4S ratios

Sample	Thiophene uptake mg/gcat	mg/m²Ni	Ni/C_4H_4S
F10	6.18	0.845	2.54
F15	7.01	0.73	2.90
F20	7.36	0.69	3.11
S1	6.38	0.68	3.17
S2	5.22	0.65	3.31
S3	3.60	0.49	4.38
S4	3.06	0.48	4.43

In order to explain the above results several computer models were developed to simulate the behaviour of the system. The simplest model which could explain all the results consisted of a pore diffusion process in series with two parallel or series rate processes for adsorption: one via a 5-site mechanism (coplanar with the surface) and the other one via a 2-site mechanism (perpendicular to the surface). A typical simulation result is shown in Fig. 2. No adjustment of parameters was required in order to get agreement between model and experiment. The effective diffusivity was calculated using a random pore-model and the rate constants were obtained by fitting the data of one experimental run; the same values were then used to simulate the uptake behaviour of all other samples which varied in crystallite size and/or loading. The fractions of the surface corresponding to 2-site and 5-site adsorption were calculated from the observed saturation stoichiometry. The model and the details of the simulation study are presented elsewhere (ref. 14).

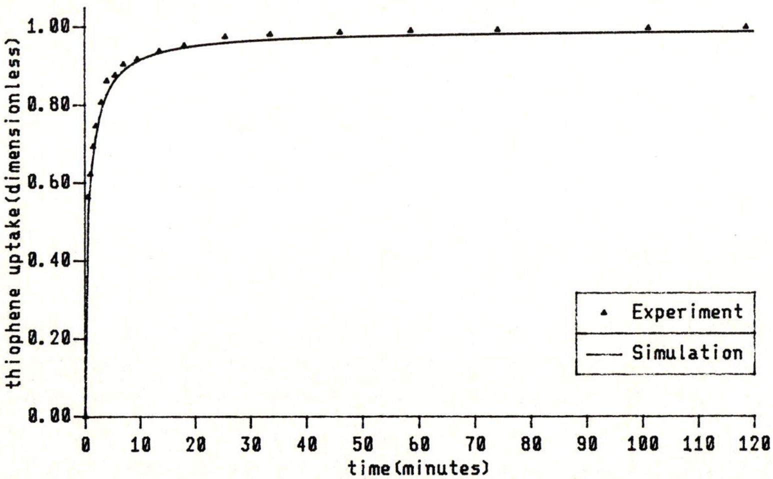

Fig. 2. Comparison of experiment and simulation for sample S2.

DISCUSSION

Since thiophene was not undergoing any decomposition at room temperature, Ni/C_4H_4S ratios such as those obtained in this study would only be possible if one assumed that thiophene was adsorbed in at least two different forms. It was postulated that a certain fraction of the incoming thiophene is adsorbed coplanar to the surface with a Ni/C_4H_4S stoichiometry of 5 and that the remaining fraction is adsorbed perpendicular via the sulphur atom and effectively poisons two nickel sites per thiophene molecule. The overall stoichiometry is determined by the extents of the two types of adsorption which in turn depends upon the fractions of the two different types of sites in the catalyst. For crystallites of 40 to 70Å, a Ni/C_4H_4S ratio of about 3 was obtained; with crystallites of 80 to 90Å, this ratio was 4.4. This would indicate that for the larger crystallites the fraction of thiophene adsorbed coplanar is substantially higher than for smaller crystallites. Other factors like crystallite shapes, their irregularity or their size distribution may also have influenced the observed uptake of thiophene but are difficult to characterize.

Coplanar adsorption, where one thiophene molecule takes up five Ni sites, is likely to take place at the central sites of the surface; perpendicular adsorption involving two Ni sites per adsorbed thiophene molecule may be occurring only at the edges and corners if coplanar adsorption is preferential over perpendicular. However, using catalyst data and assuming ideal crystallites, the geometry indicates that there are not enough edges and corners to allow for the observed Ni/C_4H_4S ratios of around 3 for samples F20, S1 or S2. On the other hand, for samples S3 and S4, the difference between the observed Ni/C_4H_4S ratios and those computed for ideal crystallites are only slightly outside the limits of experimental uncertainty.

Various hypotheses regarding the modes of thiophene adsorption and the effect of sintering are then consistent with the observed results:

1. Coplanar and perpendicular adsorption may be occurring according to the respective fractions of central surface sites, and edge and corner atoms respectively. However, it is likely that the crystallites in the unsintered and partially sintered catalysts have lattice defects which give rise to internal edges and corners on which thiophene is adsorbed perpendicularly; thus, there are more edges and corners than would be predicted from ideal crystallites. Sintering at the high temperatures of 750 and 780°C not only increases the geometric size of the crystallites, but also decreases the concentration of such defects so that the crystallites now approach regularity and ideal characteristics.

2. Perpendicular adsorption may not be limited to edges and corners, but may occur on the central surface sites as well with coplanar adsorption the preferential model at the central surface sites. Once the thiophene molecules are adsorbed coplanar, the spaces in between are filled by perpendicularly adsorbed thiophene, as these sites are no longer large enough to accommodate a coplanar species.

3. Initially, when the thiophene/hydrogen mixture is introduced, thiophene may be adsorbed in the coplanar mode and then a fraction may react irreversibly with hydrogen to form thiophane which then assumes the perpendicular position. However, if the perpendicular species is thiophane alone, then thiophene adsorption on nickel would vary with crystallite size of nickel only if there were two types of sites for thiophene adsorption on nickel: one in which thiophene can chemisorb only, and the other in which thiophene can be hydrogenated as well. The relative amounts of such sites may vary

with the crystallite size. It may also be possible that both species can exist in perpendicular mode: a fraction of the thiophene coplanarly adsorbed initially is hydrogenated to thiophane, which takes up the perpendicular position; thiophene itself may also adsorbs in the perpendicular mode at the edges and corners.

All the above hypotheses were investigated via a computer simulation of the kinetics of the adsorption process which included both physical and chemical steps. The details of the modelling study are presented elsewhere (ref. 14).

Other possible mechanisms (such as hydrogenation to butane with an adsorbed sulphur ion present; adsorption on the support or on nickel aluminate (ref. 8)) were inconsistent with the observed experimental results.

CONCLUSIONS

The experimental results have shown that thiophene adsorption on nickel is structure sensitive: the overall stoichiometric ratio of adsorbed thiophene to nickel varies with crystallite size. It is postulated that thiophene is adsorbed on nickel in two different modes: coplanar and perpendicular. In the perpendicular mode the adsorbed species is either thiophene itself or the hydrogenation product, thiophane, or both. The coplanar species appears to be adsorbed thiophene. The adsorption of the coplanar species is likely to prevail at the central sites of the surface; at the edges and corners only the perpendicular species can be adsorbed because of geometric restrictions. The perpendicular species may also be present in the spaces between coplanarly adsorbed thiophene. The coplanar species may be undergoing hydrogenation to thiophane which then assumes the perpendicular position and results in adsorption of more thiophene, presumably in the perpendicular mode. There was no evidence of hydrodesulphurisation of thiophene at room temperature.

REFERENCES

1. G.D. Lyubarskii, L.B. Avdeeva and N.V. Kul'kova, Kinetika i Kataliz, 3 (1962) 123-132.
2. K.H. Bourne, P.D. Holmes and R.C. Pitkethly, 3rd Int. Congr. on Catalysis, North Holland, 1954, pp.1400-1415.
3. T. Viveros-Garcia, Ph.D. Thesis, London University, U.K, 1985.
4. H.S. Weng, G. Eigenberger and J.B. Butt, Chem. Eng. Sci. 30 (1975) 1341-1351.
5. G.D Blyholder and D.O. Bowen, Journal of Physical Chemistry, 66 (1962), 1288-1292.
6. C.H. Rochester and R.J. Terrell, Journal of Chemical Society Faraday Transactions, 73 (1978), 596-608.
7. K. Ahmed, Ph.D. Thesis, London University, U.K., 1987.
8. K.S. Kester, E. Zagli and J.L. Falconer, Applied Catalysis, 22 (1986), 311-319.
9. C.H. Bartholomew and R.B. Pannel, Applied Catalysis, 2 (1982), 39-49.
10. K. Klier, A.C. Zettlemoyer and H. Leidheiser, Jr., Journal of Chemical Physics, 52 (1970), 589-602.
11. J.C. Tracy, Journal of Chemical Physics, 56 (1972), 2736-2747.
12. H.H. Madden, J. Küppers and G. Ertl, Journal of Chemical Physics, 58 (1973), 3401-3410.
13. H. Conrad, G. Ertl, J. Küppers and E.E. Latta, Surface Science, 57 (1976), 475-484.
14. K. Ahmed, L.S. Kershenbaum and D., Chadwick, in preparation.

THE EFFECT OF PARTIAL REDUCTION ON THE THIORESISTANCE OF Ni/Al_2O_3 CATALYSTS

D. DUPREZ and M. MENDEZ

Laboratoire de Catalyse en Chimie Organique, UA CNRS 350,

40, Av. Recteur Pineau 86022 POITIERS CEDEX FRANCE

ABSTRACT

The effect of partial reduction on the thioresistance of the metals was evaluated on two series of nickel catalysts. The first series, comprising Ni/Al_2O_3 samples with variable metal loading (2 to 12 wt %) were characterized (metal area, degree of reduction), using two different methods : chemisorption of gases (H_2, O_2) and magnetism. Despite some discrepancies between the two methods of characterisation, it can be concluded that the presence of an unreduced phase improves the thioresistance of nickel, expressed as the number of molecules of thiophen required for deactivating one atom of surface nickel. For increasing the amount of unreduced nickel, a second series of catalysts was prepared by impregnation of nickel on $NiO-Al_2O_3$ supports (pre-spinelised at 700°C). As a result, the catalysts were found to be particularly resistant to sulphur poisoning. In turn, three hypothesis were considered to interpret these results : trapping effects of sulphur by unreduced nickel species of the support, electronic effects (Ni^o-Ni^{2+} interactions) and geometric effects (dilution of the nickel surface by unreduced species). Complementary experiments (measurement of sulphur capacity by H_2S chemisorption and evolution of electronic interaction by competitive hydrogenation) were used to clarify these interpretations. Trapping effects are likely but not sufficient to account for the improvment of thioresistance, which could be due also to geometric effects.

INTRODUCTION

The presence of an unreduced phase can markedly alter the properties of metal catalysts. This behavior has been clearly demonstrated for rhodium (Ref.1,2) and cobalt catalysts (Ref.3,4) in CO/H_2 reactions and for nickel catalysts operating in the same reactions and in alcane hydrogenolysis (Ref.5) Recently, we have shown that the selectivities of alumina-supported rhodium and nickel catalysts in the steam reforming of aromatics were particularly sensitive to the reduction state of the metals (Ref.6) . The purpose of the present study was to demonstrate that partial reduction can also modify the thioresistance of the metal catalysts used in the same reactions. The chosen model has been the nickel-alumina system operating in the toluene steam reforming (TSR) at 460°C. In this study, the unreduced phase of nickel was stabilized by chemical interaction with the support and the degree of reduction was varied either by increasing the metal loading or by impregnating nickel on $NiO-Al_2O_3$ supports pre-spinelized at 700°C. The thioresistance of nickel (expressed as the number of atoms of sulphur required for deactivating one atom of surface nickel) was evaluated in TSR by using thiophen as a source of sulphur in the reactant. Complementary experiments were also performed for measuring the sulphur capacity of certain samples (H_2S chemisorption) and for estimating the electronic interaction Ni^o-Ni^{2+} (competitive hydrogenation of benzene and toluene).

EXPERIMENTAL

Materials. Rhone-Poulenc γ-alumina GFS 300 (210 m^2g^{-1}, mean pore radius 40 A, Na, Fe and Si impurities < 400 ppm, grain size 1mm) was used as a support. For simplying the nomenclature, it is referred to as alumina A. The first series of catalysts consists of Ni-Al_2O_3 samples with variable metal loading. The preparation and the characterization of this series were reported in detail elsewhere (Ref.7). Briefly, the catalysts were prepared by impregnation of alumina A with aqueous solution of nickel nitrate, dried at 120°C, then calcined at 450°C and finally reduced at 500°C. They are referred to as NixA where x is the nickel loading in wt %. This series was completed by 4% Ni catalysts prepared by exchange of the support with nickel ammonium complexes (Ref.7). These catalysts (Ni4AC1 and Ni4AC2) were not calcined prior to reduction. In order to increase the fraction of Ni^{2+} in the solids, a second series of catalyst was prepared by impregnation of pre-spinelized NiO-Al_2O_3 supports with solutions of nickel nitrate. Subsequent pretreatments (drying, calcination, reduction) are similar to those of the first series. The supports were made from standard Ni-Al_2O_3 catalysts calcined at 700°C for 14h under air stream (VHSV 500 h^{-1}). This treatment induces the formation of large amounts of nickel aluminate in a quasi-spinel structure, which is practically unreducible at 500°C. The nickel loading added to the support is invariably ca 5 wt % and the catalysts are referred to as Ni-NiO y A where y is the content of NiO in the support (15<y<25 wt%)

Catalyst characteristics. The extent of reduction R% and the dispersion of the metallic phase D% were determined in a pulse chromatographic system described elsewhere (Ref.7,8). The values of R were deduced from the oxygen uptake capacity at 500°C, assuming that Ni^o is reoxidized as NiO. The dispersion were calculated from the amounts of hydrogen chemisorbed at 25°C. The results are expressed in atoms of hydrogen per 100 atoms of reduced nickel. The first series of catalysts were also characterized by magnetic methods which allow the degree of reduction and the metallic particle sizes d_s to be estimated (Ref.7). The degree of dispersion can then be calculated from $\%D = 978/d_s$. To avoid any ambiguity, % R_c and % D_c represents the values of % R and % D determined by chromatography, whereas % R_M and % D_M are the corresponding characteristics deduced from magnetic measurements.

Poisoning studies were conducted as described in ref 9 . Toluene steam reforming (TSR) was carried out in a flow reactor at 460°C and atmospheric pressure (H_2O to toluene molar ratio of 6, weight hourly space velocity 1.2 h^{-1}). Prior to reaction, the catalyst samples were reduced for 14h at 500°C in a flow of hydrogen (VVH 3000 h^{-1}). Sulphurized feedstocks were prepared by adding known amounts of thiophen to 1l of toluene. Four grades of toluene were used containing respectively 0, 50, 100 and 250 ppmS in thiophen form.

Complementary studies:Sulphur capacity was measured by H_2S uptake at 460°C. The samples were reduced overnight at 500°C and cooled at 460°C. The sulphur capacity S_C was determined by frontal injection of a H_2S/H_2 mixture (50 ppm H_2S) monitored by a photoionization detector. The reversible part S_{rev} of adsorbed sulphur was then measured from the amount of H_2S desorbed in pure hydrogen.

Competitive hydrogenation of benzene and toluene was performed at 100°C in a flow reactor on catalyst samples reduced in situ at 500°C. The ratios of the adsorption coefficients of the toluene and of the benzene $K_{T/B}$ were deduced from the simplified method originally described by Tran Mahn Tri et al (Ref.10).

RESULTS

Preliminary investigations of the TSR kinetics on nickel catalysts

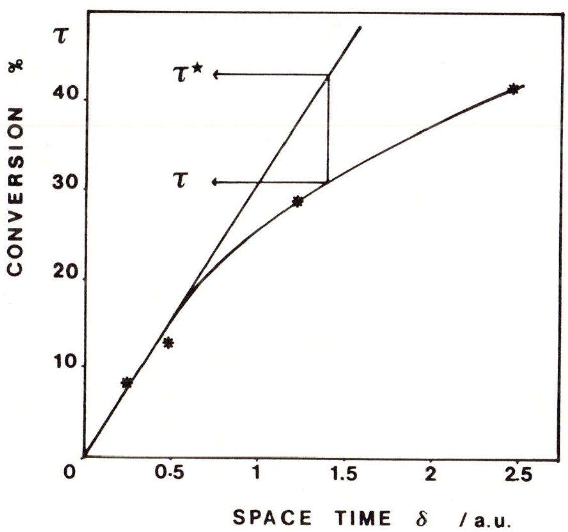

Figure 1 : Conversion versus space time plot for Ni5A at 460°C.

The deactivation curves are systematically drawn in normalized activities r/r_0, where r_0 is the initial activity and r, the activity at time t. As toluene conversions τ were obtained in the range 0-60 %, the kinetic equations of the integral reactor were applied :

$$\left.\begin{array}{ll} -(1/1-m)\left[(1-\tau)^{1-m} - 1\right] = k\, P_{Ti}\,\delta = \tau^{*} & \text{for } m \neq 1 \\ \text{and Log } (1/1-\tau) = k\,\delta = \tau^{*} & \text{for } m = 1 \end{array}\right\} (1)$$

where m is the pseudo-order with respect to toluene, k the rate constant, P_{Ti} the partial pressure of toluene at the reactor inlet and δ , the space time The pseudo-order m is defined by the simple power-law rate $r = KP_T$ which replaces, in a certain domain of P_T, the detailed kinetic equation $r = K'f(P_T, P_{H2O}, Pi)$ including the partial pressures of the products. The value of m was determined in preliminary experiments from the curves τ vs δ ; the curve correspondhg to the 5.25 % Ni/Al_2O_3 sample is shown in Fig 1. For the catalysts of these series, m = 1.9 ± 0.2. It is to note that m is quite differing from the true kinetic order n with respect to toluene determined from Log r vs Log P_T plots at low conversion. For instance, n = - 0.04 for the 5.25% Ni catalysts, in agreement with the results of Grenoble [11] . This means that the conversion is largely depending on the partial pressure of products. Thus the normalized activity r/r_0 will be taken equal to the ratio τ^*/τ_0^* determined from Eq.1.

Sulphur poisoning of $Ni-Al_2O_3$ catalysts in TSR

The catalysts of the first series are listed in Table 1. Also recorded in the table are the characteristics determined both by dynamic volumetry (chromatography) and by magnetism.

TABLE 1 : Nickel-alumina catalysts (first series) : nomenclature and characteristics

Name	Ni /wt %	Characteristics: Volumetry R_C %	D_C %	Magnetism R_M %	D_M %
Ni2A	1.93	62	2.4	47	11
Ni4A	4.35	66	5.8	48	16.3
Ni5A	5.25	72	6.7	65	16.3
Ni8A	8.1	80	6.9	76	13.8
Ni12A	11.4	92	8.0	83	15.8
Ni4AC1	3.98	79	12.5	67	25.7
Ni4AC2	4.06	84	10.2	71	23.9

The extents of reduction found by the two methods are practically similar : one may just note an overestimation by about 10% when dynamic volumetry is used. On the other hand, the relatively large discrepancies observed on the values of the metal areas have already been reported and discussed elsewhere (Ref.7). They seemed essentially related to partial reduction of nickel, since, a quite good agreement was found between volumetry and magnetism for well-reduced catalysts. In the following the metal areas obtained by the two methods will be taken into consideration to assess the validity of our conclusions.

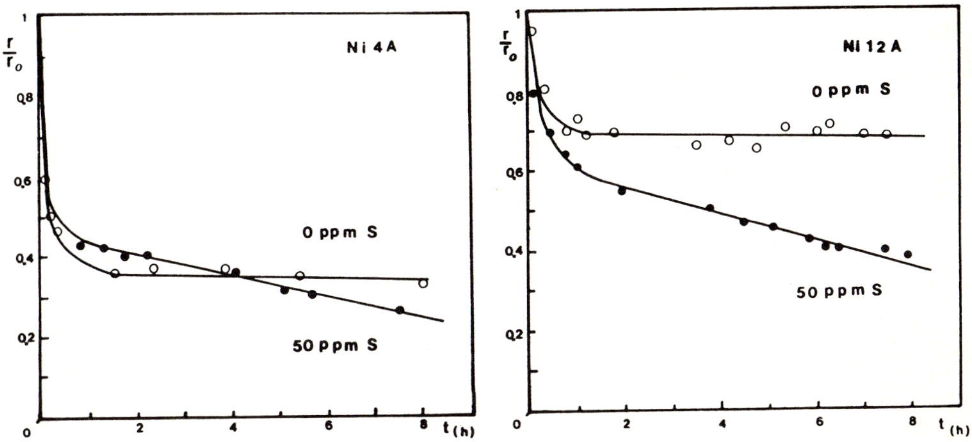

Figure 2 : Curves of deactivation for the Ni4A and Ni12A catalysts (460°C, H_2O/TOL molar ratio of 6, 50 ppmS as thiophen in the toluene).

The curves of deactivation have been drawn with pure toluene and with toluene containing 50 ppmS. The results obtained on two representative samples (Ni4A, Ni12A) are shown in Fig 2. As for rhodium catalysts (Ref.9), a sharp decrease of activity is observed during the first hour of reaction, even there is sulphur or not in the feedstock : this period of deactivation is essentially controlled by coke formation on the catalyst, which is likely to be as fast on nickel (Ref.12,13) as on rhodium (Ref.14). The presence of sulphur in toluene even can partially prevent the formation of carbon deposit (see eg. Ni4A in Fig 2.). This is a fairly general phenomenon which have already been reported for other metal-alumina catalysts in TSR (Ref.15) and for nickel in steam reforming of methane (Ref.16). After 1 hour-on-stream the activity becomes quite stable in absence of sulphur, whereas it goes on decreasing linearly with time in poisoning experiments. This allows us to determine the values S/Ni_s (amount of sulphur passed per atom of surface nickel) extrapolated to zero conversion. Two sets of values could be calculated according to the method used for determining metal areas. The results are recorded in Table 2.

Table 2 : sulphur poisoning of Ni/Al_2O_3 catalysts (first series) in TSR at 460°C with 50 ppmS : S/Ni_s ratios extrapolated to zero conversion

Catalysts	S/Ni_s (at r = 0)	
	Ni_s from volumetry	Ni_s from magnetism
Ni2A	1.25	0.38
Ni4A	0.92	0.47
Ni5A	0.61	0.28
Ni8A	0.56	0.28
Ni12A	0.35	0.18
Ni4CA1	0.49	0.28
Ni4CA2	0.62	0.32

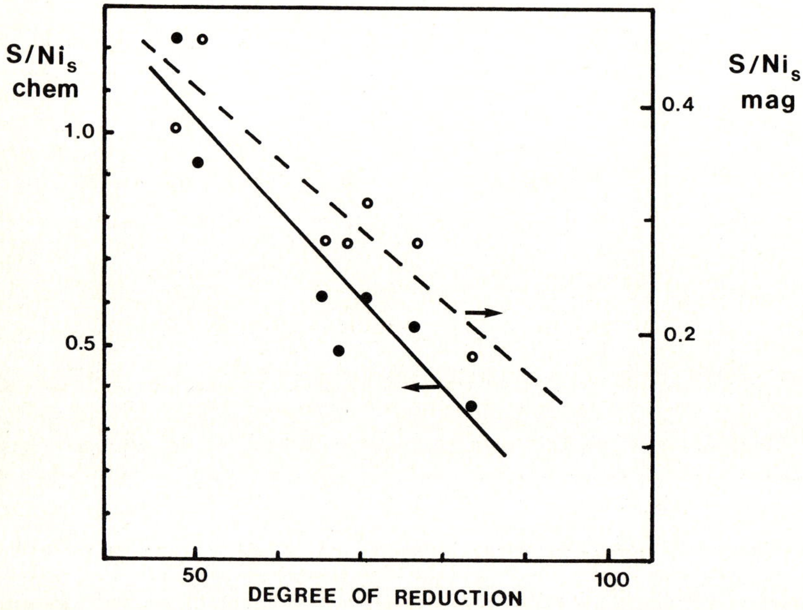

Figure 3 : S/Ni_s ratios as a function of the degree of reduction (first series of catalysts). The nickel area is determined either by chemisorption (chem) or by magnetism (mag).

No correlation could be found between the thioresistance of the catalyst and the metal dispersion : the samples prepared by exchange are relatively well-dispersed and show no particular behavior with respect to impregnated catalysts. This is not very surprising since particle size effects on the thioresistance of metals are general weak (Ref.17) or restricted to very small particles (D > 40-50%) (Ref.18). On the other hand, the presence of an unreduced phase seems to increase the thioresistance of the metallic fraction as it is demonstrated on fig 3 where are plotted the S/Ni_s ratios as a function of the degree of reduction. The same tendency is observed whatever method for determining metal areas and can thus be considered a true effect of the partial reduction of catalyst.

Sulphur poisoning of Ni-NiO-Al_2O_3 catalysts in TSR

The characteristics of the supports and of the catalysts are recorded in Table 3. Also indicated in the table are the compositions of the catalysts after reduction at 500°C. The pre-spinelized supports are partly reduced at 500°C, but the proportion of metallic nickel remains relatively low. Upon reduction at 500°C of catalysts prepared by impregnation of these supports, the added nickel is entirely reduced. In the meanwhile, a supplementary fraction of the nickel oxide of the support turns out to be reduced. This is clearly evidenced by the fact that the overall amount of reduced nickel in the catalyst (for instance, 1690 μmole g^{-1} in Ni-NiO15A) is noticeably higher than the sum of the added nickel (1003 μmole g^{-1}) and of the reduced nickel in the support (159 μmole g^{-1}).

Fig 4 shows the curves of deactivation of the Ni-NiO15A catalyst. Also represented in the figure is the own catalytic behavior of the support determined in separated experiments. sulphur poisoning is evident on the support. Nevertheless, owing to the quite low metal area, the S/Ni_s ratio amounts to a particularly high value (>5). At the same time, no sulphur poisoning can be noticed on the Ni-NiO15A within 8h-on-stream, which demonstrates the high sulphur resistance of this catalyst.

TABLE 3 : Charateristics of nickel catalysts supported on pre-spinelized NiO-Al_2O_3

SUPPORT	NiO loading wt % NiO	NiO loading μmol g^{-1}	H_C μmol $H.g^{-1}$	O_C 500 μmol O g^{-1}	% R_C
NiO15A	13.46	1802	3.7	159	8.9
NiO20A	18.77	2512	3.5	262	10.5
NiO25A	23.94	3204	6.3	789	24.6

CATALYST	added Ni wt % Ni	added Ni μmol g^{-1}	H_C μmol H g^{-1}	O_C 500 μmol O g^{-1}	% R based on added Ni	% R based on Total Ni
Ni-NiO15A	5.89	1003	87	1690	100	63
Ni-NiO20A	5.49	935	128	1650	100	51
Ni-NiO25A	4.39	748	140	1900	100	50

CHARACTERISTICS AFTER REDUCTION AT 500°C

CATALYST	reduced Ni wt % Ni	reduced Ni μmol g^{-1}	NiO wt%	NiO μmol g^{-1}	% D
Ni-NiO15A	9.9	1690	7.3	980	5.1
Ni-NiO20A	9.7	1650	12.2	1630	7.7
Ni-NiO25A	11.2	1900	14.0	1880	7.4

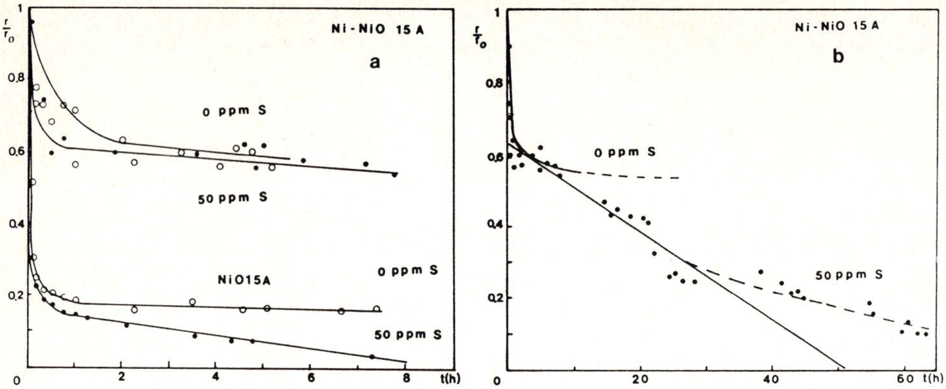

Figure 4 : Curves of deactivation for the Ni-NiO15A catalyst and the corresponding support. a-initial deactivation , b-long-time experiment.

Long-time poisoning experiments were thus performed to measure the thioresistance of the catalysts. Results are represented in Fig 4. The slow decrease of conversion (about 0.8 % h^{-1}) leads, by extrapolation, to total deactivation of catalyst at 70 h-on-stream (instead of 14 h and 27h for Ni5A and Ni12A, respectively). A similar behavior is observed on Ni-NiO20A and Ni-NiO25A catalysts (Fig 5) which are particularly thioresistant as compared to Ni-Al_2O_3 samples. S/Ni_S values recorded in Table 4 bears out that the presence of nickel oxide in the support can prevent, to a certain extent, sulphur poisoning.

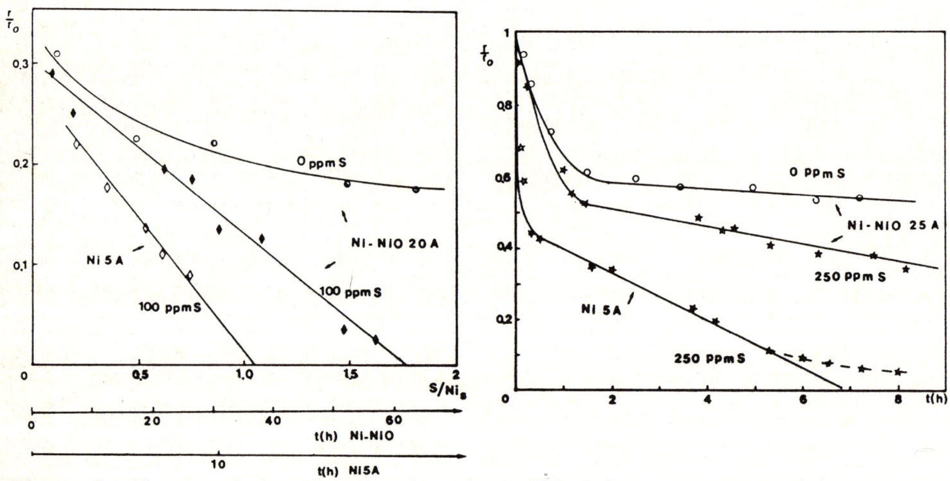

Figure 5 : Curves of deactivation for Ni-NiO20A (a) and Ni-NiO25A (b).

TABLE 4 : S/Ni_s values on nickel catalysts supported on $NiO-Al_2O_3$

CATALYST	sulphur content in toluene / ppm	S/Ni_s (at r = 0)
Ni015A	50	5
Ni-Ni015A	50	1.5
Ni5A	50	0.61
Ni12A	50	0.35
Ni-Ni020A	100	1.85
Ni5A	100	0.9
Ni-Ni025A	250	2.8
Ni5A	250	1.3

Complementary studies

Poisoning by sulphur of toluene steam reforming obeys a complex mechanism which starts very probably with the steam reforming (or the hydrogenolysis) of the molecule of thiophen into dihydrogen sulphide. These reactions are self-poisoned by sulphur and, as a rule, thiophen which entered the reactor, is not entirely converted and retained by the catalyst. To clarify this point, we have measured the sulphur capacity of the catalysts at 460°C from H_2S/H_2 mixtures. Results are reported in Table 5. For purposes of comparison, the amounts of thiophen which had entered the reactor up to total deactivation are recorded in the table.

TABLE 5 : sulphur capacities of some catalysts samples (from H_2S 50 ppm/H_2) and amounts of thiophen passed at zero conversion. Values are given in μmole S g^{-1}

Catalyst	sulphur capacity (H_2S)	Thiophen passed at r = 0
Ni015A	49	19 (50 ppmS)
Ni-Ni015A	202	130 (50 ppmS)
Ni020A	44	-
Ni-Ni020A	182	237 (100 ppmS)
Ni5A	93	27 (50 ppmS)
-id-		39 (100 ppmS)
Ni2A	22	7 (50 ppmS)

The sulphur capacity is always higher than the amount of thiophen which can deactivate the catalyst. Nevertheless the results of Table 5 bear out that the nickel supported on pre-spinelized $NiO-Al_2O_3$ possesses a high thioresistance (the amount of thiophen is relatively close to the sulphur capacity). One of the hypothesis which is involved in explaining this particular behavior of Ni-$NiOAl_2O_3$ catalysts is an electronic effect between the reduced nickel particles and the support which could be reinforced by the presence of nickel ions in the support. Competitive hydrogenation of benzene and toluene was used to evaluate these electronic interactions (Ref.19). The results obtained on selected catalysts are reported in Table 6

TABLE 6 : Competitive hydrogenation of benzene and toluene on Ni/Al_2O_3 and $Ni/NiO-Al_2O_3$ catalysts

Catalyst	$^a\ V_B^o$ mol h^{-1} g^{-1}	$^b\ V_B$ mol h^{-1} g^{-1}	$K_{T/B}$
Ni2A	2.0 10-4	0.9 10-4	5.25
Ni12A	2.9 10-3	1.4 10-3	4.28
NiO20A	4.5 10-4	1.7 10-4	6.67
Ni-NiO20A	6.4 10-3	3.5 10-3	3.63

[a] rate of benzene hydrogenation at 100°C with pure benzene
[b] rate of benzene hydrogenation at 100°C with 75% mol benzene-25% mol toluene mixtures

The presence of an unreduced phase of nickel exerts an increasing influence on the first three samples (NiO20A>Ni2A>Ni12A) in accordance with their degree of reduction. On the other hand, no electronic effect of the partial reduction can be evidenced in the Ni-NiO20A catalyst, which behaves as a well-reduced catalyst without any interaction between the reduced nickel particles and the support.

DISCUSSION

The present study shows that the sulphur poisoning of $Ni-Al_2O_3$ catalysts is influenced by the presence of an unreduced phase of nickel : the less the degree of reduction, the more resistant to poison the reduced phase. By using nickel catalysts prepared on pre-spinelized $NiO-Al_2O_3$ supports, the proportion of unreduced phase can be significantly increased and this results in a reinforced thioresistance of the catalyst. Three hypothesis may be put forward for explaining this behavior

a - the most evident reason would be that the unreduced fraction of nickel acts as a sulphur trap protecting the metallic nickel. Values recorded in Table 5 show that the supports (NiO15A and NiO20A)possess a significant sulphur capacity. Nevertheless, it is very likely that an important fraction of sulphidable NiO in the support will be reduced in the final catalyst (the added nickel induces a supplementary reduction of the support, see Table 3) so that the capacity of the support to trap sulphur is significantly less in the catalyst than

in the bare support. Moreover the amount of thiophen required for deactivating the Ni-NiO15A catalyst, for instance, is largely higher than the sum of the amounts of sulphur necessary for poisoning the support NiO15A and the catalyst Ni5A which contains the same quantity of nickel added to support than Ni-NiO15A. Accordingly, the trapping effect of the support is likely but not sufficient to explain the high resistance to sulphur of the Ni-NiOAl_2O_3 catalysts.
b - the second reason which may be invoked for explaining the effect of partial reduction on the thioresistance of nickel is an electronic interaction between Ni^o centers of the metallic particles and Ni^{2+} species of the unreduced phase. In the same way as these interactions are able to inhibit ring opening in aromatic hydrocarbons (Ref.20), they can also decrease the ability of the metal to operate thiophen conversion in the conditions of steam reforming. Nevertheless, the results obtained in competitive hydrogenation are rather in contradiction with this hypothesis : nickel deposited on NiO-Al_2O_3 supports behaves as it was well-reduced, without interaction with the support.

c - the third reason would be due to geometric effects resulting from dilution of the metallic surface by unreduced species of nickel. This hypothesis has been put forward for explaining the discrepancies between volumetry and magnetism when metal areas were attempted to be measured on partially reduced Ni/Al_2O_3 catalysts (Ref. 7). H_2S chemisorption was recommended by Rostrup-Nielsen (Ref. 21) for measuring nickel surface areas. If we compared the values of chemisorbed H_2S on Ni2A and Ni5A (Table 5) and the metal areas determined both by volumetry and by magnetism (Table 1), we can note that the sulphur capacity is rather close to the surface area measured by magnetism. This supports the dilution hypothesis, given that Ni^{2+} species can chemisorb H_2S but not hydrogen. Accordingly, the main effect of dilution should be an inhibition of thiophen steamolysis, because it is hardly conceivable that the presence of unreduced species can decrease the sulphur coverage on the reduced nickel. Thiophen conversion is very sensitive to presulphidation of the metal catalysts. This has been shown in hydrogen reforming catalysts (Ref. 22) and remains probably true for steam conversion. As a rule thiophen conversion require the presence of special sites on which hydrocarbons are also hydrogenolyzed. When these sites are poisoned by sulphur atoms, thiophen hydrogenolysis (or steamolysis) is severely inhibited. The same effect should result from the presence of Ni^{2+} species on the nickel surface. The lack of precise data concerning the rate of thiophen hydrogenolysis or steamolysis on partially reduced Ni/Al_2O_3 catalysts does not allow to conclude definitively. This requires further studies for bearing out interpretation.

ACKNOWLEDGMENTS

We are indebted to the Societe Nationale Elf Aquitaine for financial support and we wish to thank Drs GUEGUEN and BOUSQUET (SNEA Solaise) for helpful discussions and constant interest converning this work. Thanks are due to Dr MARECOT for sulphur capacity measurements and to Dr S. PROBST for competitive hydrogenation measurements.

REFERENCES

1 P.R. Watson and G.E. Somorjai, J. Catal. 72 (1981) 347.
2 F.G.A. Van der Berg, J.H.E. Glezer and W.M.H. Sachtler, J. Catal. 93 (1985) 340.
3 R.C. Revel and C.J. Bartholomew, J. Catal. 85 (1984) 78.
4 S.H. Moon and K.E. Yoon, Appl. Catal. 16 (1985) 289.
5 P. Turlier, H. Praliaud, P. Moral, G.A. Martin and J.A. Dalmon, Appl. Catal. 19 (1985) 287.
6 a G. Delahay, Thesis, Lille 1984
b D. Duprez and G. Delahay, submitted for publication.
7 D. Duprez, M. Mendez and J.A. Dalmon, Appl. Catal. 21 (1986) 1.
8 D. Duprez, J. Chim. Phys., 80 (1983) 487.
9 D. Duprez, M. Mendez, G. Delahay and J. Bousquet Nouv. J. Chim., 9 (1985) 545.
10 Tran Mahn Tri, J. Massardier, P. Gallezot and B. Imelik in "Metal-support and metal-additive effects in catalysis" (B. Imelik et al, Eds), Lyon, 1982. Stud. Surf. Sci. Catal., Elsevier Publ. 11 (1982) 141.
11 D.C. Grenoble, J. Catal. 51 (1978) 203.
12 C.H. Bartholomew in "Catal. Rev. Sci. Eng." (H. Heinemann and J.J Carberry eds) M. Dekker Publ., New York Vol 24 (1982) p 67.
13 C.A. Bernardo, I. Alstrup and J.R. Rostrup-Nielsen J. Catal. 96 (1985) 517.
14 D. Duprez. M. Mendez and J. Little, Appl. Catal., 27 (1986) 145.
15 a J. Bousquet, D. Duprez and M. Mendez, Proc. 8 th Ibero-Amer. Symp. Catal., La Rabida (Spain) 1982. Vol 2 p 839.
b M. Mendez, Thesis, Poitiers (1983).
16 J.R. Rostrup-Nielsen, J. Catal. 85 (1984) 31.
17 C.R. Apesteguia, T.F. Garetto, C.E. Brema and J.M. Parera, Appl. Catal. 10 (1984) 291.
18 J. Barbier, P. Marecot, L. Tifouti, M. Guenin and R. Frety, Appl. Catal. 19 (1985) 375.
19 Tran Thanh Phuong, J. Massardier and P. Gallezot, J. Catal. 102 (1986) 456.
20 G. Delahay and D. Duprez, unpublished results.
21 J.R. Rostrup-Nielsen in "Steam Reforming Catalysts" Teknisk Forlag, Copenhagen (1975).
22 R.W. Coughlin, A. Hasan and K. Kawakami, J. Catal. 88 (1984) 163.

B. Delmon and G.F. Froment (Editors), *Catalyst Deactivation 1987*

DEACTIVATION OF A SUPPORTED COPPER CATALYST IN THE INDUSTRIAL ANILINE PLANT

B. DVOŘÁK[1], J. PAŠEK[1], P. PAVLAS[2] and Z. HEJDA[2]

[1]Department of Organic Technology, Institute of Chemical Technology, Prague 166 28 (Czechoslovakia)

[2]Moravian Chemical Works, Ostrava 709 03 (Czechoslovakia)

ABSTRACT

The influence of macromolecular carbon deposits, catalytic poisons, sintering, and destruction of pellets both on the deactivation and life of a copper catalyst used for the selective gas-phase catalytic reduction has been discussed. The catalyst applied in an industrial tube non-isothermic reactor is deactivated mainly by carbon deposits and sintering. The contribution of catalytic poisons is in fact negligible if their concentration in the processed raw material is lower than 0.5 ppm. It has been proved that the support composition, the presence of poisons, and the amount of 1,3-dinitrobenzene in the raw material can have the major influence on the formation of carbon deposits. The catalyst sintering occurs nearly exclusively in the starting period of the operational cycle. The slow destruction of pellets has a positive influence on the catalyst life.

INTRODUCTION

In contrast to most catalytic processes the catalyst consumption in aniline production is approximately ten times higher and fluctuates between 0.5 and 2.0 kg/t. The magnitude of this consumption is thus one of the criteria characterizing the standard of an aniline process technology.

In the discussed case the aniline production is based on the gas-phase hydrogenation of nitrobenzene on the copper supported catalyst of BASF, type R 3-11. The catalyst is applied both in a tube and an adiabatic reactors connected in series. The deactivation of the catalyst in the tube, non--isothermic, watter-cooled reactor is the subject of this study. From previous research work "(refs. 1-2)" the catalyst has already been known to be deactivated in this process by three parallel routes:

(i) contamination of the surface by macromolecular carbon deposits

(ii) poisoning of the active surface by chlorine and sulphur compounds contained in the raw material

(iii) sintering of primary copper crystallites.

The direct influence of the reaction mixture on the crushing strength of catalyst pellets is a specific property of the investigated process.

RESULTS AND DISCUSSION

Contamination of the catalyst by macromolecular carbon deposits

In the course of the aniline process carbon substances are formed and deposited on the surface of the catalyst. An average amount of these substances in the deactivated catalyst ranges from 12 to 23 mass % C being dependent on the factors discussed further. Carbon deposits are not distributed equally both along the length of the tube and in the catalyst pellet. The axial concentration profile of carbon in the catalyst bed is demonstrated in Fig. 1. The radial concentration profile of carbon decreases from the external surface of the pellet towards its centre.

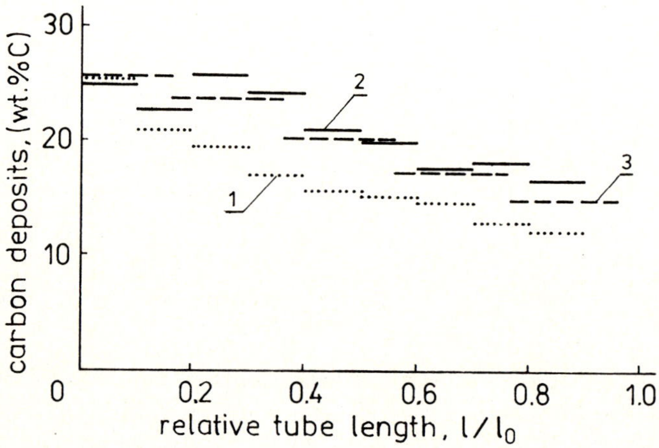

Fig. 1. Dependence of an average axial concentration profile of carbon in a catalyst bed on the period of its operational exposition.

The mechanism of the formation of these deposits which have the character of organic sludges has not been known to date. The average molecular mass of the deposits ranges from 900 to 10,000. These substances consist mainly of carbon and nitrogen in the ratio of C/N = 6 to 8. This ratio indicates that these substances are formed by a chain of benzene nuclei mutually linked with nitrogen atoms. For example, the aniline black has a similar structure.

Substances of this type can be formed by the oxidative effect of nitrobenzene on aniline or on intermediates raised by nitrobenzene reduction and the following condensation of these substances. The shape of the axial concentration profile of carbon in the catalyst bed (see Fig. 1) is in accordance with this idea. Experiments have proved that the contaminants are not formed in the gas-phase but exclusively on the catalyst surface. A different explanation of the deposits formation is introduced by Sada et al. "(ref. 3)". In his opinion, diphenylamine and carbazole are supposed to be carbon deposit precursors. From our point of view, these substances take part in the contamination of the catalyst surface but they are not, the main source of the deposits. It is aniline that has proved to be the dominant substance detected by the pyrolytic chromatography of sludges isolated from the catalyst. Unexpectedly, the rate of the deposits formation was the lowest in the catalyst producing the greatest amount of diphenylamine in nitrobenzene hydrogenation.

The influence of both the reaction conditions and the type of the catalyst on the rate of contamination of its surface was studied under laboratory conditions. The results obtained are given in Tables 1 and 2.

TABLE 1
The influence of experimental conditions and catalytic poisons on the rate of copper catalyst deactivation

Experiment number	Variable experimental cond.	Conversion (%) initial	final	Final relat. activity	Carbon deposits (mass % C)
1	standard experiment (a)	96.5	79.4	0.47	2.49
2	$T_L = 200^oC$	95.7	70.5	0.37	1.87
3	$u = 0.182$ m/s	94.8	77.3	0.48	2.40
4	$u = 0.865$ m/s	99.1	84.8	0.43	2.74
5	0.5 mass % DNB in nitrobenzene	96.9	65.1	0.30	3.13
6	thiophene (b) in nitrobenzene	92.9	46.3	0.29	3.82
7	aniline hydrochloride in NB (c)	92.6	55.8	0.35	3.89

The experimental conditions are identical in all experiments (see a) except for the variable condition.
(a) $T_L = 160^oC$, H_2/NB = 25, duration of the experiment 44 hours, velocity of reaction mixture flow u = 0.5 m/s; T_L - temperature of cooling bath, NB - - nitrobenzene, DNB - 1,3-dinitrobenzene
(b), (c) concentration of sulphur and chlorine in deactivated catalyst: 0.05 mass % of S and 0.1 mass % of Cl.

The influence of the reaction temperature on the rate of contamination of the catalyst by carbon deposits is surprising. The increase of the cooling bath temperature by 50 K led to the decrease of the average carbon amount in the catalyst bed by 25 %. It means that in the temperature interval (433-473 K) the rate of contamination decreases with increasing temperature. The dependence observed can be interpreted e.g. in the following way: the formation of both aniline and carbon deposits proceeds via a common precursor P in two parallel reactions (scheme 1) with different activation energy. If $E_1 > E_2$, increasing of reaction temperature depresses carbon deposits formation.

TABLE 2

The influence of the support of a copper catalyst on the rate of carbon deposits formation

Experiment number	Support	Conversion (%) initial	final	Relative activity (a)	Carbon deposits (mass % C)
1	silica	96.5	79.4	0.47	2.49
8	Mg-silicate	93.2	81.2	0.60	2.49
9	$ZnO-Cr_2O_3$	97.7	85.7	0.54	0.61

Experimental conditions are identical with those of the standard experiment - Table 1.
(a) activity at the end of the experiment related to the initial activity.

$$\text{Nitrobenzene} \xrightarrow{H_2} P \begin{cases} \xrightarrow{E_1} \text{Aniline} \\ \xrightarrow{E_2} \text{Carbon deposits} \end{cases} \qquad (1)$$

From this point of view the desirable increase of the average temperature in the catalyst bed can be easily attained in an industrial reactor (by the temperature of the bath, the excess of hydrogene etc.). Such a change leads, however, to an irreversible catalyst deactivation because the rate of copper sintering increases.

The increase of the linear flow velocity of the reaction mixture had an accelerating effect on the rate of catalyst contamination. The observed dependence can be explained in terms of the increase of nitrobenzene surface concentration resulting from a shift of the hydrogenation reaction from the transition region to the kinetic one.

The artificially elevated concentration of 1,3-dinitrobenzene in nitrobenzene has unambiguously proved the well-known fact "(ref. 4)" that this common component of technical nitrobenzene increases the rate of catalyst deactivation. In the Czechoslovak technology of aniline production the concentration of 1,3-dinitrobenzene in the fed nitrobenzene is decreased down to 0.005 mass % in a rectification evaporator.

Surprisingly the greatest increase of the rate of carbon deposits formation was caused by the presence of catalytic poisons (S and Cl) in the fed raw material. The increase of undesirable carbon deposits seems to occur in such cases when the applied perturbance causes a decrease in the rate of the principal reaction.

As already mentioned, the deposits formation is a catalyzed process. The catalyst (BASF, type K 3-10) the copper component of which is dispersed on the $ZnO-Cr_2O_3$ type of support is "highly selective" because it does not catalyze carbon contaminants formation. As discussed further, a great disadvantage of this catalyst is a rapid destruction of its pellets in the reaction mixture. In accordance with the present state of knowledge, chromic oxide hinders the carbon deposit formation. A higher toxicity, much higher price and lower effectiveness of the copper dispersion stabilization are its disadvantages as compared with the supports based on SiO_2 or $SiO_2-R_xO_y$ (R = Mg, Ca, Mn).

Catalyst poisoning

Great sensitivity of copper to the poisoning with sulphur compounds the central atom of which contains free electron pairs is a well-known fact "(ref. 5)". One of such contact poisons is thiophene which is the main sulphur impurity of the cokery origin benzene used in the production of nitrobenzene in Czechoslovakia.

The sensitivity of the copper catalyst (Usiness de Melle, type Cu/kieselguhr) to poisons on the sulphur base was tested as early as the hydrorefining of benzene started in Czechoslovakia. It was found out that the concentration of 0.4-0.5 mass % of sulphur in the catalyst results in its total deactivation "(ref. 1)". Another quantitative illustration of the influence of sulphur on the properties of the copper catalyst (BASF, type R 3-11) is given in experiment N^{o} = 6 in Table 1. The comparison of the result of this experiment with the result of a standard one (N^{o} = 1) shows that after the adsorption of 0.05 mass % of sulphur, the activity of the catalyst decreased by 70 %. The sulphur poisoning is accompanied by the carbon deposits contamination of the catalyst surface. The rate of their deposition increased by 50 % in comparison with the standard experiment. The quantitative take-up of sulphur was confirmed by balance of sulphur concentration in both the processed raw material and the deactivated catalyst. In such a case, knowing the WHSV, it was possible to determine the admissible maximum of sulphur concentration in nitrobenzene which has not a dominant effect on the life of the catalyst. Sulphur concentration in nitrobenzene lower than 1 ppm was in accordance with this demand.

After a series of successful operational cycles in an experimental pilot plant unit with an output of about 1 t per hour a rapid deactivation of the catalyst occured repeatedly. During this period nitrobenzene containing 0.3-0.4 ppm of sulphur was processed. A detailed analysis of the catalyst bed in several tubes proved that the catalyst had not been poisoned by sulphur but contaminated by macromolecular carbon deposits in a short period of time. More than a twofold increase of the amount of carbon deposits could not be explained by any change of technological conditions. Their influence on the rapid deactivation was examined simultaneously (see the discussion of the results of model laboratory experiments - Table 1).

Later on we were informed by the producer that nitrobenzene had been accidentally contaminated by 2,4-dinitrochlorobenzene and for a long period by chlorobenzene. Experiment N^{o} = 7 (Table 1) clearly proved a great influence of chlorine impurity in nitrobenzene (presented in the form of aniline hydrochloride) on the catalyst deactivation. In contrast to the standard (44 hours) experiment, this experiment had to be interrupted for a low activity of the catalyst after 30 hours. In the course of this time 0.1 mass % of chlorine was taken up on the catalyst surface. An analysis of the catalyst bed poisoned in this way showed that the amount of carbon deposits in it had increased by 60 % as compared to the non-poisoned one.

Additionally, the presence of chlorine was proved in samples of deactivated catalysts applied in the pilot plant unit during 4 years. The concentration of these contaminants in the processed raw material was determined afterwards from the average content of chlorine and sulphur in catalysts from individual operational cycles. Their influence on the rate of deactivation of particular catalyst batches applied in individual operational cycles was quantified. The poison effect is expressed by the correlation between the total content of poisons (S and Cl) in the raw material and a specific catalyst consumption in corresponding adequate operational cycle (Fig. 2).The correlation

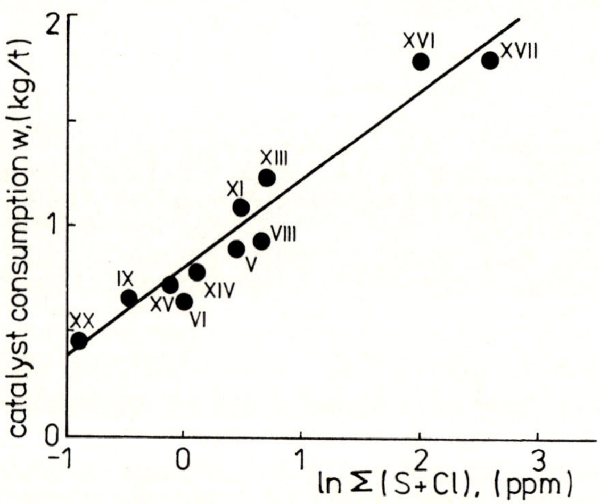

Fig. 2. Dependence of the specific catalyst consumption on the concentration of poisons in fed nitrobenzene.

is described by the following equation:

$$c_{cat}(kg/t) = \frac{\ln \Sigma (S + Cl)}{2.26} + 0.79 \qquad (2)$$

From the extrapolation of the present results it can be concluded that the poisoning of the copper catalyst (BASF, type R 3-11) is totally screened by deactivation due to carbon deposits and sintering when the total content of poisons (Cl, S) in nitrobenzene is lower than 0.5 ppm.

Sintering

The exact determination of the contribution of coalescence, or may be of sintering, of active copper crystals to the deactivation of the catalyst in the aniline process is not easy. The total decrease of activity reaching as much as 95 % is due, apart from coalescence, also to other, already discussed, processes. Their influence in the catalyst deactivated in a pilot plant unit cannot be, however, separated from the discussed influence of sintering.

The only method practically used for the estimation of the sintering effect on the activity of a catalyst deactivated under operational conditions is the X-ray line-broadening. The method is based on the determination of the difference between the average size of copper particles of a fresh and a deactivated catalysts. The decrease of the specific copper surface area is in structurally insensible reactions proportional to the change of the activity caused by sintering. The disadvantage of this method is, however, that the determined (average) particle diameters do not reflect the real change of an effectively utilized surface but they only describe the changes linked to the growth of copper crystals, or more accurately, to the growth of the size of its coherent areas.

The average size of copper particles in the samples of industrially deactivated catalyst R 3-11 (see Table 3) was determined. The samples were taken from the region of their highest integral thermal exposition. WHSV and the total decrease of the activity is practically the same for all the samples, however, there are differences in the rate of their deactivation and time of their operational exposition. During the operational exploatation the value of "the average size of copper particles" increases approximately two times which corresponds roughly to a 50 % decrease of the specific copper surface area (see the results summarized in Table 3). The magnitude of this change is independent of the period of operational exposition of the catalyst and is influenced neighter by the total rate of deactivation (samples 2 and 10), nor by the changes in the regime of the technological process. An important fact has been found out: the increasing growth of the copper particle sizes is reached particularly in the initial phase of the operational cycle. In the

TABLE 3

Average magnitude of the coherent area of copper crystallites in samples of an operationally deactivated catalyst (BASF, type R 3-11)

Sample number	Operational cycle	Dimensionless Coordinate (a) l/l_0	Time of operational exposition	Magnitude of Cu coh. area (nm)
1	VI	-	0	13.9
2	VI	0.22-0.33	3008	29
3	VIII	0.22-0.33	1923	28
4	IX	0.22-0.44	2665	24
5	XI	0.22-0.33	1340	30
6	XIII	0.22-0.44	1398	25
7	XIV	0.22-0.44	2295	24
8	XV	0.22-0.44	2257	38
9	XVI	0.27-0.33	680	31
10	XVI	0.22-0.33	880	28
11	XVI	0.11-0.33	1040	26

(a) axial coordinate of a sample in the reactor tube.

further course of the cycle the size of particles does not practically change. In the starting period of the operational cycle the temperature maximum reaches about 360^{0}C lasting for several tens of hours. Thus, it is quite clear that the sintering of copper crystallites in the catalyst at this temperature is a very fast process. This conclusion is in accordance with the results of "copper sintering" determined in a number of supported catalysts under laboratory conditions. The time dependence of "copper sintering" in the catalyst (BASF, type R 3-11) is demonstrated by curves in Fig. 3. The results of a sintering study of other copper catalysts are the object of our further research work "(ref. 6)". The rate of sintering was examined by determining the changes of the specific copper surface by the method of decompositive N_2O adsorption described by Dvořák "(ref. 7)".

The surface sintering and the poisoning make impossible the catalyst reactivation by burning carbon deposits. Controlled burning of organic deposits and the following reduction of the catalyst result in a 30 % restoring of the initial activity. The results of the X-ray line-broadening analysis showed that the average size of copper particles before and after reactivation does not practically change. From this it follows that the burning of deposits controlled by partial pressure of oxygen does not lead to secondary sintering of primarily sintered copper crystallites. Apart from this the pellets destruction limiting the life of a catalyst in many cases does not allow the reactivation of the deactivated copper catalyst.

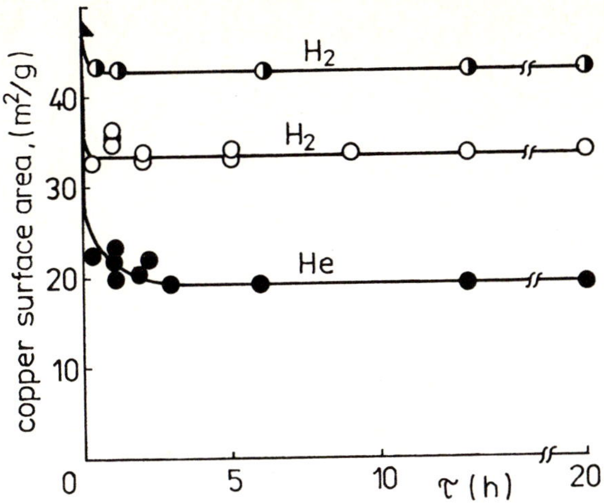

Fig. 3. The dependence of the specific copper surface area of the catalyst (BASF, type R 3-11) on the atmosphere, temperature and the time-on-stream.

Pellets destruction

An important criterion for the choice of a catalyst for the aniline process is the mechanical strength of its pellets. During the testing of a great number of commercial copper catalysts it was observed that most catalysts gradually lose the mechanical strenght of pellets, their consistence is affected and eventually they become totally destructed and disintegrate eighter into roughly grained particles or into powder. The velocity of the pellet destruction decreases with the increasing value of their initial mechanical crushing strength. The chemical composition of the support has a decisive effect on the stability of the mechanical strength.

Under the aniline process conditions, catalysts for the low temperature conversion of CO (BASF, K 3-10 type; CCE, C 18 and C 18 HC types) had an extremely low mechanical strength. This strongly decreased mechanical strength is a specific property of the aniline process (redox atmosphere, enhanced carbon deposits formation) while these catalysts have been applied without any significant changes in the LT gas shift conversion process for 2 or 3 years. Of the three LT shift catalysts the pellets of the catalyst (CCE, C 18 HC type) was the most rapidly destructed. Reciprocal relationship between the mechanical strength of pellets and the amount of ZnO in the catalysts is supposed to explain the cause of the low mechanical strength of these catalysts.

Of the active copper catalysts, only copper chromite ones resist practically any change of mechanical crushing strength in the aniline process. Copper catalysts with the support based on Mg, Ca and other silicates have relatively good mechanical strength of pellets.

Fast pellet destruction limits the life of the catalyst but a partial or even controlled destruction on the contrary prolongs the catalyst life. Due to low effectiveness of the utilization of the inner surface of the pellets and the sterical blocking of pore mouths by macromolecular carbon contaminants and poisons, a slow continuous destruction of pellets compensates for the decrease of the catalyst activity.

The mechanism of the pellet destruction has not been discovered yet, but the destruction is known to be localized in the areas identical with those of the carbon deposits. The axial concentration carbon profile and its time dependence (see Fig. 1) correlates to the axial distribution of the pellet destruction in the tube.

The mass concentration of the fraction of the destructed pellets (grain size < 2 mm) in half-a-meter long layers in the reactor tube characterizes the extent of the destruction. Thus, we can say that the destruction is initiated either by a strong redox effect on copper or by the disturbance of pellet cohesion by expansion of organic sludges.

It has been proved that both the pellet destruction and the hydrodynamic resistence of the catalyst bed in the tube are concentrated into a relatively short initial layer. The pressure drop, exceeding the upper limit, in a tube reactor can be quite easily decreased by the sucking of a narrow layer of the destructed pellets. This makes it possible to prolong the catalyst life by up to 40 % "(ref. 8)".

REFERENCES

1 B. Dvořák and J. Pašek, Chem. Prům., 18 (1968) 288-293.
2 J. Černý, V. Pexidr and J. Pašek, Chem.-Ing.-Tech., 43 (1971) 683-687.
3 M. Sada, T. Zinna, Y. Otsuka, T. Ohrui and E. Niihama, Ger. pat. 2320658.
4 K.H. Gharda and C.M. Sliepcevich, Ind. Eng. Chem., 52 (1960) 417-420.
5 E.B. Maxted, J. Chem. Soc., Part. III (1949) 1987-1991.
6 B. Dvořák, A. Hudec and J. Pašek, "in preparation".
7 B. Dvořák, A. Hudec and J. Pašek, "J. Catal., in press".
8 P. Pavlas, R. Rozinek, J. Lubojacký and K. Bancíř, Czech. pat. 211 923 (1981).

B. Delmon and G.F. Froment (Editors), *Catalyst Deactivation 1987*

STRUCTURE SENSITIVE DEACTIVATION OF SUPPORTED PALLADIUM CATALYSTS: CARBON MONOXIDE POISONING OF METHYLCYCLOPROPANE HYDROGENOLYSIS

C. L. M. JOYAL AND J. B. BUTT

Ipatieff Laboratory and Department of Chemical Engineering
Northwestern University, Evanston, IL 60201 (USA)

ABSTRACT

The hydrogenolysis of methylcyclopropane has been used as a probe reaction to investigate the structure sensitivity of the deactivation of a series of well characterized Pd/SiO_2 catalysts by carbon monoxide. Catalysts ranging from 5 to 75 percent metal exposed have been characterized as to CO and H_2 chemisorption, and the hydrogenolysis turnover frequency determined at 298°C as a function of CO coverage and percent exposed. It is found that CO chemisorption is structure sensitive on the lower percentage exposed materials, and that relatively low levels of CO on the catalyst alter the structure sensitivity of the hydrogenolysis reaction.

INTRODUCTION

The chemisorption stoichiometry of small molecules has been noted to be structure sensitive on certain supported metal catalysts (refs. 1,2) with both metal particle size and morphology playing a role. This has obvious implications to catalyst poisoning (refs. 3-7). We have recently examined series of Pt/SiO_2 and Pt/Al_2O_3 catalysts for structure sensitivity in the CO poisoning of methylcyclopropane (MCP) hydrogenolysis. In the case of Pt/SiO_2, poisoning greatly altered both the magnitude and pattern of structure sensitivity (ref. 7), however for Pt/Al_2O_3 only more moderate changes were observed (ref. 8). The present study with Pd/SiO_2 extends this to a system of considerably greater complexity, since β-hydride formation (itself structure sensitive) is possible with Pd, and CO bonds in both linear and bridged forms (variable with surface coverage).

METHODS

Catalysts

The Pd/SiO_2 catalysts were prepared by ion exchange of $Pd(NH_3)_4(NO_3)_2$ onto 80-100 mesh Davison 62 silica gel. Metal loadings were typically 2 wt% or less; details of preparation are given by Pitchai et al. (ref. 9). The results of chemisorption characterization of these materials are given in Table 1.

TABLE 1

Chemisorption Characterization of the Pd/SiO_2 Catalysts

Catalyst[a]	Wt% Pd	$\bar{D}_h$[b], %	$\bar{D}_{CO}$[c], %
7.1-$PdNO_3$	1.91	6.64 ± 0.3	3.3 ± 0.2
13.8-$PdNO_3$	2.09	—	—
29.3-$PdNO_3$	2.09	24.4 ± 2.2	17.7 ± 0.8
49.8-$PdNO_3$	1.56	47.5 ± 2.8	35.0 ± 1.4
65.5-$PdNO_3$	2.09	60.6 ± 2.4	47.4 ± 3.5
79.1-$PdNO_3$	0.49	70.3 ± 3.0	53.5 ± 2.5[d]

[a]Designation from (ref. 9)

[b]Percentage exposed from hydrogen chemisorption/desorption

[c]Percentage exposed from CO chemisorption/desorption except for [d]adsorption

Chemisorption Procedure

Chemisorption and reaction data were obtained with an experimental unit combining a pulse chemisorption section with a differential reactor unit (ref. 7). All experiments employed a "standard pretreatment" consisting of exposure to oxygen at 300°C for 30 min, purging with inert for 15 min, and heating in inert to 450°C and maintaining for 1 h. At the end of this sequence the catalyst was cooled to room temperature in inert for CO chemisorption, or 60°C (to avoid hydride formation) for H_2 chemisorption. For reaction studies the catalyst was cooled in inert, the bed fluidized if desired, and a known amount of CO pulsed over the bed at 25°C before cooling to 0°C and contacting with the reaction mixture (~ 16:1/H_2:MCP).

RESULTS AND DISCUSSION

Carbon Monoxide Chemisorption

To determine an average CO to palladium surface atom (Pd_s) stoichiometry at saturation coverage, the D_h from hydrogen chemisorption is used as a direct measure of the number of Pd_s. It is reasonable for chemisorption above 60°C to use H/Pd_s of unity; conditions of the present work are such that no hydride phases are formed during any of the chemisorption experiments (ref. 10). For the CO chemisorption measurements a CO/Pd_s ratio of unity was assumed with the understanding that such analysis was for comparative purposes only. As indicated in Table 1, the value for the 79.1% catalys is only from adsorption; here desorption values were either lower than adsorption values, or multiple desorption peaks were observed. This last is possibly due to dissociation of CO, which has been reported at relatively mild (<550 K) temperatures (refs. 11-13).

Further investigation of this point is provided by examining how H_2 uptake is affected by CO and H_2 adsorption/desorption cycles and regeneration. After an initial determination of D_h several adsorption/desorption cycles were run where the surface was partially covered by CO, then saturated with H_2 before desorption. A final determination of D_h was then carried out. This final D_h was the same as the initial value for the low D_h catalysts, but significant decreases were observed for the 65.5 and 79.1% samples, as shown in Table 2. Refs. (14-16) give evidence obtained by a variety of means for the existence

TABLE 2
Effect of adsorption/desorption cycles of coadsorbed CO and H_2 and regeneration on D_h

Catalyst	$\bar{D}_{h-A/D}$, % (before CO)	$\bar{D}_{h-A/D}$, % (after CO)	$\bar{D}_{h-A/D}$, % (after regeneration)
65.5-$PdNO_3$	59.6 ± 1.5	44.8 ± 1.5	55.9 ± 2.7
79.1-$PdNO_3$	67.5 ± 2.1	37.0	—
	69.7 ± 1.4	56.2 ± 1.3	66.0 ± 1.0

of carbon on the surface of supported Pd after room temperature CO chemisorption and desorption up to 675-775 K for relatively high percentage exposed catalysts, ≫ 40%. Thus it is quite possible that surface carbon from disproportionation blocks H_2 adsorption sites. Carbon blocking of CO adsorption upon cycling has also been reported (refs. 14,15), however we observed no such effect. The regeneration values, as shown in Table 2, are obtained by normal H_2 chemisorption after the cycled materials have been resubjected to standard pretreatment. As can be seen, both catalysts essentially recover full adsorptive capacity.

We attribute the results of the adsorption/desorption cycle experiments on D_h to CO disproportionation, which is apparently structure sensitive since only the smaller particles of Table 2 show this effect (particles below 65.5% show no effect of adsorption/desorption cycles). A detailed study of this, however, would be complicated since the disproportionation leading to deposition of surface carbon can be variable dependent upon factors such as temperature, surface coverage, etc. There is also some evidence of hydrogen-assisted CO dissociation in these two highest percent exposed catalysts; the details, while not of direct import here, are of interest in understanding the overall behavior of highly dispersed Pd and are discussed elsewhere (ref. 17).

CO/Pd_s Stoichiometry

The chemisorption results, expressed in terms of D_h and D_{CO}, serve to determine actual CO/Pd_s values for the series of catalysts at saturation

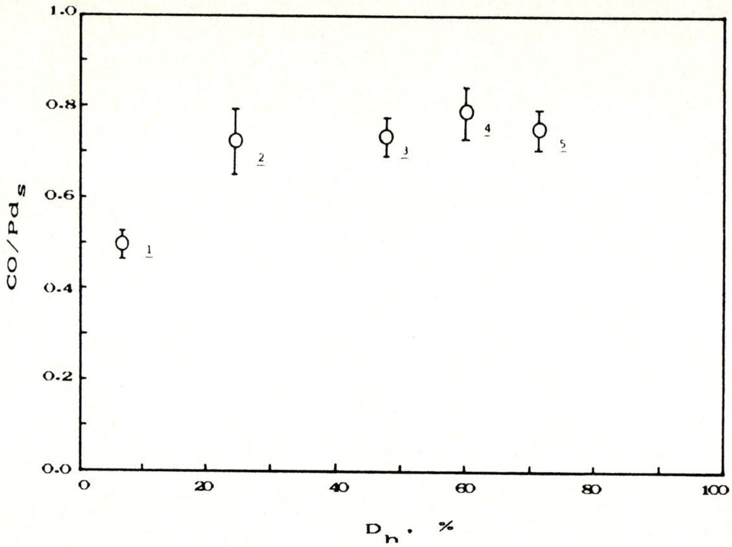

Fig. 1. Relationship between CO/Pd_s and D_h for the Pd/SiO_2 series.

coverage, as shown in Figure 1. There is a significant variation for the lowest D_h catalyst, where the CO/Pd_s ratio of ~ 0.5 is indicative of purely bridge bonded CO. The other catalysts (CO/Pd_s ~ 0.75) are suggestive of a mixture of linear and bridge bonded species and there is no significant trend for high D_h toward any limit.

There is divergence in the literature on this question of CO/Pd_s stoichiometry. Good agreement for CO/Pd_s of unity is reported in refs. 18 and 19, while others report prevalent bridge bonding or large particles with the amount of linear bonding increasing as particle size decreases (refs. 14, 20). While specifics of this undoubtedly depend upon catalyst preparation and pretreatment, our results accord with the latter view, and specific ratios from Figure 1 are used in interpretation of the reaction data.

MCP Reaction Studies

If one wishes to have a direct measure of activity vs. extent of poisoning (i.e., surface coverage of poison), the poisoning technique should be carefully considered since ideally both inter- and intraparticle gradients should be avoided. In the extreme of fixed bed poisoning and rapid uptake the CO contacts the bed as a moving front so that a portion of the bed is completely deactivated (100% coverage) and the remaining catalyst is unpoisoned (coverage ~ 0%). The CO/Pd_s ratio determined from chemisorption can be used to calculate directly the number of poisoned surface atoms. Figure 2 illustrates that turnover frequencies, N_t (sec^{-1}), for a fixed bed poisoned catalyst agree well with those of an unpoisoned catalyst when calculated on the basis of available surface atoms, but are considerably less when based on the total Pd_s in the total bed.

Fluidized bed poisoning with a 1.5% CO in Ar mixture eliminates the interparticle gradients of the fixed bed and should give an overall more uniform poison distribution. The initial activity is considerably lower for the fluidized bed poisoned catalyst, as shown in Figure 3. This may be due

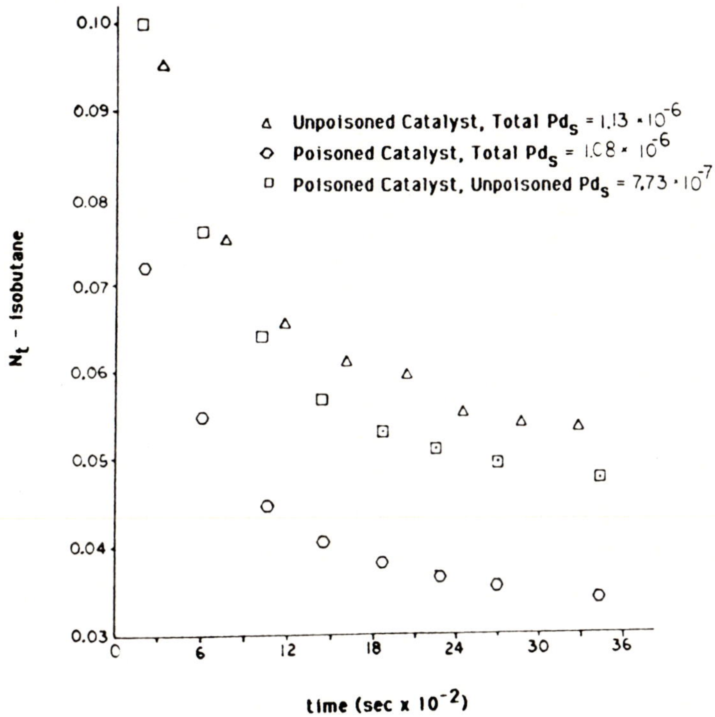

Fig. 2. Fixed bed poisoning results for D_h = 29.3%, surface coverage of CO = 28%.

to a larger number of bridge-bonded CO molecules at the lower (uniform) coverage level (N_t is on a per surface atom basis, so backmixing is presumably accounted for). It is apparent from the comparison that in cases where there is rapid uptake of poison such experiments should be carried out in a fluid bed environment.

Some typical fluidized bed poisoning results are shown in Figure 4.

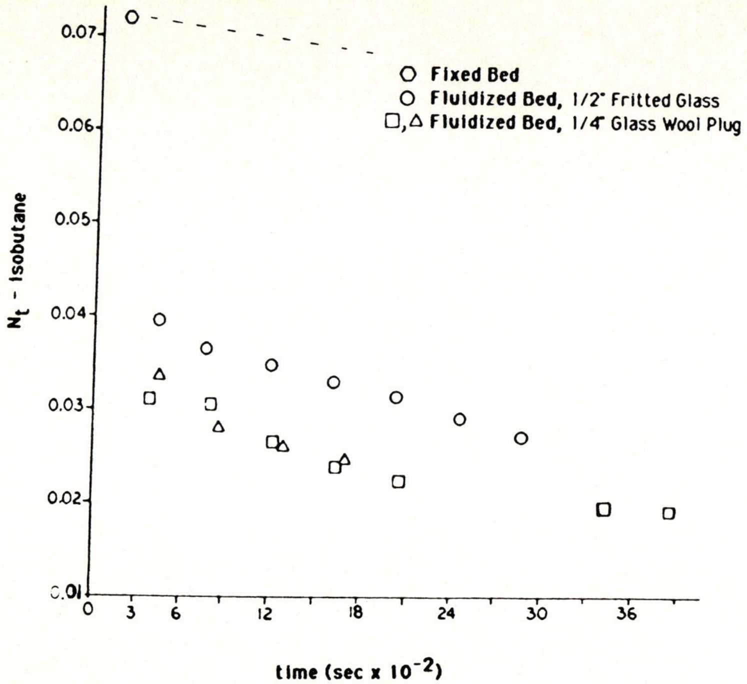

Fig. 3. Comparison of fixed and fluidized bed poisoning results for D_h = 29.3%, surface coverage of 28%.

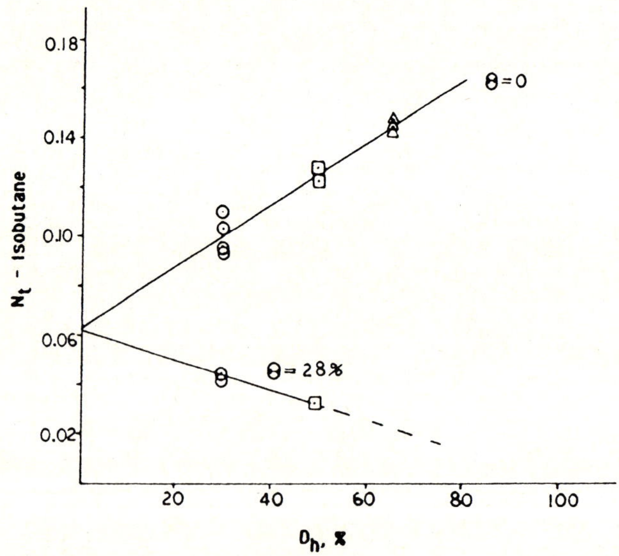

Fig. 4. Changes in the structure-sensitive pattern of MCP hydrogenolysis upon CO poisoning.

Here it is seen that even low levels of CO on the catalyst reverse the structure sensitive pattern of MCP hydrogenolysis from increasing N_t with D_h to decreasing with D_h. The larger particle sizes (smaller D_h) maintain higher activity upon poisoning to the same extent of surface coverage. This is of interest, since larger particles form β-hydride under these reaction conditions (ref. 10), which is reported to decrease hydrogenolysis activity. Bucur (ref. 21) reports that adsorbed CS_2 inhibited the formation and decomposition of hydride in Pd thin films; here the adsorbed CO appears to act in a similar manner to inhibit hydride formation in the Pd/SiO_2. Additional experiments at low coverage levels (θ = 2 - 20%) will be helpful in interrelating the compensating effects of poisoning and hydride formation on MCP activity.

Only a few examples of structure-sensitive deactivation have appeared in the literature (refs. 22-24). In particular Barbier et al. (ref. 24) report that benzene hydrogenation on Pt/Al_2O_3 is transformed from a structure-insensitive to structure-sensitive reaction upon ammonia poisoning. In that case the smaller particles deactivated more rapidly via site blocking and there was an increased resistance to poisoning with increasing metal particle size.

CONCLUSIONS

The CO/Pd_s ratios for this series of Pd/SiO_2 catalysts, determined at saturation coverage, depend upon percent metal exposed with the stoichiometric coefficient significantly less for low D_h catalysts. The CO/Pd_s does not approach unity, nor is there any noted trend in this direction for very high D_h materials.

The CO surface reaction is also structure sensitive, with disproportionation occurring in the vicinity of 575 K on high percentage exposed materials, but not on low. A hydrogen-assisted dissociation also appears significant for high percentage exposed catalysts, distinct from direct disproportionation. The onset of these as a function of particle size has not been determined precisely, but is within the region of 50 to 70 percent exposed.

A comparison of fixed and fluidized bed poisoning modes shows clearly that the latter is to be preferred in a case such as the present where the uptake of poison is rapid and irreversible. Low levels of CO coverage are seen to reverse the structure sensitivity of MCP hydrogenolysis on Pd/SiO_2, with larger particles retaining a higher activity upon poisoning.

ACKNOWLEDGMENT

C. L. M. Joyal acknowledges the fellowship support of Procter and Gamble and J. B. Butt that of the Alexander von Humbuldt-Stiftung. Additional funding was provided by the Stauffer Chemical Co. and the Mobil Foundation, Inc.

REFERENCES

1 F. J. C. M. Toolemar, A. G. T. M. Bostein and V. Ponec, J. Catal., 82 (1983) 35.
2 T. Uchijima, J. M. Herrmann, Y. Inoue, R. L. Burwell, Jr., J. B. Butt and J. B. Cohen, J. Catal., 50 (1977) 464.
3 T. A. Dorling, M. J. Eastlake and R. L. Moss, J. Catal., 14 (1969) 23.
4 J. Schlatter and M. Boudart, J. Catal., 24 (1972) 482.
5 G. A. DelAngel, B. Coq and F. Figureas, Nouv. J. Chim., 7 (1983) 173.
6 V. K. Shum, J. B. Butt and W. M. H. Sachtler, J. Catal., 96 (1985) 371.
7 I. Onal and J. B. Butt, J. Chem. Soc., Faraday Trans. I., 8 (1982) 1887.
8 P. H. Otero-Schipper, W. A. Wachter, J. B. Butt, R. L. Burwell, Jr., and J. B. Cohen, J. Catal., 50 (1977) 494.
9 R. Pitchai, S. S. Wong, N. Takahashi, J. B. Butt, R. L. Burwell, Jr. and J. B. Cohen, J. Catal., 94 (1985) 478.
10 R. K. Nandi, R. Pitchai, S. S. Wong, J. B. Cohen, R. L. Burwell, Jr., and J. B. Butt, J. Catal., 70 (1981) 298.
11 R. W. Joyner and M. W. Roberts, J. Chem. Soc., Faraday Trans. I, 70 (1974) 1819.
12 G. G. Low and A. T. Bell, J. Catal., 57 (1979) 397.
13 E. Gillet, S. Channakhone and V. Matolin, J. Catal., 97 (1986) 437.
14 S. Ichikawa, H. Poppa and M. Boudart, J. Catal., 91 (1985) 1.
15 S. Ichikawa, H. Poppa and M. Boudart, ACS Symp. Series, 248 (1984) 439.
16 D. L. Doering, H. Poppa and J. T. Dickinson, J. Vac. Sci. Tech., 17 (1980) 198.
17 C. L. M. Joyal and J. B. Butt, J. Chem. Soc., Faraday Trans. I (in press).
18 J. Turkevich and G. Kim, Science, 169 (1970) 873.
19 G. Chen, W. Chou and C. Yen, Appl. Catal., 8 (1983) 389.
20 G. Gubitosa, A. Berton, M. Camia and N. Pernicone in G. Poncelet, P. Grange and P. A. Jacobs (Editors), Preparation of Catalysts, III, Elsevier Science Publishing, Amsterdam, 1983, p. 431.
21 R. V. Bucur, J. Catal., 70 (1981) 92.
22 R. Maurel, G. LeClercg and L. LeClercg, Bull. Soc. Chim. Fr., (1972) 491.
23 S. Fuentas and F. Figueras, J. Catal., 54 (1978) 397.
24 J. Barbier, A. Morales, P. Marecot and R. Maurel, Bull. Soc. Chim. Belge, 88 (1979) 569.

B. Delmon and G.F. Froment (Editors), *Catalyst Deactivation 1987*

THE ROLE OF CRYSTALLITE STRUCTURE ON MECHANISMS OF COKE AND SULPHUR POISONING IN CATALYTIC REFORMING

J. BISWAS[1], G.M. BICKLE, P.G. GRAY and D.D. DO

Department of Chemical Engineering, University of Queensland, St. Lucia, Qld., 4067, Australia.

[1]Kon./Shell Laboratorium, P.O. Box 3003, 1003 AA Amsterdam, The Netherlands

ABSTRACT

The activity of typical platinum-based catalysts is dependent on the surface crystallite configuration. Although the ensemble requirement determines the reaction pathway the coordination of metal atoms in the crystallite i.e. face or corner atoms, has some influence on reaction selectivity; the electron deficient character of corner atoms makes these atoms more active for certain reactions. Sulphur is shown to preferentially bond irreversibly to the face atoms of a platinum crystallite, which is in a sulphided state under industrial conditions. Thus the mechanism of further sulphur poisoning is reversible attachment to crystallite corner atoms. The corner atoms are also found to be coke free due to high coke cleaning rates there, as well as steric influences. The coke deposition during long-term reformer operation (20 wt%) is found to be on the alumina; however the observed deactivation in octane yields is due to the change in nature of coke (gradual grafitization) on the metal sites of the catalyst. Thus, two types of coke are distinguished on the metal sites; one being easily removed by hydrogen, the other less readily; they are labelled reversible and irreversible (graphitic) coke. Hydrogen limits the mutual site deactivation rate by removal of the reversible and irreversible coke types by catalyzed hydrogeneration and hydrogasification, respectively. In addition to coke removal by hydrogen, hydrogenolysis of coke precursors serves to limit catalyst deactivation. The enhanced activity maintenance of platinum-iridium is due to high rates of hydrogenolysis and hydrogasification. In the case of platinum-rhenium catalysts the graphitization rate of metallic coke is sterically hindered by the preferential sulphidation of rhenium atoms.

INTRODUCTION

The reforming of petroleum naphthas is carried out over bifunctional catalysts which consist of a single metal or a combination of metals dispersed on an acidic support such as alumina or silica-alumina (ref. 1). At temperatures near 770K, such catalysts simultaneously promote metal- and acid-catalyzed conversions of saturated hydrocarbons to aromatics. During the 1950's and 1960's, conventional platinum on alumina. Catalysts were employed exclusively in commercial units, however in the last decade and a half there has been a gradual replacement by catalysts containing platinum and a second element such as rhenium, tin or iridium, which gives improved stability (ref. 2).

The three most important aspects of the application of these heterogeneous catalysts are activity, selectivity and life. The life or the stability of activity and selectivity is dictated by the possibility of sintering, poisoning or coking. The latter two forms of chemical deactivation are caused by the deposition of feed stream impurities (such as sulphur) and formation of surface residues (coke) by side reactions respectively. Under industrial conditions, a large part of the surface area of the metal component of the catalyst is covered by coke (ref. 3) and sulphur (ref. 4), which detrimentally affect the activity and stability of metal and acid functions of modern monometallic and bimetallic catalysts. Therefore it is timely to examine the effects of sulphur and coke on the atomic level in an attempt to relate fundamental observations in surface science to industrial experience. The purpose of this paper is to discuss the following aspects:

(i) The influence of metal crystallite structure and associated geometric effects on reforming reactions

(ii) Similarities between sulphur, coke, and additive nonmetals on selectivity of Pt/Al_2O_3 reforming catalysts

(iii) The role of sulphur in catalytic reforming and the influence of crystallite configuration

(iv) Mechanisms of coking deactivation and the role of coordination effects.

ROLE OF CATALYST SURFACE MORPHOLOGY ON ACTIVITY AND SELECTIVITY

Coordination Effects

Typical industrial reforming catalysts have the metal dispersed on the surface of the support as small crystallites, usually in the size range 8 - 100Å in diameter. Crystallite corner atoms have a coordination number (number of nearest neighbour atoms) of 4, edge atoms 6 or 7, and atoms on the face of the plane, 8 or 9. Work by van Hardefeld and Hartog (ref. 5) demonstrated two important points:

(a) Low coordination surface atoms - corner atoms, edge atoms ($i < 7$) - are present in significant proportions only in crystallites of sizes $d < 40$Å. Large crystallites consist almost exclusively of face atoms

(b) Corner atoms predominate on the surface of extremely small crystallites ($d < 10$Å).

These surface atoms differ from bulk atoms of the crystallite in that they have an incomplete set of neighbours. The extra valencies of these surface atoms are taken up by adsorbates and reactants, and one can imagine that atoms in different surroundings display distinct adsorption and reaction properties, ie. the stereo chemistry of corner atoms can be quite different from face atoms due to energetic effects (ref. 6). These effects are amplified by the finding that corner atoms are electron deficient compared to face atoms (ref. 7).

Blakely and Somorjai (ref. 8) showed with metallic single crystals that flat faces have a significantly lower activity that terraces, since atoms in step, kink and corner sites exhibit a higher degree of coordinative unsaturation. These effects are partly responsible for the fact that crystallite faces are efficient in C - C bond breakage, while C - H and H - H bond scissions are more effective on crystallite and edges (ref. 9), eg. several atomic ligand sites necessary for cyclization are available on corner atoms of low coordination number. Table 1 lists coordination requirements for typical reforming reactions.

TABLE 1

Reaction Site Requirements on Platinum Crystallites (ref. 49)

Reaction	Example Compound	Generic Reaction Mechanism Code	Crystallite Size Range (where mechanism dominant)	Effect of* Increasing Dispersion on Rate	Minimum Ensemble Requirement	Coordination Requirement
Hydrogenolysis	1. Methyl-cyclopentane	non-selective cyclic	< 20 Å	-	1	corner
		bond shift	full range	-	1	corner
		selective cyclic	> 25 Å	-	2	corner and face
	2. Alkanes		small	+	1	corner
			large	-	3	face
Isomerization	1. 3-Methyl-pentane	non-selective cyclic	< 20 Å	+	1	corner
		bond shift	full range	-	1	corner
		selective cyclic	> 25 Å	-	2	corner and face
	2. 2-Methyl-pentane	non-selective cyclic	12-200 Å	+	1	corner
		bond shift	12-200 Å	-	1	corner
Dehydrocyclization (with 1,5 closure)	Hexane	non-selective cyclic	small	+	1	corner
		bond shift	small	+	1	corner
		selective cyclic	large	-	2	corner and face
Ring Enlargement (after 1,5 closure)	Methylcyclopentane		full range	negligible	1	corner and face
Dehydrocyclization (with 1,6 closure)	Heptane		full range	negligible	1-2	corner and face (higher on corners)
Dehydrogenation	Alkanes Naphthene		full range	negligible	1	corner and face
Self-poisoning	Alkanes		> 10 Å	-	2	face

* + means increase of rate
- means decrease of rate

Ensemble Requirement

The ensemble requirement is the minimum required number of contiguous surface atoms of the element able to form bonds with the end adsorbate. This definition accepts the conjecture that for a specific reaction mechanism, the required active centre on the catalyst surface can be either a single metal atom or an ensemble of several adjacent atoms (see Table 1).

The Similar Roles of Alloying, Sulphur and Coke

The surface geometry of a Pt/Al_2O_3 catalyst shows an intimate relationship between ensemble size, selective poisoning by an additive and deactivation by carbonaceous fragments (ref. 10):

(i) Alloying with inactive metal (tin)

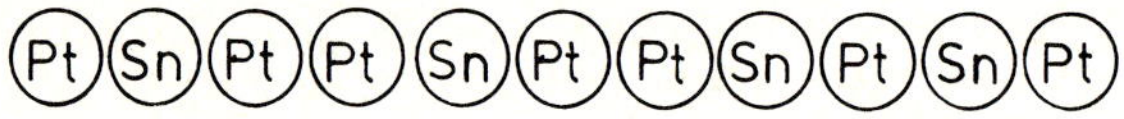

(ii) Poisoned by Sulphur

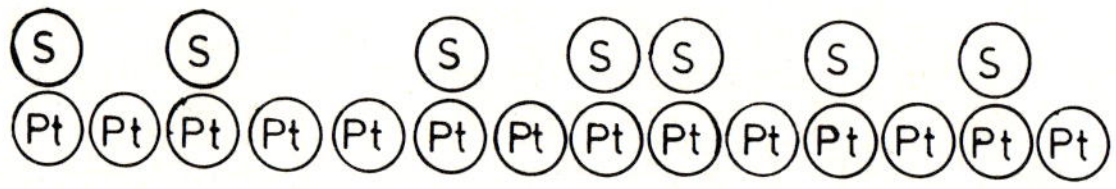

(iii) Deposits of Coke

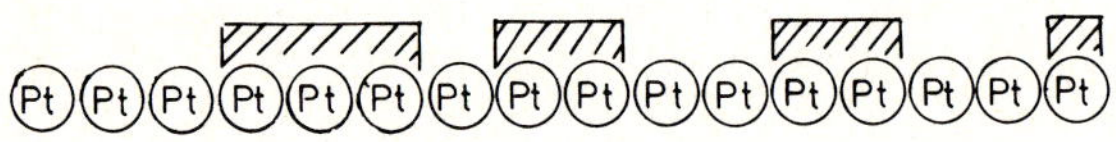

In each case, the result is a dilution in the number of large active ensembles of platinum. This causes a decrease in hydrogenation rate (refs.11 - 13) and leads to an enhancement of all reactions running as through dehydrogenation eg. 1, 6 dehydrocyclization and isomerization. Thus, two types of coke are distinguished on a reforming catalyst; the initial deposition on the metal, which is necessary to transform the cracking catalyst into an aromatization catalyst, and the detrimental long term coking (ref. 14); this initial deposition (2 wt %) is seen to occur over a period of 2 minutes to 2 hours depending on the pressure (ref. 14). After this initial deposition the quantity of coke on the metal is seen to be constant over the length of the reformer cycle (refs. 14 - 16).

COKING OF REFORMING CATALYSTS

The most remarkable progress made in improving reforming catalysts is due to the use, with platinum, of metal additives commonly called 'promoters'. The additives used can be grouped into two types (ref. 14):

(a) additives such as iridium and unsulphided rhenium which decrease the overall coke deposit rate

(b) additives such as germanium, tin or sulphided rhenium, for which the overall coking rate is at least equivalent, if not higher, than that observed with Pt alone.

Even though the overall coke depositions are higher than Pt/Al_2O_3 for case (b), the deactivation rate is less than Pt/Al_2O_3. Hence, a distinction is made between coke deposition and deactivation mechanisms, which are not necessarily interrelated. Four points of note are

(i) the metal component controls the octane improvement reactions (paraffin dehydrocyclization) (ref. 17)

(ii) the majority of the deposited coke is on the alumina

(iii) high coke producing bimetallic catalysts may have greater resistance to coke deposition compared to Pt/Al_2O_3

(iv) after the lineout period the coke content on the metal component is constant over the reforming cycle.

It is concluded the only possible mechanism for the deactivation of the octane improvement function of a reforming catalyst, must be due to the alteration in structure of coke initially deposited during the 'lineout' period (ref. 18).

Bimetallic catalysts reduce the rate of this alteration of metallic coke by different mechanisms depending on the additive component. Firstly, the mechanisms of metal and acid site coking must be distinguished as a prerequisite to a model showing the mechanism of coking deactivation resistance of different bimetallic catalysts.

Mechanism of Coke Formations on the Model

Figure 1 shows a typical model for production of coke on platinum.

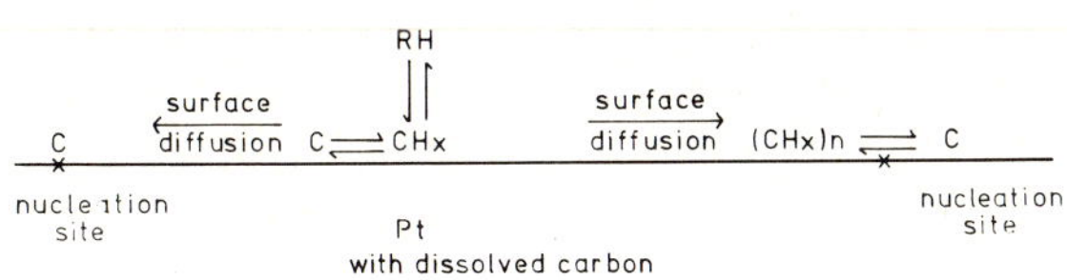

Fig. 1. Model for the production of carbon on Platinum (ref. 19)

A series of fragmentation reactions and successive dehydrogenation reactions leads to the formation of carbon atoms and these atoms (or partially hydrogenated intermediates) may combine to form more toxic coke deposits. The coke deposits are found to have, initially, a hydrogen content of about 1.0 - 1.5 hydrogen atoms per surface carbon atom (ref. 18), and hydrogen transfer with species on the surface that produce gaseous products is easy. Removal of this hydrogen by successive fragmentation (hydrogenolysis) and dehydrogenation leads to a more graphitic form of coke (this also involves migration to a nucleation site where the irreversible deposit grows); reorganisation can also be included by increasing temperature. The fraction of the metal site carbonaceous overlayer which is graphitic is shown in Figure 2 for cyclohexane dehydrogenation on Pt/Al_2O_3. This discussion introduces the concept of reversible (partially

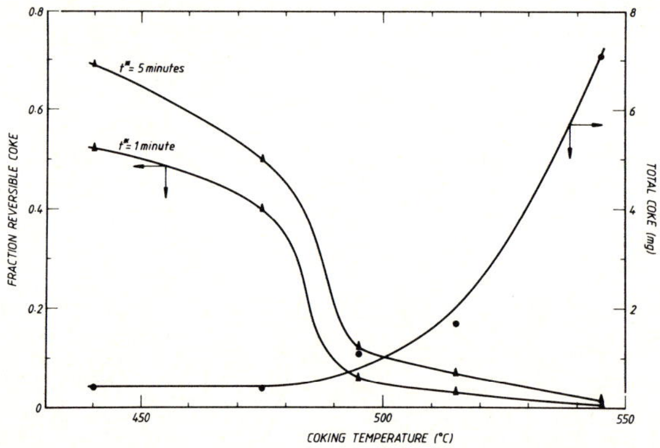

Fig. 2. Effect of temperature of operation on fraction of reversible coke on metal [TGA; Calculation of C_{rev} conducted at T_C; all samples coked for 2 hours in H_2] (ref. 14)

hydrogenated) and irreversible (graphitic) coke, one being easily removed by hydrogen and the latter less readily. Other mechanisms suggested in the literature for metal site coking also indicate there are different types of coke on the surface (ref. 19 - 21). The routes are based on polymerization reactions occurring on the metal surface.

These mechanisms, outlining different types of coke on the surface of the metal, are in agreement with the postulated theory that the deactivation of a reforming catalyst is due to a change in the nature of metallic coke (ref. 22). This is verified in Figure 3 which shows the formation of an initial deposit of coke during the 'running in' period. After this 'lineout' period the quantity of coke in this metal sites does not change, but the coke gradually becomes more graphitic with time on-stream, slowly encapsulating the atoms on the crystallite. Eventually the catalyst is spent when the metal component is covered by this graphitic structure (ref. 23, 24).

A mathematical model has been formulated to quantitatively describe these deactivation processes (ref. 23). The rate of graphitization is determined by computing effects of coking and coke removal by catalytic hydrogenation and hydrogasification (Figure 4).

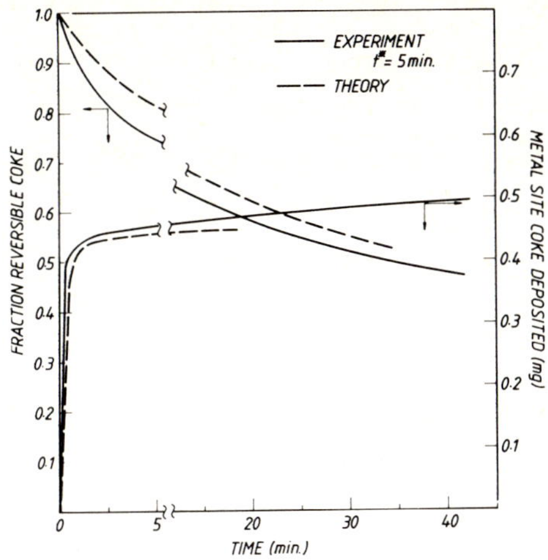

Fig. 3. Comparison of theory with experimental observations of initial deposition and further graphitization of coke [TGA, T_c = 480°C] (ref. 14)

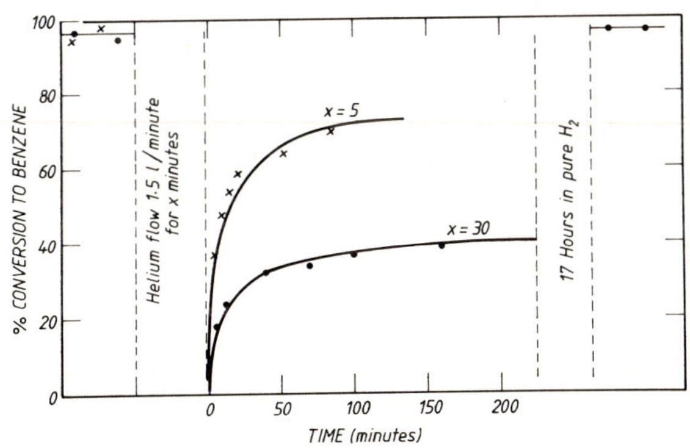

Fig. 4. The effect of helium carrier on the activity recovery of cyclohexane conversion for a Pt/Al_2O_3 catalyst initially in a cyclohexane/hydrogen stream where x denotes time length in the cyclohexane/helium stream. [Fixed Bed, WHSV = 30, H_2/HC = 5, T = 480°C, P = 1 atma] (ref. 14)

Location of Coke on Metal Crystallites

The previous discussion suggests that the initial deposition of coke is on the metal crystallites (ref. 25) and the quantity does not change much with time (within experimental error). Based on this fact, there are a few experimental results which give a hint to the location of coke on the metallic site of a heterogeneous crystallite:

(a) Coke forming reaction requires the formation of multiply bonded species similar to hydrogenolysis of cyclopentane (ref. 26), thus requiring high coordination number metal atoms and large ensembles (> 3).

(b) Small crystallites have greater coke resistance (ref. 26).

(c) Initial coke deposition causes a sharp decrease in the hydrogenolysis activity of a catalyst (ref. 9, 12, 21) which is caused by both ensemble and site selective effects:

(i) The ensemble effect has been discussed earlier for hydrogenolysis, where deposited coke fragments reduce the probability of occurrence of ensembles of required size. A similar argument may be used for the coking reaction itself because of the similar site requirement (Table 1).

(ii) The site selective effect is due to the preferential coking of the most active sites on the metal surface. Different active sites on the metal have different chemistries, observed as different heats of adsorption, the most active ones being the face atoms of metal crystallites, which preferentially coke first (ref. 21).

(d) Hydrogen catalyzed coke removal rates are highest on corner and edge sites (ref. 27)

(e) Corner and edge sites are difficult to cover by a continuous graphitic layer due to steric effects (ref. 28).

These results suggest the coke is partially deposited preferentially on the face atoms of metallic crystallites, although corner atoms are partially covered by coke. This is in agreement with single crystal studies (ref. 8) where it is shown the low coordination number corner sites are the longest surviving on platinum crystallites. Ponec (ref. 28) suggests a model of a working crystallite surface almost always covered by a continuous layer of 'coke', with only the corner atoms of intrinsically high activity in H-H and C-H bond breaking serving as portholes for molecules arriving at the surface from the gas phase and for molecules desorbing from the surface.

Deactivation Mechanism for Bimetallic Catalysts

The deactivation study using Pt/Al_2O_3 shows

(i) observed deactivation in aromatic yields is due to graphitization of the initial coke deposition on the metal component of the catalyst, rather than the larger coke deposit on alumina;

(ii) hydrogen acts as a cleaning mechanism where it cleans the metallic reversible and graphitic cokes by catalytic hydrogenation and hydrogasification respectively;

(iii) the graphitization process is accelerated by high temperatures but is inhibited by high pressures, which limit 'deep dehydrogenation' reactions involved in the mechanism.

The improved stability of Pt-Re/Al_2O_3 is due to a number of effects (note that Pt-Re is presulphided in industry):

(i) the rhenium-sulphur bond sterically hinders graphitization (ref. 22) of the carbonaceous overlayer which exists on catalyst metal sites under industrial conditions

(ii) sulphidation of rhenium is similar to dilution of platinum in an inactive matrix (ref. 29) e.g. tin. The ensemble effect due to sulphidation causes a reduction in coke formation on the metal sites (ref. 30) due to the inability of multiple bond formation which is a prerequisite for metal site coking (ref. 26). However, the isolation of these platinum atoms causes a dramatic lowering in the hydrogenolytic activity of these catalysts (where hydrogenolysis usually destroys coke precursors for acid site coking), hence carbon is more quickly deposited on the acid support (ref. 16). The ensemble effect explains the improved stability of Pt-Sn catalysis.

(iii) the ensemble effect discussed in (ii), i.e. the rhenium and sulphur bond, dilutes the number of large Pt ensembles, also causes inhibition of the graphitization of coke which is a structure sensitive reaction (ref. 31).

The difference in metal site coke quality on Pt/Al_2O_3 and Pt-Re/Al_2O_3 (less graphitic coke) catalysts was experimentally verified (ref. 32).

The improved activity and stability of Pt-Ir/Al_2O_3 is due to three reasons:

(i) hydrogenolytic activity of Ir serves to destroy some coke precursors (ref. 33);

(ii) the lower rate of dehydrogenation of iridium (ref. 33) also serves to restrict the reaction from reversible to irreversible coke

(iii) the ability of Ir to lower the formation of firmly bonded unreactive coke precursors by hydrogenation and gasification (ref. 34).

Thus the coke content of these catalysts is far less than Pt and Pt-Re.

In addition to the mechanisms above, Volter (ref. 12), proposes a drain-off model (see Figure 5).

THE ROLE OF SULPHUR

According to Schultze (ref. 35), the valency of adsorbed sulphur on a metal

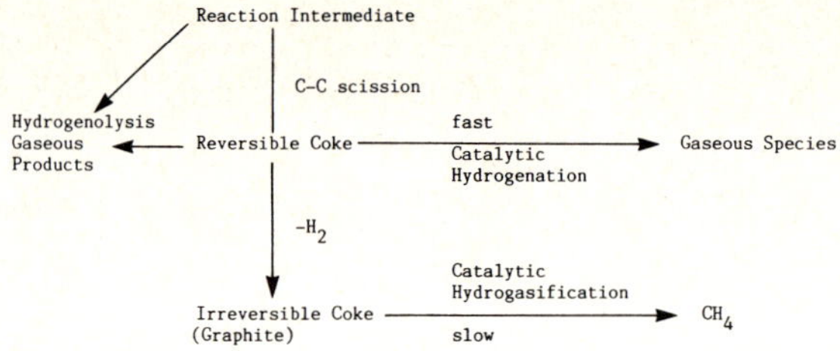

Fig. 5. Interaction of coke deposition and removal mechanisms.

introduced as sulphide ion, can be estimated by the difference between the electron affinity of the metal (2.12eV for Pt) and that of sulphur (2.08eV).

$$M + S^{2-} \longrightarrow M - S^{(-2+\gamma)} + \gamma e^-$$

The lower this difference, the more covalent the chemisorption bond. When the disparity between electronic affinities increases, the chemical bond tends to be polarized. For platinum, the affinity is similar to that of sulphur, hence the Pt-S chemisorptive bond is essentially covalent (ref. 36, 37), i.e. the bond length equals the sum of the covalent radii of the metal and sulphur (ref. 38). The chemisorption of sulphur on metallic catalysts clearly depends on the electronic properties of the catalyst and the adsorption of an electron acceptor compound such as sulphur must be promoted on metals of low electronic affinities (ref. 39) i.e. deficiency in electrons can explain the reduced aptitude of a metal for adsorbing an acceptor compound such as sulphur. This principle is of fundamental importance when analyzing the location of sulphur adsorption on platinum crystallites.

The effect of sulphur additions on catalyst activity is shown in Table 2 (ref. 40). The experiments show that whether Pt/Al_2O_3 is presulphided or not, the existence of trace amounts of sulphur in typical industrial feeds will cause the activity of the catalyst to reduce to that of a sulphided Pt/Al_2O_3 catalyst. This occurs irrespective of the mode of sulphur addition ie. before, during or after the lineout region. Noting the fact that negligible coking occurs on the metal sites of presulphided Pt/Al_2O_3 (ref. 41) it can be deduced that coke formation (as well as cyclopentane hydrogenolysis) and sulphur adsorption take place preferentially on the same sites (ref. 40, 42-44). Specifically, these sites are the high coordination number face atoms of metal crystallites, which are in electron surplus (ref. 9).

Single crystal studies reviewed by a number of researchers (ref. 45-47), all show the stoichiometry of stably adsorbed sulphur on low index faces of platinum are in the range 0.4-0.45. This c(2x2) structure has recently been confirmed on

TABLE 2

The Effect of Mode of Irreversible Sulphur Addition and Timing of Addition on Chlorided 0.3% Pt/Al_2O_3

Catalyst[a]	Group product yields/100 moles of n-heptane feed[b]			
	n-Heptane	Isomers	Toluene	Cracked products
A	47.34	24.31	14.32	36.63
B	30.17	34.13	16.01	34.85
C	34.25	28.41	15.27	38.45
D	37.31	30.59	14.86	35.06
E	21.04	28.83	31.55	32.34

[a]The catalysts used were sulphided as follows: A, presulphided in H_2S at reduction temperature (480°C) until breakthrough is seen on wet lead acetate paper, then removal of reversible sulphur by pure H_2 flowing until no further H_2S removal is observed; B, lined out on pure n-heptane, followed by a period of n-heptane feed doped with 500 ppm sulphur (as thiophene) until equilibrium achieved then returned to pure n-heptane feed for a period long enough to remove reversible sulphur (indicated by a steady state in dehydrocyclization activity); C, as for catalyst B but using 10 ppm sulphur doped n-heptane; D, lined out on 10 ppm sulphur doped n-heptane feed until equilibrium achieved, then switched to pure n-heptane feed until steady state in dehydrocyclization activity achieved; E, lined out on pure n-heptane feed with no sulphur addition by any method.

[b]All activities quoted for the reactor conditions of T = 480°C, P = 10 atm, WHSV = 5, H_2/hydrocarbon = 10, and pure n-heptane feed.

NOTE: Lineout is the term given to initial fast coking of metal sites during first 2-3 hours of operation until pseudo steady state in dehydrocyclization activity is reached.

the face atoms of dispersed platinum crystallites (ref. 48). Thus it can be concluded that at typical reforming temperatures (500°C), a stable, saturated sulphur layer contains about an S atom per two surface Pt atoms.

On the basis of the above discussion, we unambiguously state the following theory:

'Due to the high stability of sulphur on crystallite face atoms of high coordination number, small concentrations of sulphur in industrial feeds (0-20 wt ppm) will cause complete deactivation of uncoked face atoms. Hence the activity of a Pt/Al_2O_3 catalyst under industrial conditions is due to the activity of corner atoms of low coordination number which are more sulphur and coke resistant. Any sulphur in the feed will deactivate these corner atoms by an equilibrium relation'.

Hence, we would expect greater sulphur tolerance of an on-line industrial catalyst at high pressures, where adsorbed sulphur levels are lower on the corner sites, due to the equilibrium relationship (p_{H_2S}/p_{H_2}).

REFERENCES

1 M.J. Sterba and V. Haensel, Ind. Eng. Chem. Prod. Res. Dev., 15 (1976) 3-17.
2 B.C. Gates, J.R. Katzer and G.C.A. Schuit, Chemistry of Catalytic Processes, McGraw Hill, New York, 1979.
3 S.M. Davies, F. Zaera and G.A. Somorjai, J. Catal., 77 (1982) 439-459.
4 P.G. Menon, G.B. Marin and G.F. Froment, Ind. Eng. Chem. Prod. Res. Dev., 21 (1982) 52-56.
5 R. van Hardefeld and F. Hartog, Surf. Sci., 15 (1969) 189.
6 J.R. Anderson, K. Foger and R.J. Breaksphere, J. Catal., 57 (1979) 458-475.
7 D.F. Melius, T.H. Upton and W.A. Goddard III, Solid State Commun., 28 (1978) 501-504.
8 D.W. Blakely and G.A. Somorjai, Surf. Sci., 65 (1977) 419-442.
9 G.A. Somorjai, Adv. Catal., 26 (1977) 2-68.
10 B. Coq and F. Figueras, J. Molec. Catal., 25 (1984) 87-98.
11 P. Biloen, J.N. Helle, H. Verbeek, F.M. Dautzenberg and W.M.H. Sachlter, J. Catal., 63 (1980) 112-118.
12 J. Volter, in L. Cerveny, (Ed), Catalytic Hydrogenation, Elsevier, Amsterdam, 1986, pp. 337-373.
13 C.R. Apesteguia and J. Barbier, J. Catal., 78 (1982) 352-359.
14 J.M. Parera, N.S. Figoli, E.M. Traffano, J.N. Beltramini and E.E. Martinelli, Appl. Catal., 5 (1983) 33-41.
15 J. Barbier, Appl. Catal., 23 (1986) 225-243.
16 J.P. Franck and G. Martino, in J. Oudar and H. Wise (Ed), Deactivation and Poisoning of Catalysts, Marcel Deppar, New York, 1985, pp. 205-258.
17 V.K. Shum, J.B. Butt and W.M. Sachtler, Appl. Catal., 11 (1984) 151-154.
18 S.M. Davis, F. Zaera and G.A. Somorjai, LBL - 146II preprint, submitted to J. ACS, 1982.
19 L. Luck, S. Aeiyack and G. Maire, Proc. 8th Int. Congr. Catal., Berlin, 1984, Vol II, pp. 695.
20 A. Sarkany, H. Lieske, T. Szilagyi and L. Tote, Proc. 8th Int. Congr. Catal., Berlin, 1984, Vol II, pp. 613-623.
21 D.L. Trimm, Appl. Catal., 5 (1983) 263-290.
22 W.M.H. Sachtler, J. Mol. Catal., 25 (1984) 1-12.
23 J. Biswas, P.G. Gray, D.D. Do, submitted to Appl. Catal (1986).
24 M. Masai, S. Chimadzu, T. Sachiwa, S. Sawa and M. Mimura, in B. Delmon and G.F. Froment (Ed), Catalyst Deactivation, Elsevier, Amsterdam, 1980, pp. 261-270.
25 J. Barbier, G. Corro, Y. Zhang, J.P. Bournville and J.P. Franck, Appl. Catal., 13 (1985) 245-255.
26 E.H. van Broekhovan, J.W.F.M. Schoonhoven and V. Ponec, Surf. Sci., 156 (1985) 899-910.
27 G.A. Somorjai, Chemsitry in Two Dimensions: Surpus, Cornell University Press, Ithica, 1981.
28 V. Ponec, Adv. Catal., 32 (1983) 149-214.
29 P. Biloen, J.N. Helle, H. Verbeek, F.M. Dautzenberg and W.M.H. Sachtler, J. Catal., 63 (1980) 112-118.
30 J.M. Parera, R.I. Verdrone, C.L. Pieck and E.M. Traffano, submitted to Appl. Catal.
31 J. Jothimurugesan, A.K. Nayak, G.K. Mehta, K.N. Rai, S. Bhatia and R.D. Srivastava, AIChEJ 31 (1985) 1997-2007.
32 K.H. Ludlum and R.P. Eischens, Symp. Catal. on Metals, Div. Petrol. Chem., Am. Chem. Sco., New York Meeting, April 4 - 7, 1976, pp. 375-384.
33 A.V. Ramaswamy, P. Ratnaswamy and S. Sivasanker, Proc. 6th Int. Congr. Catal., London, 1976, pp. 855-862.
34 J.C. Rasser, PhD Thesis, Delft University, 1977.
35 J.W. Schultze, Croatica Chemica Acta, 48 (1976) 643.

36 T.E. Fischer and S.R. Kelemen, J. Catal., 53 (1978) 24-34.
37 E. Lamy-Pitara, L. Bencharif and J. Barbier, submitted to Electrochimica Acta.
38 H. Wise, J. McCarty and J. Oudar, in J. Oudar and H. Wise (Ed), Deactivation and Poisoning of Catalysts, Marcel Dekkar, New York, 1985, pp. 1-50.
39 P. Gallezot, J. Datka, J. Massardier, M. Primet and B. Imelik, Proc. 6th Int. Cong. Catal., London, pp. 696-707.
40 G.M. Bickle, J. Biswas and D.D. Do, submitted to Appl. Catal., (1987).
41 J.M. Parera, R.J. Verderone, C.C. Pieck and E.M. Traffano, submitted to Appl. Catal. (1986).
42 C.R. Apesteguia and J. Barbier, Bull. Soc. Chim de France, Nos. 5-6, Part 1, (1982) 1-165.
43 J. Barbier, A. Morales, P. Morecot and R. Morecot and R. Maurel, Bull Soc. Chim. Belg., 88 (1979) 569-576.
44 J. Barbier and I. Marecot, submitted.
45 J. Oudar, Catal. Rev. Sci. Eng., 22 (1980) 171-195.
46 C.H. Bartholomew, P.K. Agarval and J.R. Katzer, Adv. Catal., 31 (1982) 135-242.
47 Y. Berthier, M. Perdereau and J. Oudar, Surf. Sci., 36 (1973) 225-242.
47a X. Yang and I. Pang, Int. Chem. Eng., 22 (1982) 125-132.
48 G. Bergeret and P. Gallezot, J. Catal., 87 (1984) 86-112.
49 J Biswas, G.M. Bickle, P.G. Gray, D.D. Do and J. Barbier, submitted to Cat. Rev. Sci. & Eng., (1987).

B. Delmon and G.F. Froment (Editors), *Catalyst Deactivation 1987*

CARBONACEOUS DEPOSITS FORMED ON ZEOLITES HY, HZSM-20 AND H-BETA DURING THE CONVERSION OF POLYNUCLEAR AROMATICS

M. NEUBER[1], S. ERNST[2], H. GEERTS[3], P.J. GROBET[3], P.A. JACOBS[3], G.T. KOKOTAILO[1] and J. WEITKAMP[2,4]

[1]University of Karlsruhe, Engler-Bunte Institute, Richard-Willstaetter-Allee 5, D-7500 Karlsruhe (Federal Republic of Germany)

[2]University of Oldenburg, Department of Chemistry, Chemical Technology, Ammerlaender Heerstrasse 114-118, D-2900 Oldenburg (Federal Republic of Germany)

[3]Katholieke Universiteit Leuven, Laboratorium voor Oppervlaktechemie, B-3030 Leuven (Belgium)

[4]Author for correspondence

ABSTRACT

1-Methylnaphthalene was reacted over three large pore zeolite catalysts, viz. HY, HZSM-20 and H-Beta at 180, 250 and 300°C. All catalysts underwent deactivation due to the formation of carbonaceous deposits. The deposits were characterized by elemental analysis and CP/MAS-^{13}C-NMR spectroscopy. HY and HZSM-20 showed very similar catalytic behaviours: At 250 and 300°C, considerable cracking and transalkylation occurred with a simultaneous formation of coke. On H-Beta, deactivation due to coking is much less severe, and there is hardly any cracking. All these observations can be accounted for by somewhat narrower pores as measured independently by the Spaciousness Index. MAS-NMR indicates that at low temperatures, the deposits are best described by unconverted methylnaphthalene whereas at higher temperatures, condensed ring aromatics are gradually built up.

INTRODUCTION

The formation of carbonaceous deposits or coke is an undesired side reaction in almost all reactions of hydrocarbons over acid catalysts. In general, the accumulation of such deposits on the catalyst reduces its activity and deteriorates the selectivity. Coke on catalysts consists of a complex mixture of high molecular compounds built up in disproportionation, condensation and hydrogen transfer reactions [1]. Many factors can have an influence on the coke forming tendency of a catalyst and the nature of the deposits. For example, both the rate of coke formation and the nature of the carbonaceous deposits were found to depend strongly on the feed hydrocarbon [2 - 4]. In many investigations, unsaturated compounds such as olefins and aromatics were found to be much more potent coke producers than saturated hydrocarbons [2, 3].

Reaction conditions, especially temperature, have a great influence on coking. From the finding that medium pore zeolites deactivate slowly compared to large pore zeolites, Rollmann and Walsh [5 - 7] concluded that coke formation is a shape selective reaction. In medium pore zeolites, reaction steps which lead to high molecular weight deposits are inhibited, whereas they can occur in large pore zeolites.

Carbonaceous residues on acid catalysts were studied by means of a large variety of experimental techniques [1]. The determination of the H/C atomic ratio of the coke enables a first insight into the coke composition. More detailed information on its nature can be obtained by spectroscopic methods, e.g., by infrared spectroscopy [3, 8] or cross-polarization/magic angle spinning ^{13}C nuclear magnetic resonance (CP/MAS-^{13}C-NMR) spectroscopy [4, 9].

In the present study, 1-methylnaphthalene (1-M-Np) was reacted over three large pore zeolites, viz., HY, HZSM-20, and H-Beta. Methylnaphthalenes are often considered to be typical coke precursors. The zeolites employed possess similar effective pore widths since their Spaciousness Indices [10] are close together. It was the objective to investigate whether such subtle differences in the effective pore widths can influence the deactivation due to coking. The carbonaceous deposits formed from 1-methylnaphthalene were characterized by elemental analysis and CP/MAS-^{13}C-NMR spectroscopy.

EXPERIMENTAL

Zeolite Beta was obtained in an attempt to synthesize ZSM-20 according to a recipe described by Valyocsik [11]. The latter zeolite could be obtained by modifying this recipe. The detailed procedure for the synthesis of pure ZSM-20 has been given elsewhere [12]. After hydrothermal synthesis, the zeolites were filtered, washed with distilled water and dried at 120°C. To remove the organic template, Beta and ZSM-20 were calcined in air at 400°C for 3 days and 540°C for 1 day, respectively. It was ascertained by X-ray powder diffraction that none of the zeolites was contaminated by other crystalline phases. NaY was purchased from Union Carbide Corp. (Tarrytown, N.Y., USA). All zeolites were transferred to the NH_4^+-forms by ion exchange with 0.5 n NH_4Cl solution under reflux conditions. The Si/Al-ratios of the zeolites Y, ZSM-20, and Beta were 2.4, 4.8, and 10, respectively. They were pressed binder-free, crushed and sieved. The particle size of 0.2 - 0.3 mm was used for the catalytic runs.

The catalytic experiments were conducted in a flow-type apparatus from glass with a fixed bed reactor. The catalysts were activated in-situ in flowing nitrogen at 400°C for 6 h. The purity of 1-M-Np amounted to 99.4 %, the main impurity was 2-M-Np (0.5 %). The partial pressures of N_2 and 1-M-Np and the modified residence time (W/F_{1-M-Np}) were 100 kPa, 2.0 kPa, and 110 g · h/mol, respectively. Reaction temperatures were 180, 250, and 300°C. After 11 h, the catalysts were purged with N_2 at reaction temperature until the purge gas was free from hydrocarbons. The deactivation behaviour was monitored by automatic on-line sampling. The reaction products were analyzed by high resolution capillary glc.

Elemental analysis for H and C in the coke deposits was carried out in a modified combustion apparatus [4]. It was designed in such a manner that hydrogen originating from the carbonaceous deposits could be discriminated from inorganic hydrogen, e.g., of adsorbed water or acid OH-groups. A detailed description of this experimental technique will be published soon [13].

The CP/MAS-^{13}C-NMR spectra of the coked zeolites were recorded on a Bruker MSL 400 Fourier transform spectrometer with a magnetic field of 9.4 Tesla and a ^{13}C frequency of 100.6 MHz. The rotor was from ZrO_2 and a spinning rate of 4.5 or 5.0 kHz was used for all experiments. The ^{1}H-pulse, the ^{13}C-pulse, the ^{1}H-^{13}C contact time, and the high power decoupling time were 3 μs, 5 μs, 1 ms, and 20 ms, respectively. The recycle time was 3 s. For all experiments, equal volumes of used zeolites were loaded in the rotor. Chemical shifts are given with respect to an external standard of liquid tetramethylsilane (TMS). Spinning side bands resulting from the chemical shift anisotropy of aromatic hydrocarbons are denoted by S.

RESULTS AND DISCUSSION

Conversion curves of 1-methylnaphthalene on the three zeolite catalysts are depicted in Fig. 1. All zeolites undergo deactivation. At 180°C, their deactivation behaviour is very similar. At 300°C, H-Beta deactivates much slower than both HY and HZSM-20.

In Figures 2 - 4, the product yields are shown for zeolite HY, HZSM-20 and H-Beta, respectively. At low reaction temperature, isomerization of 1-methylnaphthalene into 2-methylnaphthalene is the predominant reaction. This is true for HY and HZSM-20 while on H-Beta at 180°C, isomerization of 1-M-Np is completely free from any side reaction. On HY and HZSM-20, some transalkylation into dimethylnaphthalenes and naphthalene takes place.

At a reaction temperature of 300°C, the differences in product yields are even more pronounced. In the beginning of an experiment, the yield of 2-methylnaphthalene passes through a maximum. During this stage, 1-M-Np and 2-M-Np are in thermodynamic equilibrium (39 % 1-M-Np and 61 % 2-M-Np at 300°C [14]), i.e., the apparent maximum in $Y_{Iso.}$ is trivial. On HY and HZSM-20, the yields of products formed by transalkylation are as high as 30 % in the beginning. Furthermore, cleavage of one aromatic ring takes place initially on HY and HZSM-20 to a considerable extent of ca. 30 %. At 300°C, these two zeolites suffer from

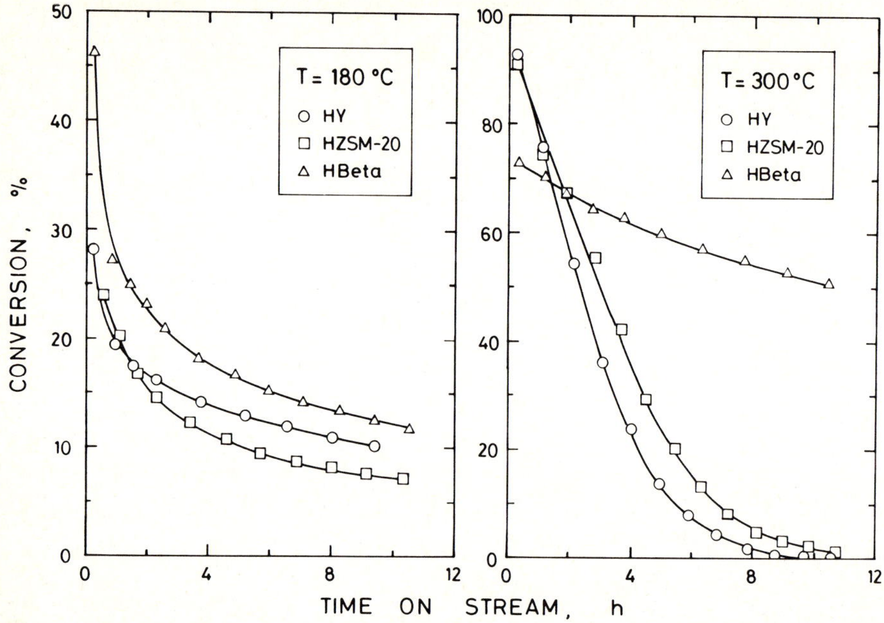

Fig. 1. Conversion of 1-methylnaphthalene in dependence of time on stream at 180°C and 300°C.

severe deactivation. After several hours on stream, hardly any reaction except isomerization occurs.

In contrast, H-Beta is remarkably stable at 300°C. Initially, it is less active than both HY and HZSM-20, but due to its low rate of deactivation, it is by far the most active catalyst after several hours on stream (s. Fig. 1). Virtually no cracking and very little transalkylation are observed on H-Beta in the beginning (s. Fig. 4).

At a reaction temperature of 250°C, the catalytic behaviour of the three zeolites was similar as at 300°C. There again, H-Beta showed a remarkable selectivity for isomerization of 1-M-Np to 2-M-Np.

Up to now, neither the crystallographic structure of zeolite ZSM-20, nor the one of zeolite Beta have been published. It has been claimed [11] that ZSM-20 resembles faujasite in certain structural aspects. Indeed, their Spaciousness Indices, i.e., the ratios of rates of formation of i-butane and n-butane during hydrocracking of a C_{10}-naphthene, e.g., butylcyclohexane, were found to be 20 for ZSM-20 and 21 for zeolite Y [10]. Zeolite Beta possesses a Spaciousness Index of 18 [10] which indicates that its effective pore width is

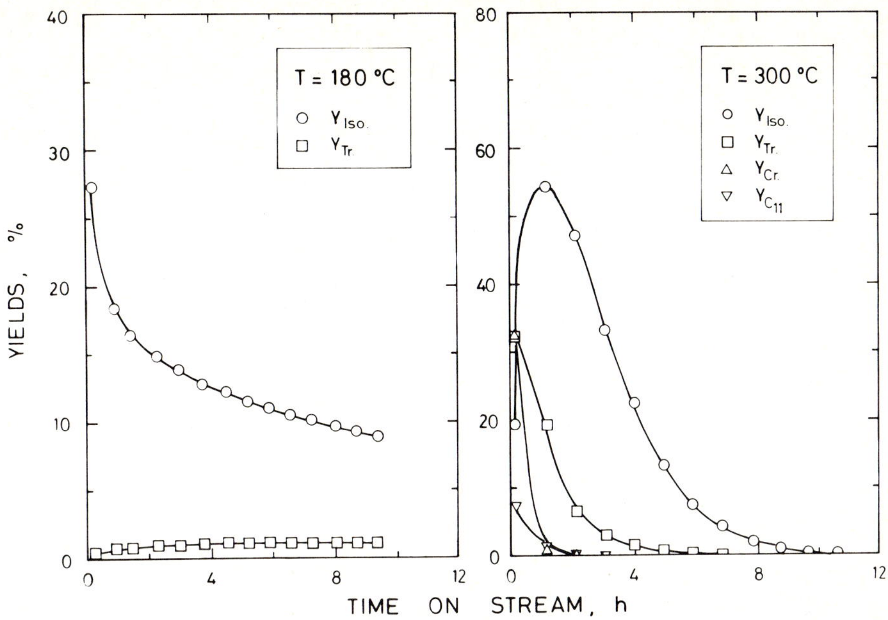

Fig. 2. Reaction of 1-methylnaphthalene on zeolite HY ($Y_{Iso.}$, $Y_{Tr.}$ and $Y_{Cr.}$ designate yields of products formed by isomerization, transalkylation and cracking, respectively. $Y_{C_{11}}$ is the yield of unidentified hydrocarbons with 11 carbon atoms, except 1-M-Np and 2-M-Np).

somewhat lower than those of ZSM-20 and Y. In principle, the same conclusions were drawn from the results of another catalytic test reaction for probing the effective pore width, viz. isomerization and hydrocracking of n-decane [15]. The high selectivity of zeolite Beta can, therefore, be best explained in terms of its narrower pores: The bimolecular transition state required for transalkylation of the bulky methylnaphthalene can probably not be accommodated inside the channel system of zeolite Beta. Isomerization, by contrast, can proceed via a monomolecular transition state.

It is a straightforward assumption that the low rate of deactivation of zeolite Beta has the same origin. Presumably, disproportionation and/or condensation reactions to high molecular coke require too bulky transition states. In HY and HZSM-20, there is enough free space for transalkylation and cracking of 1-M-Np to take place. The formation of cracked products which possess higher H/C ratios than the feed hydrocarbon requires the simultaneous formation of hydrogen deficient components inside the zeolite. Thus, the severe deactivation of HY and HZSM-20 at 300°C can be attributed to a rapid formation of coke in the beginning of the experiment when the rate of cracking is high.

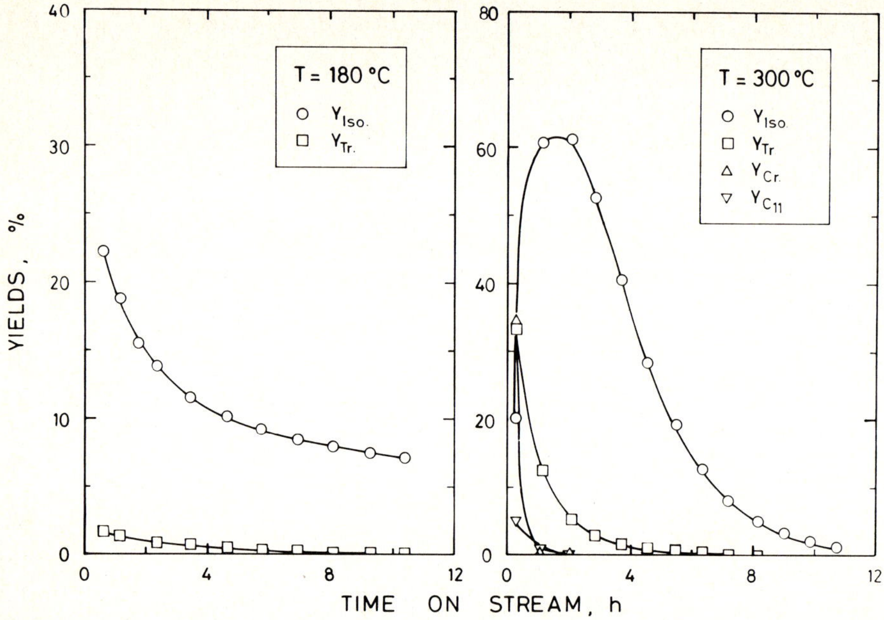

Fig. 3. Reaction of 1-methylnaphthalene on zeolite HZSM-20 (see Fig. 2 for explanation of the symbols).

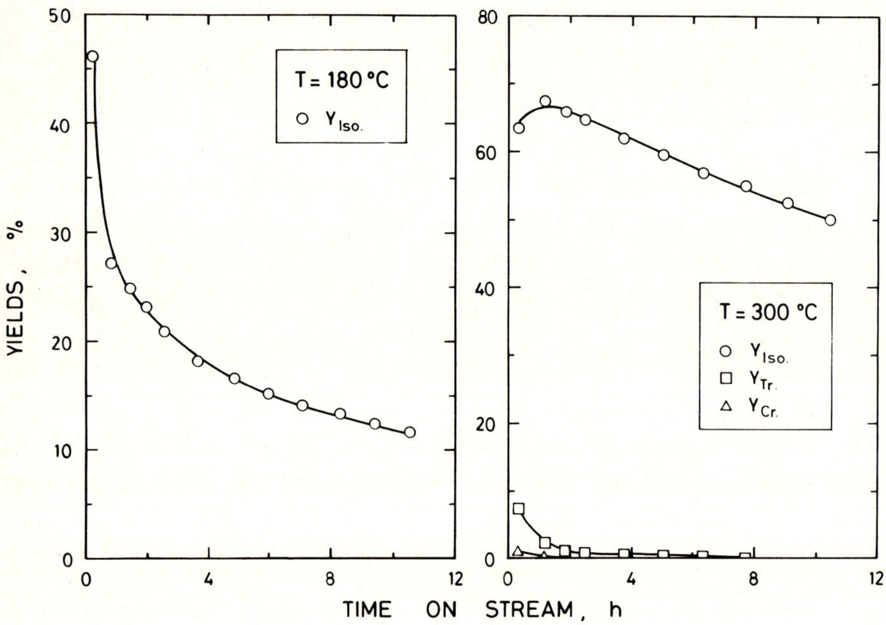

Fig. 4. Reaction of 1-methylnaphthalene on zeolite H-Beta (see Fig. 1 for explanation of symbols).

At 250°C, expectedly, the rate of cracking as well as the rate of deactivation were less for both zeolites than at the higher reaction temperature. This confirms the close connection between coke formation and cracking in the reaction of 1-M-Np.

In Table 1, the results of the elemental analyses, viz. coke loadings of the used zeolites and H/C atomic ratios of the carbonaceous deposits are given.

TABLE 1
Coke loadings L and H/C atomic ratios in the coke on the used zeolite catalysts.

T, °C		180	250	300
HY	L, wt.-%	18.2	a)	a)
	H/C	0.87	a)	0.42
HZSM-20	L, wt.-%	6.4	24.5	26.4
	H/C	0.81	0.63	0.60
H-Beta	L, wt.-%	3.8	7.4	7.3
	H/C	0.91	0.80	0.78

a) not determined

At 180°C, the coke loadings of the used zeolites differ drastically from each other. On HY, it amounts to more than 18 wt.-% which is close to the value found earlier on LaY in experiments with a variety of feed hydrocarbons [4]. Much lower coke loadings are detected at 180°C on HZSM-20 and H-Beta. Interestingly, the H/C ratios of the carbonaceous deposits formed at 180°C are similar and not very different from the one of the feed hydrocarbon ($C_{11}H_{10}$, H/C = 0.91). As a good approximation, therefore, the residual organic matter held on the acid zeolites at 180°C can be described as strongly adsorbed methylnaphthalene. The large differences in the amount of organic matter held by the zeolites at 180°C appear to correlate with their Al contents, at least qualitatively. Hence, the L values measured at 180°C seem to reflect the strength of interaction between the zeolites and the polynuclear aromatic sorbate.

At elevated reaction temperatures, the carbonaceous deposits are getting more deficient in hydrogen. This is particularly true for zeolite HY. The results from elemental analysis indicate that on HY and, to a lesser extent, on HZSM-20, highly condensed polynuclear aromatic deposits are formed. H-Beta, again, shows a distinctly different behaviour: Even at 300°C, the H/C ratio of the organic deposits is relatively high (0.78) and not too far from the one of the feed. It is, moreover, interesting to notice that at 300°C, the amount of coke held in zeolite H-Beta is less than one third of the amount retained by HZSM-20. All these findings correlate well with the slow deactivation of H-Beta (Fig. 1) and the low selectivities for transalkylation and cracking (Fig. 4).

Selected CP/MAS-^{13}C-NMR spectra of the used zeolites are shown in Fig. 5. The ^{13}C-spectra of the samples used at 180°C are best interpreted by methylnaphthalene adsorbed on the zeolites, in agreement with the results from the catalytic experiments and the elemental analyses. The band at 19 ppm can be

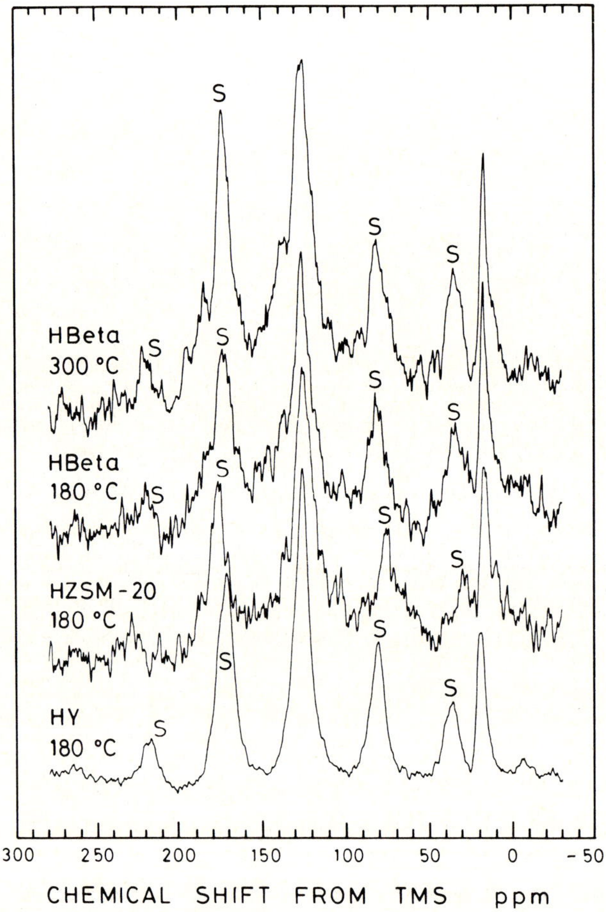

Fig. 5. CP/MAS-^{13}C-NMR spectra of carbonaceous deposits on HY, HZSM-20 and H-Beta used in the conversion of 1-methylnaphthalene (S denotes spinning side bands).

attributed to methyl groups attached to an aromatic ring, whereas the band at 127 ppm arises from carbon in the aromatic nuclei [16]. Peak positions are equal for all three zeolites. The signal/noise ratio of the coke spectrum of HY is significantly higher than the one for the other zeolites. This is a consequence of the higher carbon content of HY (this conclusion can immediately be drawn since equal volumes of the zeolites were loaded to the MAS-NMR-rotor). Thus, the high coke loading of HY found by elemental analysis is nicely confirmed by CP/MAS-^{13}C-NMR spectroscopy.

The NMR-spectrum of H-Beta coked at 300°C does not differ substantially from the spectra of the zeolites used at 180°C. The band at 127 ppm has now broadened. No further information on the nature of the coke can be deduced from this broad signal since the carbon shifts reported for naphthalene, phenanthrene, anthracene and pyrene in the liquid state vary between 125 and 131 ppm [16, 17]. Again, the peak at 19 ppm is indicative of methyl groups attached to aromatic nuclei. Relative to the band at 127 ppm, its intensity has slightly diminished, so only relatively few methyl groups disappeared during coke formation from methylnaphthalene. As a whole, the results of ^{13}C-NMR spectroscopy along with the results of elemental analysis show that the coke structure can be satisfactorily described by partially methylated polynuclear aromatics with a limited number of condensed aromatic rings.

CONCLUSIONS

The catalytic data suggest that transalkylation of 1-methylnaphthalene is inhibited within the pores of zeolite H-Beta because of transition state shape selectivity. Therefore, condensation and disproportionation reactions and hydrogen transfer reactions which lead to hydrogen deficient high molecular carbonaceous deposits cannot occur in this zeolite. Indeed, the structure of coke in H-Beta does not change very much with reaction conditions and exhibits typical features of the feed hydrocarbon, even at a relatively high reaction temperature of 300°C. At the same time, the rate of deactivation is remarkably low.

If the reaction pathways via bulky intermediates can proceed, e.g. in HY and HZSM-20, a hydrogen deficient coke is built up at high reaction temperatures, accompanied by the formation of light cracked products. Both zeolites deactivate very fast. Reaction temperature then has a distinct influence on the composition of the carbonaceous deposits.

It is a striking result that only small differences in the effective pore widths of large pore zeolites, as indicated by the Spaciousness Index [10], lead to quite different results in the catalytic behaviour of a zeolite and the structure of the coke.

At low reaction temperatures, coke may consist mainly of adsorbed feed molecules. The Si/Al ratio of the zeolites, viz. the density of Al and therefore of active sites, has a great influence on the amount of adsorbed species. The high loadings with carbonaceous residues, viz. 18 % on HY at 180°C even after purging with N_2, points to very strong sorbate-zeolite interactions.

Though the coke formed during the catalytic conversion of 1-M-Np will not vary very much in its chemical nature, valuable information can be obtained by combined application of elemental analysis and CP/MAS-^{13}C-NMR spectroscopy. ^{13}C-NMR spectroscopy is very useful for elucidating the nature of the coke [4] (viz. paraffinic, aromatic) and gives information about structural aspects, e.g. whether or not an aromatic coke is alkylated.

ACKNOWLEDGEMENTS

Jens Weitkamp, Stefan Ernst and Marita Neuber acknowledge financial support by the Federal Ministery of Research and Technology of the Federal Republic of Germany (BMFT), the German Science Foundation (DFG), Fonds der Chemischen Industrie (FdChI) and Max-Buchner-Forschungsstiftung (MBFSt). Marita Neuber moreover acknowledges a scholarship within the frame of Landesgraduiertenförderung Baden-Württemberg. George T. Kokotailo gratefully acknowledges the Humboldt Senior US Scientist Award 1985.

REFERENCES

[1] E.E. Wolf and F. Alfani, Catal. Rev.-Sci. Eng. 24 (1982) 329-371.
[2] W.G. Appleby, J.W. Gibson and G.M. Good, Ind. Eng. Chem., Proc. Des. Dev. 1 (1962) 102-110.
[3] P.E. Eberly, Jr., C.N. Kimberlin, Jr., W.H. Miller and H.V. Drushell, Ind. Eng. Chem., Proc. Des. Dev. 5 (1966) 193-198.
[4] S. Maixner, C.Y. Chen, P.J. Grobet, P.A. Jacobs and J. Weitkamp, Proc. 7th International Zeolite Conference, Y. Murakami, A. Iijima, and J.W. Ward (Editors), Kodansha, Tokyo, and Elsevier, Amsterdam, 1986, pp. 693-700.
[5] L.D. Rollmann, J. Catal. 47 (1977) 113-121.
[6] D.E. Walsh and L.D. Rollmann, J. Catal. 49 (1977) 369-375.
[7] L.D. Rollmann and D.E. Walsh, J. Catal. 56 (1979) 139-140.
[8] F. Fetting, E. Gallei and P. Kredel, Ger. Chem. Eng. 7 (1984) 32-38.
[9] E.G. Derouane, J.P. Gilson and J.B. Nagy, Zeolites 2 (1982) 42-48.
[10] J. Weitkamp, S. Ernst and R. Kumar, Appl. Catal. 27 (1986) 207-210.
[11] E.W. Valyocsik, Europ. Patent Appl. 12572, assigned to Mobil Oil Corp., June 25, 1980.
[12] S. Ernst, G.T. Kokotailo, and J. Weitkamp, Zeolites, in press.
[13] J. Weitkamp, S. Maixner, C.Y. Chen and C. von Branconi, Chem.-Ing.-Tech., submitted for publication.
[14] D.R. Stull, E.F. Westrum, Jr. and G.C. Sinke, The Chemical Thermodynamics of Organic Compounds, J. Wiley and Sons, New York, Sydney, Toronto, 1969, p. 390.
[15] J.A. Martens, M. Tielen, P.A. Jacobs and J. Weitkamp, Zeolites 4 (1984) 98-107.

[16] J.B. Stothers, Carbon-13 NMR Spectroscopy, Organic Chemistry, A Series of Monographs, Vol. 24, Academic Press, New York, London, 1972, p. 90-100.
[17] E. Breitmaier and W. Voelter, Carbon-13 NMR Spectroscopy. High-Resolution Methods and Applications in Organic Chemistry and Biochemistry, 3rd Ed., VCH-Verlagsgesellschaft Weinheim 1987, p. 266.

B. Delmon and G.F. Froment (Editors), *Catalyst Deactivation 1987*

OXYGEN INDUCED FOULING IN A XYLENE ISOMERIZATION REACTOR BED

W.T. KOETSIER[1] AND J. VAN LEENEN[2]

[1]BASIC CHEMICALS TECHNOLOGY; EXXON CHEMICAL HOLLAND B.V.
P.O. BOX 7225; 3000 HE ROTTERDAM; THE NETHERLANDS.

[2]ALFA-LAVAL N.V.; STROOMBAAN 4; AMSTELVEEN; THE NETHERLANDS.

ABSTRACT

The causes for the plugging of a xylene isomerization reactor have been studied in a pilot plant program. Two contaminants in the feed to this reactor, namely O_2 and diphenylmethane isomers, were the main cause for the formation of coke. Furthermore the presence of small Fe containing particulates contributed to this plugging process. Once the recommendations to prevent the presence of these contaminants had been implemented plugging has not been observed anymore over the last four years of operation.

INTRODUCTION

During 1979-1981 our Aromatics plant periodically experienced pressure drop build-ups across the bed of the xylene isomerization reactor (the isoformer). These pressure drop build-ups resulted in severe throughput limitations leading each time to a shut-down of the unit for a period of 6 to 12 days.

The deposition of foulings on top and within the first two feet of the reactor bed was identified as the main cause for this bed plugging. Several techniques were tried to clean up the reactor bed and to reduce the pressure drop again.

A coke burn reduced the pressure drop by only 50 % and was therefore not sufficient.

A sieving of the complete reactor bed removed all the foulings, but it had the disadvantage of breaking and pulverizing a small fraction of the catalyst particles. Moreover, it was time consuming and required a shut-down of the unit for a period of at least 12 days.

The installation of a two foot guard bed on top of the catalyst bed was considered as the preferred technique to solve this problem. Each time the pressure drop across the reactor bed became too high, the whole guard bed was replaced and the top of the catalyst bed was vacuum cleaned. This procedure could be completed in about 7 days.

However, shutting-down the unit each half year for a period of 7 days is undesirable from the standpoint of both operations and economics. After the third shut-down we decided to start a research program in order to get an understanding of the actual causes leading to the deposition of foulings on top of the reactor bed. This program resulted in three recommendations which were implemented in 1981/1982. Since that time our unit has been operating without any increase in pressure drop across the reactor bed.

The results of our investigations and the basis for our recommendations are summarized below.

SEVERAL UNFORESEEN SHUT-DOWNS REQUIRED

When bed plugging was observed for the first time in 1979, we decided to do a full oxygen burn. This burn reduced the pressure drop by only 50 %. The reactor was opened and several samples were taken from the top of the guard bed for which gamma-alumina extrudates were used.

These samples contained a highly magnetic dust. This dust was loosely adhering to the outer-surface of the alumina extrudates and could be removed almost completely by sieving. As this dust was present to a depth of two feet, it was considered as the main cause for the pressure drop build-up.

The reactor was unloaded, the whole charge was sieved and it was put back into the reactor.

Six weeks after start-up the pressure drop started to increase again rapidly. Within two weeks another shut-down was required. The cause for this pressure drop build-up was different from that observed two months earlier. There were no carbonaceous deposits present. We assumed that the cause was the accumulation of catalyst fines somewhere in the bottom of the bed. Therefore a charge of fresh catalyst was installed.

Seven months later the pressure drop had reached a level where a third shut-down was required. The top of the reactor bed again contained a lot of deposits. It was vacuum cleaned and again a guard bed was installed.

We decided to check whether this dust originated from a source upstream of the reactor (e.g. the furnace tubes or the heat-exchangers) and had been carried over into the reactor bed. Fouling of heat-exchangers is a well known phenomenon in the oil industry.

The heat-exchangers were opened for inspection. The feed side of the last two heat-exchangers was almost completely fouled with a friable flakey coke sitting in between the tubes. Since these flakes could be broken and pulverized easily, it could have caused a flow of dust particles in the feed to the reactor.

These heat-exchangers had not been opened and cleaned for almost three years. We expected that a proper cleaning of these two heat-exchangers would give us at least another two years of uninterrupted operation. However, the unit experienced a rise in pressure drop much earlier than predicted, and the reactor bed needed to be cleaned again 7 months later.

It was difficult to explain why a layer of deposits was observed so quickly within the first two feet of the reactor bed. The fouling phenomenon was much more severe than we had foreseen.

As we could not give an acceptable explanation for this fouling behaviour, we decided to set up a thorough investigation of all the potential causes which could lead to the deposition of carbonaceous deposits.

ANALYSIS OF DEPOSITS

The heat-exchanger deposits were subjected to analyses done at EXXON laboratories:

- GC analyses on a OV-275 column of a $CHCl_3$ extract (8 wt %) showed primarily alkylnaphthalenes (82 wt %) and alkylbenzenes (17 wt %)
- IR-analysis on $CHCl_3$ extract confirmed aromatic nature and showed the presence of the functional oxygen containing groups.
- Elemental analysis on C, H, N, S and O gave the following atomic ratio:

$$C : H : N : S : O = 16 : 10 : 0.2 : 0.2 : (1-2)$$

- The results of high resolution MS analyses of the volatile fraction are summarized in Table 1.

TABLE 1

MS ANALYSES OF VOLATILE FRACTION OF HEAT-EXCHANGER DEPOSITS

	Sample 1 (ppm)	Sample 2 (ppm)
1-Ring Aromatics	65600	77900
2-Ring Aromatics		
- $C_{16}H_{16}$ dimers	560	180
- $C_{16}H_{18}$ dimers	380	140
3-Ring Aromatics	200	50
4-Ring Aromatics	20	10
Oxygen compounds	2450	1870
Thiophenes	170	110
Total volatiles :	69400	80200

SIGNIFICANCE OF DEPOSITS ANALYSES

Although the xylenes and alkylbenzene predominate in the volatile analysis, there is a notable amount of 3 and 4 ring aromatics. These components would not be expected to be present in the isoformer feed to any extent, and therefore the polynuclear aromatics must have been formed at the temperature range at which the last two heat-exchangers had been operating, namely 200°C - 270°C.

Moreover the presence of oxygenated compounds in relatively large amounts is highly significant. These include very high boiling phenols, oxides, carboxilic acids... etc., which most certainly are formed by the presence of dissolved oxygen-induced oxidation of the side chain methyl groups.

The presence of nitrogen can be attributed to alkylamines which are used as corrosion inhibitors in the benzene and toluene fractionators, two columns which are located upstream of the xylene isomerization reactor.

The presence of sulphur probably originates from the decomposition of sulfolane used in the extraction unit.

ISOFORMER FEED CONTAMINANTS

The next step in our investigations was to find a clue for the mechanism of forming the carbonaceous deposits.

We expected that the contaminants which are present in the isoformer feed play an important role in this coking process. An analysis of the isoformer feed identified the following components which were potentially responsible for this fouling process:

- Small Fe/Fe-oxide/Fe-sulfide particles originating from isoformer feed tankage;
- dissolved oxygen in amounts of 15 wppm;
- C_9-aromatic components such as isopropylbenzene in amounts of 1000 wppm; and
- a "heavy aromatic residue" in an amount of 1 to 5 wppm.

The T.N.O. laboratory in Rijswijk, the Netherlands, analyzed the composition of this "heavy aromatic residue". The characteristic GC spectrum showed a total of 30 peaks. The components which were identified by MS are summarized in Table 2.

TABLE 2

GC-MS ANALYSIS OF ISOFORMER FEED RESIDUE

Type of component	Molecular weight
xylenes	106
C_3 -, C_4 - and C_5 benzenes	120,134,148
cyclohexyl benzene	160
cyclohexyl toluene	174
cyclohexyl xylenes	188
C_8 - and C_9 - benzenes	190-204
The following diaryl aromatics	
C_{14} H	182
C_{15} H	196
$C_{16}H_{18}$	210
$C_{17}H_{20}$	224
$C_{18}H_{22}$	238
and the following oxygenates	
C_8H_8O	120
$C_8H_{10}O$	122
$C_{16}H_{16}O$	224
$C_{17}H_{18}O$	238
$C_{18}H_{18}O$	252

The oxygen content of several isoformer feed residues varied between 0.5 wt % and 1 wt %.

Considering these observations we decided to start a pilot plant program to unravel the role of dissolved oxygen and these heavy aromatic components in forming the non-volatile "coke".

PILOT PLANT PROGRAM

For this pilot plant program we prepared two different xylene solutions:

A: one solution which contained 10 mg of "heavy aromatics residue" per liter xylenes

B: one which was free of heavy aromatics.

Experiments with solution A

Solution A was split in two fractions. At a temperature of 100°C air was purged through one of these fractions for several hours. The other fraction was purged with nitrogen. A sample was taken from each fraction to get sufficient "heavy aromatics residue" for a GC-MS analysis.

Each fraction was processed in a pilot unit reactor. The liquid was pumped at a rate such that the residence time in the reactor was equal to the residence time of the liquid in a heat-exchanger. The pilot plant reactor temperature was set at 150°C, 200°C, 250°C and 300°C. The products were collected and slowly distilled to get the residue. The results are summarized in Table 3.

TABLE 3

RESULTS PILOT-PLANT EXPERIMENTS

pilot-plant temp. °C	wppm residue	colour residue	appearance residue
Fraction saturated with air:			
150	18	dark yellow	liquid
200	13	brown	liquid
250	27	brown	solid
300	50	black	solid/wax
Fraction saturated with nitrogen:			
150	8	light yellow	liquid
200	8	yellow	solid
250	9	yellow	solid
300	13	brown	solid

These results demonstrate the effect of the presence of oxygen. Considerably more "coke" is formed in the oxygen-saturated fractions than in the nitrogen saturated fraction. The nature of the residue in both cases was also quite different. At each processing temperature the oxygen containing fraction produced a darker residue.

Finally these residues were subjected to a TGA analyses. Each residue of the N_2-containing fraction evaporated almost completely as the temperature of the TGA unit increased above 400°C. The residues from the O_2-containing fraction did not completely evaporate, even at a temperature as high as 700°C. The last 10 % of this residue appeared to be really "hard coke". These results confirmed the indigenous role of oxygen.

The GC-MS analysis of the "residue" revealed that the same spectrum of components were present as tabulated in Table 2.

The following interesting observations were made:

- of the C_{16} isomers with a molecular weight of 210 two different types of components were identified, namely (1) diphenylmethane; and (2) diphenylethane derivatives.
- there was also a C_{16} aromatic present with a molecular weight of 208. This component was identified as a dehydrodimethyl-phenanthrene.

<u>Experiments with solution B</u>

Solution B which did not contain any type of heavy aromatics was also saturated with air and processed in the unit, but 250°C only. A GC analysis of this residue identified only 7 specific components which were all of a diphenylethane type.

A TGA analysis of this residue showed that this residue evaporated almost completely at a temperature of above 400°C. Apparently less hard coke was formed.

DISCUSSION

The following two mechanisms can explain the formation of a "coke" residue:

<u>1. Via diphenylmethane derivatives</u>

A variety of diphenylmethane derivatives having 13 - 19 carbon numbers had been identified in the isoformer feed residue. The carbon in between the two phenyl groups is very susceptible to oxygen:

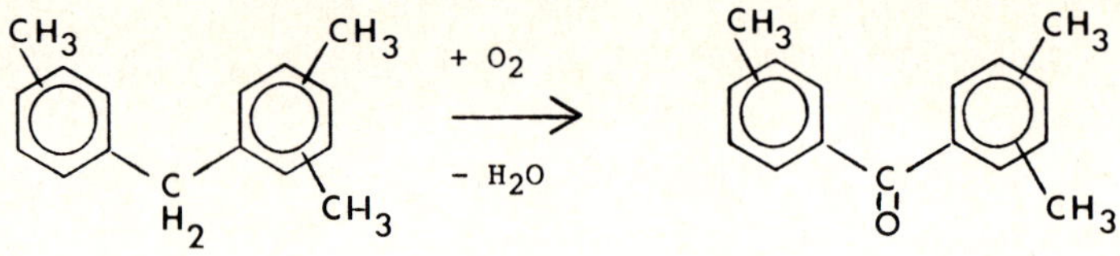

This oxidation seems to occur easily under the conditions of the xylene isomerization feed. The analyses of the O_2 contaminated feed revealed that when C_{16}, C_{17} and C_{18} biphenylmethanes are present even in amounts of less than 1 wppm, the corresponding oxygenates are formed.

Karl Elbs (lit. 1) showed that the o-methylated benzophenones are converted into polynuclear aromatics:

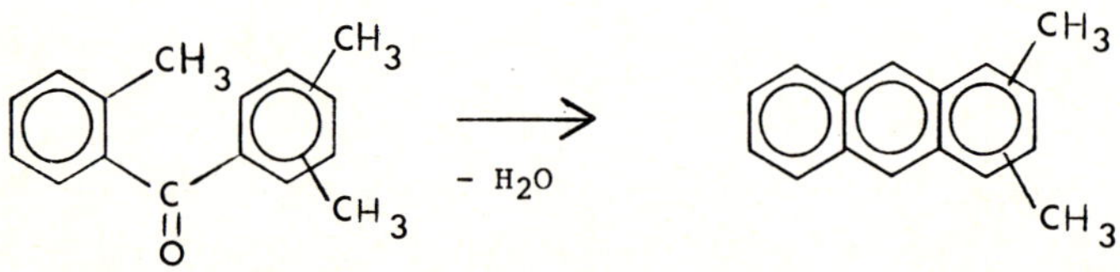

These polynuclear aromatics react much more readily with radicals than mononuclear compounds. And it is likely that there will be radicals present; the isoformer feed already contained 1000 wppm of isopropyl-benzene. This component is easily converted into an hydroperoxide, which acts as a radical initiator.

The radical substitution of anthracenes occurs preferentially at the 1 - and 2 - positions:

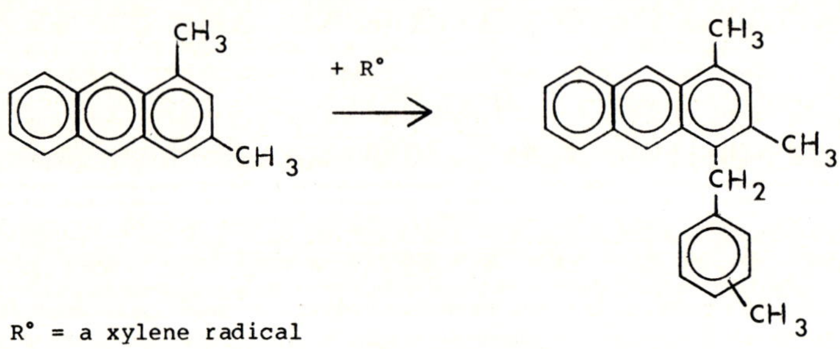

where R° = a xylene radical

Once these components are obtained, the formation of higher polynuclear aromatics follows the same route:

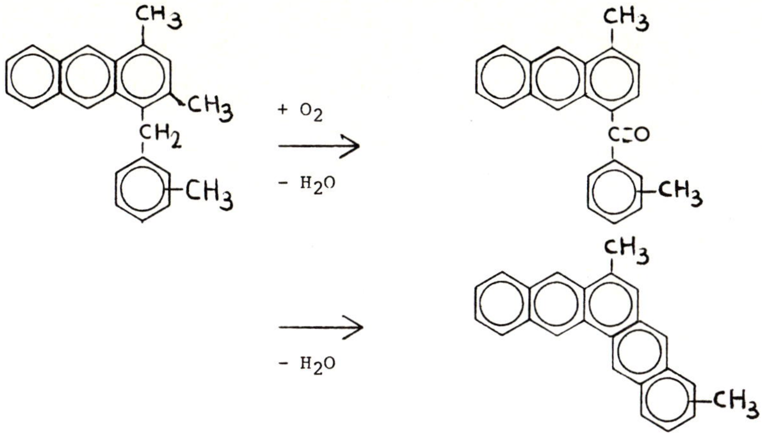

The benzopyrene components which are now obtained have an atomic ratio of C : H of 24 : 18. This is close to what has been analyzed in the coke.

2. Via diphenylethane derivatives

In the absence of diaryl aromatics the O_2 converts xylene molecules into diphenylethane molecules and as a dehydrodimethyl phenanthrene was identified in the residue from the pilot plant experiments, the following reactions seems to occur:

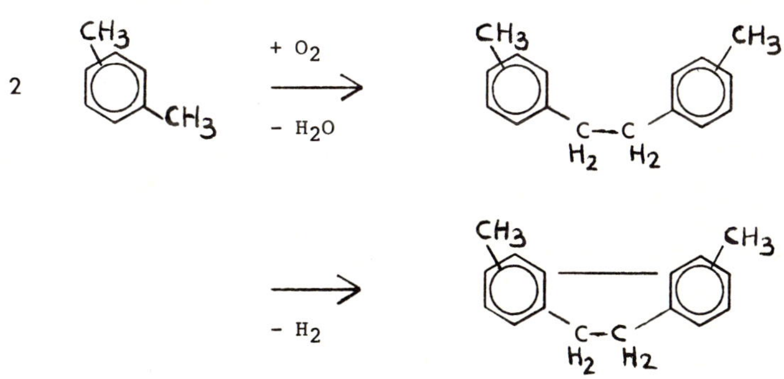

In case this phenanthrene derivative is dehydrogenated to anthracene derivatives further polymerization to coke is likely as has been explained under 1.

RECOMMENDATIONS - ACTIONS

Based on the results of our investigations we recommended that the following three main contributors of the fouling process to be eliminated from the isoformer feed:

- O_2
- "heavy aromatics", and
- Fe particulates

The elimination of O_2 required an investigation to identify the place where O_2 leaked into the feed. Once these leaks were eliminated the O_2 content in the isoformer feed dropped from 15 wppm to below negligible levels.

The elimination of "heavy aromatics" required a different feed preparation and fractionation changes.

An isoformer feed filter was installed to clean up in small particulates in the feed from all.

These changes were implemented in 1981/1982. As of that date the isoformer has been running without any significant increase in the pressure drop across the reactor bed.

ACKNOWLEDGEMENTS

We would like to express our gratitude to all the people who contributed to this program. Dr. D.J.M. van der Vleugel who proposed the coking mechanism. Mr. R.J. Philippe (EXXON, Machelen) and Mr. R.I. Botto and Mr. T. Aczel (EXXON Synthetic Fuels Research, Baytown) for their analytic support and Dr. P.J.W. Schuyl (Technical University, Delft) for the GC-MS analyses. In particular, we appreciate the valuable discussions we had with the representatives of Mobil Research and Development Corporation and with Prof.Dr.Ir. H. van Bekkum who encouraged us to publish these results.

REFERENCE

1. E. Clar, Polycyclic Hydrocarbons Volume 1 (1964) Academic Press, page 176-179.

B. Delmon and G.F. Froment (Editors), *Catalyst Deactivation 1987*

COKE FORMATION MECHANISM FROM OLEFINS OR DIOLEFINS UNDER CATALYTIC CRACKING CONDITIONS(1)

B. MERCIER DES ROCHETTES(*), C. MARCILLY(**), C. GUEGUEN and J. BOUSQUET(***)

* present address : Centre de Recherches SHELL, 76530 Grand-Couronne (France)

** E.N.S.P.M., B.P. 311, 92506 Rueil-Malmaison (France)

*** Centre de Recherches ELF-Solaize, B.P. 22, 69360 St Symphorien d'Ozon (France)

ABSTRACT

The formation of coke precursors has been studied from various simple olefinic and diolefinic molecules.

- Carbonaceous products are formed through a complex sequence of several reactions including hydrogen transfer and cyclodimerization which are essential.
- Two different routes are proposed for the latter : the classical Diels-Alder cyclodimerization which is probably the faster one and another route which involves spiro-compounds intermediates.

INTRODUCTION

In the catalytic cracking of petroleum fractions, carbonaceous materials gradually accumulate on the catalyst surface. This deposit lowers the cracking activity and must be periodically removed by burning. Since coke is a major parameter of the heat balance of an FCC unit, factors leading to its formation are of great industrial importance.

In view of the wide range of reactions occurring in catalytic cracking, the formation mechanism of coke precursors is difficult to establish even when working with pure compound feeds (1, 2, 3, 4, 5). However, when looking for molecules responsible for coke formation, partially unsaturated hydrocarbons such as olefins and diolefins are among the best candidates because they are less stable, therefore more reactive, than their more or less saturated equivalents such as paraffins, naphtenes or aromatics. This fact is well-known in catalytic reforming where the addition of unsaturated naphtenes (cyclopentenes and cyclopentadienes) to the feedstock greatly increases the coke formation (6, 7). This was also shown a long time ago in catalytic cracking by Greensfelder et al. (8).

The present investigation deals with the role played in coke formation, under catalytic cracking conditions, by various kinds of unsaturated molecules which can each act at the same time as a hydrogen donor or acceptor :

(1) This work is a part of the Ph. D. Thesis of B. MERCIER DES ROCHETTES submitted to E.N.S.P.M on Nov. 1983.

- Three simple olefinic molecules : a linear one, 1-hexene (1 HE) and two cyclic ones, cyclopentene (CPE) and cyclohexene (CHE).
- Two simple diolefins : cyclopentadiene (CPD) and methylcyclopentadiene (MCPD).

Some complementary results have been obtained by studying the tetraline transformation.

EXPERIMENTAL METHODS

1. Apparatus and test procedure

The apparatus used in the present study and described in detail in reference 9, is a M.A.T. unit modified to study model molecules.

The reactant fed by a syringe pump is first vaporized and then mixed with a dry nitrogen flow in a preheating section upstream of the reactor. The catalyst fills up a ring-like space 2.5 mm wide and 30 to 100 mm long. A special sampling device is placed at the outlet of the reactor. It is composed of four microvalves heated at 150°C in an independent furnace. During the catalytic test, these valves are closed, one after the other at given times on stream (t = 3, 5, 10, 20 and 35 minutes), thus isolating the gaseous products in a cylindric volume of about 100 µl. Before analysis the closed valves can, if necessary, be maintained overnight at 150°C without any heavy product condensation. All the products are thus retained in a gaseous phase. Each valve is then quickly transferred into a heated injection device of a GIRDEL 300 gas chromatograph equipped with a 152 ft CP sil 8 quartz column and a flame ionisation detector. The eluted products are identified either with chromatographic standards or by gas chromatography - mass spectroscopy (GC-MS) coupling.

As a classical material balance cannot be achieved with such equipment, the validity of the test is checked by means of carbon and hydrogen balances on all products sampled in the valves.

2. Material

All hydrocarbon reactants were Merck pure grade 1-Hexene (1 HE), cyclopentene (CPE), cyclopentadiene (CPDE), cyclohexene (CHE), methylcyclopentadiene (MCPDE) and tetraline (TET). Prior to use, they were all percolated through a silica gel column.

An industrial equilibrium fluid cracking catalyst containing 15 wt % of a rare earth zeolite dispersed in a silica-alumina matrix was used. It contained 0.3 wt % of coke and 1220 ppm Ni + V (250 + 970) and had a surface area of 66 $m^2 g^{-1}$. Prior to use, it was calcined overnight in the reactor under flowing nitrogen at 550°C.

3. Experimental conditions of catalytic tests

Runs were carried out under different conditions according to the type of molecule. The partial pressures were 18 KPa (0.18 bar) for all olefinic and diolefinic hydrocarbons and 25 KPa (0.25 bar) for tetraline TET. Other conditions were :

- 1-Hexene (1 HE) : = 400°C, contact time (reverse of the gaseous reactant hourly space velocity) τ = 1 to 10 seconds.
- Cyclopentene (CPE) : θ = 300 to 450°C, τ = 2 to 14 s.
- Cyclohexene (CHE) : θ = 300 to 450°C, τ = 1 to 10 s.
- Cyclopentadiene (CPD) : θ = 370°C, τ = 5 to 22 s.
- Methylcyclopentadiene (MCPD) : θ = 370°C, τ = 1 to 18 s.
- Tetraline (TET) : θ = 350 to 450°C, τ = 9 s.

RESULTS

Preliminary runs showed that hydrogenolysis and hydrogenation-dehydrogenation reactions due to Ni or V metals deposited on the catalyst could be ruled out.

1. Evolution of conversion and yields versus time on stream

- From 1 HE, the products obtained were 2 and 3 HE, isohexenes IHE (molar yields of IHE were between 10 and 16 %), HA and the isohexanes IHA (yields of HA + IHA were between 1 and 1.6 %), cracked products C_5^- (1 to 1.7 %) including essentially C_3, C_4 and C_5 hydrocarbons, methylcyclopentane MCPA (0.3 to 0.5 %), cyclohexane CHA (< 0.2 %), benzene BZ (< 0.2 %) and heavy products essentially composed of alkyl- benzenes ABZ (< 0.5 %). No CHE, no methylcyclopentene MCPE, no heavy products with more than 10 carbon atoms were detected.

  Isomerization of 1 HE into 2 and 3 HE (n HE) being very fast, the global conversion of HE was defined as :

$$X \quad 100 - \sum_{n=1}^{3} (\text{mol \% n HE})$$

  The conversion was about 28 % at t = 3 mn and decreased gradually down to 14 % at t = 35 mn. All yields decreased with conversion. The coke content of the used catalyst was less than .7 wt %.

- From CPE (Fig. 1), two main types of hydrocarbon were obtained :
  - a C_5 cut comprising CPA and cyclopentadiene (CPD)
  - a C_{10} cut composed of methylindanes (MIDA), methylindenes (MIDE), decaline (DEC), tetraline (TET), naphtalene (NAP) and alkylbenzenes (ABZ 10) (0.05 to 0.6 %).

  The amount of C_4 light products was less than 0.1 mol %.

  No cyclopentylcyclopentane was detected. Complementary analyses by GC-MS coupling clearly showed the presence of traces of dicyclopentadiene DCPD and of tricyclodecane TCD (saturated equivalent of DCPD) in the C 10 cut and of dimethylfluorenes and methylanthracenes in a C_{15} cut (trimers) which is a minor cut (< 0.15 wt/%). G.C.-M.S. coupling has also shown that MIDA have about 50 % of their methyl groups on the aromatic cycle and the other 50 % on the five-member ring.It is interesting to note that the CPD yield increases with time on stream whereas the yields of all the other products decrease.

After 40 mn of feed injection, the percentage of coke on the catalyst was only 0.76 wt %.

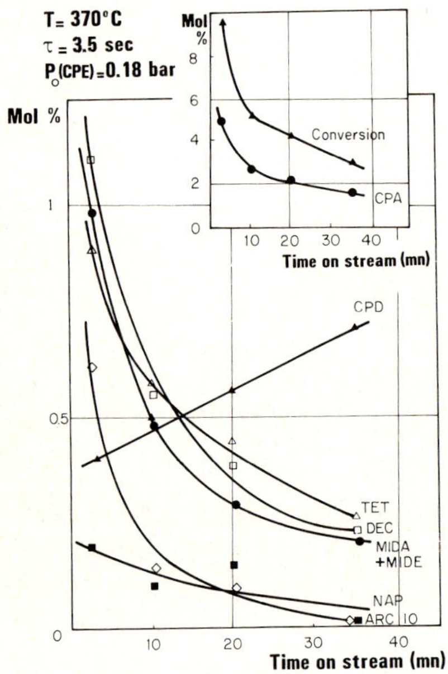

Fig. 1. Yields of products versus time on stream from CPE.

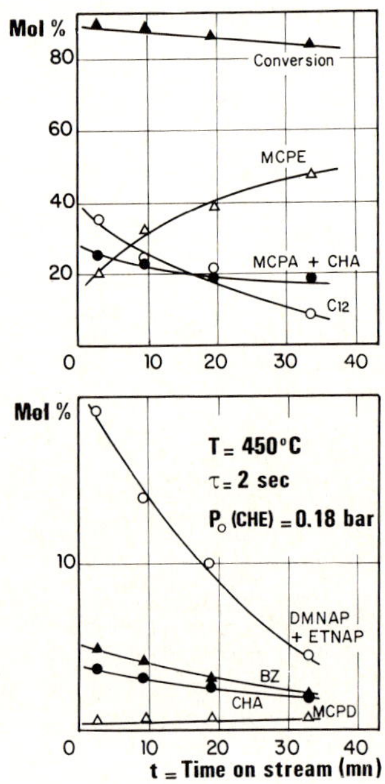

Fig. 2. Yields of products versus time on stream from CHE.

- From CHE (Fig. 2), as in the case of CPE, two main categories of hydrocarbons are evidenced :
  - a C_6 cut comprising MCPE (20 to 50 %), MCPA and CHA (yields of MCPA + CHA were between 18 and 26 %), MCPD ($\simeq$1 %) and BZ (2 to 5 %)
  - a C_{12} cut which was a complex mixture of alkylindanes (TMIDA) alkylindenes (TMIDE), alkyldecalines (ADEC), alkyltetralines (ATET) and alkylnaphtalenes (DMNAP) (these alkylcompounds were essentially dimethyl or trimethyl compounds with 12 carbon atoms). It must be pointed out that traces of dimethyldicyclopentadienes (DMDCD) were evidenced by G.C.-M.S. coupling.

Light products C_5^- and heavier products between C_7 and C_{11} were both less than 3 mol %. The C_7-C_{11} cut essentially contained toluene and polymethylbenzenes. No bicyclohexene, no bicyclohexane and no biphenyl were detected.

From t = 3 mn to 35 mn, all product yield decreased but that of MCPE which sharply increased from 20 to 48 mol. %.

- From CPD, three experiments were carried out at 370°C by varying the contact time. The reactant was actually a mixture of 90 % CPD and 10 % dicyclopentadiene DCPD. Most of the products were identical to those obtained from CPE and could be classified in a C_5 cut and a C_{10} cut. The formation of a small quantity (< 2.5 %) of products with 15 Carbon atoms (trimers) was also observed. Some dimethylfluorenes and methylanthracenes were identified by G.C.-M.S. coupling. G.C.-M.S. coupling also showed that MIDA isomers have about 80 % of their methyl groups on the aromatic cycle and 20 % on the 5-member ring.

  After 40 minutes of feed injection, the coke content on the catalyst was 2.4 wt %.
- From MCPD, four experiments were carried out at 400°C by varying the contact time. The reactant was actually a mixture of about 93 % MCPD and 7 % dimethyldicyclopentadiene DMDCPD. All products formed from CHE were evidenced in these experiments. Moreover, a small quantity (< 3 %) of trimer products (C_{18} cut) was also obtained. ATET and ADEC, if produced, were not determined.
- From TET : three experiments were carried out by varying the temperature with a time on stream of 9.5. The main products were NAP and to lesser extent, MIDA (1 and 2), ABZ, DEC and C_4^-.

2) Selectivity curves : evolution of product yields versus conversion or contact time.

Yields-versus-conversion curves were obtained by varying contact time from 1 to 14 s. at constant temperature (370°C for CPE and CDP, 400°C for 1 HE, CHE and MCDP). They are presented in (Figures 3, 4, 5, 6, 7). Figure 8 shows the difference in coke formation from various reactants : CPE, CPD, CHE and MCPD.

- From 1 HE, the following hydrocarbons appeared as primary products : IHE, HA, IHA, MCPA and the main cracked products (C_3, C_4 and C_5 hydrocarbons). BZ and ABZ (except for toluene) were secondary products. Compared to other aromatics, the particular behaviour of toluene, which appeared as a primary product, was unexpected.

  At conversion lower than 20 %, the HE isomerization rate was about 15 times higher than the hydrogen transfer rate (defined as the production rate of HA + IHA).
- From CPE (Fig. 3 and 4), the following main points emerge from the overall results.
  - CPA and CPD appeared as primary products.
  - At short time on stream (3 mn), DEC, TET, MIDA, MIDE and tricyclodecane (TCD) appeared as primary products. But they were evidenced as secondary products at longer time on stream (20 mn).
  - NAP and especially trimer products, which always appeared as secondary products, were slowly formed through a succession of consecutive reactions probably including dimerizations and hydrogen transfers.

- The yields of several products went through maximum values and then decreased when conversion increased. These maximums were reached at about 2-3 % conversion for CPD, 3-6 % for MIDE and TCD. CPD appeared as one of the main intermediate product precursors for the formation of dimer compounds (C_{10}). In the same way, MIDE and TCD might be precursors for the formation of trimer compounds (C_{15}).

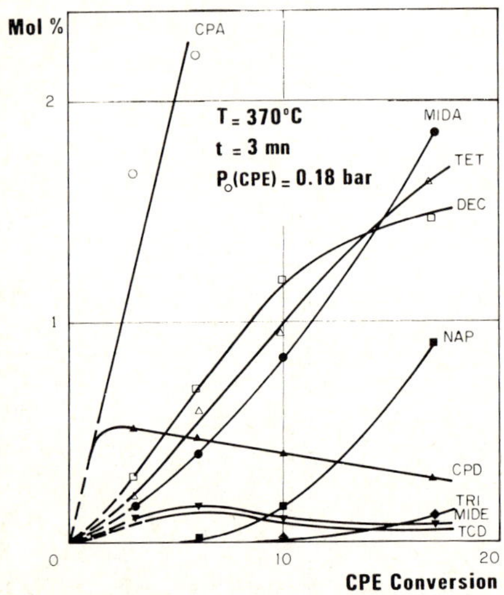

Fig. 3. Yields of products versus CPE conversion (t = 3 mn).

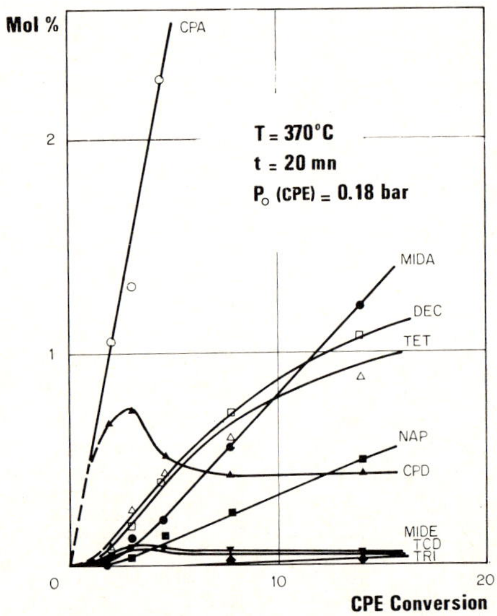

Fig. 4. Yields of products versus CPE conversion (t = 20 mn).

- Formation of DEC and TET slowed down beyond about 10 % conversion. If, on one hand, the naphteno-aromatic behaviour can be explained by its transformation into NAP via hydrogen transfer reactions, on the other hand the DEC behaviour is not easy to interpret.
- At conversion lower than 2 %, the apparent rate of CPA formation was very close to that of CPD ; this was especially obvious at t = 20 mn. So, the stoechiometry of the following hydrogen transfer reaction 2 CPE $\rightleftarrows$ CPA + CPD was met at low conversion.

From CHE (Fig. 5), the following main points were evidenced :

- MCPE, MCPA, CHA, MCPD, BZ and C_{12} dimer products appeared as primary products.
- Whatever the time on stream, the C_7-C_{11} cut and C_5^- products appeared as secondary products. The molar yields of C_1 and C_2 in the C_5^- cut were not equivalent to those of C_5 and C_4 respectively, indicating that a part of the light products were probably formed through cracking of some dimer compounds.

- MCPD yield was always less than 0.5 %. Whatever the time on stream, it reached a maximum value between 25 and 50 % CHE conversion and decreased at higher conversion.
- The hydrogen transfer reactions and dimer product formation accelerated beyond 40-50 % CHE conversion. This result, the particular evolution of MCPD, and the presence of traces of DMCPD clearly indicate that at least a part of C_{12} dimers occur through dimerization reactions involving MCPD.

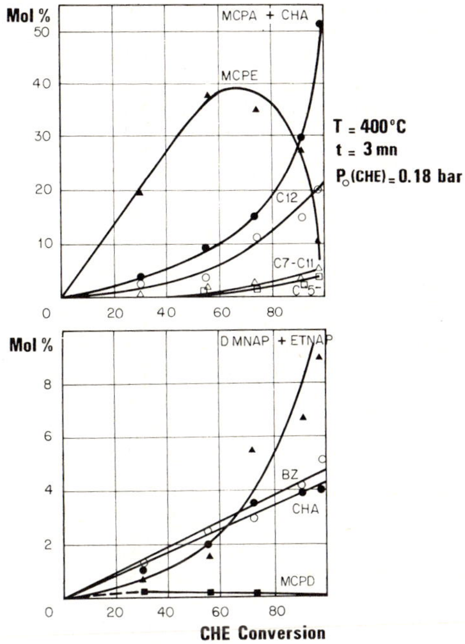

Fig. 5. Yields of products versus CHE conversion (t = 3 mn).

- CHA yields were always close to those of BZ and thus were quite different from the stoechiometry 2 of the CHE disproportionnation reaction (3 CHE $\rightleftarrows$ BZ + 2 CHA). This can be explained by the existence of other types of hydrogen transfer reaction such as :

$$CHE + 2\ MCPE \rightleftarrows BZ + 2\ MCPA$$

- At low and medium conversion (< 40-50 %), the isomerization of CHE into MCPE was about 6-8 times faster than hydrogen transfer (CHA + MCPA formation).
- As expected, the breakdown of 3, 2 and 1 MCPE in their mixture, corresponded to the thermodynamic equilibrium.

From CPD (Fig. 6), the following main conclusions can be drawn :

- Only three hydrocarbons appeared as primary products : CPE, MIDA and MIDE. All the other molecules were secondary products, their order of appearance being as follows : TET, NAP, DEC, CPA and trimers.
- Dimer products probably mainly formed from DCPD intermediates were quickly stabilized into aromatic molecules such as MIDA and then as MIDE through hydrogen transfer with CPD, leading to the formation of CPE.
- The formation rates of MIDA and above all of MIDE decreased when the conversion of CPD increased. A maximum MIDE yield was observed around 10 % conversion which corresponds to the beginning of the trimer formation. This confirms our previous observation in the case of CPE and strongly suggests that bicyclic aromatic molecules, especially indenes or alkylindenes, are probably strongly reactive intermediate molecules for coke formation.

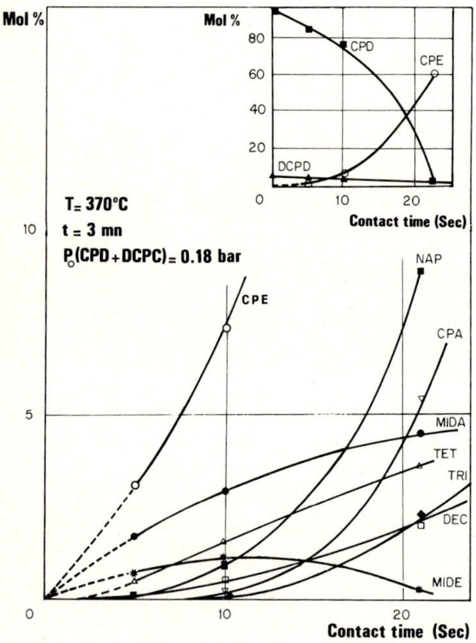

Fig. 6. Yields of products versus contact time from CPD.

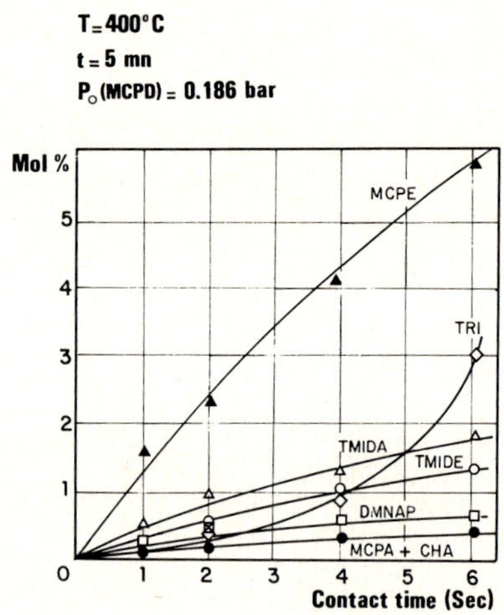

Fig. 7. Yields of products versus contact time from MCPD.

From MCPD (Fig. 7), the results were only slightly different from those obtained from CPD :

- The evolution of MCPD and DMDCPD was quite similar to that of CPD and DCPD.

- All identified products, except trimers, appeared as primary products.
- The formation rate of TMIDA, TMIDE and DMNAP decreased when the conversion of MCPD increased. So, unlike NAP, DMNAP seem to be reactive intermediate products for coke precursor formation.

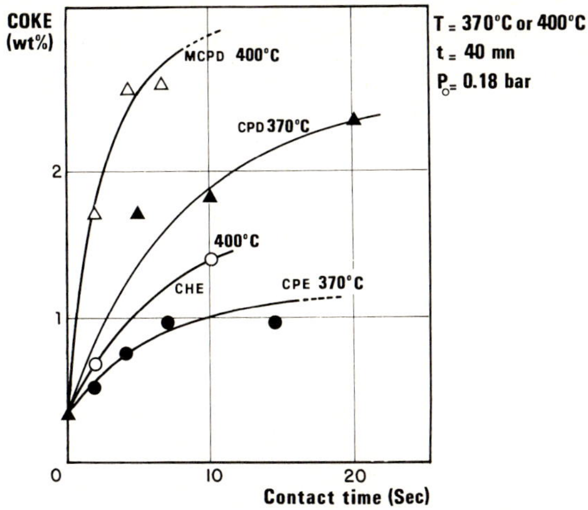

Fig. 8. Coke contents of the used catalysts from various reactants.

From TET, the following main points were evidenced :

- Isomerization of TET into MIDA (1 and 2) and hydrogen transfer producing NAP and DEC clearly appeared as primary reactions. The cycle opening of TET producing ABZ was a slow primary reaction. Dealkylation producing C_4^- light products appeared as a secondary reaction.
- At very low conversion, the DEC yield was much lower than the NAP yield (by about a factor of 3) : only 8 % of DEC was produced at 80 % conversion. The difficulty in forming DEC from TET is probably due to the resonance energy of the benzenic cycle.

DISCUSSION

Taking into account the above results, we can attempt to propose a network of reactions leading to the formation of coke precursors from the simple molecules used in the present study.

First of all, it seems clear from figures 3 to 5 that the main molecules responsible for coke precursor formation are compounds with a cyclopentadienic cycle. When the partial pressure of such compounds is high, which is the case when starting from CPE and CHE but not from 1 HE, the coke precursor formation is fast.

In the particular case of 1 HE, although noticeable formation of MCPA and CHA is evidenced, no cyclo olefins (CHE or CPE), no MCPD and therefore no heavy products with 12 carbon atoms or more were detected. The formation of BZ and ABZ which was observed, is probably the result of a dimerization reaction such as for instance the following Diels-Alder cycloaddition :

hexadiene + hexene ——> alkylcyclohexenes

These alkycyclohexenes should isomerize quickly to alkycyclopentenes and then transform, via hydrogen transfer, into alkylcyclopentadienes which should lead to heavy product formation. These heavy products are not clearly evidenced probably because they do not desorb easily from the catalysts.

As shown by our results (Fig. 3 to 5), from CPE or CHE, noticeable quantities of CPD or MCPD are present in the reaction medium (about 0.5-0.6 % for CPE and 0.2-0.3 % for CHE). As a result, the coke precursor formation is much greater from these cyclo-olefins than from 1 HE. This formation is slightly higher in the case of CPE, where a small quantity of trimers is detected, than in the case of CHE where only dimers are formed. When starting from CPD or MCPD, dimer, trimer and coke formations are much faster (Fig. 6, 7 and 8). Hereafter we will discuss the coke precursor formation from cyclo-olefins only.

1. Network of reactions

Taking into account the ready formation of DCPD or DMDCPD from CPD or MCPD (initial cyclodiolefins already contain about 8 to 10 % of the corresponding dicyclodiolefin at room temperature), these dimers are probably some of the most important intermediate molecules in the coke formation process. DCPD or DMDCPD probably further rearrange themselves through a sequence of reactions including hydrogen transfers, into various more or less saturated compounds such as DEC, TET, NAP, MIDE and MIDA. Some of these dimers, such as DCPD or MIDE (DMDCPD or TMIDE) can also react with CPE or CPD (MCPE or MCPD) to produce trimers, and so on.

The general network of reactions presented in Figure 9 is in agreement with results obtained from CPD and MCPD (Fig. 6 and 7), which show that MIDE, MIDA, TMIDE, TMIDA and DMNAP occur as primary products. These molecules and especially CPD, MCPD and some MIDE are probably key molecules for the coke precursor formation. This is suggested by Figure 6 which shows that, beyond 8-9 % conversion, the MIDE yield decreases when the trimer formation accelerates. But some MIDE and similar molecules are likely to give rise to other reactions such as isomerization and hydrogen transfer.

Polyaromatics like NAP, dimethylfluorenes and methylanthracenes (trimers) are obtained from CPE through successive hydrogen transfer reactions on the key molecules which are formed by cycloadditions and comprise 2 or 3 adjacent cycles. In turn, they may also play a role as coke precursor. However, Figures 6 and 7 show that NAP is rather unreactive compared with DMNAP. It is known that, unlike anthracene, polyaromatics with less than three linear benzene rings do not give rise to Diels-Alder cycloadditions with dienophiles, except at high pressure (11, 12). The reactivity of alkylnaphtalenes (DMNAP or ethylnaphtalenes) is not easy to explain : carbenium ions located on the alkyl groups of alkylaromatics might be formed and give rise to alkylation reactions followed by cyclization reactions. Finally, as suggested by figures 3 and 4, the dimerization and trimerization reactions appear to deactivate faster than the one producing the monomers ; as a result, the percentage of CPD increases along with the time on stream.

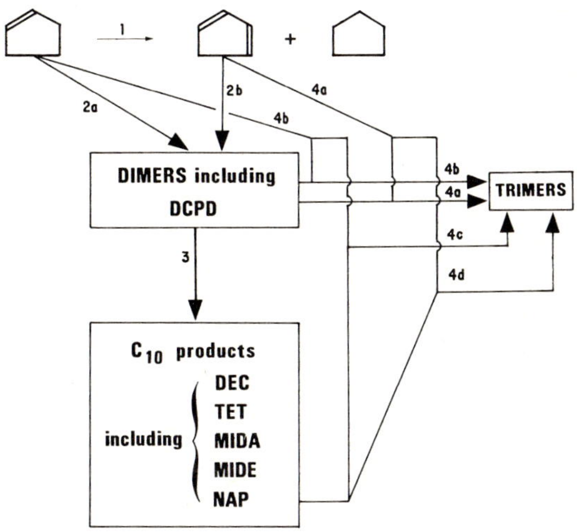

Fig. 9. General network of reactions leading to coke precursors.
(1) : hydrogen transfer
(2a) : dimerizations CPE-CPE
CPE-CPD
(2b) : dimerizations CPD-CPD
(3) : rearrangement of dimer intermediates and hydrogen transfer
(4a), (4b), (4c), (4d) : trimerizations.

2. Mechanism of dimerization

The best known way of forming a 6-carbon cycle, through dimerization of an olefin and a diolefin, is the Diels-Alder cycloaddition (10 to 21). Such a reaction can be promoted by various catalysts including acid catalysts (18, 22, 23), transition metal complexes (18, 24 to 27) and cationic radicals (18, 28, 29, 30).

The Diels-Alder cycloaddition of CPE and CPD on Bronsted acid catalyst probably comprises the following main steps : 1)protonation of CPD, 2)first C-C bond formation between CPE and CPD carbocation, 3)second C-C bond formation between both cycles,

4)Scission of the methano-bridge : taking into account the strain in the 6-member ring due to this bridge, which is similar to the strain in Norbornane or Norbornene (16), the bridge opening by B-scission is thermodynamically favored and should be fast at high temperature on a catalyst with high acidity. The resulting methyl group is linked to the 6-member ring. The final product, methyldihydroindane, can be easily and quickly stabilized into MIDA and MIDE through successive hydrogen transfer reactions. It must be pointed out that, at low conversion, the methyl group of MIDA and MIDE should be on the aromatic cycle if we accept the following likely assumption : the direct stabilization of the hexadienic cycle by aromatization is much faster than the succession of carbocation rearrangements which are necessary to transfer the methyl group from the 6-member ring to the 5-member ring. This assumption is supported by several results. According to Thomas et al. (31), the isomerization of decaline at 400°C on silica-alumina would give rise to only the dimethyl bicyclo (0, 3, 3) octane and the methyl bicyclo (0, 3, 4) nonane with the methyl groups on the 5-member ring only. Our own results on the transformation of tetraline at 400°C on REY show that the only products of isomerization are methylindanes with the methyl group on the 5-carbon cycle (methyl 1 or 2 indanes). So, according to our previous assumption, only MIDA and MIDE isomers with the methyl group on the aromatic cycle should occur as primary products.

Now, when starting from CPE, we have observed that about 50 % of the methyl groups of MIDA are on the aromatic cycle and 50 % in the 5-member ring, and that all these isomers appear as primary products. If the previous assumption is true, our results suggest that another reaction, different from the classical Diels-Alder cycloaddition, takes place from the same intermediates (CPE, CPD, MCPE, MCPD) to produce coke precursors. Such a reaction should enable the direct formation of MIDA and MIDE isomers with the methyl group on the 5-member ring.

A particular reaction proposed by Pines (32) and Criegge et al. (33) to explain the trans-octaline formation from CPE in presence of orthophosphoric acid, could be envisaged. It would imply here a spiro (4, 5) decene intermediate. Compounds such as spiroalkane, spiroalkene or spiroalkadiene species are well known (11, 17, 19, 20, 34). For instance, spiro (4, 5) decane is easily dehydrogenated into naphtalene on platinum deposited on alumina (9). Such spiro compounds would appear as intermediate polymerized species at low temperature in presence of acid catalysts (35) or in the isomerization of octohydroanthracene into octahydrophenanthrene (32, 36). The dimerization of cyclopentene via a spiro (4, 5) decene would produce octahydronaphtalene (octaline). Octaline can then undergo mainly two kinds of reaction : hydrogen transfers and isomerization of one of the 6-member rings into a 5-member ring. A succession of hydrogen transfers would lead to DEC, TET and NAP. A combination of isomerization and hydrogen transfers would produce MIDA and MIDE with the methyl group in the 5-member rings.

Starting from CPE, both the above mentionned mechanisms (Diels-Alder cycloaddition and the spiro (4, 5) decene route) could explain the particular distribution of MIDA and MIDE isomers, characterized by 50 % of the methyl groups on the aromatic cycle and 50 % on the 5-member ring (Fig. 10). But starting from CPD (which already contains some DCPD), Diels-Alder cycloaddition is probably much more likely than the other route, thereby leading to MIDA isomers with about 85 % of the methyl groups on the aromatic cycle (Fig. 10).

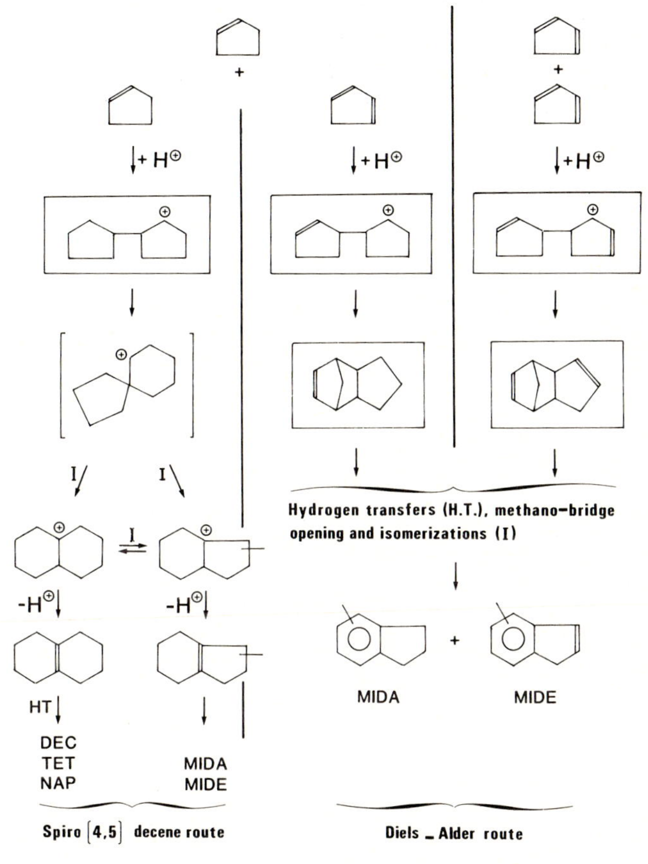

Fig. 10. The two routes for cyclodimerization from CPE.
- the Diels-Alder route.
- the spiro (4, 5) decene route.

The existence of two cycloaddition routes also enables us to explain why NAP and DMNAP respectively appear as a secondary product from CPD and as a primary product from MCPD (Fig. 6 and 7). In the first case, the only route which directly produces NAP is the minor spiro compound route (about 15 %). In the second case, DMNAP can be formed directly by both routes.

So, to summarize, the network of reactions leading to coke precursors from CPE and CPD (or CHE and MCPD) probably comprises the two different routes shown in Figure 10. In the case of interaction between 2 CPE molecules, the spiro (4, 5) decene route might be the only route. In the case of the interactions CPE-CPD or CPD-CPD, the Diels-Alder route should be more probable, but a minor spirodecene or spirodecadiene route cannot be ruled out.

CONCLUSION

Our results emphasize the important role played by cycloolefins and cyclodiolefins in coke formation. Cyclodiolefins such as cyclopentadiene or alkylcyclopentadienes and aromatic molecules such as indene or alkylindenes are among the most reactive ones.

Coke formation requires a sequence of several reactions including hydrogen transfer and cyclodimerization which are essential. The former would supply the catalyst with intermediate reactive molecules and cyclodimerization of two of these intermediate molecules would produce heavier products, thus gradually increasing the molecular weight of the coke precursors.

Our work clearly confirms the vital importance of hydrogen transfer reaction in coke formation and gives further details on coke precursor formation. Two different routes for cyclodimerization have been proposed. Cyclodimerization of cycloolefins would take place via a spiroalkene intermediate. Cyclodimerization of cyclodiolefins with either cycloolefins or other cyclodiolesins could follow both the classical Diels-Alder cyclodimerization which is probably the faster one, and the spiro compound route.

Outstanding progress has been made in the last few years with the appearance of industrial cracking catalysts specially designed to minimize hydrogen transfer and coke formation (37). Such catalysts both lead to less conversion of olefins produced by cracking and produce fewer saturated compounds, especially paraffins, thus leading to a gasoline with higher octane. A better understanding of the network of reactions, of their kinetics, and of the catalysts parameters which govern hydrogen transfer and cyclodimerization, should lead to still more progress in the future.

GLOSSARY

HE	Hexene	MIDE	Methylindene
HA	Hexane	MIDA	Methylindane
IHE	Isohexenes	DCPD	Dicyclopentadiene
IHA	Isohexane	TCD	Tricyclodecane
CPE	Cyclopentene	NAP	Naphtalene
CPA	Cyclopentane	TET	Tetraline
CPD	Cyclopentadiene	DEC	Decaline
CHE	Cyclohexene	TMIDE	Alkylindenes
CHA	Cyclohexane	TMIDA	Alkylindanes
MCPE	Methylcyclopentene	DMDCPD	Dimethyldicyclopentadienes
MCPA	Methylcyclopentane	DMNAP	Alkylnaphtalenes
BZ	Benzene	TRI	Trimers
ABZ	Alkylbenzenes		

REFERENCES

1. E. Wolf, F. Alfani, Cat. Rev. Sci. Eng. 24 (3), 1982, 329.
2. W.O. Haag, R.M. Dessau, 8th Int. Congr. Cat., Vol. II, 1984, 305-316.
3. W.G. Appleby, J.W. Gibson, G.M. Good, I.E.C., P.D.D. 1 (2) 1962, 102.
4. F. Hernandez, L. Moudafi, F. Fajula, F. Figueras, 8th Int. Congr. Cat., Vol. II, 1984, A, 447-457.
5. A. Corma, J.B. Monton, A.V. Orchilles, Appl. Cat., 16 (1), 1985, 59-74.
6. J.M. Parera, N.S. Figoli, J.N. Beltramini, E.J. Churin, R.A. Cabrol, 8th Int. Congr. Cat., Vol. II (1983), p. 593-601.
7. J. Barbier, M. Guisnet, Bull. Soc. Chim. Fr. 9-10 (1984), I 245.
8. B.S. Greensfelder, H.H. Voge, I.E.C., 37 (6), 1945, 514-520, 37 (10), 1945, 983-988, 37 (11), 1945, 1038-1043.
9. H. Ajot, B. Mercier des Rochettes, C. Marcilly, J. Bousquet, French pat. 8.211.891 (1982).
10. E.S. Gould, Mechanism and Structure in Org. Chem., Holt, Rinehart, Winston, 1959.
11. J. March, Adv. Org. Chem., Mc Graw Hill, 2nd Edn., 1977.
12. A.S. Onishchenko, Dienes Synthesis, Acad. of Sci. of the USSR, Israël Progr. for Sci. transl. 1964.
13. A.I. Konovalov, Russ. Chem. Rev., 52 (11), 1983, 1064-1080.
14. J.K. Holmes, Org. React., 4, 1948, 60-173.
15. Allen, Chem. Rev., 62, 1962, 653-664.
16. G. Malcolm Dyson, A Manual of Org. Chem., Vol. 1, Longmans, Green and Co. 1st Edn 1950.
17. W.J. Le Noble, Highlights of Org. Chem., M. Dekker Inc., 1974.
18. P. Laszlo, J. Lucchetti, L'actualité chimique Soc. Fr. Chim., Oct. 1984, 42-44.
19. G.W. Wheland, Adv. Org. Chem., J. Wiley and Sons Inc., 2nd Edn., 1949.
20. P. Karrer, Org. Chem., Elsevier Publ., 3d Edn., 1947.
21. D.J. Cram, G.S. Hammond, Org. Chem., Mc Graw-Hill Book Co Inc., 2nd Edn., 1964.
22. A. Wasserman, C.F. Blakely, J. Chem. Soc. 1961, 1946.
23. C. Kemball, J.J. Rooney, Proc. Roy. Soc., A 257, 1960, 132.
24. R.L. Funk, K.P.C. Vollhardt, J. Am. Chem. Soc., 102, 1980, 524.
25. H.T. Dieck, R. Diercks, Angew. Chem. Int. Ed. Engl., 22, 1983, 778.
26. M. Bednarski, S. Danishefsky, J. Am. Chem. Soc. 105, 1983, 3716.
27. S. Danishefsky, M. Bednarski, Tetrah. Lett., 25, 1984, 721.
28. D.J. Bellville, D.D. Wirth, N.L. Bauld, J. Am. Chem. Soc., 103, 1981, 718.
29. P. Laszlo, J. Lucchetti, Tetrah. Lett., 25, 1984, 1567.
30. R.A. Pabon, D.J. Bellville, N.L. Bauld, J. Am. Chem. Soc., 105, 1983, 5158.
31. C.L. Thomas, J. Am. Chem. Soc., 66, 1944, 1586.
32. H. Pines, the Chemistry of Catalytic Hydrocarbon Conversion, Acad. Press, N.Y., 1981.
33. R. Criegge, A. Riebel, Angew. Chem., 65, 1953, 136.
34. C.A. Buehler, D.E. Pearson, Survey of Org. Synth., Vol. 2, John Wiley and Sons, 1977.
35. V.N. Ipatieff, H. Pines, R.C. Olberg, J. Am. Chem. Soc., 70, 1948, 2123.
36. R.D. Buschick, J. Org. Chem., 33, 1968, 4085.
37. L.A. Pine, P.K. Maher, W.A. Wachter, J. Catal., 85 (1984), 466-476 and Ketjen Catal. Symp. 84, 19-28.

B. Delmon and G.F. Froment (Editors), *Catalyst Deactivation 1987* 605

DEACTIVATION AND STABILIZATION OF LATE TRANSITION METAL ZEOLITE CATALYSTS FOR ACETYLENE HYDRATION

D. KALLO and GY. ONYESTYAK

Central Research Institute for Chemistry of Hungarian Academy of Sciences, P.O.Box 17, 1525 Budapest (Hungary)

ABSTRACT

Hydration of acetylene to acetaldehyde proceeds with appropriate rates on Cu-, Ag-, Cd-, Zn-, Hg-forms of zeolites below 200 °C at atmospheric pressure. Stabilities and selectivities were studied for two sets of catalysts: for Cd-forms of A-, X-, Y-zeolites, mordenite, clinoptilolite, and for Cu-, Ag-, Cd-, Zn-, Hg-, Pb-clinoptilolites. A-, X-, Y-, MOR zeolites deactivate because crotonic condensation followed by the formation of carbonaceous deposits and unsaturated gaseous compounds takes place. Cu^{2+}, Ag^{+}, Hg^{2+} are reduced and the supported metals formed are inactive. The other forms of clinoptilolite are catalysts of high stability and selectivity. Activity increases in the order of Pb-<Zn-<Cd-clinoptilolite.

INTRODUCTION

Acetylene hydration can be catalyzed by transition metal ions especially by Cu^{2+}, Ag^{+}, Zn^{2+}, Cd^{2+}, Hg^{2+} which may be either in aqueous solutions or in solids in forms of oxides, phosphates, molybdates, and tungstates (refs. 1-7). In spite of the large variety of the catalytic systems investigated none of them proved to be sufficiently stable and selective. Catalyst deactivation occurs because of structural changes, formation of deposits from acetylene and/or from the product acetaldehyde. The selectivity decrease due to the formation of by-products such as unsaturated hydrocarbons, aldol condensation products, acetone etc., could not have been avoided (refs. 1, 4).

When the above late transition metal ions are introduced in zeolite X, catalysts of high activity but of rather low stability are obtained (ref. 8). By using milder reaction conditions i.e. by decreasing the reaction temperature below 200 °C and by feeding excess water the deactivation can be slowed down appreciably, and a selectivity over 99 percent can be achieved (ref. 9). The preadsorption of ammonia improves stability as it has been reported for the Cd-X (ref. 10). Nevertheless, the stability attained in this way does not satisfy the practical requirements.

The present paper deals with the investigation of zeolite catalysts of different crystal structure in different forms in order to clear up the nature of deactivation and to explore what are the criteria a stable catalyst having high selectivity has to meet.

EXPERIMENTAL

Materials

The following zeolites were used: 5-A (Serva, Heidelberg, FRG), Na-X (Strem Chemicals, USA), Na-Y (Bitterfeld, GDR), natural clinoptilolite (CLI,N) and mordenite (MOR,N) (in concentrations of 55 % and 30 %, resp., in sedimentary rocks, Tokaj Hills, Hungary). Samples were ion-exchanged three-times, each time for 8 hours, at 70 °C (in the case of silver at 25 °C) with 0.1 M solutions of the corresponding nitrate. The compositions are given in Table 1.

TABLE 1

Amount of transition metal ions in catalyst samples

Zeolite	Cd-A	Cd-X	Cd-Y	Cd-MOR	Cd-CLI	Cu-CLI	Ag-CLI	Zn-CLI	Hg-CLI	Pb-CLI
M-cont.										
mass %	21.8	21.9	12.4	2.1	4.1	1.65	4.5	1.44	1.02	7.1
meq/g	3.9	3.9	2.2	0.37	0.72	0.52	0.41	0.44	0.10	0.68
ion-ex.										
%	60	60	55	52	50	37	29	31	7	49

Acetylene was a high purity Dissous gas (ODV, Hungary). Before use acetone was removed in a trap at - 78 °C. Ammonia was reagent grade Matheson product.

Methods

Experiments were carried out in an atmospheric flow reactor containing 10 g of catalyst. For each catalyst conversions were determined under identical conditions: reaction temperature 180 °C, partial pressure of water 67 kPa, that of acetylene 33 kPa, feed rate of acetylene 50 cm^3/min. Products were analysed by GC, and material balances were established.

I.r. spectra were recorded by a Perkin Elmer Model 577 spectrometer. Metal dispersions in zeolites were determined by a Zeiss electron micriscope Model EF4.

RESULTS AND DISCUSSION

Hydrogen-, alkali-, alkaline earth-, early transition metal-forms of zeolites are inactive for acetylene hydration, whereas the late transition metal-forms are of high activity i.e. the reaction rates are in 10^{-7} mole g_{cat}^{-1} s^{-1} order of magnitude at 120-180 °C. This indicates that this type of cations are resposible for the catalytic activity.

The conversions on the most active Cd-forms of different zeolites and on different transition metal-forms of clinoptilolite are plotted against the time on flow in Figs. 1 and 2, respectively. It can be seen that the activities decrease with the exceptions of Cd-, Zn- and Pb-clinoptilolites. The selectivity on these catalysts is above 99 percent. Because the catalyst deactivation is always accompanied by side reactions (vide infra), catalysts of high selectivity are also of high stability. It is surprising that small pore Cd-CLI,N is of much higher activity than large pore Cd-faujasites, in spite of the fact that the amount of catalytically active cadmium is larger in the latter than in the former (see Table 1).

Two groups of catalysts deactivating are distinguished: (1) Cd-zeolites having no clinoptilolite structure as Cd-X, -A,-MOR; (2) unstable Ag-, Cu-, Hg-forms of CLI,N. For these two groups of catalysts different phenomena can be observed in the course of deactivation.

(a) In the case of Cd-X right after feeding the temperature increases rapidly and the stable operation of the reactor can hardly be ensured for some ten minutes. Such phenomenon is not observed for Ag-CLI,N, although in this case the conversion of acetylene in the exothermic hydration reaction is higher. Therefore, another fast exothermic reaction must proceed on Cd-X at the beginning of the experiment. The rate of this reaction decreases and after a while the reactor becomes stable. However, a slow deactivation can be observed in this period of catalyst loading, and in spite of the low level of activity sufficient stability is not attained.

(b) I.r. spectra of Cd-X and Cd-CLI,N were recorded (Fig.3.). Self supporting wafers of the samples were pretreated in vacuum at 180 °C (spectra 1). Adsorption of acetylene on the wafers was carried out at room temperature (spectra 2), then i.r. cell was evacuated at 110 °C (spectra 3) and at 200 °C (spectra 4). On

Cd-CLI,N the appearence of a band at 1708 cm^{-1} assigned to the stretching vibration of the -C=O group of adsorbed acetaldehyde indicates that acetylene reacts even at room temperature with the zeolitic water which remained in the zeolite after the pretreatment

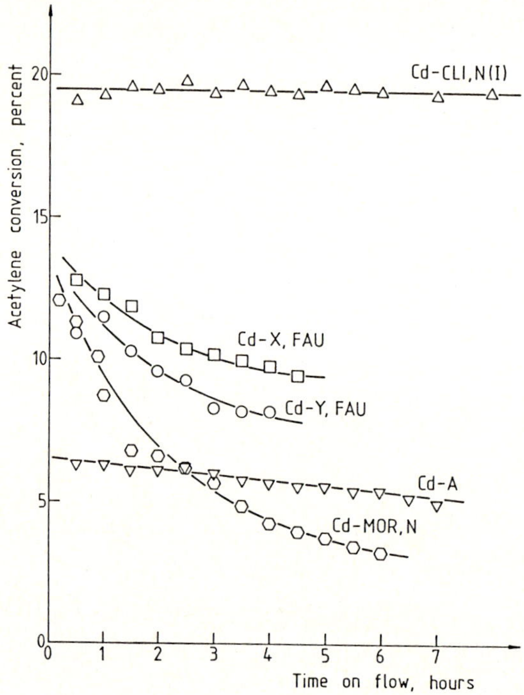

Fig.1. Activity changes of Cd-zeolites versus time on flow.

applied. In vacuum no transformations can be observed up to 200 °C, except that the intensity of the acetaldehyde band decreases to some extent owing to the desorption. Under identical conditions Cd-X behaves differently. After the admission of acetylene at room temperature the characteristic band of adsorbed acetaldehyde at 1690 cm^{-1} appears simultaneously with the -C=O stretching vibration band of crotonic aldehyde at 1635 cm^{-1}. Increasing the temperature the intensity of the 1635 cm^{-1} band increases at the expense of the acetaldehyde band intensity. The lower -C=O frequency of acetaldehyde adsorbed on Cd-X than that adsorbed on Cd-CLI,N reflects a weaker -C=O bond. In the case of Cd-X the band at 1940 cm^{-1} is assigned to adsorbed acetylene bound asymetrically.

(c) On Cd-X carbonaceous deposits with a C/H ratio of 1:0.6 and by-products as methyl acetylene, ethyl acetylene, 1-butene,

2,3-butadiene are formed during the acetylene hydration.

The amount of organic material retained by Cu- and Ag-CLI,N is four times less than in the case of Cd-X. The C/H ratio of the residue is around 2 corresponding to adsorbed acetaldehyde

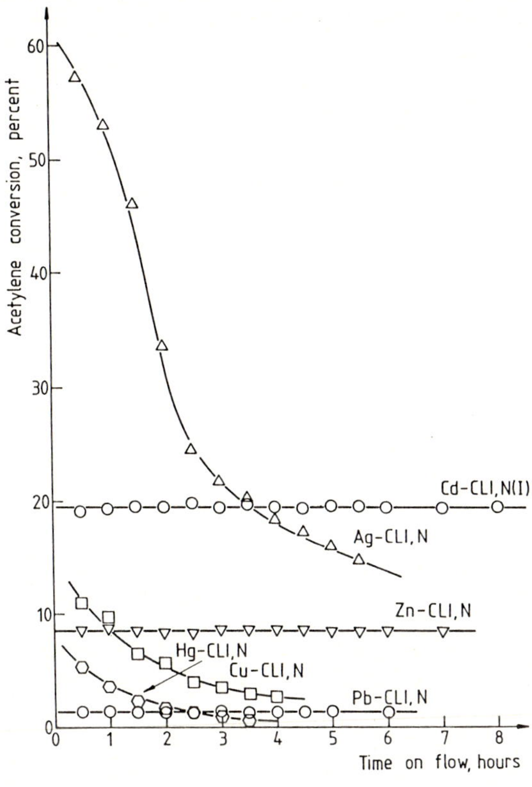

Fig.2. Activity changes of late transition metal-clinoptilolites versus time on flow.

(or acetone). The only by-product is acetone. Its formation slows down parallel with the formation of acetaldehyde. On Cu-CLI,N both products are formed with similar rates, on Ag-CLI,N the formation of acetaldehyde prevails.

These observations suggest that in the case of the first group of catalysts deactivating the very fast formation of acetaldehyde is accompanied by a very exothermic and similarly fast crotonic condensation i.e. a thermal self acceleration takes place. The cronotic condensation is catalyzed by Brønsted acid sites, which are formed by the heterolytic dissociation of

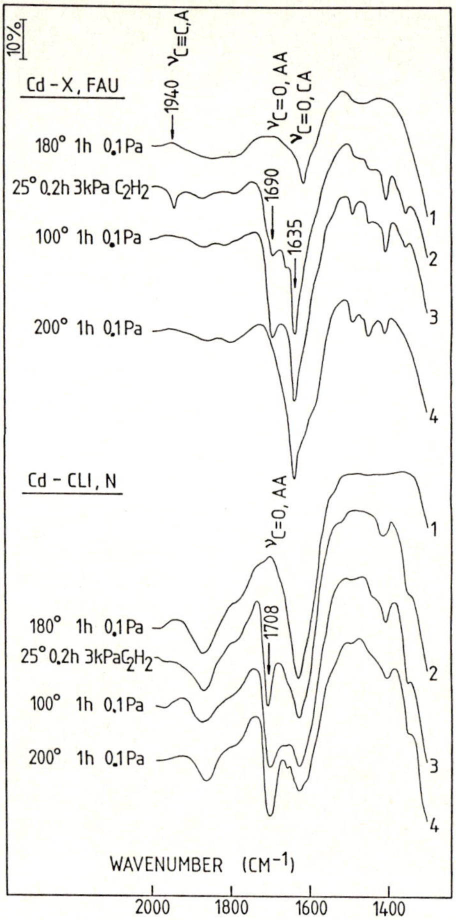

Fig.3. I.r. spectra of acetylene, acetaldehyde, crotonaldehyde adsorbed on Cd-X and Cd-CLI,N.

water in the electrostatic field of Cd^{2+} (ref. 10). In the period of fast deactivation the increase of catalyst temperature is very considerable. It is very probable that higher local overheating occurs resulting in carbonization of the deposits and in the formation of gaseous by-products richer in hydrogen than the reactant acetylene. When most of the active sites are already blocked and a rather low activity level is attained, the deactivation becomes slower.

These undesirable secondary reactions do not proceed on Cd-, Zn- and Pb-CLI,N. Most probably this is the result of the specific nature of the clinoptilolite structure. From this aspect the following features may be of importance: (i) In its pores with diameters of less than 5 Å the condensation of acetaldehyde may be sterically hindered. (ii) In connection with other transformations it was shown that the acidic OH groups generated by bivalent cations are not catalytically active (ref. 11), presumably they are in positions inaccessible for most reactants. (iii) The -C=O bond in acetaldehyde is less weakened i.e. less activated by adsorption on Cd-CLI,N than on Cd-X. Accordingly the interaction of acetaldehyde with Cd-CLI,N is as weak as with Ca-X being totally inactive for aldol condensation (ref. 12).

In the case of Ag-, Cu-, Hg-CLI,N the condensation of acetaldehyde can be disregarded. The residues on the surface correspond to adsorbed acetaldehyde and acetone. The latter is a usual by-product of acetylene hydration (ref. 1). Not the formation of carbonaceous deposits seems to be responsible for deactivation. The formation of carbides is also prohibited under reaction conditions because of thermodynamic reasons. It turns out, however, that the stable Cd-, Zn-, Pb-forms contain cations of metals of large negative standard potentials whereas the standard potentials of metals in deactivating Ag-, Cu-, Hg-forms are large positive values. Therefore, the latter cations can easily be reduced to metals. In the case of Hg-CLI,N mercury drops leave the reactor during the hydration. Since metallic silver and copper are not volatile, they remain on the catalyst. Deactivated samples were exhaustively ion-exchanged for NH_4^+ in order to remove ionic silver or copper. Most of the silver or the copper remained in the catalyst samples indicating high degree of reduction. Metal particles in sizes of a few times ten of nanometers have been detected on the electron micrographs of deactivated Ag- and Cu-CLI,N.

The reason of deactivation of Ag-, Cu-, Hg-clinoptilolites is the reduction of cations to metals, which are inactive for acetylene transformations even in high dispersity as they are formed on the zeolite support.

Cd-, Zn-, Pb-clinoptilolites are catalysts of high stability and selectivity for hydration of acetylene, since in the structure of clinoptilolite conditions for deposit formation are not favourable, the catalytically active cations accelerating the formation of acetaldehyde exclusively are not reduced.

REFERENCES

1 J.W. Coppenhaver and M.H. Bigelow: Acetylene and Carbon Monoxide Chemistry. Reinhold, New York, 1949.
2 S.A. Miller, Chem. Proc. Eng. 3 (1968) 75.
3 R.M. Fid, Trudy Inst. Khim. Nauk Akad. Nauk. Kazakh. SSR, 5 (1969) 81.
4 J. Marton, Gy. Zollner, Gy. Levai, A. Tatraaljai and Gy. Balint, Kem. Tud. Oszt. Kozl. (Comm. Chem. Dep., Hung. Acad. Sci.), 12 (1959) 441.
5 V.G. Govorov, SU Pat 1 055 737 (1983).
6 Yu.A. Gorin and L.M. Troitskii, Khim. Prom. (1964) 265.
7 D.B. Pisareva and B.M. Komarov, Khim. Prom. Ser. Azotn. Prom. 1979. No. 2, 13; ibid. 1980, No. 6, 14.
8 G. Gut and K. Aufdereggen, Helv. Chim. Acta, 57 (1974) 441.
9 E. Detrekoy, D. Kallo and Gy. Onyestyak, Hung. Pat. 178 931 (1978)
10 E. Detrekoy, Gy. Onyestyak and D. Kallo, React. Kinet. Catal. Lett., 15 (1980) 443.
11 D. Kallo, in.D. Kallo and H.S. Sherry (Editors), Proc. 2nd Int. Conf. on Natural Zeolites, Budapest, Hungary, Aug. 12-16., 1985. Akademiai Kiado, Budapest, 1987. No 48 (in press).
12 E. Detrekoy, D. Kallo, in R. Sersale, C. Colella and R. Aiello (Editors), Recent Progress Reports and Discussion, 5th Intern. Conf. on Zeolites, Naples, Italy, June 2-6, 1980, Giannini, Naples 1981, pp. 176-179.

B. Delmon and G.F. Froment (Editors), *Catalyst Deactivation 1987*

HIGH STEAM STABILITY OF ZSM-5 TYPE ZEOLITES CONTAINING ALKALINE EARTH METALS

T. SANO[1], K. SUZUKI[1], H. OKADO[2], K. FUJISAWA[3], K. KAWAMURA[4], S. IKAI[5], H. HAGIWARA[1] and H. TAKAYA[1]

[1]National Chemical Laboratory for Industry, Yatabe, Ibaraki 305 (Japan)

[2]Maruzen Petrochemical Co. Ltd., Hatchobori, Chuo-ku, Tokyo 104 (Japan)

[3]Nippon Petrochemical Co. Ltd., Uchisaiwai-cho, Chiyoda-ku, Tokyo 100 (Japan)

[4]Idemitsu Petrochemical Co. Ltd., Marunouchi, Chiyoda-ku, Tokyo 100 (Japan)

[5]Ube Industries Co. Ltd., Kasumigaseki, Chiyoda-ku, Tokyo 100 (Japan)

ABSTRACT

In order to examine the dealumination of the framework of H-ZSM-5 type zeolites containing alkaline earth metals, which yields high selectivities to light olefins in methanol conversion at high temperatures, the characteristics of the steamed zeolites were investigated by means of ^{27}Al MASNMR, FT-ir, TPD of NH_3 and methanol conversion. It was found that the dealumination of the framework of the H-ZSM-5 type zeolites is greatly inhibited due to alkaline earth metals occluded and that the rate of the dealumination has a second-order dependence on the amount of the framework aluminiums.

INTRODUCTION

The conversion of methanol to hydrocarbons over acidic catalysts has been extensively investigated. High selectivities to light olefins such as ethylene and propylene are attained at high temperatures over highly siliceous zeolites [1-5]. It is well known that under low reaction temperatures the formation of carbonaceous deposits or coke is mainly responsible for the deactivation of the zeolites used in the conversion of organic substrates. However, when the zeolites are used in a moisture-rich atmosphere such as is encountered in methanol conversion under high reaction temperatures, the deactivation of the zeolites has been considered to be attributed to the structure degradation by dealumination with water as well as the coke deposition. Therefore, in order to extend the catalyst life of the zeolites used in methanol conversion under high reaction temperatures, their resistance to steaming as well as that to coking must be much improved.

Recently, we have found that the H-ZSM-5 type zeolites containing alkaline earth metals, especially calcium, are effective in the production of light olefins from methanol at high temperatures (500-600 °C) and that the catalyst stability of the zeolites is considerably higher than that of a conventional

H-ZSM-5 [6-9]. Subsequently we have studied the dealumination of the framework of the H-ZSM-5 type zeolites containing alkaline earth metals and describe our results in this paper.

EXPERIMENTAL

Catalyst preparation

The H-ZSM-5 type zeolites containing alkaline earth metals (M-H-ZSM-5, M:alkaline earth metals) were synthesized as follows. Certain amounts of aluminium nitrate, colloidal silica, and alkaline earth metal acetate were added to a stirred mixture of tetrapropylammonium bromide and sodium hydroxide in a solution. The resultant hydrogel, with the composition of 0.025 MO • 0.1 R• 0.052 Na_2O • 0.005 Al_2O_3 • SiO_2 • 40 H_2O (R:tetrapropylammonium bromide), was then transferred into a 300 ml stainless steel autoclave and stirred at 150-160 °C under an autogeneous pressure for 15-24 h. After the crystallization of the zeolites, the autoclave was rapidly cooled; the precipitated crystals were then filtered off, washed thoroughly with deionized water, dried at 120 °C, and calcined at 500 °C for 16 h in order to remove the organic base occluded in the zeolite framework. The zeolites thus obtained were protonated in a 0.6 N hydrochloric acid solution and calcined in air at 500 °C for 6 h. Some analytical data of the zeolites are given in Table 1.

TABLE 1

Characteristics of the H-ZSM-5 type zeolites containing alkaline earth metals

Zeolites	Atomic ratios[a]		BET surface areas[b]
	Si/Al	Alkaline earth metal/Al	(m^2 g^{-1})
H-ZSM-5	120		342
Mg-H-ZSM-5	94	0.89	336
Ca-H-ZSM-5	117	1.63	341
Sr-H-ZSM-5	93	1.29	301
Ba-H-ZSM-5	90	1.35	301

[a]Determined by X-ray fluoresence spectrometry.
[b]Measured by using single point N_2 adsorption at -196 °C.

Steaming

Steaming was carried out using an atmospheric pressure flow system at 600 °C in a 100% steam for 2.5 g of the charged zeolite (14-28 mesh pieces). The rate of the addition of water was 3 ml h^{-1}.

^{27}Al Magic angle spinning nuclear magnetic resonance

High resolution ^{27}Al NMR was measured at 51.9 MHz using a JEOL FX-200 Spectometer equipped with a probe for magic angle spinning (MAS). The spectra were obtained for 0.33 g of the various zeolites in Delrin bullets spinning at about 3.5 kHz, using 4.6 μs pulses. The chemical shifts in ppm were obtained with respect to $Al(H_2O)_6^{3+}$ as an external reference.

Fourier transform infrared spectroscopy

The powdered zeolites were placed in thin-walled ampules with a diameter of 8 mm and then evacuated to about 10^{-6} Torr at 500 °C for 2 h. Diffuse reflectance infrared spectra were measured at room temperature using a Digilab FTS-60 Spectrometer equipped with an evacuable, heatable chamber. The spectra were taken at 2 cm^{-1} resolution for 1000 scans.

Temperature-programmed desorption of ammonia

The temparature-programmed desorption (TPD) spectra of NH_3 on the zeolites were obtained using a conventional TPD apparatus. A thermal-conductivity detector was employed for the detection of desorbed NH_3 molecules. The measurement was performed from 100 to 600 °C at a heating rate of 10 °C min^{-1} in helium as a carrier gas (20 ml min^{-1}) for 0.30 g of the charged zeolites.

Methanol conversion

Methanol conversion was carried out at 600 °C and LHSV=4 h^{-1} in an atmospheric pressure flow system. Each zeolite of 14-28 mesh pieces was packed into a quartz tube reactor of a 10 mm inner diameter. The zeolite charged was 1 ml and was retained by quartz wool at almost a center of the reactor. Methanol and argon as a carrier gas were fed in 50/50 mol%. The flow rate of the carrier gas was 40 ml min^{-1}. The products obtained were automatically analyzed utilizing a TCD and FID type auto gas chromatograph (Yanaco AG-1000TFH) with columns of Porpack T, Porpack Q, MS-13X, OV-17, PEG-20M and Squalane. In the calculation of the methanol conversions and carbon-based selectivities the concentration of argon was used as an internal standard.

RESULTS AND DISCUSSION

The prepared H-ZSM-5 type zeolites containing alkaline earth metals (M-H-ZSM-5) had a well-defined H-ZSM-5 zeolite structure, as demonstrated by their X-ray powder diffraction pattern and scanning electron micrograph. As shown in Table 1, the amounts of alkaline earth metals occluded in the zeolites were more than those of the alkaline earth metals which would be introduced by a conventional ion-exchange method. Recently, several investigators have reported that under basic conditions the highly siliceous ZSM-5 zeolites exhibit intracrystalline cation exchange capacity of more than a framework tetrahedral aluminium content [10-12]. It has been considered that the occluded silicate ions, trapped OH^-, or SiO^- groups are responsible for the cation exchange regardless of an aluminium content. Therefore, the presence of alkaline earth metals in M-H-ZSM-5 in more than an equivalent mole of aluminium can be explained in a similar reason described above.

Figure 1 shows the diffuse reflectance FT-ir spectra of hydroxyl groups of the various zeolites. The spectrum of H-ZSM-5 was characterized by two well-defined peaks at 3605 and 3730-3740 cm^{-1}. The low-frequency hydroxyl has been assigned to an acidic bridged OH of Si(OH)Al, while the high frequency hydroxyl to terminal SiOH or extraframework silica gel. The broad peak at near 3500 cm^{-1} is attributable to hydrogen bonding adjacent hydroxyl groups [13,14]. On the other hand, except for Mg-H-ZSM-5, the intensities of the peaks at 3730-3740 and near 3500 cm^{-1} as well as the peak at 3605 cm^{-1} for M-H-ZSM-5 were very weak. It may be considered that the drastic decrease in the intensity of the peak at 3605 cm^{-1} is due to the decrease in the amount of Si(OH)Al by the introduction of alkaline earth metals. The comparatively weak intensities of the peaks at 3730-3740 and near 3500 cm^{-1} may also be responsible for the modification with alkaline earth metals, the Al independent cation exchange as described before, although this can not be interpreted in detail at the present stage.

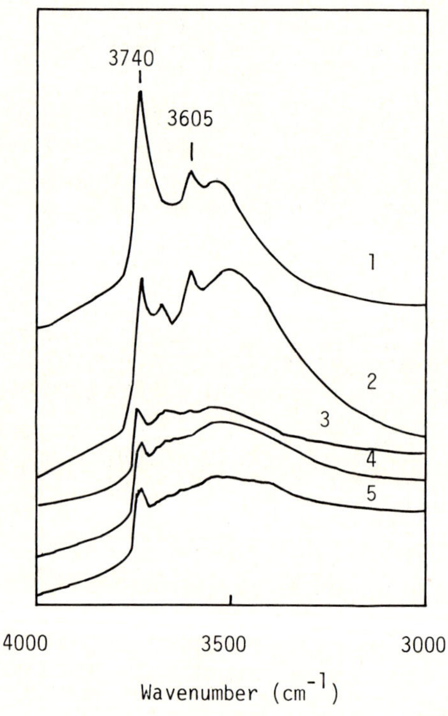

Fig. 1 Diffuse reflectance FT-ir spectra of various zeolites
(1)H-ZSM-5, (2)Mg-H-ZSM-5, (3)Ca-H-ZSM-5, (4)Sr-H-ZSM-5, (5)Ba-H-ZSM-5.

In order to examine the dealumination of the framework of M-H-ZSM-5, they were steamed at 600 °C and characterized by means of ^{27}Al MASNMR, FT-ir, TPD of NH_3 and methanol conversion. The amounts of the framework (tetrahedrally coordinated) aluminiums in the steamed zeolites were determined from the spectra of ^{27}Al MASNMR. As has already been reported, the ^{27}Al MASNMR spectrum of the conventional H-ZSM-5 has one peak at about 53 ppm assigned to the framework aluminiums [15]. The ^{27}Al MASNMR spectra of various M-H-ZSM-5 have one peak at about 53 ppm similarly to H-ZSM-5. Figure 2 shows the relationship between the time of steaming and the intensity ratio (x100) of the 53 ppm peaks (the steamed zeolites to the corresponding unsteamed zeolites). The rapid decay curve was obtained for H-ZSM-5, whereas the slow decay curve for Ca-H-ZSM-5. The order of the intensity ratios of M-H-ZSM-5 at the steaming time of 7 days is Ba-H-ZSM-5 > Sr-H-ZSM-5 > Ca-H-ZSM-5 > Mg-H-ZSM-5 > H-ZSM-5, indicating a great stability of Ba-, Sr- and Ca-H-ZSM-5 for steaming. From these results, it was found that the release of tetrahedrally coordinated aluminiums from the framework of the zeolites is depressed by the presence of alkaline earth metals to a different degree.

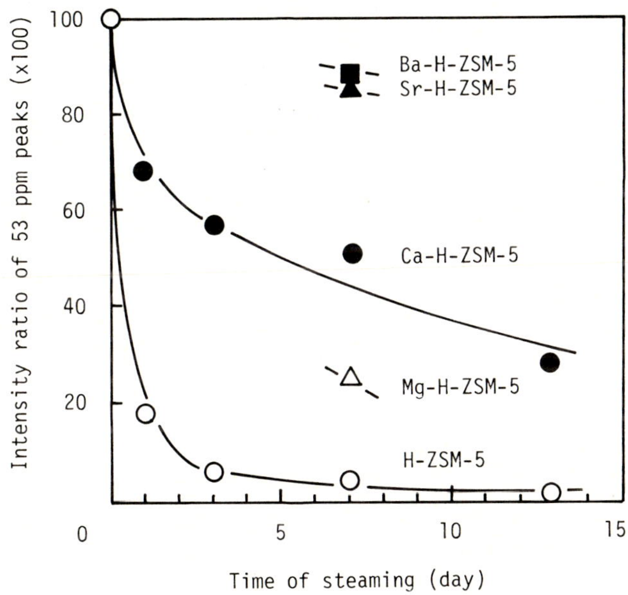

Fig. 2 Relationship between the time of steaming and the intensity ratio of 53ppm peak.

Figure 3 shows the diffuse reflectance FT-ir spectra of hydroxyl groups of the steamed zeolites. In the case of H-ZSM-5, the intensity of the peak at 3605 cm^{-1} assigned to Si(OH)Al from a framework silicon and aluminium markedly decreased with the increase in the steaming time. On the other hand, in the case of Ca-H-ZSM-5, the intensity of the peak at 3605 cm^{-1} decreased in a similar manner, while the intensity of the peak at 3660 cm^{-1} hardly changed even after the steaming for 13 days. From the facts that the intensity of the peak at 3660 cm^{-1} increases with the amounts of both calcium and aluminium, and that the peak disappeares after pyridine adsorption, we have considered that the hydroxyl groups assigned to the peak at 3660 cm^{-1} are new weak acidic sites formed by Si(OH)Al with calcium [8,9]. Therefore, it may be concluded that the steam stability of the framework aluminiums modified with calcium is considerably higher than that of the conventional framework aluminiums.

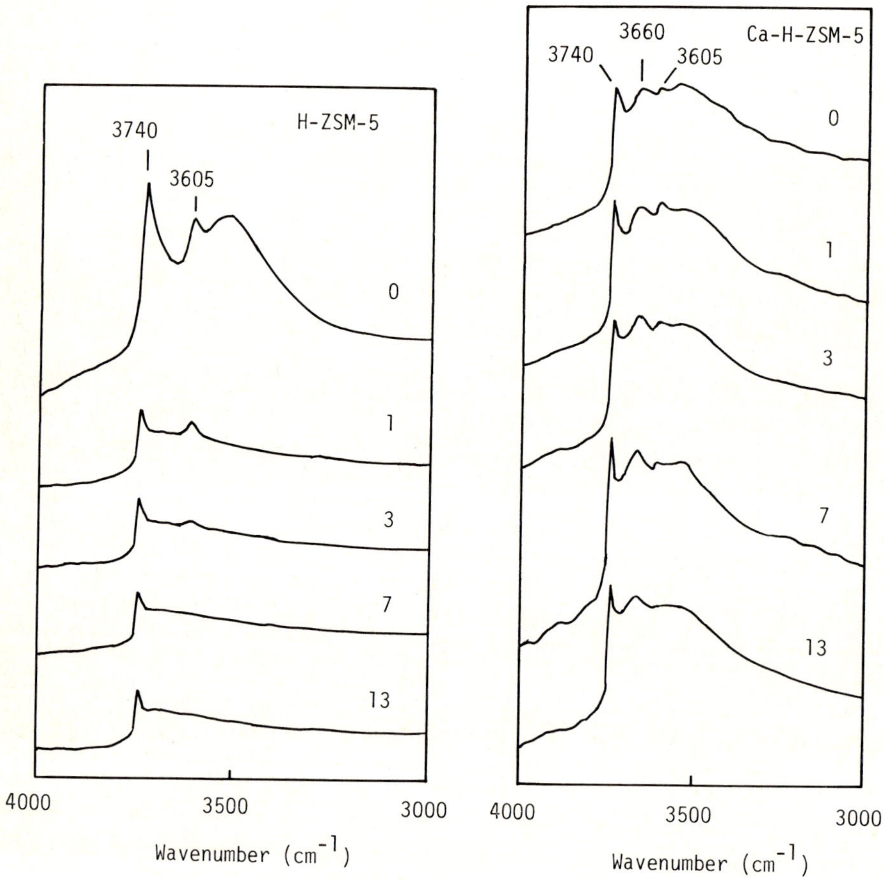

Fig. 3 Diffuse reflectance FT-ir spectra of various steamed zeolites
Arabic numbers in Fig. denote the steaming time (day).

An increase in the intensities of the peaks at 3730-3740 and near 3500 cm^{-1} is presumed by dealumination with water, as it is considered that maximum four

SiOH are created by the removal of one aluminium atom. Nevertheless, the intensities of the peaks at 3730-3740 and near 3500 cm^{-1} for H-ZSM-5 decreased with the steaming time, while those for Ca-H-ZSM-5 hardly changed. These results were very puzzling phenomenons. Although the exact interpretation for this phenomenom could not be given at the present stage, we consider as follows. The decrease in the peak intensities is possibly corresponding to that in the amount of SiOH by a transformation of SiOH to Si-O-Si species (2SiOH $\longrightarrow$ Si-O-Si + H_2O). It is easily assumed that the transformation hardly occurs when the SiOH groups are isolated from each other. From the fact that the peak intensities for both H-ZSM-5 and Ca-H-ZSM-5 remained unchanged even after evacuation at 500 °C for 1 day, the SiOH groups present in the zeolites before steaming seem to be located in some distance. As a matter of fact, the steaming enhanced the transformation in the case of H-ZSM-5. Therefore, we propose the following mechanism of the transformation under the steaming, in which the hydration of Si-O-Si to give SiOH and the dehydration of SiOH to Si-O-Si are repeated. No decrease of FT-ir intensities for Ca-H-ZSM-5 indicates that the transformation hardly proceed on the zeolite, whose acid strength is weaker than that of H-ZSM-5. The transformation could be greatly promoted by a strong acid which catalyzes the cleavage of Si-O-Si bond by hydration.

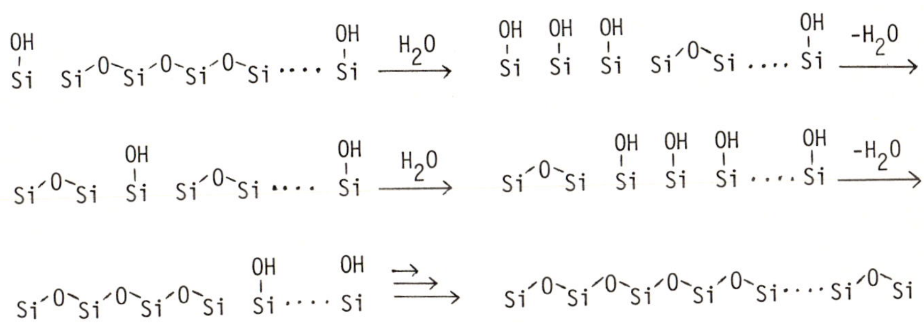

It is reasonable to considered that the rate of the dealumination is first-order dependent on the amount of the framework aluminiums in a zeolite. The rate of the dealumination is expressed by the following equation,

$$-dA/dt=k_1 \cdot A \quad (1)$$

where A is the amount of the framework aluminiums, t is a steaming time, and k_1 is a first-order rate constant. The cleavage of Si-O-Al bond with water in the dealumination is similar to that of Si-O-Si bond. Therefore, if it is assumed that the acid amount is propotional to the amount of the framework aluminiums and that the acid catalyzes the cleavage of Si-O-Al bond in the dealumination, the following equation is given.

$$k_1=k_2 \cdot A \quad (2)$$

The rate of the dealumination is consequently given from the above equations (1) and (2) as follows.

$$-dA/dt=k_2 \cdot A^2 \qquad (3)$$

Integrating the equation (3), we have

$$[(A_0/A)-1]=A_0 \cdot k_2 \cdot t \qquad (4)$$

where A_0 is the initial amount of the framework aluminiums and k_2 is a second-order rate constant. Figure. 4 is plots of the ^{27}Al NMR data from the equation (4). For both H-ZSM-5 and Ca-H-ZSM-5, the linear relationships were obtained, supporting the second-order dependence of the rate of the dealumination on the amount of the framework aluminiums. It was confirmed that the acid catalyzes the cleavage of Si-O-Al bond in the dealumination. In Table 2 are summarized the rate constants, $A_0 \cdot k_2$. These results indicate that the rate of the dealumination for M-H-ZSM-5 is greatly depressed due to the presence of alklaine earth metals.

TABLE 2

The rate constants of various zeolites

Zeolites	$A_0 \cdot k_2$ (day^{-1})
H-ZSM-5	4.0
Mg-H-ZSM-5	4.0×10^{-1}
Ca-H-ZSM-5	1.9×10^{-1}
Sr-H-ZSM-5	2.6×10^{-2}
Ba-H-ZSM-5	1.9×10^{-2}

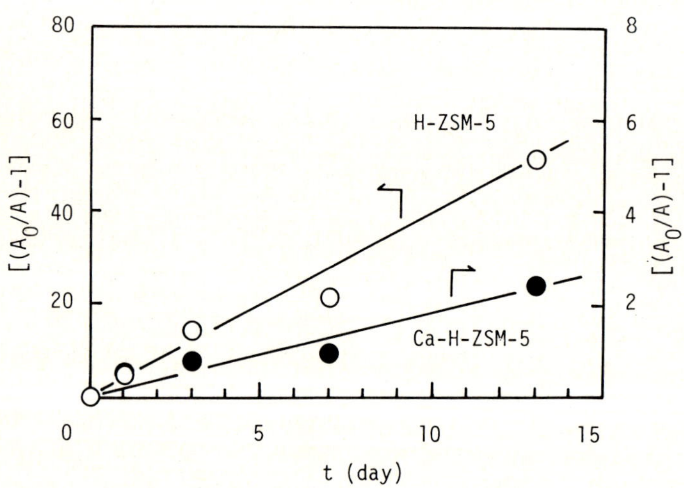

Fig. 4 Relationship between $[(A_0/A)-1]$ and t.

The typical TPD spectra of NH_3 from H-ZSM-5 and Ca-H-ZSM-5 before and after the steaming are illustrated in Fig. 5. The TPD spectra from H-ZSM-5 exhibited the two fairly sharp peaks at about 220 and 450 °C. On the other hand, the two peaks of the TPD spectra from Ca-H-ZSM-5 are broad. The total amounts of desorbed NH_3 decreased with an increase in the steaming time for both H-ZSM-5 and Ca-H-ZSM-5. However, the amount of the desorbed NH_3 from Ca-H-ZSM-5 on a steaming time decreased much gradually compared with that from H-ZSM-5. As a part of the desorbed NH_3 might originate from physically adsorbed one, the total amounts of the desorbed NH_3 are not necessarily proportional to the amounts of acid sites with which aluminiums in zeolites are concerned. Nevertheless, the relationships between the steaming time and the amount of the desorbed NH_3 from both H-, Ca-H-ZSM-5 are content with those between the steaming time and the ^{27}Al NMR intensity ratios. This result also suggests that the dealumination of the framework of Ca-H-ZSM-5 is strongly inhibited by the presence of calcium.

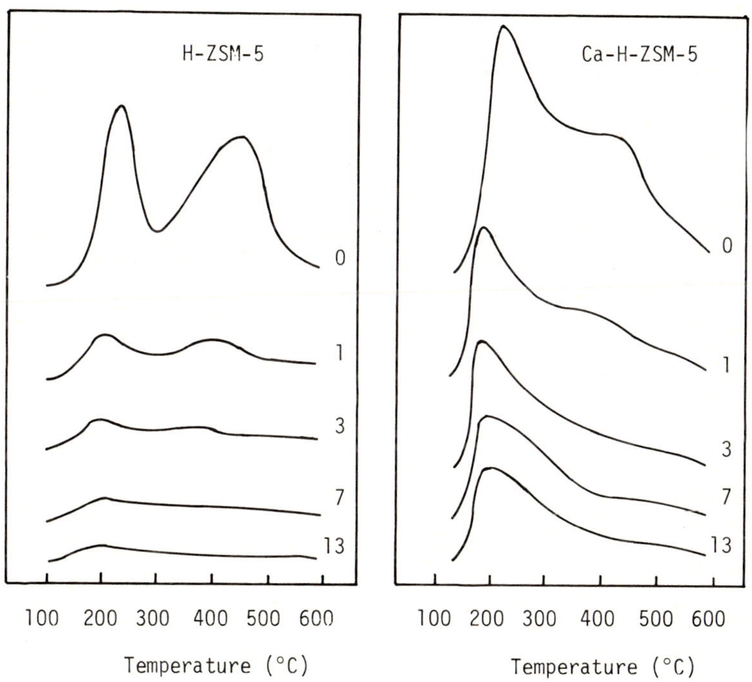

Fig. 5 TPD spectra of NH_3 from various steamed zeolites
Arabic numbers in Fig. denote the steaming time (day).

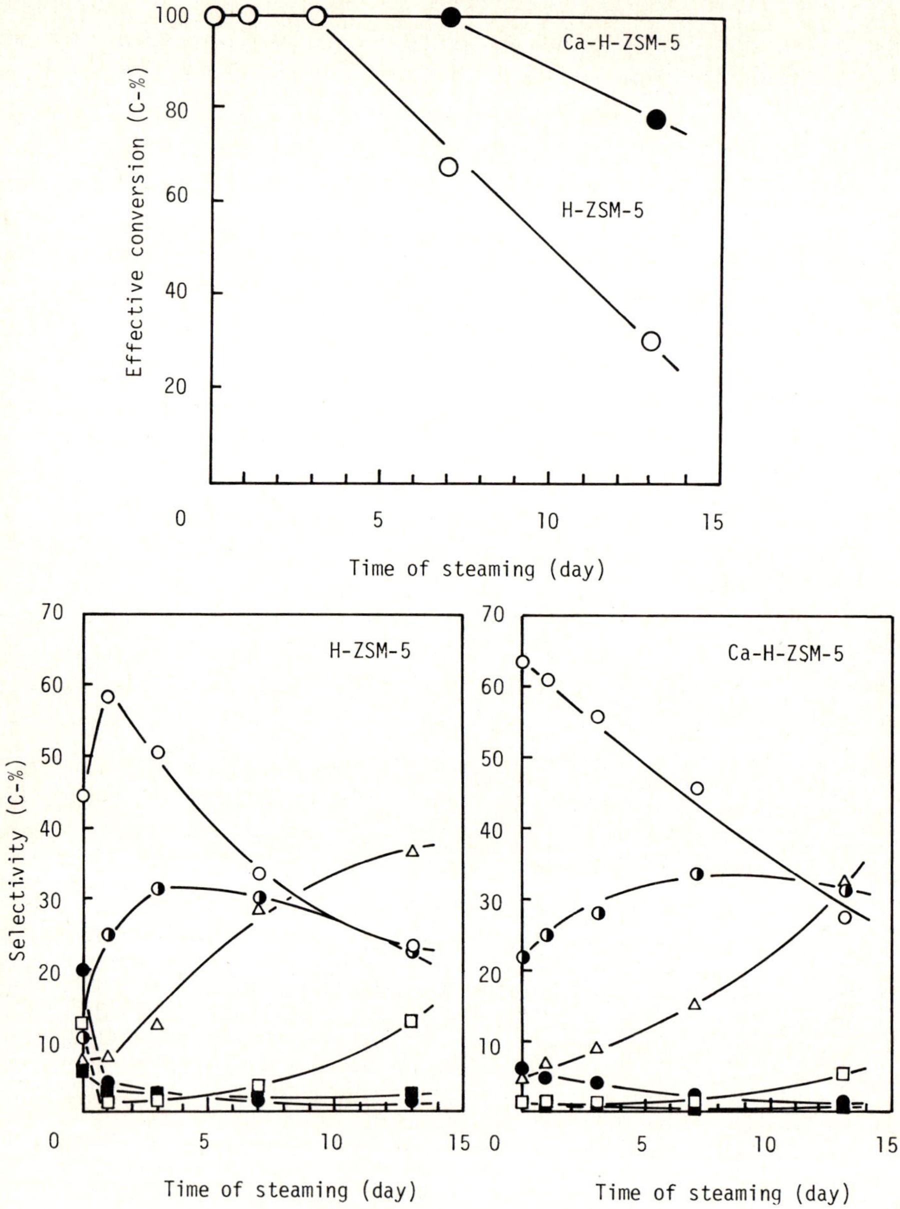

Fig. 6 Effect of steaming on the catalytic activity and the product selectivity in methanol conversion

Reaction conditions : $CH_3OH/Ar=1/1$, Temp.=600 °C, LHSV=4 h^{-1}

Effective conversion=100 – (methanol+dimethyl ether)yield

○ : $C_2H_4+C_3H_6$ ◑ : $C_4H_8+C_5H_{10}$ □: CH_4

■ : (C_2-C_5) paraffins ● : BTX △: C_6^+ .

The high steam stability of M-H-ZSM-5 is also supported by the results of methanol conversion over the various steamed zeolites (Fig. 6). The steaming affected both the catalytic activity and the product selectivity. The effective conversion, 100 - (methanol+dimethyl ether)yield, of H-ZSM-5 markedly decreased with an increase in the steaming time, while that of Ca-H-ZSM-5 slightly decreased, indicating the higher catalyst stability for steaming. However, the difference in the catalytic activity between H-ZSM-5 and Ca-H-ZSM-5 was not much, though there was the remarkable difference in the amount of the framework aluminiums after steaming as shown in Fig. 2. That the acid strength of H-ZSM-5 is considerably stronger than that of Ca-H-ZSM-5 seems to contribute to the difference in effective conversion. In the case of H-ZSM-5, the selectivity changed drastically at an early steaming time and varied gradually with the steaming time. On the other hand, in the case of Ca-H-ZSM-5, the selectivity changed gradually with the steaming time. The rapid change in the selectivity of H-ZSM-5 may be responsible for that in the amount of the framework aluminiums.

From all of the above results, it was found that the dealumination of the framework of H-ZSM-5 zeolites is strongly inhibited by adding alkaline earth metals and the rate of the dealumination is second-order dependent on the amount of the framework aluminiums. It was indicated that the dealumination is promoted by the strong acid which catalyzes the cleavage of Si-O-Al bond by hydration. However, the limited data of the present work could not clarify the essential role played by the alkaline earth metals and a further study is now progress. An similar improvement in the steam stability was achieved by maintaining a substantial number of metal cationic sites in the zeolites, for example, by the addition of Co or Cu [16-17].

This work is a part of the "C_1 Chemistry Project", a National Research and Development Program of the Agency of Industrial Science and Technology, Ministry of International Trade and Industry (M.I.T.I.), Japan.

References

1 W. W. Kaeding and S. A. Butter, J. Catal., 61 (1980) 155
2 G. Chen and J. Ling, China-Japan-U.S. Symposium on Heterogeneous Catalysts, Dalian, China, (1982) A010C
3 C. D. Chang, C. T -W. Chu and R. F. Socha, J. Catal., 86 (1984) 289
4 D. E. 2,935,863
5 D. E. 3,304,479
6 U. S. Pat. 4,544,793
7 H. Hagiwara, K. Kawamura, T. Sano, Y. Shiomi, T. Miyamoto, M. Fujimoto, Y. Yasumoto and H. Takaya, Chem. Express, 1 (1986) 439
8 H. Okado, H. Shoji, K. Kawamura, Y. Kohtoku, Y. Yamazaki, T. Sano and H. Takaya, Nippon Kagaku Kaishi, (1987) 25
9 H. Okado, T. Sano, K. Matsuzski, K. Kawamura, K. Hashimoto, H. Watanabe and H. Takaya, Nippon Kagaku kaishi, in press
10 S. G. Fegan and B. M. Lowe, J. Chem. Soc. Chem. Commun., (1984) 437

11 A. W. Chester, Y. F. Chu, R. M. Dessau, G. T. Kerr and C. T. Kresge, J. Chem. Soc. Chem. Commun., (1985) 289
12 G. L. Woolery, L. B. Alemany, R. M. Dessau and A. W. Chester, ZEOLITES, 6 (1986) 14
13 N. Y. Topose, K. Pedersen and E. G. Derouane, J. Catal., 70 (1981) 41
14 P. A. Jacobs and R. van Ballmoos, J. Phys. Chem., 86 (1982) 3050
15 C. A. Fyfe, J. M. Thomas, J. Klinowski and G. C. Gobbi, Angew. Chem. Int. Ed. Engl., 22 (1983) 259
16 P. A. Jacobs and H. K Beyer, J. Phys. Chem., 83 (1979) 1174
17 Eur. Pat. Appl. 18,117

B. Delmon and G.F. Froment (Editors), *Catalyst Deactivation 1987*

POISONING AND PASSIVATION OF AMMONIA SYNTHESIS CATALYST AT VARIOUS TEMPERATURES

A.V. KRYLOVA, N.V. NEFEDOVA and T.M. PEEV*

D.I.Mendeleyev Chemical Technological Institute, Moscow, USSR

* Institute of Chemical Engineering, Burgas, Bulgaria

ABSTRACT

The mechanism of interaction of catalytic poisons (oxygen, carbon oxide and dioxide, water vapours and their mixtures) with the ammonia synthesis catalyst has been studied in a wide range of temperatures (550 ÷ -195°C) by using chemisorption, isotopic methods, γ-resonance spectroscopy, non-stationary catalysis, derivatography, and others. It has been found that the poisoning of ammonia synthesis catalyst at intermediate catalysis temperatures ($\leq$ 400°C) is intensified, in particular, due to the presence of non-hydrated forms of oxygen-containing compounds on the surface. The results obtained were used for developing the routes of reactivation of poisoned catalysts as well as effective express methods for the elimination of catalyst pyrophoricity (stabilization) at various temperatures (below the catalysis temperature, intermediate and regular reaction temperatures).

INTRODUCTION

Oxygen and oxygen-containing compounds (H_2O, CO, CO_2) are well known poisons of the ammonia synthesis catalyst. It is customary to assume that due to the presence of excessive oxygen all oxygen-containing compounds in the process of synthesis rapidly pass into H_2O, which is usually confirmed by the equivalent poisoning effect of 100 ppm O_2 and CO_2 or 200 ppm CO and H_2O. However, not all experimental data on poisoning can be interpreted in terms of this approach. A more detailed consideration of the reasons for the well-known phenomenon of the enhanced poisoning effect of oxygen-containing poisons at intermediate catalysis temperatures ($\leq$ 400°C) was of interest, especially in the context of the search for low temperature ammonia synthesis catalysts. The phenomenon of mild surface oxidation at the temperatures much lower than those of the reaction (20 ÷ 95°C) have for a long time been used to eliminate pyrophoricity-passivation [1] , which can be regarded as a particular case of reversible surface poisoning. Recently the possibility of using the reversible poisoning of ammonia synthesis catalyst by oxygen, CO_2 and mixture of oxidizers (CO_2, H_2O, O_2) has been proposed for the elimination of pyrophoricity (stabilization) over a much wider range of temperatures, for example, by air treatment at -83 ÷ -195°C and above 400°C, by CO_2 and mixtures of oxidizers ($CO_2 + H_2O$, $CO_2 + H_2O + O_2$) at the temperature from -78°C to -17°C and from 100°C to 500°C [2-6] .

In the present paper the results obtained in the study of the interaction of oxygen, oxygen-containing poisons (CO, CO_2, H_2O and their mixtures) with the catalyst at various catalysis temperatures with respect to their poisoning effect upon the reaction and the use of the reversible catalyst poisoning effect for the elimination of pyrophoric properties have been compared.

EXPERIMENTAL METHODS

All the experiments were performed by using the standard CA-IB industrial passivated catalyst. The grains of industrial samples were ground in an air flow and a fraction 1-2 mm was separated. The sample of the catalyst (0.2-4 g) was reduced in a hydrogen flow at the usual space velocity of 5000 h^{-1} at a stepwise temperature increase and was kept for 1-3 hours, with the final reduction temperature being equal to 500-530°C. Adsorption and desorption of oxygen-containing compounds at various temperatures were studied in a pulse chromatography installation in helium and hydrogen flows using the method of regeneration of sorption sites [7] . For that purpose sorption was carried out until the saturation with pulses reached the range 0.1 - 1 cm^3 at 20°C, the velocity of the carrier-gas being 20-100 cm^3/min (as a rule, the partial pressure of the adsorbate did not exceed 25 mm of m.c.). Then the catalyst with the adsorbed gas was heated in the carrier gas flow for certain time up to 50°C, then cooled down and the second adsorption was carried out at 20°C. Using the same procedure heatings were further carried out successively at much higher temperatures (100, 150, 200, 300, 400, 500°C), Each heating was followed by cooling down to 20°C and measuring the adsorption. The value of the gas adsorption after each heating made it possible to determine the number of sorption sites regenerated at the temperature of heating. Comparison of regeneration of the sites in a helium flow with that in a hydrogen flow alowed one to identify and consider separately the processes of desorption, thermal decomposition and hydration of the adsorbate. The same installation was used for studying the effect of the poisons upon the non-stationary catalysis. The reaction was carried out by feeding the pulses of another reagent into nitrogen or hydrogen flows or the pulses of the nitrogen-hydrogen mixture into a helium flow. The ammonia formed was absorbed by water and titrated with sulphuric acid. Regular oxygen pulses were introduced into the carrier gas flow to study the poisoning. The catalysts were also treated with poisons in a flow-type installation in a flow of purified and dried nitrogen containing admixtures of oxygen, carbon dioxide, mixtures of helium and water vapours, mixtures of carbon dioxide and water vapours or oxygen, mixtures of nitrogen with oxygen and water vapours and mixtures of oxygen, carbon dioxide and water vapours of various composition. The rate of the interaction of the catalyst with the oxidizer was characterized by a temperature increase (pyrophoric heating) ΔT, °C. Homomolecular and heteromolecular oxygen exchanges were studied with the use of O^{18} isotope in stationary circulation installation linked with a mass-spectrometer. The phase composition of the catalysts treated with different oxygen-containing compounds as well as their resistance to disintegration of the surface layers were determined by using -resonance spectroscopy and derivatography.

I. Interaction of the Catalyst with Poisons at Various Temperatures. Reactivation of Poisoned Catalysts

Fig. 1 and 2 show the temperature dependences of the part of chemisorption sites of O_2, CO and CO_2 regenerated in the flows of H_2 and He. Analysis of the dependences has resulted in a probable model of the poisoning process of the catalyst at different temperatures. In all the cases a higher extent of regeneration of sites in hydrogen(curves 1,3) is indicative of the fact that the processes of poisons hydration play a decisive role only at high reaction temperatures. In fact, chemisorbed oxygen and carbon dioxide are completely hydrated on the catalyst surface only at 500°C, while under the experimental conditions a complete hydration (a hundred per cent hydration) of CO is not observed even at 500°C. At lower temperatures (even at 400°C) a considerable part of metallic centres is poisoned by strongly bonded non-hydrated forms of poisons interaction (O_2, CO_2, CO) with the catalyst. It should be noted that during the ammonia synthesis, i.e., in the presence of hydrogen, the catalyst will react with a mixture of poisons with water vapours which result from hydration of the poison, for example, such mixtures as $O_2 + H_2O$, $CO_2 + H_2O$, etc. A simultaneous effect of $CO_2 + H_2O + O_2$ and other mixtures is also possible. The fact that the poisons cannot be removed from the surface in a helium flow even at 500°C show that they may strongly interact with the catalyst resulting in the formation of chemical compounds.

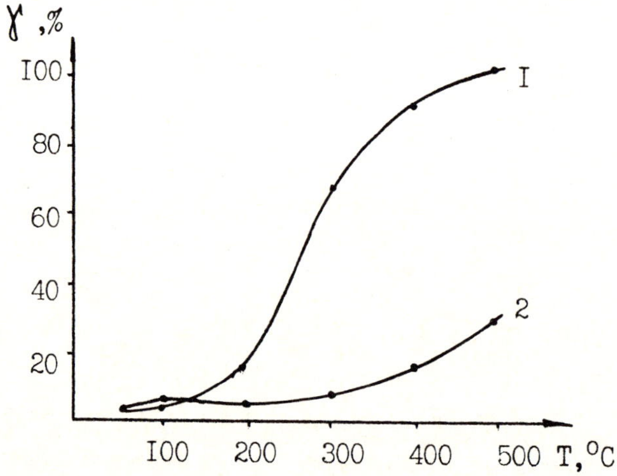

Fig. 1. Rate of regeneration of chemisorption sites of O_2 in H_2(1) and He (2)

The possible types of surface compounds of various poisons with the catalyst have been studied in the experiments on treatment of the reduced catalyst in a hydrogen-free flow of poisons at various temperatures. Fig. 3 and Table 1 show the Mössbauer spectra of the catalysts treated by the above-described procedure as well as the samples of phase composition specified by the data on the spectra. The data given show that the action of poisons CO_2 and O_2 at 350°C identically results in the formation of very close amounts of magnetite, while at 400°C, unlike O_2, the interaction of CO_2 may result in the formation of both magnetite and carbide. It should be noted that with the increase of the temperature from 350 to 400°C the degree of iron oxidation in O_2 decreases, while it sharply increases in CO_2. These data permit to conclude that similar compounds can be formed on

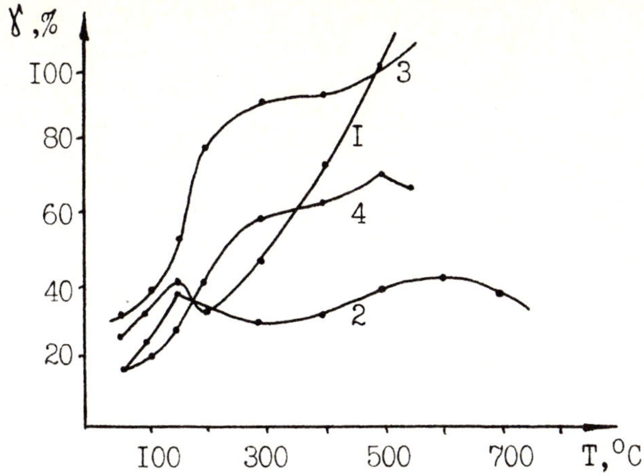

Fig. 2. Rate of regeneration of chemisorption sites of CO and CO_2 in H_2(1,3) and He (2,4)

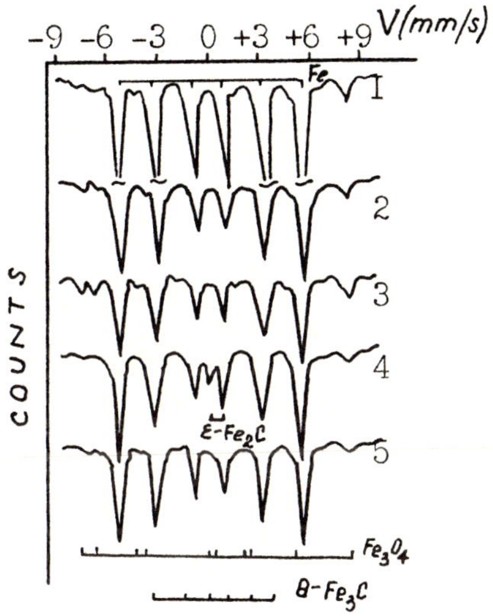

Fig. 3. Mössbauer spectra of the CA-IB samples treated with various poisons (the numbers of the curves correspond to those given in Table 1)

the surface and poison the catalyst during the synthesis since the rate of hydration of the poisons and these compounds is not sufficiently high at intermediate temperatures. The catalysts treated with a mixture of O_2+H_2O exhibited much higher degree of oxidation (at 350°-17% Fe_3O_4, at 400°-33%), than those treated with O_2 only (at 350°C-10% Fe_3O_4, at 400°-8%). Also there can be observed different effect of the increasing temperature: O_2 decreases the oxidation of iron, a mixture of O_2 + H_2O

TABLE 1

Phase Composition of CA-IB Catalyst Samples Treated with Various Poisons

Temperature of treatment	Poison	α-Fe	Fe_3O_4	θ-Fe_3C	ε-Fe_2C	Temperature of the protective layer destruction
350°C	1% O_2+2.4% H_2O	83	17	-	-	
	CO_2	90	10	-	-	108
	CO_2+2.4% H_2O+ + 1% O_2	78	18	4	-	91
	CO_2+1.4% H_2O	86	6	-	13	
	1% O_2	89	11	-	-	90
400°C	1% O_2+2.4% H_2O	67	33	-	-	
	CO_2	52	28	20	-	143
	CO_2+2.4% H_2O+ +1% O_2	44	43	13	-	
	1% O_2	82	8	-	-	

sharply increases it. At 350° the interaction of a mixture of CO_2 + H_2O with the catalyst results in a decrease of the rate of magnetite formation from 10 to 6 % with the simultaneous formation of the carbide phase ε-Fe_2C in the catalyst. Addition of another poison (O_2) to the same mixture increases the amount of magnetite formed, decreases the content and changes the form of carbide. Hence, the effect of the poison mixtures upon the catalyst is complicated and is not always of additive character.

Thus, the nature and the amount of the compounds formed depend not only on the interaction of poisons with the catalyst but also upon the nature and composition of the poison mixture. Analysis of the curves of thermal regeneration of sorption sites and spectral data given with an account of the literature results concerning the study of interaction of poisons with the catalyst carried out by other methods permit to conclude that at intermediate catalysis temperatures ($\leq$400°C) the poisoning by different poisons should be of individual character for each particular poison due to the blocking of various sites, different changes in the electronic properties of the surface, different temperature dependences and the nature of the surface compounds which are formed upon the interaction of the catalyst with the poisons and their mixtures with the vater vapours. The lower the reaction temperature, the less the hydration rate of the poisons and the greater is the contribution of the individual mechanism of poisoning by each particular poison. The results obtained allowed one to develop the routes for reactivation of the catalysts poisoned by the poisons (studied at intermediate temperatures) based on the increasing of the catalyst temperature for hydrogenation of the forms of the strong interaction of poisons with iron in the catalyst. The routes of reactiovation take into account the temperature and composition of the poisoning mixture which determine the probable composition of the surface compounds of the catalyst.

At the intermediate synthesis temperatures the catalyst exhibited an ability to considerably adsorb the reaction product, ammonia, which, in our opinion, also can poison the process as the temperature decreases [7]. The implementation of the reaction along the pulse route made it possible to increase the conversion of the reagents, the effect becoming more pronounced as the temperature decreased, and at 200°C the effect increased more than 10^2 times [8]. Implementing the ammonia synthesis through chromatographic route [8] no oxygen poisoning of the catalyst was observed (see Table 2), which indicates a possibility of a decreased poisoning effect of oxygen upon the transition to certain non-stationary routes of the reaction implemen-

TABLE 2

Effect of Oxygen upon the Rate of Reagent Conversion (α) in Chromatographic Regime at V_{pulse}/V_{cat} = 0.125*

Temperature, °C	NH_3.% in the absence of oxygen			NH_3.% in the presence of oxygen		
	H_2 in a N_2 flow	N_2 in a H_2 flow	ABC** in a He flow	H_2 in a N_2 flow	N_2 in a H_2 flow	ABC** in a He flow
450	3.7	3.4	1.7	3.8	3.3	1.9
300	3.2	3.0	1.5	3.0	3.1	1.5
200	2.7	2.2	1.2	2.6	2.4	1.4

* The ratio of the pulse volume to the catalyst volume.

** $3H_2 + N_2$

tation. The result can be interpreted by the poison adsorption at the most active catalyst sites with the subsequent displacement of ammonia and removal of the poison during the intervals between the pulses.

2. Peculiarities of Interaction of the Catalyst with Oxygen during Passivation. The Use of Effects of Reversible Poisoning by Oxygen-containing Poisons for Elimination of Pyrophoricity (Stabilization) of the Catalyst

Comparison of interaction of oxygen with the catalyst at various temperatures (of poisoning and passivation) was carried out by means of the method of isotopic exchange [9] . Homomolecular and heteromolecular oxygen exchange was studied by using a reduced sample obtained after keeping it in oxygen at various temperatures as well as a sample in the oxide form. Fig. 4 and 5 show examples of kinetic dependences thus obtained. Homomolecular exchange was observed on the samples treated in a nitrogen-oxygen mixture in the temperature range between -78 ÷ 80°C. Exchange kinetic curves (Fig.4) are described by the equation of the first order, though these curves do not pass across the beginning of the coordinates. Therefore the reaction rates were calculated against the linear part of the curves. The activation energy of the exchange calculated with respect to the rate constants was equal to 8.5 kJ/mol.

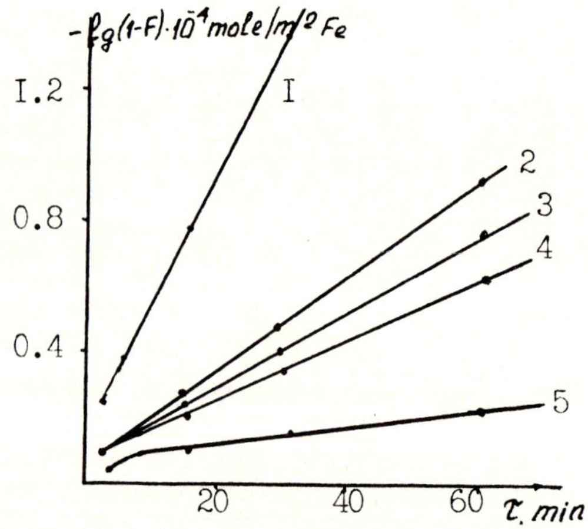

Fig. 4. Kinetics of the homomolecular exchange on the passivated catalyst: 1 - 4 - 293 K, 5 - 195 K

The exchange reaction proceeds at low temperatures due to the presence of passivated catalysts of weakly-bonded forms of non-oxide oxygen on the surface. In the course of a series of subsequent experiments the catalyst activity in the exchange decreased (curves 1-4, Fig.4), which indicates a gradual transition of weakly-bonded oxygen into strongly-bonded ones. The heteroisotopic exchange was also observed on the passivated catalysts at -78 ÷ 20°C. The number of molecules participating in a heteroexchange calculated by a change in isotope content was 0.1-0.5 . 10^{19} molecules/m^2Fe.

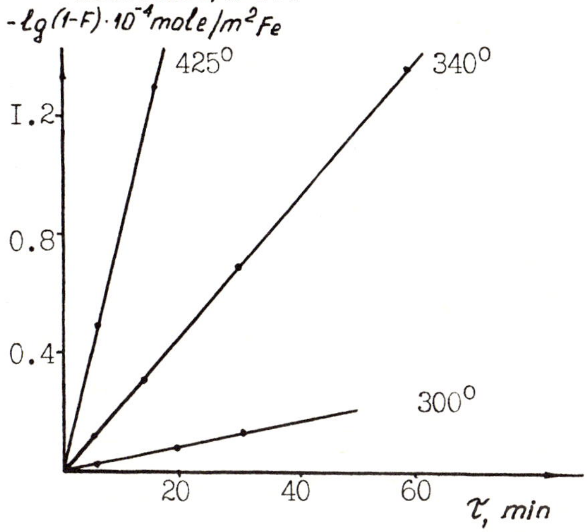

Fig. 5. Kinetics of the isotopic exchange on the oxidized catalyst

The fact that weakly-bonded oxygen was adsorbed on the metallic surface was confirmed by the absence of low-temperature exchange reaction on the catalysts in an oxide form. Homomolecular exchange on the catalysts in an oxide form (magnetite form) takes place at a noticeable rate only at 300°C. The exchange kinetics (Fig.5) was described by the equation of the first order. The exchange was followed by absorption of oxygen and according to the data on the chemical analysis by oxidizing a portion of Fe(II) into Fe(III). The activation energy of the reaction in the temperature range between 300 and 500°C was equal to ~125 kJ/mol and was close to the temperature known from the literature data for Fe_2O_3. Heteroexchange is observed in the same temperature range. Exchange on the catalysts partially oxidized at 300-500°C proceeded with the characteristics obtained for the sample in an oxide form.

Therefore, the forms of interaction of the catalyst with oxygen at the temperatures of synthesis and passivation (20°C) are different. At the synthesis temperatures oxide oxygen is formed. It was found that passivated catalysts contain weakly-bonded oxygen which occupies 5-10% of the metallic sites of the surface and slowly passes into strongly-bonded oxygen. The total amount of oxygen absorbed upon passivation is equal, according to our data, up to 10 molecular layers on the metallic surface; the most part of oxygen is strongly bonded (oxide, strong chemisorption), embraces near-surface layers and the whole passivating layer appears to be non-homogeneous.

The lengthy passivation process was due to a slow transition of weakly-bonded oxygen into strongly-bonded one and insufficient stability of the protective structure was explained by the fact that the sites of weak adsorption were unprotected, these sites can be covered by the molecules of competing adsorbates of water or even hydrogen in the process of passivation [2] and serve as initiating sites of oxidation upon the contact of the catalyst with air.

It follows from the results obtained that stable protective structures in the conditions of passivation are not formed as a result of slow transition of weakly-bonded oxygen into strongly-bonded one on the sites and a high rate of oxygen diffusion into the catalyst volume leading to a bulk structure of the passivating layer. Therefore, it was feasible to choose such conditions of stabilization under which the formation of weakly-bonded oxygen does not occur and rate of interaction of oxygen with the surface considerably increases the rate of oxygen diffusion into the catalyst volume. Such conditions appear to be high concentration of oxygen in the gas phase which provides high concentration of oxygen on the surface and low temperature which provides a decrease of the diffusion rate, or high temperature at which, as shown previously [6] in Fig. 6 the oxidation degree of the catalyst by oxygen decreases. The study of interaction of the catalyst with air at low temperatures, in fact, allowed one to identify the range of temperatures providing the formation of strong protective structures which help eliminate pyrophoricity. These structures are formed on the catalysts studied in the range of temperatures from -195° to -83°C. The studies resulted in an express method of low temperature stabilization of the pyrophoric catalyst which practically provides instantaneous formation of the stable protective layer. Elimination of the weak chemisorption of oxygen due to interaction with oxygen at high temperature served as a basis for effective high-temperature (≪400°C) stabilization of pyrophoric systems with air and oxygen [2,3] .

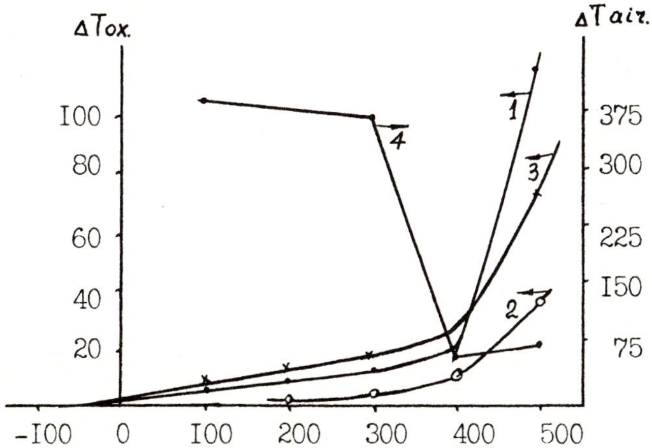

Fig. 6. Dependence of the value of pyrophoric heating of the CA-IB catalyst upon the temperature of the oxidation start in the flows: 1 - CO_2, 2 - H_2O, 3 - CO_2 + H_2O + O_2, 4 - air.

The dependences obtained in the study of reversible interaction of other poisons with the catalyst at various temperatures provided a basis for the development of stabilization of the catalysts by carbon dioxide and mixtures of oxygen-containing poisons at intermediate and low temperatures.

Fig. 6 lists the temperature dependences of pyrophoric interaction of the catalyst with oxygen (air), water vapours, carbon dioxide and mixtures of poisons, these dependences being determined with respect to increasing temperatures of the catalyst upon the reaction of pyrophoric oxidation (ΔT_{ox}). Comparison of the curves indicates a sharp difference between the action of oxygen and other oxidizers in the region of regular and intermediate (≤ 400°C) synthesis temperatures. At regular temperatures very small amount of oxygen interacts with the catalyst, while carbon dioxide, water vapours and oxidizers mixtures, on the contrary, intensively oxidize the catalyst iron. At the temperatures below 400°C and especially below 300°C, on the contrary, the interaction of all the poisons with the catalyst, except oxygen, is slight. In accordance with these data it was found that the Mössbauer spectra of the catalyst treated with air or oxygen at 200-300°C indicate the maximum concentration of magnetite, while after the treatment at 500°C the samples contain hardly identified traces of oxides [6] .

It has been mentioned that comparison of the properties of the catalysts treated with an individual oxidizer of their mixtures shows the effects of non-additivity of the mixtures action. After treatment with certain poisons under definite conditions the pyrophoric ammonia synthesis catalysts did not exhibit any pyrophoricity upon contact with air, i.e., they stabilized. At certain temperatures of interaction the synergistic effect is observed. It means that when H_2O and CO_2, for example, do not stabilize the catalyst (300°C), a mixture of these poisons readily stabilizes the catalyst at any temperature above 100°C. The new effective express methods of stabilization of the catalysts with carbon dioxide and the oxidizers mixtures at various temperatures ranging from -78 to 500°C were based on the series of the results obtained with respect to the interaction of the catalyst with CO_2 and the oxidizers mixtures [5] .

The derivatograms given in Fig. 7 indicate that the catalysts stabilized with CO_2 at intermediate temperatures are more resistant to oxidation in the air than those passivated by means of the traditional method.

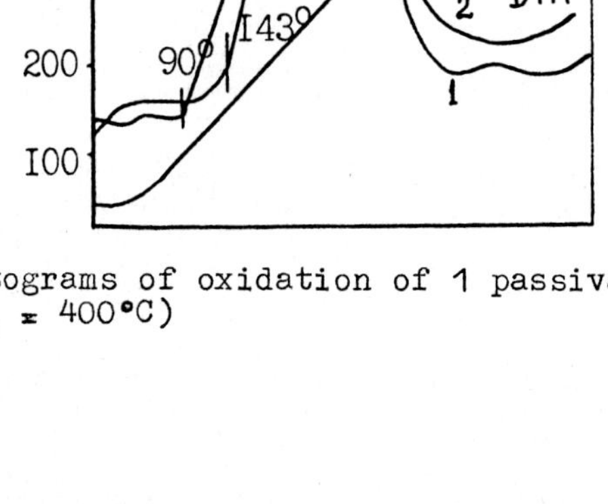

Fig. 7. Derivatograms of oxidation of 1 passivated, 2 stabilized CO_2 (T_0 = 400°C)

Thus, it follows that the peculiarities of interaction of the ammonia synthesis catalyst with CO_2, H_2O and their mixtures which are different from the peculiarities found upon interaction of the catalyst with O_2 demonstrated the possibilities of effective elimination of the catalyst pyrophoricity at intermediate and low temperatures. Reversibility of the surface poisoning upon stabilization is confirmed by the fact that after activation the catalytic activity is preserved in the reaction mixture at regular temperatures of the reaction [5] .

In general, the study performed have shown the complexity of the processes of interaction of various oxygen-containing poisons and their mixtures with the catalyst surface under the reaction conditions at intermediate temperatures. Under these conditions each of these poisons or their mixtures can interact with the catalyst according to an individual mechanism. The individual character of interaction is confirmed by various regimes of effective stabilization of the pyrophoric catalyst with different poisons or their mixtures and it should be taken into account when a certain route of regeneration of poisoned catalysts is chosen.

REFERENCES

1 Catalyst Handbook with Special Reference to Unit Processes in Ammonia and Hydrogen Manufacture, Wolfe Sci. Book, London. 1970, 222 pp.
2 A.V.Krylova, G.A.Ustimenko and N.S.Torocheshnikov, in G.Poncelet, P.Grange and P.A.Jacobs (Ed.), Proc. 3rd Int. Symp. Preparation of Catalysts III, Louvain-la-Neuve, Belgium, September 6-9, 1982, Elsevier, Amsterdam, 1983, pp.441-450.
3 A.V.Krylova, G.A.Ustimenko, N.V.Nefedova, T.M.Peev and N.S. Torochechnikov, Appl.Catal., 20 (1986) 205-213.
4 A.V.Krylova, N.V.Nefedova, T.M.Peev, T.M.Stoilova, Kinetika i Kataliz, 27 (1986) 520.
5 A.V.Krylova, N.V.Nefedova and N.S.Torocheshnikov, B.Delman (Ed.), Proc. 4th Int.Symp. Scientific Bases for the Preparation of Heterogeneous Catalysts, Louvain-la-Neuve, Belgium, September 1-4, A7, Elsevier, Amsterdam, 1986, Preprint of paper A7, pp. 1-10.
6 A.V.Krylova, T.M.Peev, G.A.Ustimenko, Kinetika i Kataliz, 27 (1986)
7 A.V.Krylova, A.A.Veselkova, N.S.Torocheshnikov, Proc. All-Union Conference on Mechanism of Catalytic Reactions, Moscow, USSR, 1978, Nauka, pp 226-233.
8 A.V.Krylova and N.S.Torocheshnikov, in O.V.Krylov (Ed.), Proc. 4th All-Union Conference on the Mechanism of Catalytic Reactions, Moscow, USSR, April 19-22, 1986,part II,pp.188-192.
9 A.V.Krylova, L.A.Kasatkina, V.V.Morozov, Proc.All-Union seminar"Isotopic methods in studying the catalysis mechanism" Novosibirsk, USSR, 1980, preprint of paper 33, pp. 1-4.

B. Delmon and G.F. Froment (Editors), *Catalyst Deactivation 1987*

CONTROL OF CATALYST DEACTIVATION CAUSED BY COKING IN METHANOL TO AROMATICS CONVERSION ON Ga- AND Zn-ION-EXCHANGED H-ZSM-5 BY ADDITION OF OTHER ALCOHOLS

T. INUI, M. TAKAKI, T. HAGIWARA, and M. YOSHIKAWA

Department of Hydrocarbon Chemistry, Faculty of Engineering, Kyoto University, Sakyo-ku, Kyoto 606 (Japan)

ABSTRACT

In order to relax catalyst deactivation by coking during synthesis of aromatic-rich gasoline from methanol on ZSM-5 type catalyst, effects of additives to both the feed and catalyst were investigated. In cyclohexanol conversion, in spite of the marked increase in selectivity to aromatics compared with in methanol conversion, coking of the catalyst bed was restrained almost comparative with that in the methanol conversion. When a mixture of methanol and cyclohexanol was converted, the selectivity to aromatics was obtained by a simple average of the selectivity in single component conversions. On the other hand, the catalyst deactivation become minimum with around the equimolal mixture of the feed, and this tendency become more evidently on Zn-ion exchanged H-ZSM-5. The cause of these phenomena was discussed.

INTRODUCTION

In Mobil's MTG process, the methanol conversion on H-ZSM-5 is performed under moderate pressure and recyclic feed of light hydrocarbon products, and aromatic-rich gasoline of high octane-number is obtained with about 85% selectivity. However, when this reaction is conducted under atmospheric pressure and one-pass operation, the yield of gasoline and the content of aromatics decrease markedly (refs. 1 and 2).

Recently, Langner (ref. 3) studied on influence of small amounts of alcohols on the duration of the induction periods for the formation of hydrocarbons from methanol on an NaH-Y zeolite catalyst at considerably low temperature, and found that only 1% addition of alcohols such as ethanol, propanol, 2-cyclohexene-1-ol and cyclohexanol exhibited striking effect that the induction periods were shortened markedly, especially in the case of cyclohexanol, however, the detail of the product distribution was not described.

More recently, we found that the following effects of additives on the methanol conversion (ref. 4). Addition of a small concentration (1 – 5%) of ethylene and propylene to the methanol feed remarkably accelerated the methanol conversion, and the yield of gasoline increased with increasing concentration of the lower olefins added. Passage of 2% ethylene before the methanol conversion caused a steep increase in methanol conversion to hydrocarbons without co-delivery of ethylene, and the yield of gasoline was approximately proportional to the duration of the ethylene pretreatment. Furthermore, addition of only 0.03% of alcohols such as isopropanol and allyl alcohol reduced the induction period which is observed in methanol conversion on H-ZSM-5 at low temperature range, and the gasoline selectivity increased from 45.9% to 55.2% in the case of allyl alcohol addition. The conversion reaction of these alcohols on a silica gel having a moderate solid acidity demonstrated the formation of lower olefins and oxygenates. These incipient products are presumed to be incorporated in the chain propagation or autocatalysis which has been confirmed by several authors (refs. 5-8).

Another potential to increase aromatics in the gasoline fraction from methanol conversion would be in improvement of catalyst property. It has been known recently that Ga and Zn components increase the yield of aromatics from light hydrocarbons (refs. 9-15).

However, the problem lies in a close relation between coke formation and aromatic hydrocarbons in the products. It is considered that coke deposit on zeolite catalysts during the methanol conversion originates mainly from aromatics and advances *via* formation of fused-ring aromatics (ref. 16). Although H-ZSM-5 exerts the longest catalyst life for the methanol conversion among various zeolites (refs. 3 and 17), when much aromatics are contained in the product, the problem of deactivation by coke formation would be serious.

In this study, in order to search a solution to reduce catalyst deactivation in the synthesis of aromatic-rich gasoline, the effect of additives to the methanol feed and modification of H-ZSM-5 catalyst upon the catalyst deactivation were investigated.

EXPERIMENTAL

Catalyst

Two kinds of H-ZSM-5 having Si/Al atomic ratio 40 designated as (1) and (2) were used. H-ZSM-5(1) and H-ZSM-5(2) were prepared by the method 2 and method 4 described in our previous paper (ref. 18), respectively. The preparation methods were based on the method appeared in a patent literature (ref. 19), but were modified in composition of the solutions, pretreatment of the precursor, and hydrothermal crystallization condition. Na-ZSM-5 form was converted to H-ZSM-5 form by repeated treatment with 1 M NH_4NO_3 solution at 80°C for 1 h, followed by washing with water at room temperature and drying overnight at 100°C. It was then calcined in air at 540°C for 3.5 h. Ion exchange for H-ZSM-5 by Ga and Zn ions was carried out by the procedure shown in Fig. 1. The resulting powder was compressed by tablet machine, and the tablet was crashed to 8 - 15 mesh pieces to provide the reaction.

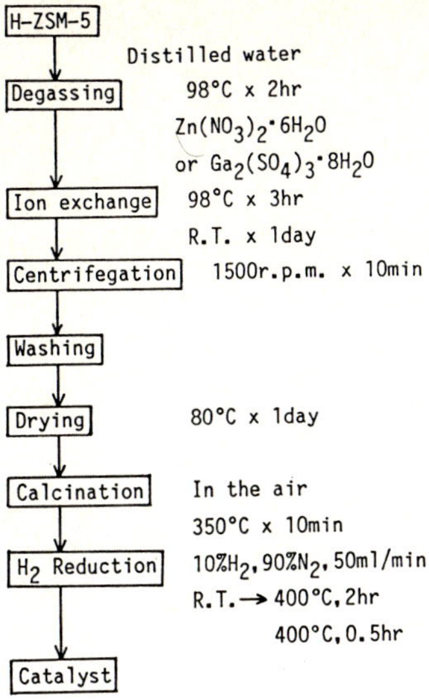

Fig. 1 Procedure for preparation of Ga- and Zn-ion-exchanged H-ZSM-5.

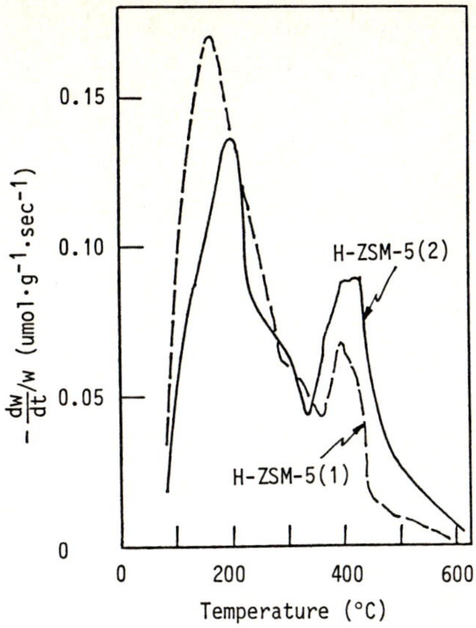

Fig. 2 Profiles of NH_3 TPD from H-ZSM-5 samples.

The physical properties of both H-ZSM-5 samples were almost same, but the acidic property was considerably different from each other. Profiles of temperature programmed desorption (TPD) of NH_3 from both samples are shown in Fig. 2. A high temperature peak for H-ZSM-5(2) which is appeared above 350°C is much larger than that of H-ZSM-5(1). The high temperature peak would correspond to strong acid sites which are responsible for the active sites for hydrocarbon formation from oxygenates (ref. 20). Therefore, H-ZSM-5(2) was expected to exhibit somewhat higher activity for formation of heavier hydrocarbons compared with that for H-ZSM-5(1).

Reaction method

Research grade reagents; methanol, ethanol, i-propanol, allyl alcohol, n-butanol, cyclohexanol, cyclohexanone, and 2-cyclohexen-1-ol, were used without further purification.

An ordinary fixed-bed continuous flow reaction apparatus was used. A 240 mg portion of catalyst was packed into a tublar reactor of 6 mm i.d.. The catalyst-bed length was 18 mm. The catalyst bed was heated from room temperature up to 450°C while flowing nitrogen gas with a space velocity of 2000 h^{-1} and maintained for 30 min at the same temperature. After this standardization for the catalyst, the reaction gas mixture of 20 mol% reactant and 80 mol% N_2 was introduced to the catalyst bed at 350°C with a space velocity of 2000 h^{-1}. All the products were analyzed by gas chromatographs equipped with integraters.

RESULTS AND DISCUSSION

Estimation of coke deposit

When non-diluted methanol vapor was fed into the catalyst-bed of H-ZSM-5(1) with a weight hourly space velocity (WHSV) 11.43 h^{-1} at 350°C, the methanol conversion to hydrocarbons maintained 100% for 22.4 h. After that time on stream, methanol conversion and hydrocarbon formation began to decrease rapidly, and compensatingly, dimethyl ether formation increased. The color of catalyst bed had changed to black. The total hydrocarbons formed until the time on stream at which the methanol conversion began to decrease corresponded to 256 g of methanol fed per one gram catalyst. When methanol vapor is diluted with N_2 to 20 mol% and is fed with a space velocity 2000 h^{-1}, if the coke deposit is proportional to the amount of converted methanol, catalyst deactivation is presumed to be detected at 215 h on stream. In fact, the color of all the catalyst bed changed to light gray within 1 h on stream, however, any distinct dark color zone was not detected and the color did not change during the measurement at least for several hours. By this catalyst, measurement of catalyst deactivation in methanol conversion needs much time, but comparison of deactivation degree for a wide spread source of coke formation would be suitable.

On the other hand, H-ZSM-5(2) which has the stronger acidity produced more aromatics from methanol than H-ZSM-5(1) as described later. In this case, a distinct black zone formed at the inlet side on the catalyst bed and the length of the black zone increased with time on stream, and for example, the percentage of coking zone of the catalyst-bed length could be estimated as 22%. This catalyst was consider to be suitable for quick measurement of catalyst deactivation, and was applied to observe deactivation by the coking zone in co-conversion of methanol and other oxygenates.

Conversion of single component

Eight kinds of alcohol and cyclohexanone were converted on H-ZSM-5(1) at 350 °C. In every case, the conversion to hydrocarbons was maintained 100% at least one hour on stream. Distribution of the products expressed by C-mol% at one hour on stream are shown in Fig. 3. Lower olefins are differentiated by shadowing, but olefin components in C_5 - C_7 aliphatic hydrocarbons are not shown and included in each section in the figure. In order to understand more precisely, the selectivity to aliphatics and aromatics for the data of Fig. 3 are plotted on Fig. 4 and 5, respectively.

In general, methane and ethane were not produced, indicating that dealkylation from alkylated aromatics and prominent hydrogenolysis of heavier hydrocarbons would not occur under the reaction condition. These types of reaction occur on an H-ZSM-5 at higher temperature condition and Pt-ion-

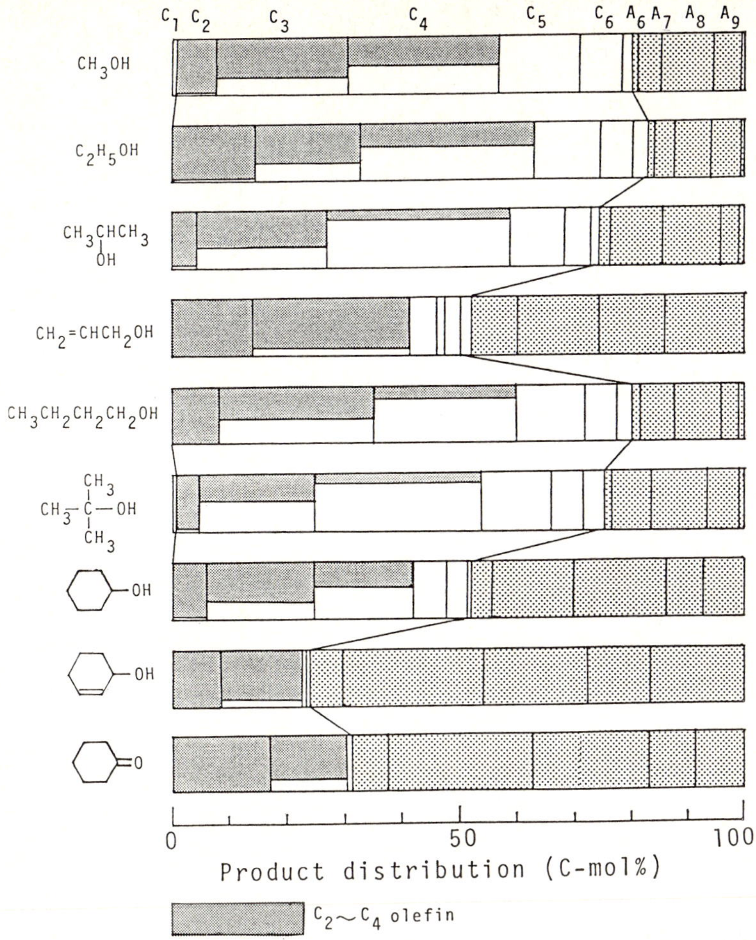

Fig. 3 Distribution of products from different kinds of alcohol and ketone. Catalyst, H-ZSM-5(1), Feed gas mixture, 20 mol% oxygenates and 80% N_2, GHSV 2000 h^{-1}, Temperature 350 °C, Time on stream 1 h.

exchanged H-ZSM-5 or H-Ga-silicate (refs. 21 and 22). As can be seen in Fig. 3, selectivity to ethylene for the conversion of secondary and tertiary alcohols; i-propanol, cyclohexanol and t-butanol, were smaller than that for primary alcohols; methanol ethanol, allyl alcohol and n-butanol. Saturated alcohols such as methanol, ethanol, i-propanol, n-butanol and t-butanol afforded much C_3 and C_4 hydrocarbons (Figs. 3 and 4). Aliphatics of C_5, C_6 and C_7 were also produced from these alcohols, but the selectivity decreased in this order and the sum of these three kinds of hydrocarbons were comparable to C_3 or C_4 hydrocarbons (Figs. 3 and 4). Ratio of paraffins in C_3 and C_4 hydrocarbons for secondary and tertiary alcohols(i-propanol and t-butanol) were larger than those for primary

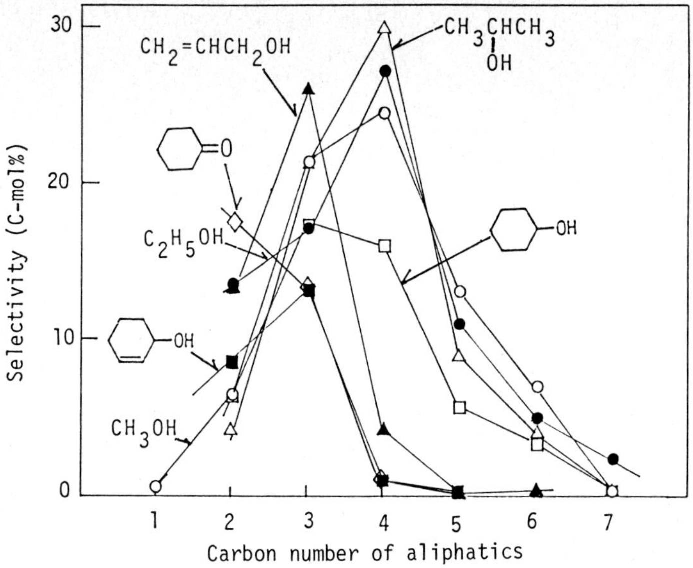

Fig. 4 Selectivity to aliphatic hydrocarbons from various alcohols of H-ZSM-5(1).

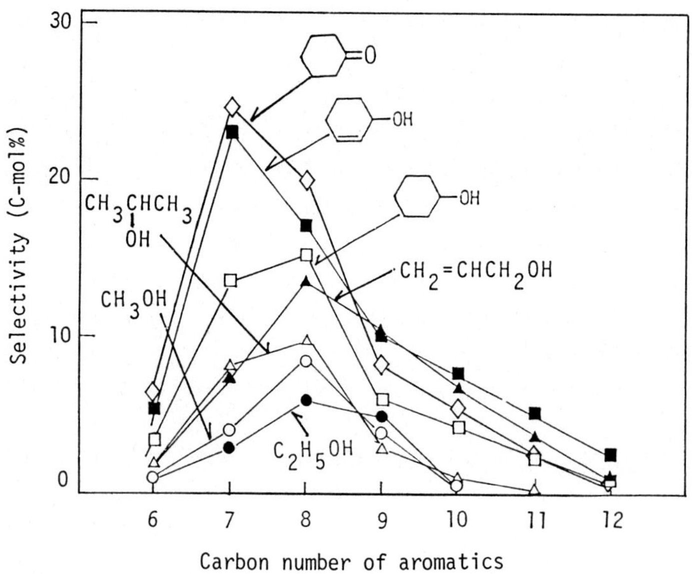

Fig. 5 Selectivity to aromatic hydrocarbons from various alcohols on H-ZSM-5(1).

alcohols; methanol, ethanol and n-butanol (Fig. 3). In the case of allyl alcohol, propylene was the major product among aliphatic hydrocarbons and the selectivity to C_5 - C_7 aliphatics were small (Figs. 3 and 4). Distribution feature of C_2 - C_7 aliphatics in cyclohexanol conversion was in middle range between allyl alcohol and saturated aliphatic alcohols (Figs 3 - 5).

Selectivity to aromatic products presented as A_n from saturated aliphatic alcohols were not large (about 25%) and occupied mainly by A_6 - A_9 in which A_6 i.e. benzene was very little. On the other hand, selectivity to aromatics from unsaturated aliphatic alcohol (allyl alcohol) and alcohols having six-membered ring hydrocarbon (cyclohexanol) was large. An alcohol which has both parts of olefinic and six-membered ring (2-cyclohexene-1-ol) afforded the largest selectivity to aromatics (76%) among oxygenates tested. The largest among aromatics was toluene and the second was xylenes. Furthermore, distribution of aliphatic hydrocarbons from 2-cyclohexene-1-ol was quite different from other alcohols, namely most of them were ethylene and propylene, and C_4 and C_5 aliphatic hydrocarbons were very little. The product distribution from cyclohexanone was similar to that of 2-cyclohexene-1-ol, although ethylene was almost twice.

The hydrogen/carbon ratio of dehydrated form of these oxygenates are classified into three degrees as follows;

Group 1, H/C = 2; methanol, ethanol, i-propanol, n-butanol, t-butanol
Group 2, H/C = 1.66; cyclohexanol,
Group 3, H/C = 1.33; allyl alcohol, 2-cyclohexene-1-ol, cyclohexanone.

Evidently, these classes i.e. the degree of unsaturation are closely related to the product distribution. The oxygenates which have lower saturation degree and cyclic part in the molecular structure afford much aromatics and light olefins, however, the degree of deactivation by coking was also larger with this order.

It has been concluded by many authors (refs. 1 and 23, for example) that the reaction pass in going from methanol to hydrocarbons is represented by the following scheme (1).

$$2CH_3OH \underset{+H_2O}{\overset{-H_2O}{\rightleftharpoons}} CH_3OCH_3 \xrightarrow{-H_2O} C_2 - C_5 \text{ olefins} \longrightarrow \begin{array}{l}\text{paraffins}\\ \text{aromatics}\\ \text{cycloparaffins}\\ C_6\text{+ olefins}\end{array} \qquad (1)$$

Judging from the similarity of the reaction products from the alcohols of Group 1, these alcohols take a common reaction pathway. This has been pointed out previously by Chang and Silvestri (ref. 1).

One of the most intrinsic properties of H-ZSM-5 is its strong acidity which enables to afford aromatics from lower olefins *via* cyclization and dehydrogenation. However, this ability inevitably accompanies with formation of light paraffins by hydrogen transfer that hydrogenation of light olefins with hydrogen generated from the aromatization pass (refs. 22 - 24). The light paraffins thus produced are stable for consecutive conversion to aromatics at the moderate reaction condition, and reduce the gasoline fraction and/or content of aromatics.

It is noteworthy that in the case of oxygenates having six-membered ring, the major compounds for hydrogen transfer would be limited to the part of cyclohexene. Therefore, hydrogenated compounds by this hydrogen transfer still have a large potential for conversion to aromatics. When feed oxygenates have an unsaturated part in their molecule, this part would play a role as the acceptor of hydrogen evolved from the aromatization pass and prevent the formation of saturated aliphatics. Light aliphatic olefins would be produced as by-products by ring cleavage of unsaturated six-membered ring compounds, but these compounds still can join to the aromatization course. Allyl alcohol would be easily converted to unsaturated six-membered ring compounds, however, as can be seen in Fig. 3, much olefinic aliphatics also forms by dehydration and hydrogen transfer. In summary, the reaction pass for oxygenates having six-membered ring can be represented by the following scheme (2).

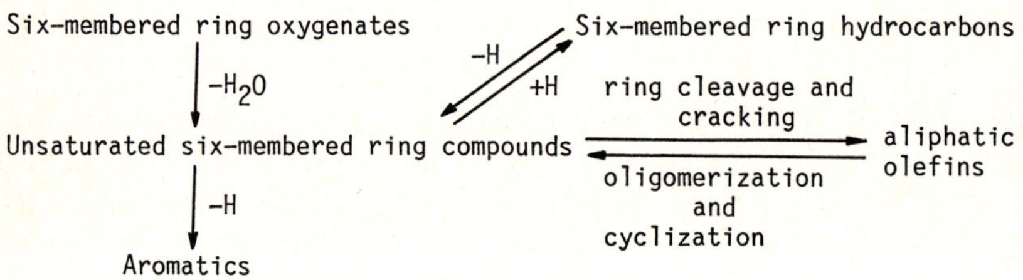

(2)

<u>Conversion of binary mixture of methanol and other unsaturated alcohols or ketone</u>

<u>(i) Conversion of methanol-allyl alcohol mixture</u>

As we reported previously (ref. 4), since addition of small concentration of allyl alcohol to the methanol feed increased aromatics in the product, influence of allyl alcohol addition was investigated using H-ZSM-5(2) as the catalyst with varying the allyl alcohol concentration.

The product distributions from various concentration-combinations of methanol and allyl alcohol are shown in Fig. 6. When allyl alcohol was solely converted, 100% conversion was maintained until 60 min and after that time on stream the conversion decreased slowly. The color of catalyst changed to black from the inlet part the catalyst bed and increased the length of the zone with increasing time on stream, and the whole catalyst bed completed to change into black. The color change by coke formation and the catalyst deactivation, which can be detected by the beginning of conversion decrease from 100% level, were synchronized in the reaction condition, especially due to the proper space velocity of the feed. No significant change in the product distribution within 60 min on stream could be observed, which was confirmed by every 20 min analysis of the products. By this reason that the catalyst was deactivated by allyl alcohol conversion until one hour on stream, all the data in Fig. 6 were compared at that time on stream.

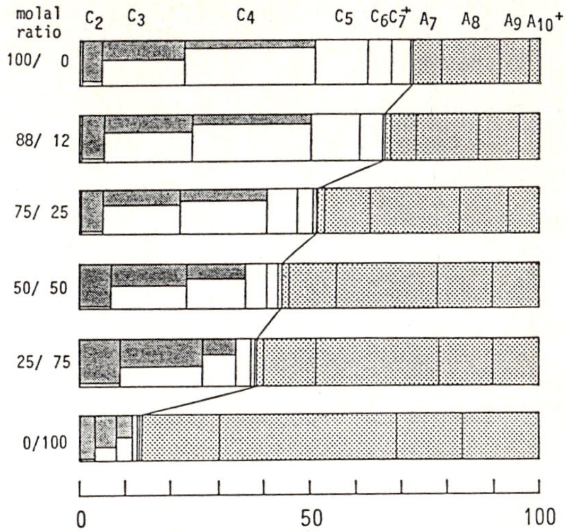

Fig. 6 Distribution of products from methanol-allyl alcohol mixture of different composition. a) molar ratio of methanol/allyl alcohol, Catalyst, H-ZSM-5(2), Reaction condition was same as shown in Fig. 3.

By comparison with methanol and allyl alcohol single component conversion in Fig. 3, the selectivities to paraffinic aliphatics and aromatic hydrocarbons in Fig. 6 are higher. This was caused by stronger acidity of H-ZSM-5(2). In Fig. 7 the selectivity to aromatics appeared in Fig. 6 and the catalyst-bed length of changing to black by coking are plotted against the concentration of allyl alcohol in the mixture of methanol and allyl alcohol. In every concentration, the conversion of the mixture was 100%. The average selectivity to aromatics for the sole-conversion of methanol and allyl alcohol is indicated by broken line in Fig. 7. The obtained data for the selectivity of aromatics is roughly along the average line. On the other hand, the ratio of coking zone at the equimolal mixture of both alcohols is seems to

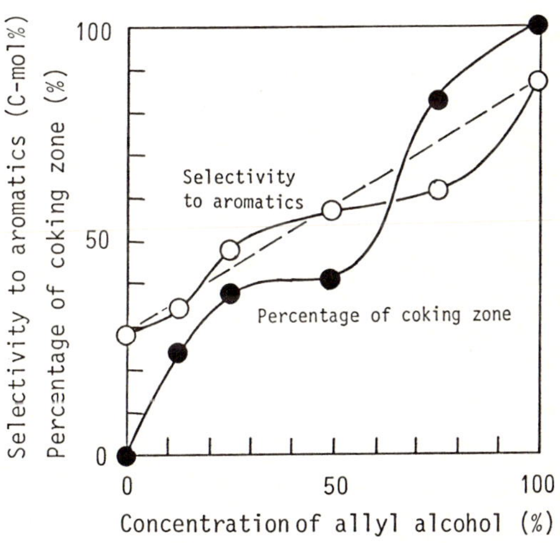

Fig. 7 Effect of allyl alcohol concentration on the content of aromatics in the product and the ratio of coking zone of the catalyst bed. Catalyst, H-ZSM-5(2), Time on stream, 1 h.

be lower than that expected from the average for both alcohols, however, it is not clear the reason of this phenomena because any special feature in the product distribution for the equimolal mixture cannot find out compared with the case of neighbour compositions. However, this tendency will appear again later in this paper.

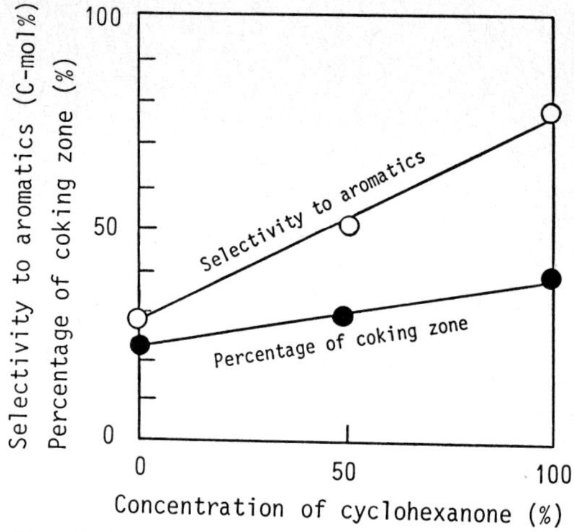

Fig. 8 Effect of cyclohexanone concentration on the content of aromatics in the product and the ratio of coking zone of the catalyst bed. Catalyst, H-ZSM-5(2), Time on stream, 6 h.

<u>(ii) Conversion of methanol-cyclohexanone mixture</u>

As described above, cyclohexanone belongs to the same group (Group 3) of allyl alcohol, but afford more aromatics, and the reaction scheme differs from that for allyl alcohol. In fact, the coking of the catalyst bed in cyclohexanone conversion was much smaller than that in the allyl alcohol conversion. Fig. 8 shows the aromatic content in the products and the ratio of coking zone of the catalyst bed at 6 h on stream. Even though 6 h on stream, the ratio of coking zone was only 37% while maintaining a high selectivity to aromatics. The time on stream until the catalyst deactivation will detect by the decrease of conversion can be presumed as 16 h by supposition that the progress of coking zone is proportional to the time on stream. This time on stream corresponds to 16 times of that in the case of allyl alcohol conversion. The aromatics content and the ratio of coking were proportional to the concentration of cyclohexanone in the feed, however, evidently the incline of the linear line for the content of aromatics is larger than that for the

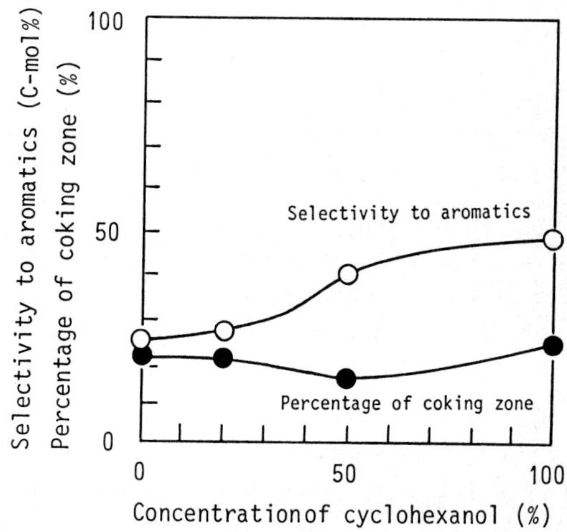

Fig. 9 Effect of cyclohexanol concentration on the content of aromatics in the product and the retio of coking zone of the catalyst bed. Catalyst, H-ZSM-5(2), Time on stream, 6 h.

ratio of the coking. This means that an aromatic-rich gasoline can be produced by the addition of cyclohexanone into the methanol feed without significant decrease of catalyst life by coking.

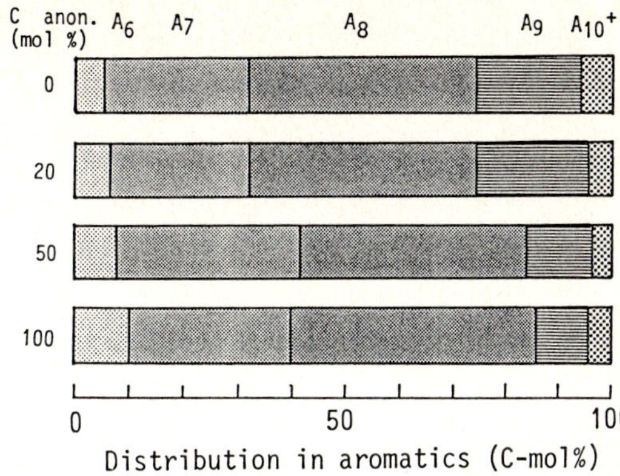

Fig. 10 Distribution of aromatics in the product of the methanol-cyclohexanol conversion.

(iii) Conversion of methanol-cyclohexanol mixture

Cyclohexanol which classified in Group 2 was used as additives to methanol. As shown in Fig. 9, when equimolal mixture of methanol and cyclohexanol was used, the content of aromatics was somewhat above the expected value by average of both solo-conversions of methanol and cyclohexanol, and the ratio of coking zone of the catalyst-bed was rather decrease compared with the solo-conversion of methanol. This was confirmed repeatedly. The distribution of aromatics in the products are shown in Fig. 10. Evidently, for the feed of equimolal mixture, distribution of aromatics shifts to light aromatics, and this interprets the longer catalyst life, suggesting that aromatics mainly toluene and xylenes formed on the catalyst surface would leave rapidly before progress to the formation of fused ring aromatics, i.e. precursor of the coke. Proper content of methanol and cyclohexanol would enhance the formation of toluene and xylenes by methylation of benzene ring.

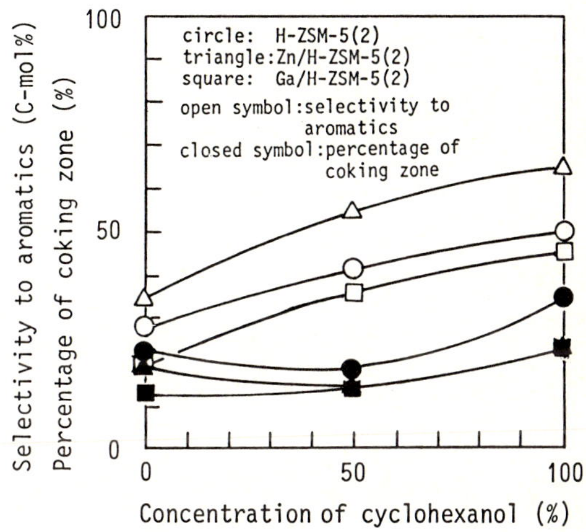

Fig. 11 Effect of ion-exchanged metal for H-ZSM-5(2) on the content of aromatics in the product and the ratio of coking zone of the catalyst bed. Feed, methanol-cyclohexanol mixture, Time on stream, 6 h.

Effect of modification for H-ZSM-5 by ion exchange

Effect of the ion exchange to H-ZSM-5(2) on the conversion of methanol and cyclohexanol mixture was studied. As shown in Fig. 11. Zn-ion-exchanged H-ZSM-5(2) exerted evident effects on the reaction compared with for non-treated H-ZSM-5(2). The selectivity to aromatics increased, and in spite of this, the catalyst coking decreased. The composition of aromatics was quite similar to that in non-treated H-ZSM-5(2). In the case of Ga-ion-exchanged H-ZSM-5(2), the catalyst coking decreased as well as that in the Zn-ion-exchanged H-ZSM-5(2), but the selectivity to aromatics was rather decreased than that in non-treated H-ZSM-5(2). The minimum coking for the equimolal mixture of methanol and cyclohexanol was consistently observed for both the ion-exchanged catalysts. The detail mechanism of the effect of Zn ion is not yet elucidated, however, the ability of Zn ion which increases aromatics and resists against coke formation must be important subject in the field of selective synthesis of aromatic-rich hydrocarbons.

REFERENCES

1 C. D. Chang and A. J. Silvestri, J. Catal., 47(1977)249-259.
2 T. Inui, T. Suzuki, M. Inoue, Y. Murakami and Y. Takegami, in P. A. Jacobs, N. I. Jaeger, P. Jiru, V. B. Kazansky and G. Schulz-Ekloff (Editors), Structure and Reactivity of Modified Zeolites, Studies in Surface Science and Catalysis, Vol 18, Elsevier, Amsterdam, 1984, 201-208.
3 B. E. Langner, Appl. Catal., 2(1982)289-302.
4 T. Inui, T. Hagiwara and J. Tarumoto, J. Jpn. Petrol. Inst., 28(1985)341-348.
5 N. Y. Chen and W. J. Reagan, J. Catal., 59(1979)123-129.
6 C. D. Chang, W. H. Lang and R. L. Smith, J. Catal., 56(1978)169-173.
7 C. D. Chang, Chem. Eng. Sci., 35(1980)619-622.
8 Y. Ono and T. Mori, J. Chem. Soc. Faraday Trans., 1, 77(1981)2209-2221.
9 P. Chu, U. S. Patent, (1978)4120910.
10 A. W. Chester and Y. F. Chu, U. S. Patent, (1982)4350835.
11 D. Dane, A. Hall and P. Harold, Eur. Patent Appl., (1982)50021.
12 T. Mole, J. R. Anderson and G. Creen, Appl. Catal., 17(1985)141-154.
13 T. Inui, Y. Makino, F. Okazumi and A. Miyamoto, J. Chem. Soc. Chem. Comm., (1986)571-573.
14 T. Inui, Y. Makino, S. Tamaya and A. Miyamoto, Chem. Express, 1(1986)451-454.
15 H. Kitagawa, Y. Sendoda and Y. Ono, J. Catal., 101(1986)12-18.
16 E. G. Derouane, in B. Imelk, C. Naccache, Y. Ben Taarit, J. C. Védrine, G. Coudurier and H. Praliaud (Editor), Catalysis by Zeolites, Studies in Surface Science and Catalysis, Vol. 5, Elsevier, Amsterdam, 1980, 5-18.
17 P. Dejaifve, A. Auroux, P. G. Gaxelle, J. C. Védrine, Z. Gaberica and E. G. Derouane, J. Catal., 70(1981)123-136.
18 T. Inui, O. Yamase, K. Fukuda, A. Itoh, J. Tarumoto, N. Morinaga, T. Hagiwara and Y. Takegami, Preprints of 8th International Congress on Catalysis, Berlin, 1984, Vol. III, 569-579.
19 C. J. Plank, E. J. Rosinski and A.B. Schwartz, U. S. Patent, (1974)1402981.
20 T. Inui, H. Matsuda and Y. Takegami, in D. Olson and A. Bisio (Editors), Proceedings of Sixth International Zeolite Conference, Butterworths, 1984, 316-324.
21 T. Inui and F. Okazumi, J. Catal., 90(1984)366-367.
22 T. Inui, A. Miyamoto, H. Matsuda, H. Nagata, Y. Makino, K. Fukuda and F. Okazumi, in Y. Murakami, A. Iijima and J. W. Ward (Editors), New Developments in Zeolite Science and Technology, Kodansha, Tokyo, 1986, 859-866; Discussion, 160-162.
23 P. Dejaifve, J. C. Védrine, V. Bolis and E. G. Derouane, J. Catal., 63(1980)331-345.
24 T. Inui, J. Jpn. Petrol. Inst., 28(1985)279-292.

B. Delmon and G.F. Froment (Editors), *Catalyst Deactivation 1987*

EFFECTS OF COKE FORMATION AND REMOVAL ON THE ACIDITY OF ZSM-5

D.M. Bibby[1], G.D. McLellan[2] and R.F. Howe[2]
[1]Chemistry Division, D.S.I.R., Private Bag, Petone, New Zealand

[2]Chemistry Department, University of Auckland, Private Bag, Auckland, New Zealand

ABSTRACT

Previous work(ref.5) used the techniques of chemisorption of NH_3 and pyridine, TPD/MS(ref.7) and IR spectroscopy to study the effect of coking on the acid sites in the zeolite ZSM-5. This work has been extended to include two other ZSM-5 samples and to study regeneration of the sites by oxidation and pyrolysis of the coke. Correlations between the loss of acid sites (as indicated by NH_3 chemisorption) and the changes in IR bands associated with silanol groups and Bronsted acid sites can be interpreted in terms of the relative Al contents and distributions in the three samples. However, pyridine chemisorption can give lower values for acid site concentrations, because of steric effects. This work confirms the deduction(ref.2) that coking is initially in the channels of ZSM-5 and occurs at a later stage at the surface of the crystals. Lengthy heat treatment to regenerate the activity of the ZSM-5 can result in some permanent loss of active sites.

INTRODUCTION

The deactivation of the zeolite ZSM-5 during methanol conversion has been attributed(ref.1) to the build-up of involatile hydrocarbon residues termed "coke", which block access to the catalytic sites. The coke is initially formed within the channels(ref.2) with little coke formation on the surface until complete deactivation has occurred (at ca. 15% coke).

The effects of coke on the acidity of ZSM-5 and the role of the acid site in coke formation have so far received little study. It has been shown(ref.3) that the amount of chemisorbed NH_3 is lower in ZSM-5 previously used for methanol conversion than it is in fresh catalyst. It has been concluded(ref.4) from calorimetric measurements that, after use, a substantial proportion of the medium- and strong- acid sites is blocked by non-aromatic residues, and that coke is also deposited on the external surface of the ZSM-5.

Previous work(ref.5) on one of the samples used here has shown that the acidity, as determined by NH_3 and pyridine chemisorption, initially falls very rapidly as coke forms. As the amount of coke increases the rate of acid site loss decreases; the acid site concentration, as shown by NH_3 chemisorption, falls to zero at ca. 15% coke.

This work extends the previous study(ref.5) and shows that the initial rapid loss of acidity with coke formation depends on the Al content of the ZSM-5 and probably on its distribution. The recovery of acidity on coke removal by both oxidation and pyrolysis has also been followed, the original acidity being regained only after oxidation above 500°C.

This work compares three different ZSM-5 zeolites, two synthesised here and one supplied by the Mobil Research and Development Corp. The acidity as a function of coke content is followed by NH_3 and pyridine chemisorption and by monitoring the intensity of the infrared (IR) hydroxyl bands corresponding to surface silanols and to Bronsted acid sites. The recovery of acidity as coke is removed is also followed.

EXPERIMENTAL

The samples used here comprised two samples (denoted "ZSM-5#2" and "ZSM-5#3") prepared at Chemistry Division using standard methods(ref.6) as well as a sample from Mobil Research and Development Corporation (denoted "Mobil"). The samples contained ca. 2.5, 1.3 and 3.2 Al/unit cell, respectively. Samples were uniformly coked in a tumbling bed reactor at 370°C with a flow of methanol in nitrogen passing over the bed of zeolite. After a predetermined time, selected to give a desired coke content, the methanol stream was cut off and the nitrogen flow was continued so that volatile products were swept from the catalyst bed before it cooled to room temperature. Coke contents were determined by combustion in a thermobalance(ref.14). The amounts of NH_3 and pyridine desorbed on thermal treatment were measured by a quantitative mass spectrometric method (TPD/MS)(ref.7) in order to avoid complications arising from the simultaneous loss of pyrolysis products from the coke.

Infrared spectra were obtained on a Nicolet 5-DX spectrometer as described previously(ref.5) with hydroxyl band heights being normalised to a zeolite overtone band at 2000 cm^{-1}.

Oxidation of the coke was carried out in a stream of dry air (100 cc min^{-1}) at 500°C.

RESULTS

Many TPD curves for desorption of NH_3 from ZSM-5 have been published (refs. 3,8-13). The relatively small differences between these probably arise from the particular experimental conditions used by different authors and from variations in Al content and distribution in the samples used. A one-to-one correlation between the number of acid sites and the number of NH_3 molecules chemisorbed in H-ZSM-5 and in other zeolites has been reported so frequently that the concentration of chemisorbed NH_3 can be taken as a measure of the acid site concentration and of the total framework Al content. The data for pyridine absorption are not as numerous and not as clear-cut. Previous work(ref.8) has shown that chemisorbed pyridine desorbs between 400°C and 700°C and that the ratio of pyridine molecules to acid sites can be less than unity. The low ratio may be due to steric hindrance if mutual interference of the relatively large pyridine molecules prevents access to some of the acid sites.

Previous work(ref.5) on the effect of coke formation on the chemisorption of NH_3 in one sample of ZSM-5 has been extended to a second sample and although the same overall trend occurs there are significant differences (Figure 1) in the rates of loss of acid sites.

The chemisorption of pyridine is shown as a function of coke for the three ZSM-5 zeolites, in Figure 2. The change in the intensity of the IR bands from the silanols at 3740 cm^{-1} and the Bronsted acid hydroxyls at 3610 cm^{-1} are shown in Figure 3. Both bands were found to decrease in intensity as the coke content increased and an additional broad band appeared at 3670 cm^{-1}. Other broad bands appeared at 3250 and 2750 cm^{-1} at 4.56 percent coke, and at 3380 cm^{-1} at 8 percent coke. However, these bands had largely disappeared at 14.4 percent coke leaving a few bands due to coke between 3100 and 2800 cm^{-1}. The normalised heights of the 3740 and 3610 cm^{-1} bands (due to silanols and Bronsted acid hydroxyls respectively) are shown in Figure 4 as a function of coke content. The chemisorption of NH_3 on pyrolysed ZSM-5#3 is shown in Figure 5 and compared to the chemisorbed NH_3 on the original coked material. The effect of coke removal, by pyrolysis, on the pyridine chemisorption is shown in Figure 6 after treatment at 650°C for 2 hours.

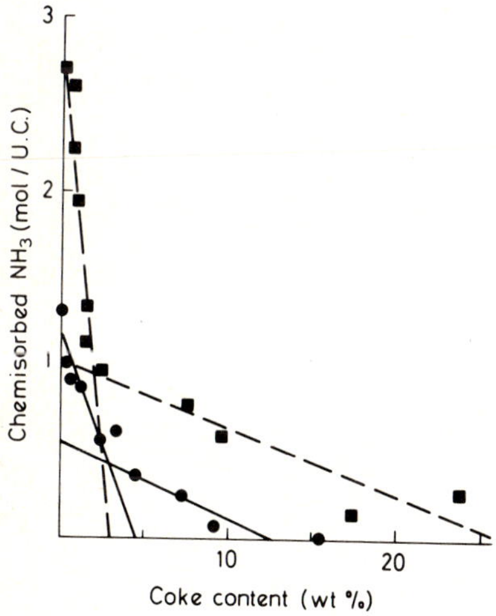

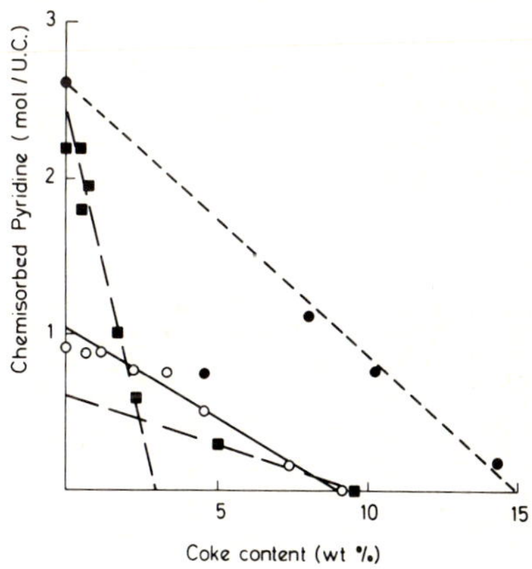

Figure 1. Molecules of chemisorbed NH_3 per unit cell versus coke content for ZSM-5#2(O) and ZSM-5#3(x).

Figure 2. Molecules of chemisorbed pyridine per unit cell versus coke content for ZSM-5#2(O), ZSM-5#3(x) and Mobil ZSM-5(•).

Oxidation of the coke at 560°C caused near complete recovery of the intensity of the 3740 and 3610 cm^{-1} bands. The time required for this complete recovery increased, however, with the starting coke content. For sample ZSM-5#2 with coke contents of 9.14 and 15.4 percent only 80 percent of the IR band intensity due to hydroxyls was regenerated by 100 minutes at 560°C. The chemisorption of pyridine confirmed these measurements. For ZSM-5#3 containing 7.42 and 11.04 percent coke regeneration at 560°C for ca. 200 minutes led to the recovery of 81 Similar results were obtained for the Mobil ZSM-5 containing 4.56 and 8.00 percent coke and regenerated for ca. 90 minutes: 92 and 87 percent of the initial pyridine chemisorption capacity was obtained, respectively, together with 85 and 90 percent of the intensity of the 3610cm^{-1} band and 70 and 80 percent of the 3740 cm^{-1} band.

Some indication of permanent loss of Bronsted acidity was found when regeneration times of 360 minutes were used on a sample containing 10.2 percent coke. The pyridine chemisorption reached a maximum of 91 percent of the original capacity as did the intensity of the band at 3610 cm^{-1}. But the intensity of the silanol band at 3740 cm^{-1} reached only 55 percent of the initial value.

DISCUSSION

The number of carbon atoms deposited as coke, per acid site blocked, can be calculated from the data in Figure 1. The initial loss of acid sites from ZSM-5#2 corresponds to ca. 17 carbons per acid site while that from ZSM-5#3 corresponds to 5-6 carbon atoms. The average size of the coke residues or

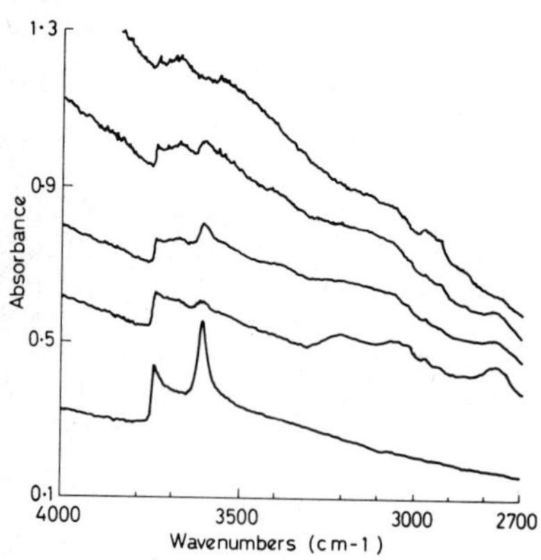

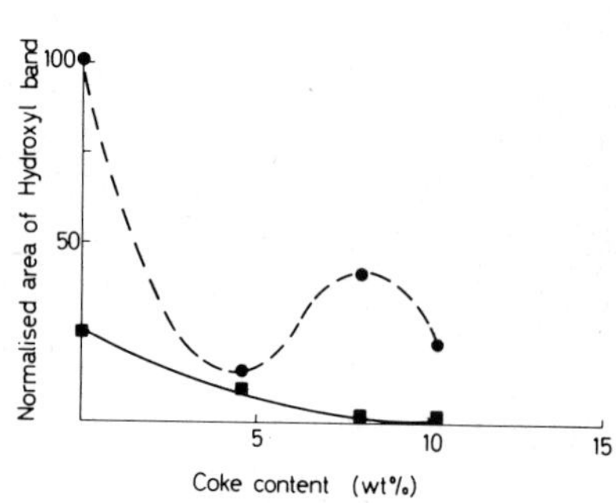

Figure 3. IR absorption spectra of Mobil ZSM-5 with (from bottom to top) 0 percent, 4.56 percent, 8.0 percent, 10.2 percent and 14.4 percent coke.

Figure 4. Integrated peak areas for the 3740 cm^{-1} silanol ( ) and 3610 cm^{-1} Bronsted (•) hydroxyl bands versus coke content for Mobil ZSM-5. Normalised to the 3610 cm-1 = 100 at 0 percent coke.

"molecules" in sample ZSM-5#3 is unlikely to be as small as C_6 which implies that each of the initial coke residues covers, or blocks, more than one site: e.g. a C_{12} residue could block 2 sites or a C_{18} residue could block 3 sites. It is acceptable, however, that the coke residue could contain 17 carbon atoms in sample ZSM-5#2 and cover one acid site only. The difference between these two samples can be explained if they are heterogeneous not only in bulk (as is known (ref.2) from their Si/Al ratios) but also on an atomic scale, with significantly more acid sites in close proximity to each other in ZSM-5#3 than in ZSM-5#2. The probability that a channel intersection can contain more than 1Al atom can be calculated assuming a Poisson distribution. Then sample ZSM-5#2 will have ca. 4 percent of the channel intersections containing 2 or more Al atoms, while for ZSM-5#3 ca. 13 percent of the channel intersections will contain 2 or more Al atoms, i.e. ca. 30 percent of the acid sites will be in close proximity. This percentage could be even greater if one assumed a non-uniform Al distribution in the bulk of the crystal.

As the coke content was increased the chemisorption of both NH3 and pyridine showed an initial rapid loss of acid sites. (Figures 1 and 2). For sample ZSM-5#3 the slope for pyridine had approximately the same value as for the initial chemisorption of NH_3, and this was followed by a similar, much slower, loss of acid sites. However, the pyridine chemisorption fell to zero at ca. 10 percent coke although there was, at this stage of deactivation, still

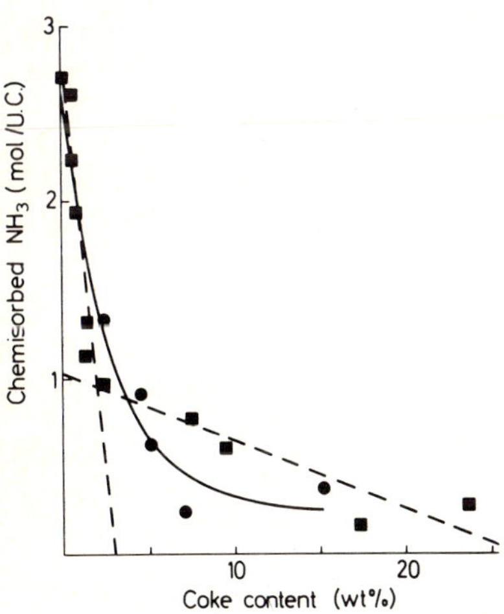

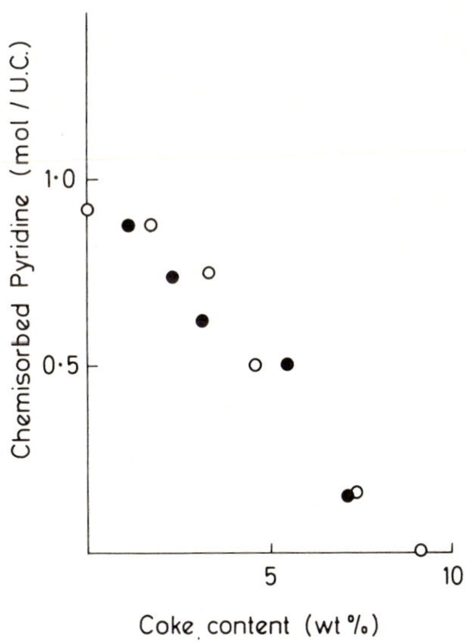

Figure 5. Molecules of chemisorbed NH_3 versus coke content for ZSM-5#3. Before (x) and after (•) pyrolysis.

Figure 6. Molecules of chemisorbed pyridine versus coke content for ZSM-5#2. Before (O) and after (•) pyrolysis.

significant chemisorption of NH_3 and also considerable methanol conversion activity. Clearly the pyridine was unable to gain access to sites still available to NH_3 and methanol molecules, presumably because of steric hindrance to pyridine diffusion through partially deactivated ZSM-5#3. In contrast, for the sample ZSM-5#2 the fall in pyridine chemisorption was relatively linear with coke (Figure 2), but also reached zero at ca. 10 percent coke. For the Mobil sample the data, though more limited, followed a similar pattern with measurable pyripine sorption up to ca. 15 percent coke.

The requirement of a larger coke "molecule" per acid site lost in ZSM-5#2, and the apparent lack of steric hindrance to pyridine in samples ZSM-5#2 and Mobil to the remaining acid sites, combine to give evidence that the Al distribution was considerably more uniform in samples ZSM-5#2 and Mobil than in sample ZSM-5#3. This more even distribution in ZSM-5#2 might be expected from the low Al content of this sample, so that there are few intersections with 2 or more Al atoms even on a purely random distribution. However, the sample from Mobil with its high Al content, must have had a very even distribution of Al with virtually one Al atom per intersection throughout the bulk of the crystal.

That the rapid loss of acid sites is not due simply to blocking of the channels (thereby preventing access by the NH_3 and pyridine bases) is shown by the loss of the normalised intensities of the IR bands at 3740 and 3610 cm^{-1} as the coke content increased. Although there is little data and the errors are significant there is clearly a rapid fall in the intensity of the Bronsted hydroxyl band at 3610 cm^{-1} for the Mobil and ZSM-5#2 samples, which indicates a strong bond between the acid proton and the coke residue. The rise in intensity of the 3610 cm^{-1} band at 8 percent coke is also reflected in the increase in pyridine absorption at that coke content for the Mobil ZSM-5 (Figure 2). This change which is observed at 8 percent coke could arise from a rearrangement of the coke in the channels as the amount of coke increases, and could be possibly related to the high level, and uniform distribution, of the Al in this sample.

Pyrolysis of the coked ZSM-5 results in the loss of H_2, CH_4, CO, CO_2 and possibly small amounts of higher alkenes, with most of the loss occurring at ca. 600°C. The maximum amount of coke lost during pyrolysis occurred at the 5 percent coke level in sample ZSM-5#2 and at the 10 percent coke level in sample ZSM-5#3; this sample showed the maximum loss of coke with 30 percent of the coke being lost. The chemisorption of NH_3 versus coke content is shown in Figure 5 before and after pyrolysis of sample ZSM-5#3 at 650°C for 2 hours.

Below ca. 4 percent coke the effect of coke on the acid sites appears less and more pyrolysed coke is needed to deactivate each acid site than unpyrolysed coke (Figure 5). Between ca. 4 and 15 percent coke the pyrolysis process apparently increases the effectiveness of the remaining coke in deactivating acid sites. In contrast the chemisorption of pyridine increased after pyrolysis.

The difference in the amount of chemisorbed NH_3 and pyridine per unit cell with coke content before and after pyrolysis suggests that considerable reorganisation of the coke occurs. Above the ca. 4 percent coke level the pyrolysed coke becomes more effective in the deactivation of acid sites as shown by the NH_3 chemisorption. Simultaneously, a reduction in the steric hindrance constraining pyridine chemisorption occurs. At the 4.5 percent coke level the number of acid sites accessible to NH_3 chemisorption fell from ca. 0.85 molecules per unit cell with unpyrolysed coke to ca. 0.75 with pyrolysed coke. In contrast the pyridine chemisorption increased from ca. 0.3 molecules per unit cell to ca. 0.55 with unpyrolysed and pyrolysed coke.

In ZSM-5#2 the mass loss of coke on pyrolysis is small and the changes observed in pyridine chemisorption are probably within experimental error (Figure 6).

The differences in behaviour of ZSM-5#2 and ZSM-5#3 possibly relate to differences in the Al distribution between the two zeolites. Evidence from the IR spectra suggest that graphitisation of some of the remaining coke occurs during pyrolysis.

The recovery of the hydroxyl IR bands at 3740 and 3610 cm^{-1} after oxidation of the coke in sample ZSM-5#2 shows that oxidation above 500°C for a few hours was necessary to obtain most of the original acid site concentration. Further work on the Mobil sample with 10.2 percent coke showed that the maximum recovery after 6 hours oxidation was 90 percent of the Bronsted hydroxyl band intensity. This was confirmed by pyridine chemisorption which showed that 91 percent of the original capacity was restored. It appears that some permanent loss of the acid sites occurred at the extended regeneration times.

CONCLUSION

The rapid reduction in the intensity of the IR band due to the Bronsted hydroxyl group with coke content, supports previous findings (refs. 2 and 5) in that the primary coke formation appears to be in the channels of the zeolite, at the acid site. The differences found here between three samples of zeolite suggest that the coke forms preferentially where acid sites are in close proximity, possibly due to a cooperative phenomenon between organic products interacting with, and at, these sites. The two samples of ZSM-5 whose Al seems to be most evenly-distributed required the lay-down of substantially more C atoms per acid site lost.

The effects of a possibly more uniform Al distribution also show on pyrolysis of the coke. In the case of ZSM-5#2, with possibly a more uniform Al distribution, pyrolysis had little effect on pyridine chemisorption. In contrast ZSM-5#3, with what appears to be a non-uniform Al distribution, pyrolysed coke was more effective at reducing NH_3 chemisorption but had less effect on pyridine chemisorption than did unpyrolysed coke.

The loss of coke during pyrolysis must arise from a range of reactions including dehydrogenation to form alkenes and aromatics, and cracking to form methane and alkenes. The formation of a more graphitised coke on pyrolysis is not unexpected and would also result in hydrogen evolution. However, this reaction to form graphitic coke would occur only on the surface of the ZSM-5 crystals or in intracrystalline voids rather than in the ZSM-5 channels due to steric constrants.

The removal of coke by oxidation is facile, at least 90 percent of the coke being easily removed. However, under some conditions the removal of the final coke residue, particularly from samples with high initial coke levels, appears to require more extreme conditions. This more refractory coke possibly includes a graphitised component as pyrolysis could well occur, even under oxidising conditions, at the high temperature used here. Since the temperatures required to remove this final small amount of coke are high enough to cause permanent deactivation these results emphasise the need to regenerate ZSM-5 at the lowest temperature possible, in order to minimise the possibility of graphitic coke formation.

REFERENCES.

1. For example, C. Chang, Catal. Rev.-Sci. Eng. 25 (1983) 1.
2. B.A. Sexton, A.E. Hughes and D.M. Bibby, J. Catal., (in press).
3. N.Y. Topsoe, K. Pederson and E.G. Derouane, J. Catal., 70 (1981) 40-52.
4. P. Dejaifve, A. Auroux, P.C. Gravelle, J.C. Vedrine, Z. Gabelica and E.G. Derouane, J. Catal., 70 (1981) 123-136.
5. G.D. McLellan, R.F. Howe, L.M. Parker and D.M. Bibby, J. Catal., 99 (1986) 486-491.
6. R.J. Argauer and J.R. Landolt, U.S. Patent 3,702,886 (1972).
7. L.M. Parker, D.M. Bibby and J.E. Patterson, Zeolites, 4 (1984) 168-174.
8. L.M. Parker, D.M. Bibby and R.H. Meinholdt, Zeolites, (in press).
9. J.R. Anderson, K. Foger, T. Mole, R.A. Rajadhyaksha and J.V. Sanders, J. Catal., 58 (1979) 114-121.
10. G.P. Babu, S.G. Hegde, S.B. Kulkarni and P. Ratnasamy, J. Catal., 81 (1983) 471-477.
11. J.G. Post and J.H.C. van Hooff, Zeolites, 4 (1984) 9-14.
12. K. Chao, B. Chiou, C. Cho and S. Jeng, Zeolites, 4 (1984) 2-4.
13. K. Scholle, A. Kentgens, W.S. Veeman, P. Frenken and G. van der Velden, J. Phys. Chem., 88 (1984) 5-8.
14. D.M. Bibby, N.B. Milestone, J.E. Patterson and L.P. Aldridge, J. Catal., 97 (1986) 493-502.

AUTHOR INDEX

STUDIES IN SURFACE SCIENCE AND CATALYSIS

Advisory Editors: B. Delmon, Université Catholique de Louvain, Louvain-la-Neuve, Belgium
J.T. Yates, University of Pittsburgh, Pittsburgh, PA, U.S.A.

Volume 1 **Preparation of Catalysts I.** Scientific Bases for the Preparation of Heterogeneous Catalysts. Proceedings of the First International Symposium, Brussels, October 14–17, 1975
edited by **B. Delmon, P.A. Jacobs and G. Poncelet**

Volume 2 **The Control of the Reactivity of Solids.** A Critical Survey of the Factors that Influence the Reactivity of Solids, with Special Emphasis on the Control of the Chemical Processes in Relation to Practical Applications
by **V.V. Boldyrev, M. Bulens and B. Delmon**

Volume 3 **Preparation of Catalysts II.** Scientific Bases for the Preparation of Heterogeneous Catalysts. Proceedings of the Second International Symposium, Louvain-la-Neuve, September 4–7, 1978
edited by **B. Delmon, P. Grange, P. Jacobs and G. Poncelet**

Volume 4 **Growth and Properties of Metal Clusters.** Applications to Catalysis and the Photographic Process. Proceedings of the 32nd International Meeting of the Société de Chimie Physique, Villeurbanne, September 24–28, 1979
edited by **J. Bourdon**

Volume 5 **Catalysis by Zeolites.** Proceedings of an International Symposium, Ecully (Lyon), September 9–11, 1980
edited by **B. Imelik, C. Naccache, Y. Ben Taarit, J.C. Vedrine, G. Coudurier and H. Praliaud**

Volume 6 **Catalyst Deactivation.** Proceedings of an International Symposium, Antwerp, October 13–15, 1980
edited by **B. Delmon and G.F. Froment**

Volume 7 **New Horizons in Catalysis.** Proceedings of the 7th International Congress on Catalysis, Tokyo, June 30–July 4, 1980. Parts A and B
edited by **T. Seiyama and K. Tanabe**

Volume 8 **Catalysis by Supported Complexes**
by **Yu.I. Yermakov, B.N. Kuznetsov and V.A. Zakharov**

Volume 9 **Physics of Solid Surfaces.** Proceedings of a Symposium, Bechyňe, September 29–October 3, 1980
edited by **M. Láznička**

Volume 10 **Adsorption at the Gas–Solid and Liquid–Solid Interface.** Proceedings of an International Symposium, Aix-en-Provence, September 21–23, 1981
edited by **J. Rouquerol and K.S.W. Sing**

Volume 11 **Metal-Support and Metal-Additive Effects in Catalysis.** Proceedings of an International Symposium, Ecully (Lyon), September 14–16, 1982
edited by **B. Imelik, C. Naccache, G. Coudurier, H. Praliaud, P. Meriaudeau, P. Gallezot, G.A. Martin and J.C. Vedrine**

Volume 12 **Metal Microstructures in Zeolites.** Preparation – Properties – Applications. Proceedings of a Workshop, Bremen, September 22–24, 1982
edited by **P.A. Jacobs, N.I. Jaeger, P. Jirů and G. Schulz-Ekloff**

Volume 13 **Adsorption on Metal Surfaces.** An Integrated Approach
edited by **J. Bénard**

Volume 14 **Vibrations at Surfaces.** Proceedings of the Third International Conference, Asilomar, CA, September 1–4, 1982
edited by **C.R. Brundle and H. Morawitz**

Volume 33 **Synthesis of High-silica Aluminosilicate Zeolites**
by **P.A. Jacobs and J.A. Martens**

Volume 34 **Catalyst Deactivation 1987**. Proceedings of the 4th International Symposium, Antwerp, September 29–October 1, 1987
edited by **B. Delmon and G.F. Froment**